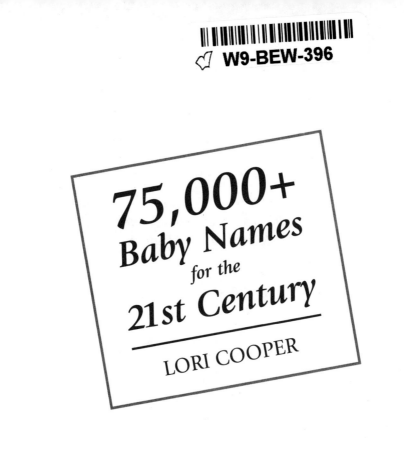

75,000+
Baby Names
for the
21st Century

LORI COOPER

Lothian
BOOKS

In memory of Betty Cooper,
Ruby Kelly and Didgie.

Thomas C. Lothian Pty Ltd.
132–136 Albert Road, South Melbourne, Victoria 3205
www.lothian.com.au

Copyright © 2001 by Lori Cooper
First Published 2001
Reprinted 2004

Distributed by NATIONAL BOOK NETWORK

National Library of Australia
Cataloging-in-Publication Data:

Cooper, Lori.
75,000+ baby names for the 21st century.
ISBN 07344 0227 9.

1. Names, Personal – Dictionaries. I. Title.
II. Title : Seventy-five thousand plus baby names for
the twentieth century.
929.4403

Cover design by David Constable
Typeset by J & M Typesetting

CONTENTS

Acknowledgements

I would like to extend my deepest appreciation to the following people for all their assistance and support and without whom this book would not have come together with such ease: Joshua, Stephanie and Duncan Marshall; John Cooper; Graeme Hearn and Kamilo and Ite Ali. Special thanks to Bill Ligakis at Acropolis Computers Wagga Wagga for your kindness, assistance and for keeping me sane.

This book is dedicated to the following: The Great Spirit and the Angel who inspired this book, Alona. Joyce and Myra Cooper; Sharon, Chloe, Christopher and Jan Hearn; Georgina Papaioanou; Josh and Cassie Dickinson; Craig Glasson for his kindness; my family and friends and my dogs Shaman-Brave-Bear (Shay-Bear) and Nebraska.

CREATIVE BABY NAMES

Modern, Traditional and Global

The aim of *75,000+ Baby Names for the 21st Century* is to give new parents a culturally diverse and imaginative range of baby names with easy-to-understand meanings and the widest array of spelling variations available. The world is increasingly becoming a cultural melting pot. The heritage of many Australians, New Zealanders, Americans, Canadians and Europeans may once have originated from simply Irish, Scottish, English, French and German stock, but as we enter the new millennium, it has become apparent that our families are now more influenced by cultural diversity. Our traditional heritage is now being influenced by Greek, Italian, Chinese, Japanese, Indian, Spanish, Koori, Maori and many other bloodlines.

This book celebrates this wonderful diversity by giving you the opportunity to reflect your family's cultural heritage in the naming of your children. In creating the contents of this book, names have been taken from 220 different languages, from large continents such as the United States of America, Australia and Africa and from small island civilisations such as Western Samoa and Fiji.

Tradition

Many parents are highly influenced by tradition. The names in the Top 50 Most Popular Female and Male Names reflect this trend. Tradition plays an important part in choosing a name for a child. Some people name their children after a much-loved grandmother, grandfather, great aunt, great uncle, from the Bible or even from royalty.

Traditional names such as Emily, Sarah, Elizabeth, Amy, Jack, Michael, Matthew and James feature prominently in classrooms around the world. This old-fashioned influence is a steady one, but keep in mind when you are choosing a name for your child that they may share a classroom with a number of children with that very same name.

Multicultural names

As a result of cultural diversity, names have lately become much more exotic. Once names such as Ann, Mary, Katharine, Margaret and Elizabeth were commonplace, but multiculturalism has brought us a greater variety of fresh names such as Georgia, Mikayla, Brianna, Tamara, Zoe, Shania, Tahlia, Denzel, Zachary and Jared.

Religion

Our spiritual beliefs also play an important part in choosing the name of a child. The Bible contains the names of a large quantity of good God-fearing men and woman as well as angels, saints, feast days and celebrations. Jewish children are often named after a beloved one who has passed over.

In Africa, a child's name may be kept a secret and first whispered to him or her before it is announced to the rest of his or her family. In some other areas of Africa, a grandparent gives the child a name at birth and after six weeks the parents will choose a name that is inspired by the birth, a relative, an event or from nature. African-Americans are now recognising their cultural heritage and are reclaiming this by naming their children traditional African names.

As they journey through life, Native Americans often change their names with each different cycle they encounter. Traditionally, babies were named after an elder, inspired by nature or feats of war and peace. Native Americans are also reclaiming their pride by choosing traditional Native American names for their children.

The Chinese also sometimes change their names as they move from babyhood, to school age, to marriage. They also give their children average names that will not attract the attention of evil spirits. The Japanese give their sons names that reflect their birth order or names that mean longevity or wealth. The girls are given names that reflect the high moral standards of the Japanese people or that come from the natural world.

Hispanic Americans like to name their children after saints. Traditionally, Greeks name the first-born child after a grandparent. Muslim boys are often named after the prophet Mohammed, which is why it is the most common name on the planet. Girls are named after virtues, positive characteristics or nature.

Middle names

A large percentage of children are given middle names. Middle names are usually inspired by a grandparent and allow the parents to follow the tradition of giving family names to their child without letting the confines of old-fashioned names hinder their child's self-esteem.

While names like Brunhilda, Wilhelmina, Winifred, Matilda, Ulfred and Vladislav might honour a much-loved family member, they may be more appropriate as middle names rather than first names. By using a middle name, parents can keep everyone happy; they can give a modern first name but still keep the family traditions alive with a middle name.

Old-fashioned names can also give a lovely flow to a more modern name. For example, Lucy Belle, Katrina May, Chantelle Elizabeth, Sophie Beth, Drew Harrison, Kyle Marcellus.

Middle names can be very handy later in life, as your child might not be happy with his or her first name. Also, in today's expanding population you can only begin to imagine how many Jessica Stevens, Sara Williams, Matthew Taylors and James Coopers there are out there. However, with the addition of a middle name, your child's name can stand out from the crowd.

For example, Sara Parker can become more imaginative with the addition of Bree: Sara Bree Parker. Troy Peters can become more imaginative with the addition of Harrison: Troy Harrison Peters.

Spelling

Your children are individuals, so why not give them names that reflect their own uniqueness? This book is especially tailored to meet the demands of parents seeking such a unique spelling for their favourite names.

For example, why not spell Rebecca Rebekka, Susanna Suzanna, Tanya Tanja, Taylor Taylah, James Jaimes, Kevin Keven or Sean Shaughn?

HOW TO USE THIS BOOK

Name   Country/ies or   Meaning/s

language of origin/s

Brielle (French) from Brie in France. (Eng) she of God.

Origin/   A form of Gabrielle, God is my strength.

Language   Breael, Breaele, Breaell, Breaelle, Breel, Breele, Breell, Breelle,

abbreviation   Briel, Briela, Brielah, Briele, Briell, Briella, Briellah, Bryel,

Bryela, Bryelah, Bryele, Bryell, Bryella, Bryellah, Bryelle

Variations of spelling the original name.

Countries of Origin

The names in *75,000+ Baby Names for the 21st Century* have originated from 220 languages. These include:

AFRICAN

Abaluhya, African, Akan, Ateso, Babara, Benin, Dutooro, Egyptian, Ethiopian, Ewe, Fanti, Ga, Ghanian, Hausa, Ibo, Kakwa, Kikuyu, Kiswahili, Lomwe, Luganda, Lunyole, Luo, Malawian, Musoga, Mwera, Ngoni, Nigerian, North African, Nyakusa, Ochi, Rhodesian, Rukiga, Rukonjo, Runyankore, Runyoro, Rutooro, Shona, Somalian, South African, Swahili, Tanzanian, Tiv, Tswana, Twi, Ugandan, Umbundu, Uset, Xhosa, Yao, Yoruba, Zimbabwean, Zulu.

NATIVE AMERICAN

Algonquin, Apache, Arapaho, Ashanti, Blackfoot, Carrier, Cherokee, Cheyenne, Chippewa, Choctaw, Comanche, Coos, Creek, Dakota, Dene, Eskimo, Fox, Hopi, Iroquois, Kiowa, Lakota, Mahona, Miwok, Mohawk, Mohegan, Moquelumnan, Native American, Navajo, Nez Perce, Omaha, Osage, Pawnee, Pomo, Ponca, Pueblo, Quiche, Sauk, Seminole, Seneca, Shoshone, Sioux, Taos, Tupi-Guarani, Watamare, Winnebago, Wyandot, Zuni.

AMERICAN
African American, American.

SPAIN & PORTUGAL
Hispanic, Old Spanish, Portuguese, Spanish.

SOUTH AMERICAN
Brazil, Incan, Laguna, Peruvian.

CANADIAN
Canadian, Native Canadian, Ojibway.

PACIFICA
Australian, Australian Aboriginal, Fijian, Hawaiian, New Zealand, Maori, Polynesian, Samoan, Tongan, Western Samoan.

EAST ASIA
Burmese, Cambodian, Chinese, Filipino, Indonesian, Japanese, Korean, Malayan, Thai, Tibetan, Vietnamese.

WEST EUROPEAN
Celtic, Cornish, Danish, Dutch, English, Finnish, Flemish, French, Frisian (Netherlandic), Gaelic, German, Gypsy, Icelandic, Irish, Italian, Manx, Middle Dutch, Middle English, Netherlandic, Norse, Norwegian, Old Danish, Old English, Old French, Old German, Old Norse, Old Welsh, Puritan, Scandinavian, Scottish, Sicilian (Italian), Swedish, Swiss, Welsh, Yiddish.

EAST EUROPEAN
Armenian, Basque, Bohemian, Bulgarian, Estonian, Hungarian, Latvian, Lettish, Lithuanian, Mongolian, Polish, Romanian, Russian, Slavic, Turkish, Ukrainian.

MIDDLE EASTERN
Afghani, Arabic, Hebrew, Hindi, Israeli, Pakistani, Pashtu, Persian, Punjabi, Sri Lankan, Syrian, Tamil, Todas, Urdu.

ANCIENT LANGUAGES

Ancient Roman (ancient Italian), Anglo Saxon (ancient British language with West German origins), Aramaic (ancient language with Syrian origins), Assyrian (ancient Semitic language), Babylonian, Breton (ancient British), Eastern Semitic (ancient language comprising of Hebrew, Arabic, Aramaic, Phoenician), Esperanto (comprised of the chief European languages), Etruscan (Italian/Roman influenced), Flemish (Belgium), Gaul (ancient Roman), Gothic (language of East German and Scandinavian origin), Greek, Illyrian (from the area of the Adriatic Sea, Yugoslavia, Albania, Greece), Latin, Old Devon, Phoenician (Syrian origins), Roman, Sanskrit (ancient Hindu), Semitic (ancient language comprising of Hebrew, Arabic, Aramaic, Phoenician), Sumerian (Ancient West Asian), Teutonic (ancient language with German and Scandinavian origins).

Abbreviations

Aba	Abaluhya	Bas	Basque
Afg	Afghani	Ben	Benin
Afr	African	Blkft	Blackfoot
Afri/Amer	African American	Boh	Bohemian
Ak	Akan	Braz	Brazil
Alban	Albania	Bret	Breton
Algo	Algonquin	Bul	Bulgarian
Amer	American	Bur	Burmese
An/Rom	Ancient Roman	Cam	Cambodian
Ang/Sax	Anglo Saxon	Can	Canadian
Apach	Apache	Carr	Carrier
Ara	Aramaic	Celt	Celtic
Arab	Arabic	Chero	Cherokee
Arap	Arapaho	Chey	Cheyenne
Arm	Armenian	Chip	Chippewa
Ashan	Ashanti	Choct	Choctaw
Assy	Assyrian	Coman	Comanche
Ates	Ateso	Cor	Cornish
Aust/Abor	Australian Aboriginal	Dak	Dakota
Austr	Australian	Dan	Danish
Bab	Babylonian	Den	Dene

Dut	Dutch	Jap	Japanese
Duto	Dutooro	Kak	Kakwa
Egypt	Egyptian	Ki	Kiowa
Eng	English	Kiku	Kikuyn
Esk	Eskimo	Kisw	Kiswahili
Esp	Esperanto	Kor	Korean
Est	Estonian	Lak	Lakota
Est/Sem	Eastern Semitic	Latv	Latvian
Ethi	Ethiopian	Lat	Latin
Etr	Etruscan	Lett	Lettish
Ewe	Ewe	Lith	Lithuanian
Fan	Fanti	Lom	Lomwe
Fij	Fijian	Lug	Luganda
Fil	Filipino	Luny	Lunyole
Fin	Finnish	Maho	Mahona
Flem	Flemish	Mal	Malayan
Fren	French	Man	Manx
Fris	Frisian (Netherlandic)	Mid/Dut	Middle Dutch
Gae	Gaelic	Mid/Eng	Middle English
Gau	Gaul	Moh	Mohawk
Ger	German	Mong	Mongolian
Ghan	Ghanian	Moq	Moquelumnan
Goth	Gothic	Mus	Musoga
Grk	Greek	N/Zea	New Zealand
Gyp	Gypsy	N/Zea/Maori	New Zealand Maori
Haus	Hausa	Nat/Amer	Native American
Haw	Hawaiian	Nat/Can	Native Canadian
Heb	Hebrew	Nav	Navajo
Hin	Hindi	Neth	Netherlandic
His	Hispanic	Ngo	Ngoni
Hop	Hopi	Nig	Nigerian
Hung	Hungarian	Nrs	Norse/Norwegian
Ice	Icelandic	Nrth/Afr	North African
Illy	Illyrian	Nya	Nyakusa
Inc	Incan	O/Dan	Old Danish
Ir	Irish	O/Dev	Old Devon
Iroq	Iroquois	O/Eng	Old English
Isra	Israeli	O/Fren	Old French
Ital	Italian	O/Ger	Old German

O/Nrs	Old Norse	Slav	Slavic
O/Wel	Old Welsh	Somal	Somalian
Och	Ochi	Sp	Spain
Oji	Ojibway	Sth/Afr	South African
Oma	Omaha	Sum	Sumerian
Osa	Osage	Swah	Swahili
Paki	Pakistani	Swed	Swedish
Pash	Pashtu	Syr	Syrian
Paw	Pawnee	Tam	Tamil
Per	Persian	Tan	Tanzanian
Phoen	Phoenician	Tao	Taos
Pol	Polish	Teut	Teutonic
Poly	Polynesian	Thai	Thailand
Pom	Pomo	Tib	Tibetan
Pon	Ponca	Tod	Todas
Port	Portugese	Tong	Tongan
Pun	Punjabi	Tswa	Tswana
Pur	Puritan	Tupi	Tupi-Guarani
Qui	Quiche	Turk	Turkish
Rhod	Rhodesian	Ugan	Ugandan
Rom	Roman	Uk	Ukranian
Roma	Romanian	Um	Umbundu
Ruk	Rukiga	Ur	Urdu
Ruko	Rukonjo	Use	Uset
Run	Runyankore	Viet	Vietnamese
Runy	Runyoro	W/Sam	Western Samoa
Russ	Russian	Wata	Watamare
Ruto	Rutooro	Wel	Welsh
S/Lan	Sri Lankan	Winne	Winnebago
Sam	Samoan	Xhos	Xhosha
Sans	Sanskrit	Yid	Yiddish
Sau	Sauk	Yor	Yoruba
Scan	Scandinavian	Yugo	Yugoslavian
Scott	Scottish	Zim	Zimbabwean
Sem	Semitic	Zu	Zulu
Shon	Shona	Zun	Zubi
Shosh	Shoshone		
Sici	Sicilian (Italian)		
Sio	Sioux		

The meaning

The meaning of the child's name is an important factor when choosing a name. Some names hold positive meanings, while others may be less positive and may impact on your child's psyche. Therefore it is important to pay attention to the meaning; after all, how would your child feel if his name meant 'dog' or that her mother died during the birth?

A large percentage of female names are inspired by nature – flowers, trees, seasons, birds, animals, precious stones and mythology. For example, Winter, Autumn, Summer, Willow, Daisy, Fawn, Ruby. The meanings of other female names can be derived from royalty, nobility, warriors, virtues, colours, looks etc.

The main male stock is inspired by royalty, nobility, warriors, nature, colours, looks, abilities, trades, characteristics and mythology etc. For example, Knight, Lancelot, Sampson.

Creating your own special original names

Why not combine names to make a unique one?

For example: Shaelea is a combination of Shae and Lea and the meaning also becomes combined 'from the fairy palace in the meadow'. African-Americans are renowned for this skill, for example Shaneisha, a combination of Shane and Aisha.

You can create your own names by adding to the end of a traditional name. For example, Ella, Elle, Isha, Ita, Itah, Lea, Lee, Lei, Leigh, Ley, Li, Lia, Liah, Lie, Ly, Lya, Lyah, Leata, Leeta, Lita, Lyta, Nita, Niyta, Ana, Anah, Ane, Ann, Anna, Annah, Anne, Ona, Onah, Ria, Rya, Rita, Ryta, Ina, Inah etc. For example, add Elle to Brie and it becomes Brielle.

Nicknames

Be wary of nicknames when choosing a name for your child. Write down every nickname variation you can think of when you have chosen a name and use them to help decide the right name. Remember, children can be very cruel to each other, so keep an open mind and explore all the possibilities. For example the nickname for Richard is Dick. The connotations of this name today are very different from what they were fifty years ago.

Initials

It is also important to keep an eye on the initials of your child's names. Together they might make up a word that is less than flattering.

For example, Daniel Ulan Douglas may seem uneventful until the initials are combined to make DUD. Winona Olivia Walker may also seem uneventful until the intials are combined to make WOW.

TOP 20 MOST POPULAR NAMES

Australian

GIRLS

	1800	1850	1900	1950	1980	1999	2000
1	Sarah	Mary	Dorothy	Linda	Sarah	Emily	Jessica
2	Elizabeth	Elizabeth	Jean	Judy	Rebecca	Jessica	Emily
3	Ann	Sarah	Mary	Susan	Amanda	Chloe	Sarah
4	Maria	Ann	Winifred	Margaret	Claire	Sarah	Georgia
5	Hannah	Alice	Marjorie	Carol	Alison	Georgia	Olivia
6	Emma	Nelly	Doris	Patricia	Elizabeth	Chelsea	Emma
7	Phoebe	Emily	Kathleen	Barbara	Kate	Emma	Chloe
8	Harriet	Edith	Bridget	Sandra	Jennifer	Olivia	Sophie
9	Ellen	Ada	Elizabeth	Jean	Lauren	Sophie	Hannah
10	Margaret	Margaret	Eileen	Diana	Michelle	Hannah	Isabella
11	Martha	Bridget	Lillian	Betty	Catherine	Tayla	Caitlyn
12	Susan	Emma	Daisy	Valerie	Amy	Amber	Grace
13	Louise	Jane	Vera	Elizabeth	Anna	Caitlin	Samantha
14	Alice	Louise	Margaret	Wendy	Melissa	Isabella	Amy
15	Catherine	Clara	Edna	Gloria	Alexandra	Courtney	Lauren
16	Rachel	Harriet	Gladys	Shirley	Belinda	Brooke	Jasmine
17	Emily	Hannah	Florence	Pamela	Erin	Amy	Zoe
18	Bridget	Ethel	Doreen	Joan	Emma	Lauren	Laura
19	Jane	Martha	Violet	Helen	Rachel	Natasha	Brooke
20	Charlotte	Ellen	Nelly	Christine	Katie	Samantha	Rebecca

BOYS

	1800	1850	1900	1950	1980	1999	2000
1	William	William	John	David	Matthew	Joshua	Joshua
2	John	John	William	Peter	James	Lachlan	Jack
3	Thomas	George	George	John	David	Matthew	Lachlan
4	George	Arthur	James	Michael	Michael	Jack	Thomas
5	James	Thomas	Ronald	Robert	Andrew	Thomas	Matthew
6	Henry	James	Robert	Alan	Chris	James	James
7	Joseph	Henry	Kenneth	Stephen	Benjamin	Nicholas	Daniel
8	Charles	Charles	Frederick	Paul	Daniel	Daniel	Nicholas
9	Robert	Samuel	Thomas	Brian	Nicholas	Jordan	William
10	Edward	Edward	Keith	Graham	Timothy	Samuel	Benjamin
11	Samuel	Alfred	Eric	Philip	Luke	Dylan	Ryan
12	Richard	Frederick	Alfred	Anthony	Robert	Jacob	Jacob
13	Alfred	Walter	Arthur	Colin	Mark	Liam	Samuel
14	Frederick	Richard	Charles	Barry	Alexander	Michael	Liam
15	Benjamin	Albert	Leslie	Ian	Stephen	Benjamin	Luke
16	David	Herbert	Dennis	Ray	Peter	Bryan	Dylan
17	Daniel	Edwin	Joseph	Trevor	Jonathon	Luke	Michael
18	Walter	David	Alan	Charles	Adam	William	Mitchell
19	Edwin	Daniel	Stanley	Thomas	Philip	Nathan	Nathan
20	Isaac	Sidney	Ernest	Patrick	Simon	Jake	Alexander

American

GIRLS

	1800	1850	1900	1950	1980	2000
1	Mary	Mary	Florence	Susan	Jennifer	Hannah
2	Ann	Elizabeth	Mary	Linda	Sarah	Emily
3	Elizabeth	Sarah	Alice	Christine	Nicole	Sarah
4	Sarah	Ann	Ann	Margaret	Jessica	Madison
5	Jane	Eliza	Elsie	Carol	Katherine	Brianna
6	Hannah	Jane	Edith	Jennifer	Stephanie	Kaylea
7	Susan	Emma	Elizabeth	Janet	Elizabeth	Kaitlyn
8	Margaret	Hannah	Doris	Patricia	Amanda	Hailey
9	Charlotte	Ellen	Dorothy	Barbara	Melissa	Alexis
10	Harriet	Martha	Ethel	Ann	Lindsay	Elizabeth
11	Betty	Emily	Gladys	Sandra	Rebecca	Taylor
12	Maria	Harriet	Lillian	Pamela	Lisa	Lauren
13	Catherine	Alice	Hilda	Pauline	Rachel	Jessica
14	Frances	Margaret	Margaret	Jean	Lauren	Ashley
15	Mary-Ann	Maria	Winifred	Jacqueline	Andrea	Samantha
16	Nancy	Louise	Lily	Kathleen	Christina	Abigail
17	Rebecca	Caroline	Ellen	Sheila	Emily	Anna
18	Alice	Charlotte	Ada	Valerie	Kristen	Alyssa
19	Ellen	Susannah	Emily	Maureen	Megan	Emma
20	Lucy	Frances	Violet	Gillian	Angela	Emily

BOYS

	1800	1850	1900	1950	1980	2000
1	William	William	John	Robert	Michael	Michael
2	John	John	William	Michael	Christopher	Jacob
3	Thomas	George	Charles	James	Matthew	Matthew
4	James	Arthur	Robert	John	David	Nicholas
5	George	Thomas	James	David	Jason	Christopher
6	Joseph	James	George	William	Daniel	Joseph
7	Richard	Henry	Samuel	Thomas	Robert	Zachary
8	Henry	Charles	Thomas	Richard	Eric	Joshua
9	Robert	Samuel	Arthur	Gary	Brian	Andrew
10	Charles	Edward	Harry	Charles	Joseph	William
11	Samuel	Alfred	Edward	Ronald	Ryan	Daniel
12	Edward	Frederick	Henry	Dennis	James	Tyler
13	Benjamin	Walter	Walter	Stephen	Steven	Ryan
14	Isaac	Richard	Louis	Kenneth	John	Anthony
15	Peter	Albert	Paul	Joseph	Jeffery	Alexander
16	Daniel	Herbert	Ralph	Mark	Adam	David
17	Francis	Edwin	Carl	Daniel	Justin	James
18	David	David	Frank	Paul	Andrew	John
19	Stephen	Daniel	Raymond	Donald	Mark	Christian
20	Jonathon	Sidney	Francis	Gregory	Nicolas	Justin

English

GIRLS

	1800	1850	1900	1950	1980	2000
1	Mary	Mary	Florence	Susan	Sarah	Jessica
2	Anne	Elizabeth	Mary	Linda	Claire	Charlotte
3	Elizabeth	Sarah	Alice	Christine	Emma	Hannah
4	Sarah	Ann	Annie	Margaret	Laura	Emily
5	Jane	Elisa	Elsie	Carol	Rebecca	Sophie
6	Hannah	Jane	Edith	Jennifer	Gemma	Samantha
7	Susan	Emma	Elizabeth	Janet	Rachel	Emma
8	Martha	Hannah	Doris	Patricia	Kelly	Chloe
9	Margaret	Ellen	Dorothy	Barbara	Victoria	Lucy
10	Charlotte	Martha	Ethel	Ann	Katharine	Kate
11	Harriet	Emily	Gladys	Sandra	Kate	Laura
12	Betty	Harriet	Lillian	Pamela	Nicola	Rebecca
13	Maria	Alice	Hilda	Pauline	Jennifer	Lauren
14	Catherine	Margaret	Margaret	Jean	Natalie	Amy
15	Frances	Maria	Winifred	Jacqueline	Hayley	Elizabeth
16	Isabel	Louise	Lily	Kathleen	Michelle	Victoria
17	Grace	Caroline	Ellen	Sheila	Amy	Caitlyn
18	Nancy	Charlotte	Ada	Valerie	Lisa	Ashley
19	Rachel	Frances	Emily	Maureen	Lindsay	Britney
20	Rebecca	Catherine	Violet	Marilyn	Samantha	Brianna

BOYS

	1800	1850	1900	1950	1980	2000
1	John	William	William	David	Christopher	Thomas
2	William	John	John	John	Matthew	James
3	Thomas	George	George	Peter	David	Jack
4	Richard	Thomas	Thomas	Michael	James	Joshua
5	James	James	Charles	Alan	Daniel	Matthew
6	Robert	Henry	Frederick	Robert	Andrew	Ryan
7	Joseph	Charles	Arthur	Stephen	Steven	Daniel
8	Edward	Joseph	James	Paul	Michael	Luke
9	Henry	Robert	Albert	Brian	Mark	Samuel
10	George	Samuel	Ernest	Graham	Paul	Michael
11	Samuel	Edward	Robert	Philip	Richard	Alexander
12	Francis	Frederick	Henry	Anthony	Adam	Christopher
13	Charles	Alfred	Alfred	Colin	Robert	Benjamin
14	Daniel	Richard	Sidney	Christopher	Lee	William
15	Benjamin	Walter	Joseph	Geoffrey	Craig	Andrew
16	Edmund	Arthur	Harold	William	Benjamin	Jake
17	Matthew	Benjamin	Harry	James	Thomas	Joseph
18	Peter	David	Frank	Keith	Peter	Anthony
19	Nicholas	Edwin	Walter	Terence	Anthony	Shaun
20	Isaac	Albert	Herbert	Barry	Shaun	Nicholas

NAMES TO WATCH FOR

Below is a list of predictions for the new millennium. Traditional names such as Emma/line, Jessica, Lucy, Sophee, Lily, James, Jack, Samuel, Harrison and Lachlan will be among the most popular names. Names that are new and will prove to be popular in time to come feature: Brianna, Georgia, Mikaela, Brandon, Brodie, Brock, Jesse and Ryan.

Name predictions for girls

Emily, Tayla, Jessica, Brianna, Emma, Brielle, Georgia, Olivia, Samantha, Chloe, Rhiannon, Cassidy, Mikaela, Jaimee, Brianne, Isabella, Heidi, Brittany, Victoria, Shania, Montana, Tammy, Tahnee, Bethanee, Amberlie, Talise, Vanessa, Chelsea, Jennilee, Kaylea, Mackenna, Poppy, Holly, Taya, Bridie, Gabrielle, Sophee, Mia, Kate, Liberty, Tianna, Jenna, Paige, Kylie, Katrina, Kiara, Kassandra, Brooke, Taylor, Keija, Portia, Natalie, Madeline, Lulani, Layla, Holly, Lexia, Liana, Laura, Krystalee, Jessica, Helaina, Grace, Erin, Teanna, Tegan-Evvron, Tiana, Trinity, Vanora, Calandra, Brenna, Arianna.

Name predictions for boys

Joshua, Jack, Brodie, Brock, James, Brandon, Jesse, Thomas, Lachlan, Ryan, Luke, Matthew, Evan, Shaughn, Grant, Kyle, Jai, Lance, Xander, Stein, Zane, Timothy, Cody, Clint, Hunter, Evander, Bryce, Fynn, Shep, Emerson, Knight, Slade, Todd, Shane, Kane, Seth, Cheyne, Presley, Sonny, Adam, Mitchell, Mackenzie, Ky, Tristan, Jasper, Garth, Kennedy, Kai, Mitchell, Jonah, Harrison, Craig, Nathaniel, Sawyer, Damon, Will, Cameron, Conner, Farley, Halen, Jarell, Garrison, Jason, Jonah, Noah, Jovan, Kacey, Kannan, Kellen, Leith, Mackenzie, Austin, Raphael, Raynor, Roman, Sam, Shamus, Tamson.

NAMES FOR ALL OCCASIONS

Nature names

Some children in the 1990s were given names inspired by the sixties and the hippie movement.

GIRLS

Breeze, Brooke, Bunny, Cherry, Coral, Crystal, Daisy, Dawn, Delta, Dove, Dusty, Fawn, Fern, Flame, Flora, Flower, Gardenia, Ginger, Holly, Honey, Hyacinth, Iris, Ivory, Ivy, Jasmine, Lavender, Lea, Lilac, Lily, Lorilkeet, Lynx, Mahogany, Misty, Moon, Ocean, Olive, Palm, Pansy, Peach, Rain, Rainbow, Raven, River, Roo, Rose, Sage, Savanna, Shade, Shelly, Silver, Sky, Star, Storm, Stormy, Summer, Sun, Sunny, Tempest, Tulip, Valley, Viola, Violet, Willow, Winter.

BOYS

Ash, Bat, Birch, Blaze, Branch, Brook, Buck, Burr, Clay, Cliff, Colt, Creek, Dale, Dell, Ford, Forest, Fox, Ginger, Glade, Hawk, Mango, Park, Pony, Rain, Ray, Reed, Ridge, River, Rush, Sage, Shade, Shadow, Sparrow, Stone, Storm, Sun, Sunny, Tempest, Thorn, Vale, Web, Wood, Woody.

Unisex names

Names that can be given to either sex come in handy if you don't know the sex of your child but are determined to give your child his or her name before the baby is born.

Aaron	Amery	Astro	Bellamy	Bjorg
Adair	Angel	Aubrey	Bennet	Blaine
Adan	Arden	Avis	Berkeley	Blair
Adrian	Ariel	Bailey	Berry	Blaise
Aidan	Asa	Bard	Beryl	Blake
Aimon	Ashley	Bardo	Bethan	Bliss
Ainsley	Asta	Beck	Beverly	Bo
Alec	Astley	Bejay	Bevin	Bobby
Alex	Astra	Bela	Billy	Bon

Bona	Conner	Dylan	Frankie	Hurley
Bowie	Cooper	Eachon	Freddy	Indiana
Bradlee	Corbin	Eavan	Fynn	Indigo
Brady	Corey	Echo	Gabe	Innes
Brae	Corin	Eddie	Gable	Isa
Brandy	Cosmo	Eden	Gabriel	Ithel
Breck	Crystal	Eirian	Gaby	Iva
Brett	Dacey	Eirwen	Gale	Jaan
Britt	Dai	Elan	Ganan	Jace
Brodie	Dakota	Eliot	Garland	Jacey
Brook	Dale	Elk	Garrie	Jackie
Cable	Dallas	Elvis	Geary	Jacoba
Cai	Dan	Elvy	Gene	Jacy
Caley	Dana	Emery	George	Jade
Calypso	Danny	Eneas	Germaine	Jae
Cam	Danyon	Engel	Gerry	Jael
Cameron	Darby	Erin	Gia	Jai
Canada	Darcy	Eskil	Gian	Jala
Carey	Darrin	Ethel	Gil	Jamaica
Carol	Daryl	Fabia	Gilen	Jamaine
Casey	Daryn	Fahey	Ginger	James Jamie
Cass	Dasha	Fallon	Glenn	Jamison
Cassidy	Dean	Farley	Gray	Jan
Cassie	Dejon	Faxon	Hadley	Janne
Catalin	Del	Findlay	Hai	Jasia
Cavan	Derry	Finlay	Halen	Jasper
Chance	Desi	Fira	Haley	Jassi
Chanel	Devon	Flame	Halian	Jay
Cheyenne	Dillion	Flannery	Harley	Jaylee
Chris	Dior	Florie	Harry	Jazz
Christian	Dodie	Fonda	Hatley	Jeri
Christmas	Dominic	Fontanna	Haven	Jess
Coby	Domino	Forrest	Hayden	Jesse
Coco	Don	Fox	Heath	Jet
Cody	Donny	Fran	Hilary	Jevan
Colby	Drew	France	Howi	Jimi
Con	Dusty	Francis	Hunter	Jo

Jodan	Kin	Mango	Oriel	Quincy
Jody	Kip	Marden	Orli	Quinn
Joey	Kit	Marlin	Oz	Rabi
Jojo	Ky	Marlow	Ozzie	Radley
Jordan	Kyle	Max	Paddy	Rae
Jordy	Lacey	Mel	Pagan	Rafa
Jovan	Lach	Michael	Paige	Rain
Jovi	Lachlan	Micki	Palmer	Raine
Jules	Lane	Mika	Paris	Rainer
Julian	Langi	Mikey	Park	Randi
Justa	Lani	Mona	Parker	Rangi
Justice	Larry	Montana	Parnel	Rani
Kacey	Laurie	Morgan	Pascal	Rapa
Kai	Leaf	Morie	Pat	Raven
Kailen	Lee	Myer	Patty	Reece
Kaine	Leif	Naal	Payton	Regan
Kala	Leslie	Nada	Paz	Remi
Kale	Liberty	Nat	Peg	Remy
Kallan	Linden	Nav	Peri	Rena
Kama	Lindley	Naylor	Perry	Rene
Kami	Lindsay	Nebraska	Petra	Renny
Kanya	Linley	Nevada	Peton	Rhody
Karey	Loa	Nicholas	Phoenix	Ria
Kasey	Lochie	Nicky	Ping	Ricca
Kassidy	Luc	Nike	Piper	Richael
Keeley	Lucian	Niki	Pirrit	Ricki
Kei	Lucky	Nikki	Pita	Rika
Kelby	Lui	Nila	Pomme	Riley
Kelly	Luke	Nita	Poni	Rin
Kelsey	Lyndal	Nova	Porsche	Ripley
Kendell	Lyndon	Nyle	Qamar	Risa
Kenya	Mackenzie	Oakley	Quamby	Risley
Kerry	Macy	Odessa	Quan	River
Kesse	Madison	Ona	Quentin	Riza
Kia	Mal	Ontario	Questa	Robin
Kim	Malory	Onyx	Quigley	Rocio
Kimberley	Mandisa	Ori	Quinby	Rodnae

Roe	Shai	Storm	Tracey	Whaley
Roma	Shane	Stormy	Trey	Whitney
Romana	Shanley	Sulley	Trilby	Wilder
Romia	Shannon	Summer	Trinity	Willmot
Romy	Sharman	Sun	Tristen	Wilmer
Roni	Sharron	Sunny	Tye	Wisia
Rori	Shawn	Tabby	Tyler	Xander
Rory	Shay	Tacey	Tyree	Xandy
Roslin	Shea	Taffy	Tyson	Xen
Roto	Shelby	Tam	Urana	Xiang
Rowan	Shelby	Tandy	Utah	Xuan
Rudy	Sheridan	Taniel	Vail	Yael
Sage	Sidney	Tao	Val	Yakuma
Sahara	Sierra	Tasmin	Valentine	Yancy
Sam	Silver	Tate	Van	Yang
Sasha	Sloan	Tatum	Varian	Yani
Sass	Sol	Taylor	Vidal	Yardley
Sawyer	Soma	Teague	Vina	Yen
Saxon	Sonny	Teddy	Vinie	Zales
Schuyler	Spark	Tempest	Vivian	Zaltana
Scooby	Sparrow	Terry	Wade	Zane
Scully	Spencer	Thorne	Walker	Zen
Sean	Stacey	Tierney	Wallis	Zephirah
Seeley	Star	Timmy	Waverley	Zerrin
Shadow	Stevie	Toby	Wendell	
Shaelea	Stone	Toni	Wesley	

Surnames as first names

There has been resurgence in using surnames as first names to imply elegance, style and sophistication. Below are some examples for both boys and girls:

Alexander	Elliot	Hayden	Kingswell	Macrea
Bailey	Emerson	Holden	Knight	Madison
Bancroft	Everton	Hubert	Lancelot	Maguire
Barclay	Falkner	Hudson	Lander	Maitland
Bentley	Farnham	Humphrey	Landon	Major
Berkeley	Filmore	Hunter	Lane	Malachi
Bilbert	Finnegan	Huntington	Langley	Manning
Bladwin	Fitzgerald	Hurley	Lawford	Mansfield
Booker	Fitzpatrick	Hutchinson	Lawrence	Marsdon
Brock	Fitzwilliam	Huxley	Lawson	Marshall
Bronson	Flannery	Ingham	Lennox	Martin
Callaghan	Fletcher	Ingram	Lester	Mason
Callum	Forbes	Irving	Leverton	Maverick
Campbell	Ford	Isaac	Leyland	Maxwell
Carson	Forest	Jackson	Lincoln	Melbourne
Cartwright	Franklin	James	Linford	Melvin
Cassidy	Fraser	Jameson	Linley	Midddleton
Chandler	Frasier	Jarrett	Livingston	Milan
Charlton	Fremont	Jefferson	Logan	Milford
Clark	Gallagher	Jordan	Lorimer	Mitchell
Clinton	Garrett	Kane	Louis	Monrow
Connor	Garrick	Keaton	Lucas	Montague
Cooper	Garrison	Keegan	Macadam	Montgomery
Craig	George	Keelan	Macallister	Morgan
Dalton	Glasson	Keenan	Macarthur	Morrison
Dawson	Grant	Kelly	Macaulay	Mortimer
Delany	Grantley	Kenley	Macbride	Morton
Denver	Hamilton	Kennedy	Maccoy	Murdoch
Dion	Hanson	Kent	Macdonald	Murphy
Donahue	Harley	Kenton	Mackenna	Murray
Douglas	Harrington	Killian	Mackenzie	Nelson
Eaton	Harrison	Kingston	Mackinley	Neville

Newell	Quigley	Sedgwick	Tennyson	Wentworth
Newland	Quillan	Sefton	Thatcher	Wesley
Newman	Quimby	Seymour	Thomas	Westbrook
Newton	Rafferty	Shannon	Thornton	Weston
Nicholas	Redford	Shaw	Torrance	Wetherby
Norman	Rhodes	Sheldon	Travis	Whalley
Norvell	Ridgeway	Shelton	Trent	Wheatley
Oakley	Riley	Sheppard	Tristan	Wheaton
Oberon	Ripley	Sheridan	Truman	Wheeler
Odell	Ritter	Sherlock	Tucker	Whitfield
Orlando	Robert	Sherwood	Turner	Whitford
Orville	Robertson	Simpson	Twain	Whitney
Oscar	Rochester	Sinclair	Tyler	Whycliff
Owen	Rockwell	Slade	Tyson	Wickam
Palmer	Roderick	Sloan	Ulric	Wilford
Parker	Rodman	Smith	Upton	Wilfred
Parnell	Rogan	Spencer	Vaughn	Wilkinson
Parrish	Roland	Stacy	Vincent	Williams
Pascal	Roman	Stafford	Wagner	Williamson
Patrick	Roscoe	Stanley	Waite	Wilson
Patton	Rossevelt	Stanmore	Walker	Wilton
Paxton	Roswell	Stanton	Wallace	Windsor
Perry	Rover	Steele	Walton	Winslow
Phelps	Rowan	Stein	Ward	Winston
Powell	Royce	Sterling	Warren	Wolfe
Prentice	Russell	Stewart	Warwick	Wright
Prescott	Rutherford	Sullivan	Watson	Wyatt
Presley	Sargent	Sydney	Waylon	Yale
Preston	Sawyer	Taggart	Wayne	Yardley
Price	Saxon	Talbot	Webster	Yates
Priestley	Scott	Tanner	Wellington	Zalman
Pryor	Scully	Tate	Wells	
Quentin	Seaton	Taylor	Wendell	

Biblical names

GIRLS

Abigail, Adah, Adina, Adria, Ahava, Aiah, Anna, Apollonia, Ariel, Bathsheba, Bernice, Beth, Bethany, Bethia, Beulah, Candace, Carmel, Cassia, Chloe, Claudis, Damaris, Deborah, Deenah, Delilah, Diana, Dinah, Eden, Elisheba, Esther, Eunice, Eve, Hadassah, Hali, Hannah, Hava, Jael, Janna, Japhia, Jarah, Jemima, Joanna, Judith, Keturah, Kezia, Leah, Lilith, Lois, Lydia, Magdalene, Mara, Marsena, Martha, Mary, Michal, Miriam Moriah, Myra, Naomi, Ophrah, Orpha Peninnah, Phoebe, Priscilla, Rachel, Rhoda, Ruth, Salmone, Samaria, Sara, Sharon, Shifra, Shobi, Susanna, Tabitha, Tamar, Thirza, Tirza, Veronica, Yedida, Zillah, Zipporah, Zorah.

BOYS

Aaron, Abel, Abiel, Abner, Abraham, Absolom, Adam, Adlai, Alexander, Alva, Amal, Amon, Amos, Amram, Andrew, Ara, Aram, Ariel, Asa, Asher, Barnabas, Bartholomew, Baruch, Ben, Benjamin, Boaz, Caleb, Cyrus, Dan, Daniel, Darius, David, Demetrius, Elam, Elazar, Ali, Alihu, Elijah, Elisha, Emanuel, Enoch, Enos, Ephraim, Esau, Ethan, Ezekiel, Ezra, Felix, Gabriel, Galieth, Garrison, Gershom, Gideon, Haran, Herod, Hillel, Hiram, Hosea, Ira, Isaac, Isiah, Israel, Jabez, Jacob, James, Japhet, Jared, Jason, Javan, Jedejiah, Jeremiah, Jesse, Jesus, Jethro, Joel, John, Jonah, Jonathon, Joram, Jordan, Jose, Joseph, Joshua, Josia, Josiah, Judah, Julius, Kenan, Laban, Lazarus; Lemuel, Levi, Linus, Lucas, Malachi, Matthew, Micah, Michael, Mordecai, Moses, Nathan, Nathaniel, Nehemiah, Noah, Obadiah, Omar, Oren, Ozni, Paul, Peter, Phares, Philip, Phineas, Raphael, Reuben, Rufus, Samson, Saul, Seth, Shiloh, Silas, Simon, Solomon, Stephen, Thaddeus, Thomas,Timothy, Tobias, Uri, Uriah, Yoav, Zachariah, Zacharias, Zalmon, Zared, Zebadiah.

Angel names

GIRLS

Alona, Ambriel (Angel of May), Anela, Anela, Angel, Angela, Angelica, Arela, Brielle, Cassiel (Angel of the Earth & Saturday), Dara (Angel of the Rain & Rivers), Dina (Angel of Wisdom & Law), Engel, Engelina, Erela, Gabriel, Gabriella, Gabrielle, Kadl (Angel of Friday), Kamali, Kannitha, Laila (Angel of Spirits at their Births), Melek, Mona, Muriel (Angel of June), Nariel (Angel of the Noon Winds), Neria (Angel of the Moon), Nitika (Angel of Precious Stones), Sachiel (Angel of Water & Thursday), Seraphina, Sofiel (Angel of Fruit & Vegetables), Solange, Tangela, Tangia, Tariel (Angel of Summer), Tevy, Tuyen, Uriel (Angel of September), Zazel (Angel of Saturn).

BOYS

Angel, Angelo, Chi, Deandelo, Engelbert, Gab, Gabela, Gabriel (Angel of Joy, Life, Truth, Mercy, Death, Resurrection, Annuciation, Holy Spirit, Prayer, Mysteries & Dreams), Gaby, Geron (Angel of Prayer), Gotzon, Hamal (Angel of Water), Inglebert, Ingram, Javan (Angel of Greece), Joel (Angel of Names), Malach, Malachy, Michael (Chief Angel, Prince of Presence, Purifier of Places & People who experience Disharmony & Evil, Angel of Repentance, Righteousness, Mercy, Sanctification & Holder of the Keys to Heaven, Oriel (Angel of Destiny), Paniel (Angel who wards off Evil), Raphael (Prince to the Second Heaven, Guardian of the Tree of Life, Angel of the Sun, the South, Evening and West Winds, Angel of Science, Knowledge, Repentance, Light & Love), Tabris (Angel of Free Will), Uriel (Angel of Writers, Teachers & Prophecy, Yael (Angel who is God's Assistant at the Throne), Yahmel (Angel of the Moon), Zachriel Angel of Memory), Zamael (Angel of Joy), Zaniel (Angel of the Zodiac).

Angels of the Months

January	Gabriel
February	Barchiel
March	Malchidiel
April	Asmodel
May	Amriel
June	Muriel
July	Murdad
August	Hamaliel
September	Uriel
October	Aban
November	Azar
December	Anael

Angels of the Winds

North	Gabriel
South	Uriel
East	Michael
West	Raphael

Angels of the Days

Monday	Gabriel
Tuesday	Zamael
Wednesday	Raphael
Thursday	Sachiel
Friday	Anael
Saturday	Cassiel
Sunday	Michael

Mythological names

GIRLS

Acantha (nymph), Anila (Goddess of the Wind), Aphrodite (Goddess of Love), Apolda, Appollonia, Ara (Goddess of Vengeance & Destruction), Artemis (Goddess of the Moon), Artemisia(Goddess of the Hunt), Aurora (Goddess of Dawn), Benton (Goddess of love), Canace, Cassandra (prophetess), Ceres (Goddess of the Harvest), Ceridwen (Goddess of Poetry), Chandra, Chasca (Goddess of Dawn), Chloris (Goddess of Agriculture), Damia (Goddess of the Forces of Nature), Dea, Deva (Goddess of the Moon), Devi (Goddess of Power & Destruction), Diana (Goddess of the Moon, Fertility & the Hunt), Dione, Eos (Goddess of Dawn), Epona (Goddess of Horses), Felicitas (Goddess of Fortune), Feronia (Goddess of Flowers), Fortune (Goddess of Luck), Freja (Goddess of Love), Hathor (Goddess of the Sky), Holla (Goddess of Fruitfulness), Isadora (Goddess of Nature, Moon & Fertility), Isis (Goddess of Nature, Moon & Fertility), Kawn Yin (Goddess of Mercy), Kiupita (Cupid), Lada (Goddess of Beauty), Ladana, Lakshmi (Goddess of Beauty & Luck), Latona, Latonia, Lea (Goddess of Canoe Makers), Lorelei (Siren), Madira (Goddess of Wine), Mahuika (Goddess of Fire), Maia (Goddess of Spring), Minerva (Goddess of Wisdom), Muse, Musette, Muisidora, Nahid (Goddess of Love), Nephthys (Goddess of the House), Nia, Norna (Goddess of Fate), Oba (Goddess ofthe Rivers), Padmavati (Goddess of Flora), Pallas (Goddess of Wisdom & Knowledge), Pandora, Panthea, Penthesilea (Queen of the Amazons), Perizada (fairy), Persephone (Goddess of Spring), Pola, Prithivi (Goddess of the Earth), Psyche, Qadesha, Quilla (Goddess of the Moon), Ran (Sea Goddess of Destruction), Rusalka (Mermaid), Sedna (Goddess of Sea Animals), Shanda, Sibena (Siren), Sirena (Siren), Tafne (Goddess of Life), Thora, Thorberta, Vedis; Venus (Goddess of Love & Beauty), Vesta (Goddess of Fire & the Home), Ziva (Goddess of Light), Zivah.

BOYS

Aries (God of War), Dionysus (God of Wine), Fudo (God of Fire &Wisdom), Heimdall, Hercules, Kaili, Manoj (Cupid), Masou (God of Fire), Mayon, Mercurina (God of Mercury), Mercury (Messenger of the

Gods), Narcissus, Oberon (King of the Fairies), Oceanus (God of the Sea),Ogun (God of War), Pitri-Pati, Raini (Creator God), Serapis (God ofFertility), Thor (God of Thunder), Zeus (King of the Gods).

Gem names

GIRLS

Adornah, Agate, Allira (quartz), Amber, Amberlie, Amethyst, Amipa (amber), Atara, Azura (lapis stone), Beryl, Carnelian Ceinwen, Chu (pearl), Coral, Cordelia, Crisiant (crystal), Crystal, Crystalin, Diamantra (diamond), Diamond, Emerald, Enya, Esme (emerald), Esmeralda (emerald), Frayruz (turquoise), Garnet, Gasparde, Gem, Gemma, Ghita (pearl), Gita (pearl), Greta (pearl), Gretchen (pearl), Gretel (pearl), Hong Ngoc (ruby), Jade, Jasper, Jem, Jet, Jetta (jet), Jewel, Jewelana, Jewelle, Jumana (pearl), Kaimana (diamond), Kalauni (crystal), Kenya, Le (pearl), Lin (jade), Lulu (pearl), Lupe (Ruby), Lupi (ruby), Maggie (pearl), Margaret (pearl), Meg (pearl), Meralda (emerald), Momi (pearl), Mya (emerald), Narooma, Ngoc, Onike (onyx), Onyx, Opal, Opalina, Opeli, Pearl, Penina (pearl), Quartz, Ratana (crystal), Ratna, Reet (pearl), Reumah (pearl), Rubina Ruby, Safaia (sapphire) Safiya (sapphire), Sapphira, Sapphire, Siete (jet), Siliva, Silver, Silvia, Sima (treasure), Siva (treasure), Smaragda (emerald), Taimani (diamond), Tama Tiara, Topaz, Topaza, Tourmaline, Treasure, Tu-Jade (jade), Turquoise, Vread (pearl).

BOYS

Arden, Bernstein (amber), Beryl, Carnelian, Casper, Cephas, Cinnabar, Crisiant (crystal), Crystal, Dar (pearl), Diamond, Emerald, Flint, Galena,Garnet, Gaso, Gasper, Hau-ngoJade, Jasper, Jashar (jewel), Kiton (crown), Koloa (treasure), Leshem, Mica, Narooma, Ngoc, Onike (onyx), Poutini, Ratan, Shovai, Tiki, (green stone), Toakase (turquoise), Trai (pearl).

Colourful names

GIRLS

Gold: Aneira, Chryseis, Cressida, Dior, Doreen, Dore, Dorena, Gilda, Golda, Goldie, Iora, Koula, Marigold, Ofira, Orabel, Oralia, Oriana, Orla, Orlena, Ortrud, Orva, Pazia, Pazice, Rukmini, Zahavah, Zehava, Zeresh, Zlatka, Zorina.

Silver: Argenta, Argyro, Arianrod, Arianwen, Eun, Gin,Gina, Hiriwa, Yin.

Bronze: Pinga.

Yellow: Gulla, Jonquil, Jonwuila, Mamo, Melinah, Nell, Nellie, Saffron, Topaz, Xanthos.

Flesh: Carna, Carnelian.

White: Albina, Alva, Beca, Bela, Bianca, Blanche, Blaniki, Candice, Ceridwen, Galanthe, Galatea, Gwen, Gwenda, Gpwendolyn, Ivory, Jenilee, Jenna, Jennie, Jennifer, Jenny, Jinny, Kolfinia, Lewanna, Livana, Marya, Moswen, Neva, Nevada, Phryne, Shalgia, Tuyet, Vianca, Zahra.

Grey: Tiba.

Orange: Moli, Morela, Tangerine.

Red: Akako, Burgundy, Carmine, Garnet, Kulokula, Mahogany, Omaira, Ruby, Rusty, Scarlett, Sorrell, Talutah.

Pink: Hong, Hue-Lan, Topaz.

Purple: Giacinta, Hyacinth, Ianthe, Indigo, Iola, Iolanda, Ione, Jacinda, Jacinta, Jakinda, Jolanda, Jolan, Juniper, Lavender, Laveni, Lilac, Mauve, Phoenix, Prunella.

Blue: Azure, Azurine, Lanu-Moana, Larmina, Mora, Teal, Thanh, Turquoise.

Green: Midori, Orna, Ornat, Ornice, Tale, Teal, Turquoise, Viridis, Vrida, Yarkona, Zayit, Zeta.

Beige: Guire, Maguir, Nelek.

Brown: Burgundy, Mahogany, Rusty, Sorrell.

Black: Ciara, Ebony, Elk, Jet, Jetta, Jette, Kala, Kara, Nerina, Nigella, Sommer.

BOYS

Gold: Aneurin, Chrysander, Chrysanthus, Chrysocomes, Chrysostom, Dory, Eurwyn, Gold, Golding, Goldwin, Grisostomo, Kane, Kin, Oro, Santerl, Sovann, Zahavi, Zeheb, Zlatar, Zlatka.

Bronze: Ardon.

Yellow: Hsuang, Mamo, Walkara.

White: Abban, Alban, Arjuna, Arnfinn, Banan, Banquo, Berwyn, Bialas, Blanco, Candide, Candido, Dwight, Elgin, Gwynne, Havgan, Heimdall, Hotah, Incencio, Ivory, Kent, Laban, Lavan, Lavaughan, Lavon, Orin, Pawhuska, Tecwyn, Weiss, White, Whitey, Whitlock, Whitman.

Grey: Gary, Gray, Grey, Pachomai, Taklishim, Tiba.

Red: Carmine, Flann, Garnet, Kizil, Lootah, Raktim, Roana, Roja, Ross, Shani.

Purple: Giacinto, Hyacinthe, Jacinto, Porfirio.

Blue: Cesar, Hinto, Neel, Nila, Wullun.

Green: Glaukos, Hewnet, Iterika, Odhran, Odran, Oran.

Brown: Baiardo, Brown, Bruno, Brunon, Cronan, Dunham, Hari, Palauni, Puluno, Rhydderch.

Black: Adham, Ashur, Aswad, Dubham, Jett, Montsho, Nero, Oreb, Palaki, Sierra, Shachor, Taman, Wattan.

Hair colour names

GIRLS

Blond Hair: Alaina, Alaine, Alana, Alanna, Alina, Aselma, Aubrey, Aubrianne, Belilanca, Bellanca, Blake, Blanca, Blanche, Blondelle, Blondie, Cainwen, Chitsa, Dior, Eavan, Eiddwen, Elvira, Fayre, Fenna, Finna, Finola, Flavia, Fulvia, Gwendolyn, Ivory, Jenilee, Jenna, Jennie, Jennifer, Jenny, Kentigerna, Madelberta, Malfrid, Marigold, McKenzie, Meinwen, Morgwen, Nyx, Ofira, Orabel, Oralia, Oriole, Orla, Orlena, Ortrud, Tsomah, Vefa, Vefeli, Veva, Vevette, Wira, Wynne, Xanthe, Xanthia, Xanthus, Zelda, Zenevieva, Zilia, Zinerva.

Red Hair: Derry, Fawn, Flanna, Flannery, Ginger, Laroux, Rufina, Russhell, Rusty.

Dark Hair: Adria, Adrian, Adriana, Adriane, Blake, Brenna, Darcy, Ebony, Eponi, Fawn, Kerri, Kerrianne, Kerrie, Kerrielle, Kerry, Laila, Leila, Maureen, Maurise, Melana, Melanie, Morena, Moriah, Morissa, Morrissa, Raven.

Grey Hair: Tiba.

BOYS

Blond Hair: Alan, Alban, Alben, Alpin, Alva, Aurek, Aurelian, Aurelius, Bain,Banning, Barra, Bellamy, Blanco, Blundel, Blunden, Bowie, Boyd, Canute, Chrysocomes, Dewitt, Dwight, Elvio, Eurwyn, Fairfax, Faxabrandr, Finbar, Findlay, Fingal, Finian, Finlay, Finn, Flavian, Flavio, Gannon, Gerwyn, Gold, Gwyn, Gwynfor, Gwpynne,

Havgan, Izod, Jin, Kefu, Kenton, Kenyon, Laban, Linus, Minkah, Morven, Moswen, Oro, Palben, Sherlock, Tecwyn, Tongatea, Venn, White, Whitey, Whitlock, Whitman, Wynn, Xanthus, Zanthus, Zlatka.

Red Hair: Ahenbarbus, Alroy, Aubin, Aubrey, Auburn, Bayard, Clancy, Darrie, Derry, Flann, Flynn, Ginger, Gough, Harkin, Kuper, Pirro, Reade, Reading, Red, Reed, Reid, Rez, Rogan, Rooney, Roshaun, Roslin, Ross, Roth, Rousse, Row, Rowan, Roy, Ruadhan, Ruff, Fuffin, Rufus, Rush, Rushkin, Ruskin, Russ.

Dark Hair: Adrian, Blake, Blakeley, Bronson, Brown, Bruno, Burnell, Colby, Colley, Corbin, Cronan, Daegan, Darkon, Dolan, Dolye, Donahue, Donnell, Donovan, Dooley, Doug, Doyle, Duane, Dubric, Duff, Dugan, Duncan, Dunham, Dwade, Dwayne, Erebus, Fineas, Jett, Kedar, Kerry, Kerwin, Kieran, Mauli, Maurice, Moore, Morey, Morrell, Morris, Morrison, Morse, Nigel, Pinchas, Sorrell, Taman, Tynan.

Grey Hair: Blandford, Ferrand, Floyd, Gray, Grey, Lloyd, Tiba.

Names for children born at special times

BORN ON DAYS

GIRLS

Born on a Tuesday: Mardi.

Born on a Wednesday: Ekva.

Born on a Thursday: Aba, Abena, Baba, Lakya.

Born on a Friday: Efia.

Born on a Saturday: Amaborn, Sanya.

Born on a Sunday: Cyraca, Domencia, Neda, Quaashie, Quirie, Sabbatha.

BOYS

Born on a Monday: Jojo, Kodwo, Kojo.

Born on a Tuesday: Bobo, Ebo, Jumaane, Kwabena.

Born on a Wednesday: Kwako, Kwakou.

Born on a Thursday: Hamisi, Khamisi, Thursday.

Born on a Friday: Coffie, Jimoh, Jumah.

Born on a Saturday: Kwame, Quaashie.

Born on a Sunday: Boseda, Cirko, Cur, Danladi, Dinko, Domingo, Kwas, Kwasi, Kwesi, Sabiti, Sisi.

CHRISTMAS NAMES

BOYS

Christmas, Noel, Yule

GIRLS

Bozenka, Latasha, Natalie, Natasha, Natividad, Nitasha, Noeline, Noeline, Noela, Noella, Noelle, Tasha, Tasia.

EASTER NAMES

BOYS

Easter, Pace, Palmiro, Pasche.

GIRLS

Palmyra, Pascal, Pascale, Pascha, Pascasia, Pasqualina, Sulgwyn.

SEASONAL NAMES FOR BOYS

Born in summer: Jimiya.

Born in autumn/fall: Kalif, Sarad, Thu.

Born during the day: Kiho, Nuru, Orjunjan, Taimab.

Born during the night: Daren, Mbita, Okon, Omolara.

Born during a storm: Kamuhanda.

SEASONAL NAMES FOR GIRLS

Born in summer: Summer, Sunny.

Born in autumn/fall: Jora, Jori, Seble, Suzuko.

Born in winter: Mashika, Winter, Winterborn.

Born in spring: Vasanta.

Born during the day: Asa, Dae, Dawn, Tassaria, Tasarla.

Born during the night: Laila, Layla, Leila, Sayo, Yoi.

Born during a storm: Taima.

Family birth order names

GIRLS

Adelpha	sister
Ayesha	youngest child
Kamea	only child
Messina	middle child
Dawatha	last child
Omega	last-born child
Primavera	first-born of spring
Lumusi	born face down
Rubena	daughter
Kaya	oldest sister
Natane	daughter
Nituna	daughter

First Born: Alula, Dede, Katina, Magara, Mina, Mosi, Ofra, Prima, Rishona, Sukoji, Winona, Wynona.

Second Born: Kakra, Poni, Secunda.

Third Born: Tertia, Triana, Trinity.

Fourth Born: Delta, Pita, Quastilla, Reba, Tess.

Fifth Born: Quincy, Quinella. Quinta, Quintana.

Sixth Born: Rokuko.

Seventh Born: Sapta, Septima.

Eighth Born: Octavia, Ottavia, Tavia.

Ninth Born: Anona, Nona.

Tenth Born: Decimus, Dixie.

BOYS

Atiu	**eldest son**
Kifeda	**only boy among girls**
Kizza	**born after twins**
Kontar	**only child**
Lumo	**born face down**
Matope	**last-born child**
Potik	**youngest child**
Okoth	**born during a storm**
Uzom	**born while travelling**
Vasant	**born in the spring**
Wekesa	**born during harvest time**
Zhong	**second brother**

First Born: Ariki, Awwal, Becher, Chaska, Ichiro, Kacancu, Kpodo, Mosi, Okpara, Omar, Premysl, Primo, So, Taha, Taro, Uno, Wynono.

Second Born: Brodie, Brody, Jiro, Kenji, Lado, Najji, Pili, Rehema, Secundus, Segundo, Tanjiro, Teiji, Zinan.

Third Born: Manzo, Mensah, Saburi, Saburo, Shelesh, Tertius, Trey, Trini, Trinity.

Fourth Born: Quadrees, Ravia, Raviya, Reba, Shiro.

Fifth Born: Goro, Kindin, Kwintyn, Laquinton, Pahkatos, Ponce, Quentin, Quincy, Quinton.

Sixth Born: Essien, Msrah, Sextus, Sisto, Sixtus.

Seventh Born: Ashon, Bay, Noah, Septimus, Seven, Severn.

Eighth Born: Octavio, Octavius, Tavey, Valu.

Ninth Born: Ennis

Tenth Born: Decimus, Kalkin.

Twin names

GIRLS

Kissa, Nashoto, Taiwo, Tamasina, Tamassa, Tameka, Tavie, Tawia, Thomasina.

BOYS

Ata, Chumo, Gemini, Kato, Kehind, Kizza, Magomu, Masaccio, Massio, Maslin, Massey, McTavish, Opio, Taiwo, Tam, Tamas, Tamson, Tavish, Thom, Thomas, Thompson, Tom, Tomkin, Tomlin, Tommy, Tse, Tuomas, Twia, Yamal, Zesiro.

Royal names

GIRLS

Queens: Basillia, Darice, Elizabeth, Gina, Hera, Hippolyta, Jaa, Juno, Kortanya, Kuini, Laa, Latania, Latanya, Malha, Malka, Malki, Milcah, Morowa, Nelia, Ningai, Queen, Queena, Queenie, Queeny, Quenna, Raine, Rane, Rani, Rania, Regan, Regina, Reina, Rexana, Rexanne, Riane, Rictrude, Rioghnach, Riona, Royanna, Saravnlya, Shebah, Tahnee, Takuhi, Tanah, Tanasha, Taneya, Tania, Tanisha, Tannis, Tanya, Tata, Tatiana, Thema, Tiana, Tu'i.

Princesses: Almira, Amira, Aricia, Brina, Bryna, Diana, Elmira, Gladys, Grace, Laricia, Latia, Latin, Loricia, Panchali, Sarah, Sade, Salette, Salliann, Sally, Sara, Saratisha, Saree, Sari, Sarice, Sarika, Sarina, Sarita, Sarolta, Sarotte, Sasa, Satara, Scotia, Serita, Shantia, Shara, Sharae, Shari, Sharna, Sharolyn, Sharon, Sharona, Sharonda, Sharon, Sirri, Sospita, Sorcha, Sydelle, Tia, Tianna, Urbi, Valentia, Xara.

Royals: Raelene, Rana, Rika, Roderica, Royale, Rula, Ryann, Rashieka, Rayann, Rayleen.

BOYS

Kings: Bahram, Balthasar, Basil, Caderyn, Gautrek, George, Henry, James, John, Khalif, King, Kinsey, Kiral, Leroy, Loe, Louis, Malik, Mansa, Melchior, Min, Mwinyl, Obadele, Oba, Raja, Ray, Reagan, Regan, Regis, Rex, Rian, Rory, Roy, Ryan, Ryne, Sakima, Sersa, Shabouh, Shah, Tatius, Tatius-Tekea, Vortigern, Wang, Xerxes.

Princes: Albert, Alvph, Amir, Baldemar, Charles, Creon, Dima, Edward, Eisonbolt, Erconwald, Garibaldo, Harry, Henry, Khan, Kumar, Mehtar, Nabil, Nouri, Prince, Royce, Sargon, Sayed, Seid, Shapoor, Sharezer, Theo, Theobald, Torna, Vladad, Vladimir, Vladislav, William, Zola.

Royals: Auguste, Augustus, Elroy, Fu Chung, Kyne, Mustafa, Pakile, Royal, Tierney.

Knights: Arthur, Chevelier, Chevy, Knight, Lance, Lancelot, Naite, Ritter, Templar, Vasilis, Yves.

Rulers: Czar, Sultan, Sum, Vlad, Waldo, Walther, Zultan.

Flower names for girls

Acacia	Burnet	Evanthe	Iris	Kulokula
Aiyana	Byrony	Fiala	Ivyivy	Kumfuda
Akasma	Camelia	Fiusa	Jacinta	Laflora
Algoma	Cassiaing	Fleur	Jakinda	Lailaka
Alyssa	Celandine	Fleurette	Japonica	Laime
Alyssum	Celyren	Fleur	Jasmina	Lala
Amarantha	Chalina	Flo	Jassi	Lamani
Amaryllis	Chantree	Floras	Jazlyn	Lanorchis
Anemone	Charo	Florences	Jessamine	Lasipeli
Angelica	Cherry	Florias	Jessenia	Latika
Anh	Chloe	Floridas	Jolanda	Laurel
Anthea	Chrissanth	Flories	Jolan	Lavender
Ardith	Chrysanthe	Florine	Jonquilah	Laveni
Arika	Chrysanth-	Flower	Jonquil	Leaf
Arnurna	emum	Floweria	Juniper	Lei
Asphodel	Chu	Garlands	Jute	Leilani
Aster	Cicely	Geranium	Kakala	Leotie
Azalea	Cinnamon	Giacinta	Kalei	Lesi
Bakula	Cleantha	Ginger	Kalepi	Lilac
Basil	Clematis	Girraween	Kalika	Lile
Bay	Cliantha	Hanako	Kamilia	Lilibeth
Begonia	Clover	Hibiscus	Kaooroo	Lillian
Berony	Cveta	Hoa	Karmel	Lilo
Biancafiore	Daffodil	Hyacinth	Kawana	Lilybelle
Blodwen	Dahlia	Ianthe	Ketifa	Lilybet
Blossom	Daisy	Ilima	Kiki	Linneah
Blum	Diantha	Iola	Kiku	Lis
Boronia	Eglantine	Iolanda	Kohia	Loiyelu

Loke	Nitza	Roannah	Siale	Vija
Lomasi	Nurita	Roesia	Sihu	Violanie
Lose	Ogin	Roisin	Siola'a	Violante
Lotus	Orvokki	Rosabelle	Smiljana	Viola
Lou	Padma	Rosa	Soleil	Violet
Magnolia	Padmani	Rosalba	Sonel	Violette
Mali	Panisi	Rosalee	Sue-Ellen	Viridis
Malva	Pansy	Rosalind	Sue	Viv
Mamo	Patya	Rosamond	Suke	Xuxa
Mansi	Peony	Roscrana	Sukey	Yalanda
Marguerite	Petunia	Roseanne	Sumalee	Yamka
Marjolaine	Philanthas	Rosedale	Susammi	Yasmine
Mausi	Polla	Rose	Susan	Yasmin
May	Pomme	Roselani	Susannah	Yelena
Meiko	Pomona	Rosemary	Susie	Yolanda
Meiying	Poplar	Rosetta	Suzette	Yola
Mejoran	Poppy	Rosie	Tafotila	Yoluta
Melantha	Posy	Rosina	Talia	Yuriko
Melia	Primrose	Rosita	Tansy	Yuri
Mignonette	Pua Fisi	Roza	Tao	Zahara
Miki	Pua	Rozelle	Tiulipe	Zahra
Minore	Pualani	Rozena	Tola	Zerdali
Minta	Raisa	Roz	Tulip	Zetta
Mohala	Raizel	Ruza	Tulsi	Zinnia
Mulga	Ran	Sabara	Umeko	Zohra
Myrtle	Rasia	Saffron	Umpima	Zoza
Nara	Reseda	Sage	Valmaimay	Zsa Zsa
Narcissa	Reyhan	Sakura	Valmamay	Zsuzsan
Narcisse	Rhoda	Sana	Vardar	Zsuzsanna
Nardoo	Rhodanthe	Sanne	Vardina	Zusa
Nerida	Rhodelia	Shaba	Vardis	Zusana
Neridah	Rhodopis	Shoshanah	Verda	Zyt
Neta	Rhody	Shoshana	Verna	
Nili	Rihana	Shoshi	Vianna	
Niree	Rita	Shoshona	Vianne	

YOUR FAVOURITE NAMES

Below is an area you can write your favourite baby names and to give family and friends a say in what name you will give your child.

Name	Origin	Meaning	Spelling Alternatives	Family Members Like/Dislike?	
For example					
Chloe	Greek	flowering; goddess of agriculture	Khloe	✓ ✓ ✓	Like Dislike
_____	____	_____	_____		Like Dislike
_____	____	_____	_____		Like Dislike
_____	____	_____	_____		Like Dislike
_____	____	_____	_____		Like Dislike
_____	____	_____	_____		Like Dislike
_____	____	_____	_____		Like Dislike
_____	____	_____	_____		Like Dislike
_____	____	_____	_____		Like Dislike
_____	____	_____	_____		Like Dislike
_____	____	_____	_____		Like Dislike
_____	____	_____	_____		Like Dislike
_____	____	_____	_____		Like Dislike
_____	____	_____	_____		Like Dislike

MOST POPULAR PET NAMES

Our pets are an important part of our families, but some people lack imagination when naming their pets. How many pets do you know named Max, Sam, King, Prince and Fluffy? From the Top 10 Most Popular Names for Cats and Dogs (see next page), it is quite apparent that there are many animals that share the same name. Therefore, this book includes some imaginative names as alternatives for your pet.

For a sweet-natured pet why not consider Rainbow, Treasure, Angel, Flower, Heaven, Truly or Faith? For those pet owners who prefer a 'tough guy' image, consider Punisher, Warrior, Brutus, Soldier, Bossman, Bear, Werewolf, Samson, Hercules or Commando.

For those with pets that leave a trail of destruction in their wake, consider Cyclone, Twister, Messer, Terror or Wrecker.

Alcohol is becoming an inspiration for many Australians; dogs named Keg, XXXX, Beer, Sambucca, Midori, Tia-Maria, Brandy, Whisky, Bundy and Cognac are not uncommon.

For a pet whose looks leave a lot to be desired (but we still love anyway), consider Yowie, Big Foot, Sasquatch, Hobgoblin or Critter. Pets with distinguishing marks may be named Jigsaw, Magpie or Measles.

For little aquatic creatures, consider Shark, Whale, Dolphin, Jaws, Pisces, Shamu, Piranha or Tuna.

For our feathered friends, consider Toucan, Vulture, Tweety, Lorikeet, Woodstock or Hawkeye.

Or if you have a pair of animals, why not consider pairing up their names too? For example: Buffy & Angel, Bonnie & Clyde, Hansel & Gretel, Sampson & Delilah, Yogi & Boo-Boo, Scooby & Scrappy Doo, Snoopy & Charlie Brown, Clark & Lois, Cleopatra & Mark Antony, Gilligan & Skipper, Mulder & Scully, Bam-Bam & Pebbles, Fred & Wilma, Barney & Betty, Bart & Lisa, Homer & Marge, Batman & Robin, Jekyll & Hyde, Kermitt & Miss Piggy, Mickey & Minnie, Donald & Daisy, Mork & Mindy, Sandy & Danny, Popeye & Olive, Romeo & Juliette, Spock & Kirk, Tarzan & Jane, Milo & Otis, Thelma & Louise, Harry & Sally, Sonny & Cher, Thor & Zeus.

Remember when choosing your pet's name that animals recognise the *sound* of their name, not their actual name/s, so keep it simple. For example, an animal is more likely to answer to Lulu than to Queen Ambrosia.

Popular dog names

	English	Australian	American
1	Max	Jessie	Maggie
2	Ben	Sam	Molly
3	Sam	Buddy	Sam
4	Charlie	Bear	Buddy
5	Holly	Max	Oscar
6	Barney	Molly	Max
7	Jake	Chloe	Bailey
8	Toby	Jack	Jake
9	Lucy	Sasha	Jack
10	Rosie	Zoe	Charlie

Popular cat names

	English	Australian	American
1	Charlie	Misty	Max
2	Oscar	Coco	Sam
3	Tiger	Simba	Simba
4	Tigger	Cleo	Milo
5	Lucy	Tom	Tiger
6	Sam	Lucky	Oscar
7	Jasper	Ginger	Kitty
8	Chloe	Kitty	Gizmo
9	Poppy	Jessie	Sandy
10	Rosie	Sooty	Lucy

Female pet names

Abigail	Belle	Chalice	Damsel	Estelle	Gidget
Adora	Bianca	Chantal	Dandelion	Faith	Gigi
Aimee	Bikini	Charisma	Daphne	Fancy	Glory
Aisha	Bimbo	Chastity	Dawn	Fantasia	Grace
Alex	Bonny	Chelsea	Dee-Dee	Fawn	Gretel
Alexandra	Brandy	Cherry	Diva	Fern	Heidi
Ally	Bridget	Chloe	Dixie	Fifi	Holly
Amanda	Buffy	Cindy	Dolly	Fleur	Honey
Amber	Buttercup	Cinnamon	Duchess	Flora	Honora
Ambrosia	Butterfly	Clarissa	Eartha	Flower	Hope
Amelia	Callista	Clementine	Ebony	Fortuna	Iris
Amethyst	Calliope	Cleo	Elle	Freya	Isabelle
Anastas	Cameo	Crystal	Elly	Gabrielle	Isis
April	Carmen	Cynthia	Elvira	Geisha	Ivy
Autumn	Cecelia	Daffodil	Emily	Gemma	Jacinta
Bambi	Celeste	Daisy	Esmeralda	Genevieve	Jade

Jemima	Laurel	Mia	Polly ia	Sunflower	Velvet
Jenny	Layla	Mimi	Angelica	Suzie	Venus
Jessie	Libby	Missy	Apricot	Tabitha	Veronica
Jewel	Lily	Mitzie	Poppy	Tammy	Violet
Jezebel	Liv	Molly	Princess	Tara	Virginia
Josie	Lucy	Noelle	Rosie	Tasha	Vixen
Joy	Madeleine	Olivia	Sally	Tia	Willow
Katie	Maggie	Opal	Samantha	Tiara	Xena
Kay	Marigold	Pandora	Sasha	Tiffany	Yolanda
Keisha	Marina	Paris	Scarlett	Tinker	Zara
Kira	Matilda	Pebbles	Sheba	Trixie	Zoe
Kizzy	Maxine	Penny	Sheena	Ursula	
Koo	Meadow	Pepper	Sirena	Valerie	
Lady	Meg	Phoebe	Sissy	Vanilla	
Lani	Melody	Pipper	Stella	Vanya	

Male pet names

Abe	Ben	Burt	Dalton	Ferdinand	Harry
Ace	Benjamin	Butcher	Damper	Fergus	Harvey
Adonis	Benji	Casanova	Demon	Fernando	Heman
Al	Benny	Cazaly	Dexter	Fetch	Herbie
Albert	Billy	Charlton	Dickens	Fitz	Hercules
Amos	Bob	Chico	Dillion	Floyd	Himbo
Andre	Bobo	Chip	Dion	Fox	Homeboy
Angus	Bogart	Chook	Dirty-Harry	Fraiser	Homer
Antonio	Bon	Chuck	Doc	Frankie	Hugh
Apollo	Bram	Churchill	Don-Juan	Fritz	Humphrey
Archie	Bro	Clark	Douglas	Garth	Isaac
Attila	Brock	Claude	Drover	Gazza	Issy
Badger	Brodie	Clay	Duke	George	Ivanhoe
Bam-Bam	Bruce	Clint	Dustin	Giorgio	Ivor
Bandit	Bruno	Cody	Edison	Godfrey	Jack
Barney	Buck	Conan	Einstein	Gramps	Jai
Baron	Bugger	Conman	Elvis	Grover	Jasper
Bart	Bumper	Cowboy	Eugene	Hamlet	Jock
Beau	Bundy	Curtis	Felix	Hans	Joey

Jonah	Larry	Mulder	Ossie	Rafferty	Seamus
Jose	Liam	Murray	Otis	Randolph	Sebastian
Julio	Lockie	Mutt-Man	Othello	Rembrandt	Shakespeare
Kane	Lothario	Napoleon	Otto	Rex	Shep
Kermit	Louis	Nash	Pablo	Rhett	Silvester
Khan	Luke	Nashville	Paddy	Roman	Spencer
King	Mack	Nelson	Peppe	Romeo	Spock
Kirk	Magnus	Norm	Pete	Roscoe	Tex
Knight	Major	Nosey	Phantom	Rover	Valentino
Kojak	Master	Nyles	Pharaoh	Ruffus	Wolf-Man
Kramer	Max	Obi	Pierre	Rupert	Zorro
Krusty	Milo	Oliver	Prince	Samson	
Laddie	Monte	Omar	Quin	Sawyer	
Lancelot	Mozart	Oscar	Quincey	Scottie	

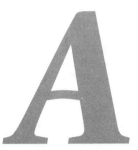

Aaliyah (African) rising.
Aaliya, Aalyya, Aalyyah, Aliya,
Aliyah, Alyia, Alyiah, Alyya, Alyyah

Aasta (Norse) love.
Aastah, Asta, Astah

Aba (Ghanaian) born on a
Thursday.
Abah, Abba, Abbah

Abbey (Hebrew) her father rejoiced.
Abbea, Abbee, Abbi, Abbie, Abea,
Abee, Abi, Abie, Abby, Aby

Abebi (Nigerian) she was asked for
and she came.
Abebea, Abeebe, Abeebee, Abebie,
Abeby

Abena (African) born on a Tuesday.
Abenah, Abina, Abinah, Abyna,
Abynah

Abequa (Chippewa) home lover.
Abequah

Abigail (Hebrew) born of a joyous
father.
Abaigeal (Ir), Abbagael, Abbagail,
Abbagale, Abbagayle, Abbegael,
Abbegail, Abbegale, Abbegayle,
Abbigael, Abbigale, Abbigayle,
Abagael, Abagail, Abagale,
Abagayle, Abegael, Abegail,
Abegale, Abegayle, Abigael,
Abigale, Abigayle, Abbygael,
Abbygail, Abbygale, Abbygayl,
Abbygayle, Abygael, Abygail,
Abygaile, Abygayl, Abygayle

Abira (Hebrew) strong, heroic.
Abirah, Abyra, Abyrah, Adira,
Adirah, Adyra, Adyrah, Amiza,
Amizah, Amyza, Amyzah

Abra (Hebrew) earthmother.
Abrah, Abria, Abriah, Abrya,
Abryah

Abriana (Italian) mother of the
multitudes. The feminine form
of Abraham.
Abrianah, Abriania, Abrianiah,
Abranna, Abriannah, Abrianne,
Abriell, Abriella, Abrielle, Abryan,
Abryana, Abryanah, Abryane,
Abryann, Abryanna, Abryannah,
Abryanne, Abryel, Abryela, Abryele,
Abryell, Abryella, Abryelle

Acacia (Greek) thorny. (Span)
honourable.
Acaciah, Acacya, Acacyah, Cacia,
Caciah, Cacya, Cacyah

Acantha (Greek) sharp, thorny;
mythical fairy.
Acanthah

Achilla (Greek) without lips. The
feminine form of Achilles.
Achila, Achilah, Achile, Achillah,
Achille, Achyla, Achylah, Achyle,
Achylla, Achyllah, Achylle

Acima (Illyrian) God gives high
praise.
Acimah, Acyma, Acymah

Acton (Old English) from the town
with acorn trees.
Actan, Acten, Actin, Actun, Actyn

Ada (Hebrew) ornament.
(Eng) prosperous. (Lat) of noble
birth.
Adah, Adan, Adda, Addah, Addi,
Addia, Addiah, Addie, Addy, Ade,
Eda, Edah, Edna, Ednah

Adair (Scottish) from the oak tree ford.
Adara, Adarah, Adare, Adaira, Adairah, Adayr, Adayra, Adayre

Adalia (Teutonic) noble; kind; cheerful. The Spanish form of Adela.
Adala, Adalah, Adaliah, Adall, Adalla, Adalle, Adallia, Adalliah, Adallya, Adallyah, Adalya, Adalyah

Adama (Nigerian) child of beauty. (Lat) of the red earth. The feminine form of Adam.
Adamma, Adamah, Adamia, Adamiah, Adamin, Adamina, Adaminah, Adamine, Adamya, Adamyah, Adamyn, Adamyna, Adamynah, Adamyne

Adanna (Nigerian) her father's daughter. The feminine form of Aidan; little fiery one.
Adana, Adanah, Adania, Adaniah, Adannah, Adannia, Adanniah, Adannya, Adannyah

Adar (Hebrew) high; fiery.
Adair, Adaira, Adairah, Adaire, Adara, Adarah, Adare, Adayr, Adayra, Adayrah

Adara (Arabic) purity. (Grk) beautiful young girl.
Adarah

Adawna (Latin) jewel-like sunrise.
Adawna, Adawnah

Adela/Adelaide (Teutonic) noble; kind; cheerful.
Adalada, Adaladah, Adalade, Adalaid, Adaliada, Adalaidah, Adalaide, Adalayd, Adalayda, Adalaydah, Adalayde, Adalgisa, Adela, Adelah, Adelaid, Adelaida, Adelaida, Adelais (Fren), Adelajda- (Pol), Adelayd, Adelayda, Adelaydah, Adelayde, Adelena,

Adeleine, Adelhaid (Ger), Adelheid (Ger), Adelia (Span), Adeliah, Adelicia (Eng), Adelin, Adelina, Adeline (Eng), Adeliz, Adeliza, Adleta, Adell, Adella (Ger), Adelle (Fren), Adelya, Adelyah, Alina, Aline, Alita, Alyna, Athelyna, Audule, Edelaid, Edelaide, Edelin, Edelina, Edeline, Edolina, Edoline

Adelinda (Teutonic) noble; serpent.
Adelindah, Adelynda, Adelyndah, Adelyne

Adelpha (Greek) sister.
Adelfa, Adelfe, Adelfia, Adelpha, Adelphe, Adelphia, Adelphya, Adelphyah

Adena (Hebrew) sensuous; delicate. (Grk) noble.
Adeana, Adeanah, Adeane, Adeena, Adeenah, Adeene, Adenah, Adenia, Adina, Adinah, Adine, Adyna, Adynah, Adyne, Dea, Dee, Dee-Dee, Dena, Denah, Din, Dina, Dinah, Dine, Dinee, Diney, Diney, Dini, Dinie, Diny, Dyn, Dyna, Dynah, Dyne, Dynee, Dyney, Dyni, Dynie, Dyny

Adesina (Nigerian) beginning of the family.
Adesinah, Adesyna, Adesynah

Adiel (Hebrew) ornament of the Lord.
Adiela, Adielah, Adiele, Adiell, Adiella, Adiellah, Adielle, Adyel, Adyela, Adyelah, Adyele, Adyell, Adyella, Adyellah, Adyelle

Adina (Australian Aboriginal) good. (Heb) voluptuous; beautiful.
Adeana, Adeanah, Adeane, Adeena, Adeenah, Adeene, Adenah, Adenia, Adinah (Is), Adine, Adyna, Adynah, Adyne, Dea, Dee, Dee-Dee, Dena, Denah, Din, Dina,

Dinah, Dine, Dinee, Diney, Diney,
Dini, Dinie, Diny, Dyn, Dyna,
Dynah, Dyne, Dynee, Dyney, Dyni,
Dynie, Dyny

Adira (Arabic) strength.
Adirah, Adyra, Adyrah

Aditi (Sanskrit) creative power;
freedom.
Aditee, Aditie, Adity, Adytee,
Adytey, Adyti, Adytie, Adyty

Adoeete (Kiowa) tall tree.

Adolpha (Teutonic) noble; fierce
wolf; hero. The feminine form of
Adolf.
Adolfa, Adolfah, Adolfia, Adolfiah,
Adolfya, Adolfyah, Adolphah,
Adolphia, Adolphiah, Adolphie,
Adolphya, Adolphyah

Adonica (Spanish) sweet.
Adonciah, Adoncya, Adoncyah

Adonia (Greek/Spanish) beautiful
woman.
Adoniah, Adonya, Adonyah

Adora/Adorabella (Latin) adorable;
beautiful.
Adorah, Adorabel, Adorabell,
Adorabelle (Fren), Adorabelle,
Adoree, Adoria, Adoriah, Adorya,
Adoryah

Adorlee (French) adorable one from
the meadow.
Adorlea, Adorleah, Adorlei,
Adorleigh, Adorley, Adorli, Adorlia,
Adorliah, Adorlie, Adorly, Adorlya,
Adorlyah

Adorna (Greek) beautiful woman.
(Lat) decorated with jewels.
Adornah, Adornia, Adorniah,
Adornya, Adornyah

Adrasta (Greek) no escape.
Adrastah, Adrastar

Adria/Adriana/Adriane (Greek)
dark; mysterious; from the
Adriatic Sea. The feminine form
of Adrian.
Adrea, Adreah, Adrean, Adreana,
Adreanah, Adreane, Adreann,
Adreanna, Adreannah, Adreanne,
Adreena, Adreenah, Adreene, Adria,
Adriah, Adrian, Adrianah, Adriane,
Adriann, Adrianna, Adriannah,
Adrianne, Adrien, Adriena,
Adrienah, Adriene, Adrienn,
Adrienna, Adriennah, Adrienne,
Adrina, Adrinah, Adrine, Adryan,
Adryana, Adryanah, Adryane,
Adryann, Adryannah

Adsila (Cherokee) flowering.
Adsilah

Aerona (Welsh) berry.
Aeronah, Aeronna, Aeronnah

Afina/Afra (Hebrew) young deer.
Afinah, Afra, Afrah, Afria, Afriah,
Afrya, Afryah, Afyna, Afynah,
Aphina, Aphinah, Aphyna,
Aphynah

Africa (Celtic) pleasant.
(Geographical) the country.
(O/Eng) beloved freedom.
Afelica (Tong), Affreeca, Affreecah,
Affreeka, Affreekah, Affrica,
Affricah, Affricka, Affryca, Affrycah,
Affryka, Affrykah, Afreeca, Afreecah,
Afreeka, Afreekah, Africah, Afryca,
Afrycah, Afrycka, Afryka, Afrykah

Afton (Old English) (Geographical)
from Afton in England.
Aftona, Aftonah, Aftone, Aftonia,
Aftoniah, Aftonie, Aftony, Aftonia,
Aftoniah, Aftonie, Aftony, Aftonya,
Aftonyah, Aftonye

Agapa (Greek) love.
Agapah

Agate (Old French/Greek) precious stone.
Agata, Agatah

Agatha/Agathia (Greek) kind; good.
Agace, Agacia, Agafa, Agafia, Agase, Agata (Ger/Span/Pol/Lith/Bret), Agathe (Eng/Ger)Fren), Agathi, Agathiah, Agathie, Agathy, Agathya, Agathyah, Ageia, Agota (Ir), Agueda, Aphte, Apka, Atka

Agave (Greek) noble.
Agava, Agavah

Aglaia (Greek) brilliant beauty.
Aglae (Fren), Aglaiah, Aglaya, Algayah, Algaye

Agnella (Greek) purity.
Agnel, Agnela, Agnelah, Agnele, Agnelia, Agneliah, Agnelie, Agnell, Agnellah, Agnelle, Agnellia, Agnelliah, Agnellie, Agnelly, Agnellya, Agnellyah

Agnes (Greek) purity.
Adneda, Agna, Agnella, Agnelle, Agnesca (Ital), Agnese (Ital), Agnessa (Rus), Agnesse, Agnessija (Boh), Agneta (Swed/Dan), Agnete, Agnetha (Swed), Agnetis, Agnetta, Agnette, Agnies (Fren), Agnieszka (Lith), Agnizika (Pol), Agnizica (Slav), Agnizka, Agnola, Aigneis (Ir), Agytha, Ameyce, Anis, Annais, Annes, Anneys, Anneyse, Annice, Annot, Annys, Ina, Ines (Span), Inesila, Inessa, Inez (Span), Nancy, Nesa, Nesta, Neziko

Agrippa/Agrippina (Latin) born with the feet first.
Agripa, Agripah, Agripin, Agripina, Agripinah, Agripine, Agrippa, Agrippah, Agrippin, Agrippinah, Agrippine, Agrypina, Agrypinah, Agrypine, Agryppina, Agryppinah, Agryppine, Agryppyna, Agryppynah, Agryppyne

Aharona (Hebrew) singing; enlightened; mountain. (Arab) messenger. The feminine form of Aaron.
Ahronit, Arnina, Arninah, Arninit, Arona, Aronah

Ahava (Hebrew) loved.
Ahavah, Ahuda, Ahuva, Ahuvah

Ahawi (Cherokee) deer.
Ahawee, Ahawie, Ahawy

Ahimsa (Hindi) peaceful.
Ahimsah, Ahymsa, Ahymsah

Ahuda (Hebrew) peaceful.
Ahudah

Ahulani (Hawaiian) heavenly shrine.
Ahulanee, Ahulaney, Ahulania, Ahulaniah, Ahulanie, Ahulany, Ahulanya, Ahulanyah

Ahyoka (Cherokee) bringer of happiness.
Ahyokah

Aida (Latin/Old French) to assist; helper. (Eng) prosperous. (Heb) ornament. (Lat) of noble birth. The Italian form of Ada.
Aidan, Aidah, Aidana, Aidanah, Aidane, Aidann, Aidanna, Aidannah, Aidanne, Ayda, Aydah, Aydan, Aydana, Aydanah, Aydanae, Aydann, Aydanna, Aydannah, Aydanne, Iraida, Iraidah

Aidan (Irish) small fire.
Adan, Adana, Adanah, Aden, Adena, Adenah, Adene, Aidana, Aidanah, Aidane, Aydan, Aydana, Aydanah, Aydane

Aileen (Irish/Greek) shining light. The Irish form of Helen.
Aila, Ailean, Aileana, Aileanah, Aileane, Ailee, Ailena, Ailenah, Ailene, Ailey (Eng), Alean, Aleana,

A

Aleanah, Aleane, Aleen, Aleena, Aleenah, Aleene, Alena, Alene (Fren), Alina, Aline, Eilean, Eileana, Eileane, Eileen, Eileena, Eileene, Eilleen, Eleana, Eleanah, Eleane, Elena, Elenah, Elene (Fren), Ileana, Ileane, Ilina, Ilinah, Iline, Illean, Illeana, Illeanah, Illeane, Illian, Illiana, Illianah, Illiane, Illianna, Illiannah, Illianne, Leana, Leanah, Leane, Lena, Liana, Lianah, Lyan, Lyana, Lynah, Lyann, Lyanna, Lyannah, Lyanne

Ailsa (Teutonic) cheerful girl.
Ailsah, Aylsa, Aylsah

Aine (Old Irish) joy; fire.
Ain, Aithne, Ayn, Ayne, Eithne, Ena, Ethene

Ainsley (Old English) from the meadow clearing.
Ainslea, Ainsleah, Ainslee, Ainslei, Ainsleigh, Ainsli, Ainslie, Ainsly, Anslea, Ansleah, Anslei, Ansleigh, Ansley, Ansli, Anslie, Ansly, Aynslea, Aynsleah, Aynslee, Aynslei, Aynsleigh, Aynsli, Aynslie, Aynsly

Airlea (English) from the airy meadow.
Airleah, Airlee, Airlei, Airleigh, Airley, Airli, Airlie, Airly

Airleas (Irish) promise.
Airlea, Airleah, Airlee, Airlei, Airleigh, Airley, Airli, Airlie, Airly, Ayrlea, Ayrleas, Ayrlee, Ayrlei, Ayrleigh, Ayrley, Ayrli, Ayrlie, Ayrly

Aisha (Swahili) life.
Aishah, Asha, Ashia, Asia, Aysha, Ayshah, Ayshia, Ayshiah, Ayshya, Ayshyah

Aislinn/Aissa (Gaelic) vision; dream.
Aislin, Aislyn, Aislynn, Aissah, Ayslin, Ayslinn, Ayslyn, Ayslynn, Ayssa, Ayssah

Aithne (Celtic) little fire.
Aythne, Eithne, Ethne

Aiyana (Native American) eternal flower.
Aiyanah, Ayana, Ayanah

Aja (Hindi) goat.
Ajah, Ajaran, Ajarana, Ajha, Ajia, Ajiah, Ajya, Ajyah

Ajei (Navajo) my heart.

Akako (Japanese) red.

Akala (Australian Aboriginal) parrot.
Akalah, Akalla, Akallah

Akasma (Turkish) white climbing rose.
Akasmah

Akela (Hawaiian) noble.
Akeia, Akeiah, Akeya, Akeyah, Akeyla, Akeylah

Aki (Japanese) autumn.
Akee, Akei, Akeia, Akeiah, Akey, Akeya, Akeyah, Akie, Aky

Akiko (Japanese) bright light.
Akyko

Akilah (Arabic) intelligent.
Akeia, Akeiah, Akeya, Akeyah, Akia, Akiah, Akiela, Akielah, Akila, Akilah, Akilka, Akilkah, Akyla, Akylah

Akili (Tanzanian) wisdom.
Akilea, Akileah, Akilee, Akilei, Akileigh, Akilia, Akiliah, Akilie, Akily, Akyla, Akylah

Akuna (Australian Aboriginal) knowing follower.
Akunah

Alaina/Alaine (Celtic) handsome;
fair, bright; happy. The feminine
form of Alain/Alan.
Alain, Alainah, Alaine, Alana,
Alanah, Alanna, Alannah, Alayna,
Alaynah, Alayne, Alina, Alinah,
Alinah, Aline, Allaina, Allainah,
Allaine, Allanna, Allannah,
Allanne, Allyna, Allynah, Allyne,
Elaina, Elainah, Elaine, Elayn,
Elayna, Elaynah, Elayne, Lain,
Laina, Lainah, Laine, Lana, Lanah,
Lanna, Lannah, Layna, Laynah

Alamea (Hawaiian) precious stone.
Alameah, Alamia, Alamiah, Almya,
Almyah

Alameda (Native American)
cottonwood. (Span) promenade.
Alamedah

Alana/Alannah (Hawaiian)
handsome; harmony; happy;
peaceful. The feminine form of
Alain/Alan.
Alain, Alaina, Alainah, Alaine
(Fren), Alainna, Alainnah, Alanah,
Alandra, Alandria, Alanna, Alarna,
Alarnah, Alayna, Alaynah, Alaynna,
Alaynnah, Allana, Allanah,
Allanna, Allannah, Allarna,
Allarnah, Allena, Allene, Allyna,
Allynah, Allyne, Allynee, Lana,
Lanah, Larna, Larnah

Alani (Hawaiian) orange tree.
Alana, Alanah, Alanea, Alanee,
Alaney, Alania, Alaniah, Alanie,
Alany, Alanya, Alanyah

Alanis (Irish/Gaelic) beautiful;
bright child.
Alanisa, Alanisah, Alanise, Alaniss,
Alanissa, Alanissah, Alanisse,
Alannis, Alannisa, Alannisah,
Alannise, Alannys, Alannysa,
Alannysah, Alannyse, Alanys,

Alanysa, Alanysah, Alanyse, Alanyss,
Alanyssa, Alanyssah, Alanysse

Alaqua (Native American) sweet
gum tree.
Alaquah

Alarice (Teutonic) wolf ruler; fierce;
hard; noble; supreme ruler of all.
The feminine form of
Alaric/Ulrick.
Alarica, Alaricah, Alaricia, Alarisa,
Alarisah, Alarise, Allaryca, Allaryce,
Alrica, Alrica, Alricah, Alriqua,
Alriquah, Alrique, Alryca, Alrycah,
Alryqua, Alryquah, Alryque

Alastrina (Scottish) the avenger. The
feminine form of Alastair.
Alastriana, Alastrianah, Alastriane,
Alastrianna, Alastriannah,
Alastrianne, Alastrina, Alastrinah,
Alastrine, Alastryan, Alastryana,
Alastryanah, Alastryane,
Alastryann, Alastryanna,
Alastryannah, Alastryanne,
Alastryn, Alastryna, Alastrynah,
Alastryne, Alastrynia, Alastryniah,
Alastrynya, Alastrynyah

Alate (Spanish) truth.
Alata, Alatah

Alaula (Hawaiian) dawn.
Alaulah

Alba/Alberta (Old English) noble;
industrious; bright; famous. The
feminine form of Albert.
Albertina, Albertinah, Albertine,
Albertyna (Pol), Albertyne, Albirta,
Albirtah, Albirtina, Albirtinah,
Albirtine, Albirtyna, Albyrtynah,
Albirtyne, Albretta, Albrette (Fren),
Alburta, Alburtah, Alburtina,
Alburtinah, Alburtine, Alburtyna,
Alburtynah, Alburtyne, Albyrta,
Albyrtah, Albyrtina, Albyrtine,
Albyrtyna, Albyrtynah, Albyrtyne,

Alvert, Alverta, Alvertah, Alvertina, Alvertine, Auberta, Aubertah, Aubertina, Aubertine, Elberta, Elbertah, Elbertina, Elbertine, Elbertyna, Elbertyne

Albina (Latin) white.
Alba, Albah, Albania (Ital), Albaniah, Albinah, Albinia (Ital), Albyna, Albynah, Albyne, Alvira, Alvirah, Aubina, Aubinah, Aubine (Fren), Aubyna, Aubynah, Aubyne

Alcina (Greek) strong-minded.
Alcie, Alcinah, Alcine, Alcinia, Alciniah, Alcyn, Alcyna, Alcynah, Alcyne, Alsina, Alsinah, Alsinia, Alsiniah, Alsine, Alsyn, Alsyna, Alsynah, Alsyne, Alzina, Alzinah, Alzine, Alzyn, Alzyna, Alzynah, Alzyne

Alda (Teutonic) old; wise; rich; a magical fairy who transformed people into trees and animals.
Aldah

Aldith (Old English) experienced fighter.
Ailith, Alda, Aldis, Alditha, Aldithah, Aldithia, Aldytha, Aldythah, Aldythia, Aldythiah, Aldythya, Aldythyah

Aldora (Old English) superior; noble gift.
Aldorah

Aleah (Old English) from the meadow.
Alea, Aleaha, Aleea, Aleeah, Alei, Aleia, Aleiah, Aleigha, Aleighah, Aleya, Aleyah, Alia, Aliah, Alya, Alyah

Aleela (Swahili) she does cry.
Aleala, Alealah, Aleelah, Aleila, Aleilah, Aleighla, Aleighlah, Aleyla, Aleylah, Alila, Alyla, Alylah

Aleena (Dutch) alone.
Alea, Alean, Aleana, Aleanah, Aleane, Alee, Aleen, Aleena, Aleenah, Aleene, Aleina, Aleinah, Aleine, Aleighn, Aleighna, Aleighnah, Aleighne, Alena, Alenah, Alene, Alina, Alinah, Aline, Alon, Alona, Alonah, Alone, Alyn, Alyna, Alynah, Alyne

Aleka (Hawaiian/German) noble.
(Grk) little truthful one. A form of Allison.
Aleaka, Aleakah, Aleeka, Aleekah, Aleika, Aleikah, Alekah, Aleyka, Aleykah

Alena (Russian/Latin) shining light. A form of Helen.
Aleana, Aleanah, Aleane, Aleena, Aleenah, Aleina, Aleinah, Aleighna, Aleighnah, Alenah, Alene, Alenka, Aliena, Aliene, Alina, Alinah, Alyna, Alynah

Aleria (Latin) eagle.
Alearia, Aleariah, Alearya, Alearyah, Aleriah, Alerya, Aleryah

Alesia (Greek) helper.
Alesiah, Alesya, Alesyah

Aleta (Latin) winged.
(Grk) wanderer.
Aleata, Aleatah, Aleeta, Aleetah, Aleita, Aleitah, Aleighta, Aleightah, Aletah, Aleyta, Aleytah, Alita, Alitah, Alouetta, Alouette, Alyta, Alytah

Alethea/Alethia (Greek) truthful one.
Alata, Alatah, Alathea, Alatheah, Alathia, Alathiah, Aletah, Aletheah, Aleathia, Aleathiah, Aleathya, Aleathyah, Aleethea, Aleetheah, Aleethia, Aleethiah, Aleethya, Aleethyah, Aleithea, Aleitheah, Aleithia, Aleithiah, Aleithya,

Alethea/Alethia cont.

Aleithyah, Aleighthea, Aleightheah, Aleighthia, Aleighthiah, Aleighthya, Aleighthyah, Altheia, Altheiah, Aletheia, Aletheiah, Alethiah, Aletta, Alettah, Alithea, Alitheah, Alethia, Alithiah, Allathea, Allatheah, Allathia, Allathiah, Allethea, Alletheah, Allethia, Allethiah, Allythea, Allytheah, Allythia, Allythiah, Allythya, Allythyah, Alythea, Alytheah, Alythia, Alythiah, Alythya, Alythyah, Allethya, Allethyah

Alex/Alexa/Alexandra/Alexis
(Greek) defender of humankind.
The feminine form of Alexander.
Alecsandra, Alecsandria, Alecsandrina, Alecsis, Alecxandra, Alecxandrah, Alecxandria, Alecxandriah, Alecxandrya, Alecxandryah, Aleczandra, Aleczandrah, Aleczandria, Aleczandriah, Aleczandrya, Aleczandryah, Alejandra (Span), Alejandrina, Alejandrine, Alejandryn, Alejandryna, Alejandryne, Aleksandra (Lith), Aleksandrina, Aleksandryne, Aleksia (Dan/Nrs), Aleksiah, Aleksis, Aleksya, Aleksyah, Aleksye, Aleksys, Alessandra, Alessandria, Alessandriah, Alessandrie, Alessandryn, Alessandryna, Alessandryne, Alex, Alexa, Alexah, Alexandria, Alexandriah, Alexandrina, Alexandrinah, Alexandrine, Alexandrovna (Russ), Alexandrya, Alexandryah, Alexia, Alexiah, Alexina, Alexinah, Alexine, Alexis, Alexyna, Alexynah, Alexyne, Alexxandra, Alexxandrah, Alexxandria, Alexxandriah, Alexxandrya, Alexxandryah, Alexzandra, Alexzandrah, Alexzandria, Alexzandriah, Alexzandrina, Alexzandrinah, Alexzandrine, Alexzandryna, Alexzandrynah, Alix, Alixandra, Alixandrah, Alixandria, Alixandriah, Alixandrina, Alixandrinah, Alixandrine, Alixzandra, Alixzandrah, Alixzandria, Alixzandriah, Alixzandrina, Alixzandryna, Alixzandrynah, Alixzandryne, Alyxandra, Alyxandrah, Alyxandria, Alyxandriah, Alyxandrya, Alyxandrah, Alyxandria, Alyxandriah, Alyxandrya, Alyxandrya, Alyxandria, Alxyandryah, Alyxzandra, Alyxzandrah, Alyxzandria, Alyxzandriah, Alyxzandrya, Alyxzandryah

Alfonsa (Spanish) ready; noble. The feminine form of Alfonso.
Alfonsia, Alfonsina, Alfonsine (Fren), Alfonsyna, Alfonsyne, Alonza, Alonzah

Alfreda (Old English) old counsellor; wise judge. The feminine form of Alfred.
Alfredah, Alfredia, Alfrena, Alfrene, Alfrida, Alfridah, Alfryda, Alfrydah, Alfrydda, Alfryddah, Elfrid, Elfrida, Elfridah, Elfridia, Elfried, Elfrieda, Elfrina, Elfrine, Freda, Fredah, Fredda, Freddah, Freida, Freidah, Freyda, Freydah, Frieda, Friedah, Fryda, Frydah, Frydda, Fryddah

Algoma (Native American) valley of flowers.
Algom, Algomah, Algome

Alice (Greek) truthful. (O/Ger) noble.
Addala, Adelice, Adelicia (O/Eng), Ailis (Ir), Aleece, Aleese, Aletta, Alicia (Ital/Span/Swed), Alicie, Aliciedik (Bret), Alicija (Pol),

Alicija, Aliedik, Alina, Aline, Alleta (Dut), Alisa (O/Ger), Alisan, Alisen, Alisha, Alisin, Alison, Alisun, Alisyn, Alisyn, Allisan, Allisen, Allisin, Allison, Allisun, Allisyn, Allyce, Allyse, Alyssa, Aliza, Alodia, Alse, Alyce, Alys, Alyse, Elice, Elise, Elisan, Elisen, Elisin, Elison, Elisun, Elisyn, Elsje, Ilyssa

Alicia (Greek) truthful.
Aleacia, Aleaciah, Aleecia, Aleeciah, Aleicia, Aleiciah, Aleisia, Aleisiah, Aleisya, Aleisyah, Aleighcia, Aleighciah, Aleighsia, Aleighsiah, Aleighsya, Aleighsyah, Alycia, Alyciah, Alycya, Alycyah, Alysia, Alysiah, Alysya, Alysyah

Alida (Greek) beautifully dressed. (Lat) little winged.
Adelita (Span), Adelim (Span), Aleda, Aledah, Aleta (Span), Aletah, Aletta (Ital), Alettah, Alette (Fren), Alidah, Alidia, Alidiah, Alita, Alitah, Alleda, Alledah, Allida, Allidah, Allita, Allitah, Allitta, Allittah, Allyta, Allytah, Alyta, Alytah, Leda, Ledah, Lita, Litah, Litta, Lyta, Lytah, Lytta, Lyttah

Alika (Nigerian) beautiful one who outshines all others. (Haw) truth.
Alikah, Aliqua, Aliquah, Alique, Alyka, Alykah, Alyqua, Alyquah, Alyque

Alima (Arabic) dancer; musician; mermaid.
Alimah, Alyma, Alymah

Alina (Slavic) bright; beautiful. (Celt) harmonious; fair-haired.
Aleana, Aleanah, Aleen, Aleena, Aleenah, Aleina, Aleinah, Aleyna, Aleynah, Alinah, Alinda, Alindah, Aline, Alyna, Alynah, Alynda, Alyndah, Alyne

Alinga (Australian Aboriginal) sun.
Alingah, Alynga, Alyngah

Alisa (Hebrew) joy.
Alisah, Alissa, Alissah, Alysa, Alysah, Alyssa, Alyssah

Alison/Allison (Irish/Gaelic) Alice's son; son of the little truthful one. (O/Ger) famous among the gods.
Aleason, Aleeson, Aleison, Aleighson, Alisan, Alisana, Alisanah, Alisen, Alisena, Alisenah, Alisin, Alisina, Alisinah, Alissa, Alissah, Alisson, Alissun, Alissyn, Alisun, Alisyn, Alisyna, Alisynah, Alisyne, Allisa, Allisah, Allisan, Allisanah, Allisen, Allisena, Allisenah, Allisin, Allisina, Allisinah, Allisine, Allison, Allisona, Allisonah, Allisone, Alliss, Allissa, Allissah, Allisun, Allisuna, Allisyn, Allysna, Allysyne, Alson, Alsona, Alsonah, Alsone, Alysan, Alysen, Alysena, Alysenah, Alysene, Alysin, Alysina, Alysinah, Alysine, Alyson, Alysonah, Alysone, Alysyn, Alysyna, Alysynah, Alysyne, Alyssa, Alyssah, Alysse, Alysun, Alysyn, Alyzan, Alyzana, Alyzane, Alyzen, Alyzena, Alyzene, Alyzin, Alyzina, Alyzine, Alyzyn, Alyzyna, Alyzyne

Aliya (Hebrew) rising.
Aliyah

Aliza (Hebrew) joy; holy and sacred to God. A form of Eliza.
Aleaza, Aleazah, Aleeza, Aleezah, Aleiza, Aleizah, Aleyza, Aleyzah, Altza, Alitzah, Alisa, Alisah, Aliza, Alizah, Alyza, Alyzah

Alina (Australian Aboriginal) moon.
Alkinah, Alkine, Alkyn, Alkyna, Alkyne

Allegra (Latin) cheerful. (Ital) lively.
Allegrah

Allira (Australian Aboriginal) the quartz stone.
Allirah, Allyra, Allyrah

Ally (Greek) little truthful one. The short form of names starting with 'Al' e.g. Allison.
Alea, Aleah, Alee, Alei, Aleigh, Aley, Ali, Alia, Aliah, Alie, Allea, Alleah, Allee, Allei, Alleigh, Alley, Alli, Allia, Alliah, Allya, Allyah, Aly, Alya, Alyah

Alma (Arabic) learned.
(Lat) nourishing; supportive.
(Span/Ital) spirit.
(Heb) young woman.
Almah, Almar, Almara, Almarah, Almaria, Almariah, Almarya, Almaryah

Almeda (Latin) goal-orientated.
Almedah, Almeta, Almetah, Almetta, Almettah

Almedha (Welsh) shapely.
Almeda, Almedah, Almida, Almidah, Almyda, Almydah, Enid, Enyd

Almeta (Latin) ambitious.
Almeda, Almedah, Almetah, Almetta, Almettah

Almira (Arabic) princess. (Eng) noble; famous. The feminine form of Elmer.
Allmera, Allmerah, Allmira, Allmirah, Allyra, Allysha, Almera, Almerah, Almeria, Almeriah, Almirah, Almina, Almine, Almyra, Almyrah, Elmera, Elmerah, Elmira, Elmirah, Elmyra, Elmyrah

Almita (Latin) kindness.
Almitah, Almyta, Almytah

Alnaba (Native American) wars fought at the same time.
Alnabah

Alodie (Old English) wealthy.
Alodea, Alodee, Alodey, Alodi, Alodia, Alodiah, Alody, Alodya, Alodyah, Elodee, Elodey, Elodi, Elodie, Elody

Aloha (Hawaiian) greetings; farewell.
Alohah, Alohalanee, Alohalaney, Alohalani, Alohalania, Alohalaniah, Alohalanie, Alohalany, Alohalanya, Alohilanee, Alohilaney, Alohilani, Alohilania, Alohilaniah, Alohilany, Alohilanya, Alohilanyah

Alona (Australian/English/Latin) solitary angel.
Alonah, Alonna, Alonnah, Halona (N/Amer), Halonah, Halonna, Halonnah

Aloysia (Teutonic) famous warrior.
Aloisia, Aloysiah, Aloyza (Pol), Aloyzah

Alpha (Greek) first born.
Alfa, Alfah, Alfia, Alfiah, Alfya, Alfyah, Alphah, Alphia, Alphiah, Alphya, Alphyah

Alta (Latin) majestic; high.
Altah, Altai, Alto

Altair (Arabic) bird.
Altaira, Altaire, Altayr, Altayra, Altayrah, Altayre

Althea (Greek) wholesome healing; healthy.
Altheah, Altheda, Althedah, Althia, Althiah, Althya, Althyah

Altsoba (Native American) war.
Altsobah

Alula (Arabic) first born.
Alulah

Alura (Old English) divine counsellor.
Alurah

Alva (Spanish/Latin) white.
Alvah

Alvera (Latin) truthful.
Alverah, Alveria, Alveriah, Alverya,
Alveryah, Alvira, Alvirah, Alvyra,
Alvyrah, Elvera, Elverah, Elvira,
Elvirah, Elvyra, Elvyrah

Alvina (Old English) beloved; wise
friend to all. The feminine form
of Alvin.
Alveana, Alveanah, Alveane,
Alveena, Alveenah, Alveene,
Alvena, Alvenah, Alvinah, Alvine,
Alvyna, Alvynah, Alvyne, Elveana,
Elveanah, Elvena, Elvenah, Elvina,
Elvinah, Elvine, Elvyna, Elvynah

Alyssa/Alyssum (Greek) sensible;
yellow flower.
Alisa, Alissah, Allissa, Allissah,
Allyssa, Allyssah, Alysa, Alysah,
Alyssah, Alysun, Alysumm, Ilisa,
Ilisah, Ilysa, Ilysah, Illissa, Illissah,
Illyssa, Illysah, Lisa, Lisah, Lissa,
Lissa, Lissah, Lysa, Lysah, Lyssa,
Lyssah

Alzena (Arabic/Persian) the woman.
Alsenah, Alsena, Alxena, Alxenah,
Alxina, Alxinah, Alxyna, Alxynah,
Alzenah, Alzina, Alzinah, Alzyna,
Alzynah

Am (Vietnamese) female; lunar.

Ama (African/French) born on a
Saturday.
Amah

Amabel (Latin) lovable.
Amabela, Amabelah, Amabell,
Amabella, Amabellah, Amabelle

Amada (Spanish) beloved.
Amadea, Amadeah, Amadee,
Amadey, Amadi, Amadia, Amadiah,
Amadie, Amadita, Amadite, Amady,
Amadya, Amadyah

Amadea (Italian) one who loves
God.
Amadeah, Amadee, Amadey,
Amadi, Amadia, Amadiah, Amadie,
Amady, Amadya, Amdyah

Amal (Arabic) hope. (Heb)
industrious.
Amala, Amalah, Amalla, Amallah

Amalea (Hebrew/English)
industrious meadow.
Amaleah, Amalee, Amalei,
Amaleigh, Amaley, Amali, Amalia,
Amaliah, Amalie, Amaly, Amalya,
Amalyah

Amaline (German) industrious.
Amalean, Amaleana, Amaleane,
Amaleen, Amaleena, Amaleene,
Amalin, Amalina, Amalyn,
Amalyna, Amalyne

Amalthea (Greek) God nourishes
her.
Amalthia, Amalthiah, Amalthya,
Amalthyah

Amanaki (Tongan) hope.
Amanakee, Amanakey, Amanakie,
Amanaky

Amanda (Latin) worthy of love.
Amandah, Amamde, Amandea,
Amandee, Amandey, Amandi,
Amandia, Amandiah, Amandie,
Amandina, Amandinah, Amandine
(Fren), Amandy, Amandya,
Amandyah, Amaranth, Amarantha,
Amaranthe, Amata (Span), Manda,
Mandah, Mandea, Mandee,
Mandey, Mandi, Mandie, Mandy

Amara (Greek) eternal beauty.
Amarah, Amargo, Amari, Amaria,
Amairah, Amarie, Amary, Amarya,
Amaryah

Amarina (Australian Aboriginal)
rain.
Amarin, Amarinah, Amarine,

Amarina cont.
Amaryn, Amaryna, Amarynah,
Amaryne

Amarinda (Greek) long-lived.
Amara, Amargo, Amarindah,
Amarynda, Amaryndah

Amaris (Hebrew) promise of God.
Amariah, Amariah, Amarisa,
Amarisah, Amariss, Amarissa,
Amarissah, Amarys, Amarysa,
Amarysah, Amaryss, Amaryssa,
Amaryssah

Amaryllis (Greek) fresh stream.
Amaryl, Amaryla, Amarylah,
Amarylis, Amarylla, Amaryllah

Amaya (Japanese) raining at night.
Amaia, Amaiah, Amayah

Amayeta (Native American) berry.
Amayetah

Ambel (Latin) lovable.
Amabel, Amabela, Amabelah,
Amabele, Amabell, Amabella,
Amabellah, Amabelle, Amebela,
Amebelah, Amebele, Amebell,
Amebella, Amebellah, Amebelle,
Amibel, Amibela, Amibelah,
Amilbele, Amibell, Amibella,
Amibellah, Amibelle, Amybel,
Amybell, Amybella, Amybella,
Amybelle

Amber (Egyptian) light.
(O/Fren) the amber jewel.
(Arab) jewel. (Gae) fiery.
Ambar, Ambarlea, Ambarlee,
Ambarlei, Ambarleigh, Ambarley,
Ambarli, Ambarlina, Ambarline,
Ambarlie, Ambarly, Amberlea,
Amberlee, Amberlei, Amberleigh,
Amberley, Amberli, Amberlia,
Amberliah, Amberlie (Fren),
Amberlina, Amberline,
Amberly, Amberlyah, Ambur,

Amburlea, Amburlee, Amberlei,
Amburleigh, Amburley, Amburli,
Amburlia, Amburliah, Amburlie,
Amburlina, Amburline, Amburly,
Amburlya

Ambrosia (Polish/Greek) divine
immortal. The feminine form of
Ambrose.
Ambrosa, Ambrosah, Ambrosia
(Grk), Ambrosiah, Ambrosina,
Ambrosine (Fren), Ambrosyn,
Ambrosyna, Ambrosyne, Ambroyze
(Pol), Ambrozin, Ambrozina,
Ambrozinah, Ambrozine,
Ambrozyn, Ambrozyna,
Ambrozyne

Amelia (Teutonic) hard-working.
Amala, Amalah, Amalburga,
Amalea, Amaleah, Amalee,
Amaleigh, Amaleta, Amalia
(Ger/Span/Dut), Amali, Amalie,
Amalita, Amalitah, Amelie (Fren),
Amelija (Lith), Amelina, Amelinda,
Amelindah, Ameline (Fren),
Amelita, Amelitah, Amelynda,
Amelyndah, Amilia, Amiliah,
Amilina, Amiline, Amilinda,
Amiline, Amilita, Amilitah,
Ammilina, Ammiline, Amylia,
Amyliah, Amylya, Amylyah,
Emelin, Emelina, Emeline, Emelita,
Emelitah, Emmelina, Emmeline,
Emmilyn, Emmilyna, Emmilyne

Amelinda (Latin/Spanish) beautiful
beloved.
Amalinda, Amalindah, Amalynda,
Amalyndah, Ammalyn, Amalynn,
Amalynne, Amelindah, Amelind,
Amelynda, Amelyndah, Amerlinda,
Amerlindah, Amerlynda,
Amerlyndah, Amerlyn, Amerlynn,
Amerlynne, Amilindah, Amilindah,
Amilynda, Amilyndah, Amilyn,
Amilynn, Amilynna, Amilynne

America (Latin) freedom.
(Geographical) the country.
Amarica, Amaricah, Amaricka,
Amarika, Amarikah, Amelika
(Tong), Americah, Americka,
Amerika, Amerikah, Ameriqua,
Ameriquah, Amerique, Ameryca,
Amerycah, Americka, Americkah,
Ameryka, Amerykah, Ameryqua,
Ameryquah, Ameryque

Amethyst (Greek) beneficent; wine;
purple-coloured gem.
Amathist, Amathista, Amathiste,
Amathista, Amathysta, Amathyste,
Amathistia, Amethist, Amethista,
Amethiste, Amethistia, Amethysta,
Amethyste, Amethystia,
Amethystiah, Amethystya,
Amethystyah

Amice (Latin) beloved.
Amata, Amatah, Amica, Amicah,
Amicia, Amiciah, Amisa, Amisah,
Amise, Amisia, Amisiah, Amyca,
Amycah, Amysa, Amysah, Amysia,
Amysiah, Amysya, Amysyah

Aminta (Greek) protector.
Amintah, Aminte, Amintee,
Amintey, Aminti, Amintie, Aminty,
Amynta, Amyntah, Amynti,
Amyntie, Amynthy, Minta, Mintah,
Mynta, Myntee, Myntey, Mynti,
Myntie, Mynty

Amipa (Tongan) amber stone.
Amipah

Amira (Arabic) princess.
Amirah, Amyra, Amyrah

Amita (Hebrew) truthful.
Ameeta, Ameetah, Amitah, Amyta,
Amytah

Amitola (Native American)
rainbow.
Amitolah

Amity (Latin) friendly.
Amitee, Amitey, Amiti, Amitie,
Amity, Amytee, Amytey, Amyti,
Amytie, Amyty

Amlike (Hindi) mother.
Amilkah, Amylka, Amylkah

Ammu (Arabic) beloved aunt.
Amu

Amorel (Gaelic) dweller by the sea.
Amorela, Amorelah, Amorell,
Amorella, Amorellah, Amorelle

Amorette/Amorita (Latin) beloved.
Amoreta, Amoretah, Amorete,
Amoretta, Amorettah, Amorette,
Amorit, Amoritah, Amoritt,
Amoritta, Amoritte, Amoryta,
Amorytah, Amoryte, Amorytt,
Amorytta, Amorytte

Amrita (Spanish) little love.
Amritah, Amritta, Amritte, Amryta,
Amrytah, Amryte, Amrytta,
Amryttah, Amrytte

Amy (Latin) beloved friend.
(Fren) to love.
Aime, Aimee, Aimey, Aimi, Aimia,
Aimiah, Aimie, Aimy, Aimya,
Aimyah, Amata (Ital/Swed/Span),
Amatah, Ame, Amee (Eng), Amei,
Amey, Ami, Amia, Amiah, Amie
(Eng), Amice, Amie, Amii, Amina,
Aminah, Amine, Amity, Amorett,
Amoretta, Amorette, Amorita,
Amoritta, Amorittah, Amoritta,
Amoritte, Amoryt, Amoryta,
Amorytah, Amoryte, Amorytt,
Amorytta, Amoryttah, Amorytte

An (Chinese) peaceful.
Ann

Ana (Hawaiian/Spanish/Hebrew)
God is gracious. A form of
Hannah.
Anah, Anci (Hung), Anezka
(Czech), Ania (Pol), Aniah,

Ana cont.
Annaka, Annalie (Finn), Anneka (Swed), Annika, Anniki, Annikki, Annus, Annushka

Anaba (Native American) she has returned from battle; warrior.
Anabah

Anais (Hebrew) graceful.
Anaiss, Anays, Anayss

Anala (Hindi) fine.
Analah

Anamosa (Sauk) baby deer; white in colour.
Anamosah

Ananda (Hindi) bliss; joy.
Anandah

Ananke (Greek) necessity.
Anank

Anastasia (Greek) resurrection; springtime.
Anastacia, Anastaciah, Anastacya, Anastacyah, Anastas, Anastase, Anastasee, Anastasie (Fren), Anastatia, Anestasia, Anastassia, Anastazia, Anastziah, Anastazya (Pol), Annestas, Annestasia, Annestassia, Anstace, Ansteece, Ansteese, Anstes, Anstey, Anstice (Eng), Anstice (Grk), Anstis, Natassia, Natassja, Nastasya, Nastenka, Nastia, Naztasia, Naztasiah, Nastya, Nastyenka, Natasha, Nitasse, Stacee, Stacey, Staci, Stacie, Stacy, Stassee, Stassey, Stassi, Stassie, Stassy, Tas, Tasa, Tasi, Tasia, Tasie, Tasy

Anatolia (Greek) eastern.
Anatola, Anatolah, Anatoliah, Anatolya, Anatolyah, Annatola, Annatolah, Annatolia, Annatoliah, Annatolya, Annatolyah

Ancelin (Latin) land; the knight's spear attendant. The feminine form of Lancelot.
Ancelina, Ancelinah, Anceline, Ancelyn, Ancelyna, Ancelynah, Ancelyne

Anchoret (Welsh) beloved.
Anchorett, Anchoreta, Anchorette

Ancilla (Latin) attendant.
Ancillah, Ancilee (Fren), Ancillee, Ancillia, Ancilliah, Ancyla, Ancylah, Ancylla, Ancyllah

Andra (Old Norse) a breath.
Andrah

Andria/Andriana (Latin/Greek) strong; brave; courageous. The feminine form of Andrew.
Aindrea (Ir), Anderea, Andra, Andrah, Andreana, Andreanah, Andreane, Andreann, Andreanna, Andreannah, Andreanne, Andree (Fren), Andreean, Andreeana, Andreeanah, Andreeane, Andrel, Andrela, Andrelah, Andrell, Andrella, Andrellah, Andrelle, Andretta, Andrette, Andria, Andriah, Andrian, Andriann, Andrianna, Andriannah, Andrianne, Andrina, Adrinah, Andrya, Andryah, Andryan, Andryana, Andryanah, Andryane, Andryann, Andryanna, Andryannah, Andryanne, Andryane

Aneira (Welsh) honourable; gold.
Aneirah, Aneyra, Aneyrah

Aneko (Japanese) oldest sister.

Anela (Hebrew) angel.
Anelah, Anella, Anellah

Anemone (Greek) wind; flower.
Annemone

Anga (Tongan) nature; shark.
Angah

Angel/Angela/Angelina/Angeline
(Greek) messenger of God;
angel. The short form of
Angela/Angelique.

Agnola, Aindrea (Ir), Ancela (Pol),
Angel, Angele (Fren), Angelica
(Ger), Angelika (Ger), Angelin,
Angelina (Eng), Angelinah,
Angeline, Angeliqua, Angeliquah,
Angelique (Fren), Angella,
Angellah, Angelle, Angelita (Swed),
Angiola (Ital), Angelo (Tong),
Aniela (Ital/Pol), Anja, Anjah,
Anjal, Anjala, Anjalah, Anjel,
Anjela, Anjelah, Anjella, Anjelle,
Anjelle, Engel, Engela, Engelah,
Engele, Engelchen, Engelica,
Engelika, Engell, Engella, Engellah,
Engelle, Engelyca, Engelycka,
Engelyka, Engeliqua, Engeliquah,
Engelique, Enjel, Enjela, Enjelah,
Enjele, Enjell, Enjella, Enjellah,
Enjelle, Enjelliqua, Enjelliquah,
Enjellique, Enjellyca, Enjellycah,
Enjellycka, Enjellyka, Enjellyqua,
Enjellyquah, Enjellyque

Angelo (Tongan) angel.
Anjelo, Engelo, Enjelo

Angeni (Native American) spirit.
Ange, Angee, Angeenee, Angeeni,
Angeenie, Angeeny, Angenia,
Angey, Anjee, Anjeenee, Anjeeney,
Anjeeni, Anjeenie, Anjeeny,
Anjeenia, Anjeeniah, Anjeenie,
Anjeeny, Anjeenya, Anjeenyah,
Anjena, Anjenah, Anjenee,
Anjeney, Anjeni, Anjenie, Anjeny

Angharad (Welsh) well-loved.
Anchoret, Anchorett, Anchoretta,
Anchorette, Ancret, Ancreta,
Ancrett, Ancretta, Angharad,
Ankerita, Ingaret, Ingarett,
Ingaretta, Ingarette

Anh (Vietnamese) flower.

Ani (Hawaiian) beautiful.
Anee, Aney, Aneya, Aneyah, Ania,
Aniah, Anie, Any, Anya, Anyah

Ania (Polish/Hebrew) God is
gracious. A form of Hannah.
Ana, Anah, Aniah, Anya, Anyah

Aniela (Hebrew) graceful. The
Polish form of Anna.
Anielah, Aniella, Anielle, Anniela,
Annielah, Anniella, Anielle, Anyel,
Anyela, Anyele, Anyell, Anyella,
Anyellah, Anyelle

Anika (Scandinavian/Swedish/
Hebrew) graceful. A form of Ann.
Anica, Anicah, Anikah, Aniqua,
Aniquah, Anyca, Anycah, Anyka,
Anykah, Anyqua, Anyquah

Anila (Hindi) God of the wind.
Anilah, Anilla, Anillah, Anyla,
Anylah, Anylla, Anyllah

Anisah (Arabic) friendly.
Anisa, Anisah, Annisa, Annisah,
Annissa, Annissah, Annysa,
Annysah, Anysa, Anysah, Anyssa,
Anyssah

Anita (Hebrew) graceful.
Anitta, Anittah, Anitte, Annita,
Annitah, Annite, Annitt, Annitta,
Annittah, Annitte, Annyta, Annytah,
Annytta, Annyttah, Annytte

Anja (Russian) graceful. A form of
Ann.
Ania, Aniah, Anjah, Anya, Anyah

Ann/Anna/Anne (Hebrew) graceful.
The short form of names starting
with 'Ann' e.g. Annelise.
Ana (Span), Anah, Anais, Anaisa,
Anca (Boh), Ancika, Ane, Anee,
Aney, Aneta, Anezka, Ani, Ania,
Aniah, Anica, Anita (Span), Anitra,
Anje (Dut), Anjuska (Rus), Anka
(Serv), Anna (Eng/Ger/Ital/Dut/
Dan/Swed), Annabel, Annabela,

Ann/Anna/Anne cont.

Annabelah, Annabele, Annabell,
Annabella, Annabelle, Annah,
Annali (Swis), Annchet, Annchetta,
Anne, Annebel, Annebela,
Annebelah, Annebele, Annebell,
Annebella, Annebellah, Annebelle,
Annee, Annechet, Anney, Anneke
(Dut), Annerl (Bav), Annetta,
Annette (Fren), Annica (Ital),
Annice (Eng), Annichet, Anje
(Dut), Anni, Annia, Anniah, Annie,
Annika (Rus/Swed/Lith), Annike,
Annis, Anno, Annusia (Rus),
Annora, Annore, Annot, Annusche
(Let), Annucschka (Rus), Anny,
Annya, Annyah, Annze (Lith),
Ansel, Antje, Anyanusia (Pol/Grk),
Anuska, Anya, Hana, Hanah,
Hanna, Hannah, Hanni, Hannie,
Hanny, Ineka, Naatje, Nan, Nana,
Nance, Nancee, Nancey, Nanci,
Nancie, Nancy, Nanetta, Nanette
(Fren), Nann, Nanneli, Nanni,
Nanon, Nillion, Nina, Ninetta,
Ninette, Nita (Span), Nona,
Nonah, Ona, Onah, Panna,
Pannah, Panni, Pannie, Panny,
Vanjuscha, Vanka, Vanni, Vannie,
Vanny, Zaneta, Zanetta, Zanette

Annabella (Latin/French) graceful;
lovable. (Heb/Lat) graceful,
beautiful woman.
Anabel, Anabela, Anabelah,
Anabele, Annabel, Annabell, Anna-
Bell, Annabella, Anna-Bella,
Annabellah, Anna-Bellah,
Annahbel, Annah-Bel, Annahbell,
Annah-Bell, Annahbella, Annah-
Bella, Annahbelle, Annah-Belle,
Annebel, Annebela, Annebelah,
Annebele, Annebell, Annebella,
Annebellah, Annebelle, Annibel,
Annibela, Annibelah, Annibele,
Annibell, Annibella, Annibellah,

Annibelle, Annybel, Annybela,
Annybelah, Annybele, Annybell,
Annybella, Annybellah, Annybelle

Anneka (Hebrew) graceful. The
Dutch/Swedish form of Anna.
Annekah

Annelise (German) graceful
satisfaction.
Analisa, Analise, Anetta, Annaliese,
Annalisa, Annalise, Annalyce,
Annalyca, Annalys, Annalysa,
Annalyse, Anneliese, Anneliesel,
Annelys, Annelysa, Annelyse

Annette/Annetta (French) little
graceful one. A form of Anne.
Anet, Aneta, Anetah, Anete, Anetra,
Anetrah, Anett, Anetta, Anett,
Anetta, Anette, Annet, Annettah

Annina (Hebrew) graceful.
Anina, Aninah, Anninah, Annyna,
Annynah, Anyna, Anynah

Annis (Greek) complete.
Anis, Anys, Annys

Annisa (Hebrew) graceful.
Anisa, Anisah, Anise, Annis,
Annise, Anniss, Annissa, Annisse,
Annys, Annysa, Annyse, Annyss,
Annyssa, Annysse

Annmarie (Hebrew) graceful;
wished-for child.
Anmaree, Anmari, Anmaria,
Anmariah, Anmarie, Anmary,
Anmarya, Anmaryah, Annmaree,
Annmari, Annmaria, Annmariah,
Annmarie, Annmary, Annmarya,
Annmaryah

Annona (Greek) roman goddess of
the yearly crop.
Anona, Anonah, Anona, Anonah,
Annona, Annonah, Annonia,
Annoniah, Annonya, Annonyah

Annora (Greek) shining light.
(Lat) honour. The Old English
form of Eleanor/Helen.
Anora, Anorah, Anoria, Anoriah,
Annorah, Annoria, Annoriah,
Annorya, Annoryah, Anorya,
Anoryah

Anona (Latin) annual crops; ninth
born child. (Eng) pineapple.
Anonah

Anselma (Old Norse) warrior
possessing divine protection. The
feminine form of Anselm.
Anselmah, Anzelma, Anzelmah,
Selma, Selmah, Xelma, Xelmah,
Zelma, Zelmah

Anthea (Greek) flowery.
Anthe, Antheah, Anthia, Anthiah,
Anthya, Anthyah

Antoinette/Antonia (French)
priceless. The feminine form of
Anthony.
Antonee, Antoney, Antonett,
Antonetta, Antonette, Antoni,
Antonia, Antoniah, Antonias,
Antonica, Antonicah, Antonie
(Ger), Antonietta (Ital), Antoninas,
Antonnia, Antonniah, Antonya
(Lith), Antonyah, Toinetta,
Toinette, Toynetta, Toynette,
Tuanetta, Tuanette

Anya (Hebrew) graceful. The
Russian form of Anna.
Anyah

Anzu (Japanese) apricot.

Aolani (Hawaiian) heavenly cloud.
Aolanee, Aolaney, Aolania,
Aolaniah, Aolanie, Aolany,
Aolanya, Aolanyah

Apanie (Australian Aboriginal)
water.
Apanee, Apaney, Apani, Apany

Apex (English) summit.
Apexx

Aphra (Hebrew) female deer, doe;
dust.
Afra, Afrah, Aphrah, Ayfara, Ayfarah

Aphrodite (Greek) goddess of love.
Afrodita, Afrodite, Aphrodita,
Aphrodyta, Aphrodytah, Aphrodyte

Apolda/Apoline (Greek) sunlight.
Apoldah, Apollina, Apollinah,
Apolline, Apollyn, Apollyna,
Apollynah, Apollyne, Appolina,
Appolinah, Appoline, Appollina,
Appollinah, Appolline, Appollyn,
Appollyna, Appollynah, Appollyne

Aponi (Native American) butterfly.
Aponee, Aponey, Aponie, Apony

Appollonia (Greek) sunlight.
Abbelina, Abbelinah, Abbeline,
Abeloona, Apolda, Apoldah,
Apolinarya, Apoline, Apollonia,
Apolloniah, Appolina, Appolinah,
Appoline, Apolonia, Apoloniah,
Apolonie, Appollonia, Appolloniah,
Appollonya, Appollonyah

April (Latin) born in the month of
April.
Aprel, Aprela, Aprelah, Aprella,
Aprelle, Aprila, Aprilah,Aprilett,
Apriletta, Aprilette, Aprill, Aprilla,
Aprillah, Aprille, Apryl, Apryla,
Aprylah, Apryll, Aprylla, Aprylle,
Avril, Avrilett, Avriletta, Avrilette,
Avryl, Avryla, Avrylah, Avryle,
Avryll, Avrylla, Avryllah, Avrylle,
Avryllett, Avryletta, Avryllettah,
Avryllette

Aquene (Native American) peace.
Aqueen, Aqueena, Aqueene, Aquene

Ara (Arabic) rainmaker. (Grk) altar;
the Greek goddess of vengence
and destruction.
Arae, Arah, Aria, Ariah, Arya, Aryah

Arabella (Latin) asked for; beautiful altar. (Ger) eagle heroine.
Arabe, Arabel, Arabela (Span), Arabelah, Arabell, Arabellah, Arabelle (Fren/Ger), Araminta, Aramintah

Arachne (Greek) spider.

Arctic (English) from the Arctic.
Arctica, Arcticah, Arcticka, Artickah, Artika, Artikah, Artyca, Artycah, Artycka, Artyckah, Artyka, Artykah

Ardeen/Ardelia (Latin) glowing.
Ardeana, Ardeanah, Ardeane, Ardeena, Ardeenah, Ardeene, Ardina, Ardinah, Ardine, Ardyn, Ardyna, Ardynah, Ardyne

Ardella (Latin) ardent; warm; enthusastic; desired.
Adra, Adrah, Ardeen, Ardeena, Ardeene, Ardel, Ardela, Ardelah, Ardele, Ardelia, Ardeliah, Ardell, Ardella, Ardellah, Ardelis, Ardelisa, Ardelise, Ardena, Ardenah, Ardene, Ardin, Ardina, Ardinah, Ardine, Ardis

Arden (Old English) from the valley of eagles.
Ardan, Ardana, Ardane, Ardeen, Ardeena, Ardeene, Ardena, Ardene, Ardin, Ardina, Ardine, Ardun, Ardyn, Ardyna, Ardyne

Ardis (Latin) eager.
Adisa, Adisah, Ardiss, Ardissa, Ardisse, Ardyce, Ardyse, Ardyssa, Ardyssah

Ardith (Hebrew) field of flowers.
Ardath, Ardis, Ardisa, Ardise, Ardiss, Ardissa, Ardisse, Ardyce, Ardys, Ardysa, Ardyse, Ardyth, Ardythe, Aridatha, Arydatha

Arella (Hebrew) angel; messenger of God.
Arela, Arealah, Arellah, Ariel,

Ariela, Arielah, Ariella, Ariellah, Arielle, Arien, Ariena, Arienah, Ariene, Arienna, Arienne, Arkee, Arkey, Aryel, Aryela, Aryelah, Aryell, Aryella, Aryellah, Aryelle, Orelia, Orelie, Orella, Orellah, Orelle, Orellia, Orelliah, Orellya, Orellyah

Areta/Aretha (Greek) the best.
Areata, Areatah, Areatha, Areathah, Areathia, Areathiah, Areeta, Areetah, Areetha, Areethah, Areethia, Areethiah, Areta, Aretah, Arethia, Arethiah, Aretta, Arettah, Arette (Fren), Aritha, Arithah, Arytha, Arythah, Arythia, Arythiah, Arythya, Arythyah, Retha, Rethah

Arethus (Greek) virtuous ruler.
Arethea, Aretheah, Arethia, Arethiah, Arethious, Arethius, Arethyus

Argenta (Latin) silver.
Argentah, Argentia, Argentiah, Argentina, Argentinah, Argentine, Argentya, Argentyah, Argentyn, Argentyna, Argentynah, Argentyne

Argyro (Greek) silver.
Argiro

Aria (Italian) melody; song.
Ari, Ariah, Ariann, Arianna, Ariannah, Arianne, Arya, Aryah, Aryan, Aryana, Aryanah, Aryane, Aryann, Aryanna, Aryannah, Aryanne

Ariadna/Ariadne (Greek) holy.
Adriadna, Ariadnah, Ariana, Arianah, Ariane, Arianna, Ariannah, Arianne, Aryadna, Aryana, Aryanah, Aryane, Aryann, Aryanna, Aryannah, Aryanne

Ariana (Latin) holy.
Ariadna, Ariadnah, Ariadne, Arianah, Arianna, Ariannah,

Ariane, Arianne, Arihana, Arihanah, Arihanna, Arihannah, Aryan, Aryana, Aryanah, Aryane, Aryann, Aryanna, Aryannah, Aryanne

Arianwen (Welsh) silver/white. (Eng) white friend.
Arianwena, Arianwenah, Arianwin, Arianwina, Arianwinah, Arianwyn, Arianwyna, Arianwynah, Aryanwen, Aryanwena, Aryanwenah, Aryanwin, Aryanwina, Aryanwinah, Aryanwyn, Aryanwyna, Aryanwynah

Arica (Scandinavian) ruler. A form of Erica.
Aricah, Aricca, Ariccah, Aricka, Arika, Arikah, Arikka, Arikkah, Ariqua, Ariquah, Aryca, Arycah, Arycca, Aryka, Arykah, Arykka, Arykkah, Aryqua, Aryquah

Aricia (Greek) princess of Athens.
Ariciah, Arycia, Aryciah, Arycya, Arycyah

Ariel/Ariella (Hebrew) lioness of God.
Aeriel, Aeriela, Aerielah, Aeriell, Aeriella, Aeriellah, Aerielle, Ariela, Arielah, Ariell, Ariella, Ariellah, Arielle, Aryel, Aryela, Aryelah, Aryele, Aryell, Aryella, Aryellah, Aryelle

Arietta (Italian) melody.
Ariet, Arieta, Arietah, Ariete, Ariett, Ariettah, Ariette, Aryet, Aryeta, Aryetah, Aryete, Aryett, Aryetta, Aryettah, Aryette

Arika (Australian Aboriginal) waterlily.
Arica, Aricah, Aricka, Arickah, Arikah, Ariqua, Ariquah, Aryca, Arycah, Arycka, Aryckah, Aryka, Arykah, Aryqua, Aryquah

Arleana/Arlene/Arline (Irish/Gaelic) promise. The feminine form of Arlen.
Arlana, Arlanah, Arlea, Arleah, Arlee, Arleen, Arleena, Arleene, Arlein, Arleina, Arleine, Arleigh, Arlena, Arlenah, Arlene, Arleta, Arletah, Arlete, Arletta, Arlettah, Arlette, Arleyne, Arlien, Arliena, Arlienah, Arliene, Arlin, Arlina, Arlinah, Arlind, Arlinda, Arlindah, Arline, Arluena, Arluenah, Arluene, Arlyn, Arlynna, Arlynne

Armida (Latin) little armed warrior.
Armidah, Armyda, Armydah

Armide (Greek) sorceress.
Armidea, Armidee, Armidia, Armidiah, Armydea, Armydee, Armydia, Armydiah, Armydya, Armydyah

Armilla (Latin) warrior who wears a bracelet in battle.
Armila, Armilah, Armillah, Armyla, Armylah, Armylla, Armyllah

Armina (Teutonic) warrior.
Armeda, Armedah, Armedia, Armediah, Armida, Armidah, Armidia, Armidiah, Armin, Armina, Arminah, Arminda, Armindah, Armine, Armini, Arminie, Armyn, Armyna, Armynah, Armyne, Ermina, Erminah, Ermine, Ermyn, Ermyna, Ermynah, Ermyne

Arminda (Latin) of high degree.
Armin, Armindah, Arminde, Armyn, Armynd, Armynda, Armynde

Armine (Teutonic) noble warrior. (Lat) high ranking. (Heb) faithful. The feminine from of Herman.
Armina, Arminah, Arminee, Arminey, Arminel (Corn),

Armine cont.
Arminella, Arminelle, Armyn, Armyna, Armynah, Armyne

Arnalda (Teutonic) strong; powerful like an eagle. A feminine form of Arnold.
Arnoldah

Arnelle (Latin/French/Teutonic) strong; powerful like an eagle. A feminine form of Arnold.
Arnel, Arnela, Arnelah, Arnele, Arnella, Arnellah

Arnette (Latin/English/Teutonic) strong; powerful like an eagle. A feminine form of Arnold.
Arnet, Arneta, Arnett, Arnetta, Arnette

Arnhilda (German) eagle warrior.
Arnhylda

Arnina (Hebrew) enlightened singing. The feminine form of Aaron.
Arninah, Arnine, Arnona, Arnonah, Arninah, Arnyna, Arynyah

Arnurna (Australian Aboriginal) blue waterlily.
Arnurnah

Aroona (Australian Aboriginal) running water.
Aroon, Aroonah

Arora (Australian Aboriginal) cockatoo (parrot).
Arorah

Arrow (English) arrow-like.
Arro

Artemis (Greek) the moon goddess.
Artema, Artemah, Artemisa, Artemise, Artemys

Artemisia (Greek) belonging to Artemis, the Greek goddess of the hunt.
Artemisiah, Artemysia, Artemysiah, Artemysya, Artemysyah

Artha (Hindi) wealthy. (Celt) noble strength. (Wel/Scott) bear. The feminine form of Arthur.
Athrah

Artis (Irish) noble. (Wel/Scott) bear. (Ice) follower of Thor; thunder. (Eng) rock.
Artisa, Artise, Artina, Artinah, Artine, Artrice, Artis, Artysa, Artyse, Artyna, Artynah, Artyne, Artryce, Artys, Artyse

Aruna (Sanskrit) dawning light.
Arunah

Arva (Latin) country pastures; the seashore.
Arvah

Asa (Japanese) born in the morning. (Heb) healer.
Asah

Aselma (Gaelic) fair-haired.
Aselmah, Selma, Selmah

Ash (English) ash tree.

Asha (Persian) truth. (Swa) life.
Ashah

Ashanti (Swahili) life; tribal name.
Ashanta, Ashantah, Ashantae, Ashantee, Ashantey, Ashantia, Ashantie, Ashauntee, Ashaunti, Ashauntia, Ashauntiah, Ashuntie, Ashaunty, Ashauntya, Shauntyah

Ashia (Arabic) life.
Asha, Ashah, Ayshia, Ayshiah, Ayshya, Ayshyah

Ashira (Hebrew) wealthy.
Ashirah, Ashyra, Ashyrah

Orelee, Orelia, Oreliah, Orelie,
Orla, Orlah

Aurora (Latin) Greek goddess of the
dawn.
Aurorah, Aurore (Fren), Aurure,
Ora, Orah

Austine (Latin) little majestic one.
Austina, Austinah, Austyna,
Austynah, Austyne

Autumn (Latin) autumn, fall.
Autom, Autum

Ava (Greek) eagle. (Lat) bird-like.
Arva, Arvah, Avah

Avalon (Latin) island.
Avalona, Avalonah, Avaloni,
Avalonia, Avaloniah, Avalonie,
Avalony, Avalonya, Avalonyah

Avanga (Tongan) bewitched.
Avangah

Avara (Sanskrit) the youngest child.
Avarah, Avaria, Avariah, Avarya,
Avaryah

Aveline (Teutonic) hazelnut.
Avalean, Avaleana, Avaleanah,
Avaleane, Avaleen, Avaleenah,
Avaleene, Avalina, Avaline, Avalyn,
Avalyna, Avalynah, Avalyne,
Avelean, Aveleana, Aveleanah,
Aveleane, Aveleen, Aveleena,
Aveleenah, Aveleene, Avelina,
Avelyn, Avelyna, Avelynah, Avelyne

Avena (Latin) oats.
Avenah, Avene

Avera (Hebrew) transgressor; to go
beyond.
Averah

Averil (Old English) boar battle.
Avaril, Avarila, Avarile, Averill,
Avarilla, Avarille, Averila, Averilah,
Averill, Averilla, Averille, Averyl,
Averyla, Averyle, Averyll, Averylla,

Averylle, Eberhilda, Everild,
Everilda, Everildah

Avery (Old French) confirmation.
Avaree, Avarey, Avari, Avarie, Avary,
Averee, Averey, Averi, Averie

Avice (Teutonic) sanctuary in battle.
(Lat) bird-like. (O/Fren) warrior.
Aveza, Aveze, Avicia, Avis, Avise,
Avyce, Avyse, Avys

Avis (Teutonic/Old English)
sanctuary in battle.
Amice, Aveis, Aves, Avice, Avicia,
Avison, Havoise

Aviva (Hebrew) fresh; springtime.
Abibi, Abibit, Auvit, Avivah, Avrit,
Avivah, Avivi, Avivie, Avivit, Avyva,
Avyvah

Avoca (Irish) sweet valley.
Avocah, Avocka, Avockah, Avoka,
Avokah

Avoka (Tongan) avocado.
Avoca, Avocah, Avocka, Avockah,
Avokah

Avril (Old English) born in April;
boar warrior woman. The French
form of April.
April, Aprill, Apryl, Apryll, Averill,
Averilla, Averille, Avril, Avrill,
Avrilla, Avrille, Avryl, Avryla,
Avrylah, Avryle, Avryll, Avrylla,
Avryllah, Avrylle

Awee (Navajo) baby.

Awena (Welsh) poetry.
Awenah

Aya (Hebrew) swift bird.
Aia, Aiah, Ayah

Ayanna (Hindi) innocent.
Ayania, Ayaniah, Ayannah

Ayasha (Persian/Swahili) life.
Aiasha

Ayesha (Arabic) youngest child.
Aisha, Aishah, Ayeshah, Ayeshia,
Ayeshiah

Ayita (Cherokee) first to dance.
Ayitah

Ayla (Hebrew) oak tree.
Aylah, Aylana, Aylanah, Aylanna,
Aylannah, Aylea, Aylee, Ayleena,
Aylena, Aylene

Aza (Arabic) comforting.

Azalea (Old English) flower.
(Grk) dry earth.
Azaleah, Azalee, Azalei, Azaleigh,
Azaley, Azali, Azalia, Azaliah,
Azalie, Azaly, Azalya, Azalyah

Azariah (Hebrew) God aids; blesses.
Azaria, Azarya, Azaryah

Azelia (Hebrew) helped by God.
Azena, Azenah, Azeliah, Azena,
Azenah, Azene, Azeta, Azetah, Azete

Aziza (Arabic) beloved.
Azizah

Azubah (Hebrew) abandoned.
Azuba

Azura/Azure/Azurine (Persian) blue
lapis stone.
Azora, Azorah, Azurah, Azure,
Azurina, Azurine, Azuryn, Azuryna,
Azurynah, Azuryne

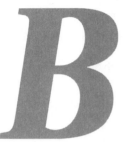

Bab (Arabic) dweller at the gateway.
The short form of Babette/Barbara;
little Barbara; little stranger.
Babb

Baba (African) born on a Thursday.
Aba, Abah, Babah

Babe (Latin) stranger. The short
form of Barbara/Babette.
Babea, Babee, Babey, Babi, Babie,
Baby, Bebe, Bebea, Bebee, Bebey,
Bebi, Bebia, Bebiah, Bebie, Beby,
Bebya, Bebyah

Babette (Greek) little Barbara; little
stranger.
Babet, Babeta, Babetah, Babett,
Babetta, Babettah

Bailey (Old French) bailiff; sheriff's
officer. (Mid/Eng) from the outer
castle wall meadow.
Bailea, Baileah, Bailee, Bailei,
Baileigh, Baili, Bailia, Bailiah,
Bailie, Baily, Baylea, Bayleah,
Balylee, Baylei, Bayleigh, Bayley,
Bayli, Baylia, Bayliah, Baylie, Bayly

Baka (Hindi) crane.
Bakah

Bakana (Australian Aboriginal)
view; lookout; guardian.
Bakanah, Bakanna, Bakannah

Bakula (Hindi) flower.
Bakulah

Balbina (Latin/Italian) little one who stammers.
Balbinah, Balbine, Balbyna, Balbynah, Balbyne

Bambalina (Italian) little girl.
Bambalinah, Bambaline, Bambalyn, Bambalyna, Bambalyne, Bambee, Bambi, Bambia, Bambiah, Bambie, Bamby

Bambi (Italian) little.
Bambea, Bambee, Bambia, Bambiah, Bambie, Bamby, Bambya, Bambyah

Bambra (Australian Aboriginal) mushroom.
Bambrah

Bandi (Middle Eastern) prisoner.
Banda, Bandah, Bandee, Bandey, Bandia, Bandiah, Bandie, Bandy, Bandya, Bandyah

Banjora (Australian Aboriginal) koala.
Banjorah

Baptista (Latin) one who baptises.
Baptisa (Ital/Grk), Baptissa, Baptiste (Fren), Baptysa, Baptysah, Baptyse, Baptyssa, Baptysse, Baptysta (Pol), Battista, Bautista

Bara (Australian Aboriginal) dawn; sunrise.
Barah, Barra, Barrah

Barb/Barbara/Barbie (Latin) stranger. (O/Eng) thorn.
Babet, Babett, Babetta, Babette, Babita, Babitta, Babitte, Babrischa, Barba (Span), Barbarina, Barbary, Barbea, Barbe (Ger/Fren), Barbee, Barbel (Ger), Barbet, Barbett, Barbett, Barbetta, Barbette, Barbey, Barbi, Barbica (Slav), Barbita, Barbie, Barbola, Barbora (Boh/Lith), Barbraa (Dan), Barbra

(Dan), Barbro (Nrs), Barbule (Lett), Barbutte (Lith), Barbchen (Ger), Barica (Illy), Barka, Varvara (Slav), Vavina (Slav), Vavinah, Vavyna, Vavynah, Vavyne

Barika (Swahili) successful.
Barikah, Baryka, Barykah

Barite (Australian Aboriginal) girl.
Barita, Baritah, Baryta, Barytah, Baryte

Barra (Hebrew) chosen.
Bara, Barah, Bari, Barra, Barrah

Barran (Irish) little hill top.
Baran, Barana, Baranah, Barean, Bareana, Bareanah, Bareane, Baren, Bareen, Bareena, Bareenah, Bareene, Barein, Bareina, Bareinah, Bareine, Bareyn, Bareyna, Bareynah, Bareyne, Barin, Barina, Barine, Barreen, Barreena, Barreenah, Barreene, Barrin, Barrina, Barrinah, Barrine, Barryn, Barryna, Barrynah, Barryne

Barri (Irish) spear; marks person. The feminine form of Barry.
Barea, Baree, Barey, Bari, Barria, Barriah, Barry, Barrya, Barryah, Barya, Baryah

Basha (Polish) stranger; unknown.
Bashah, Barsha

Basia (Hebrew) God's daughter.
Bashia, Bashiah, Bashya, Bashyah, Basiah, Basya, Basyah

Basillia (Greek) royal; majestic one; queen like; the herb basil. The feminine form of Basil.
Basila, Basilah, Basile, Basilla, Basillah, Basilie, Basyla, Basylah, Basyle, Basyll, Basylla, Basyllah, Basylle, Bazila, Bazilah, Bazile, Bazill, Bazilla, Bazillah, Bazille, Bazillia, Bazilliah, Bazilie, Bazyla, Bazylah, Bazyle, Bazyll, Bazylla, Bazyllah, Bazylle

Basima (Arabic) smiling.
Basimah, Basyma, Basymah

Bathanny (Australian Aboriginal) good day.
Bathanea, Bathaneah, Bathanee, Bathaney, Bathani, Bathania, Bathaniah, Bathanie, Bathannee, Bathanney, Bathanni, Bathannia, Bathanniah, Bathannie, Bathany, Bathanya, Bathenee, Batheney, Batheni, Bathenie, Batheny, Bethanee, Bethaney, Bethani, Bethanie, Bethannee, Bethenney, Bethenni, Bethennie, Bethenny

Bathilda (Teutonic) warrior.
Bathild, Bathildah, Bathilde, Bathyld, Bathylda, Bathyldah, Bathylde

Bathsheba (Hebrew) seventh daughter; promise.
Batsheva, Batshevah, Sheba, Shebah

Bathshua (Hebrew) daughter of wealth and prosperity.
Bathshuah

Batul (Arabic) little palm-tree shoot.
Batula, Batulah

Bayo (Yoruba) founder of joy.
Baio

Bea/Beatrice (Latin) she brings joy and happiness.
Beatriks (Russ), Beatrix (Ger/Span), Beatriz (Span), Beatryx, Beatryz, Bee, Bei, Bey, Beitris (Scott), Blazena, Venedict, Venetia, Venetiah, Venetya, Venetyah

Beata (Latin) happy; blessed.
Beatah, Beeta, Beetah, Beita, Beitah, Beyta, Beytah

Beca/Becky (Slavic/Hebrew) white. The short form of Rebecca, bound; tied; faithful.
Becah, Becca, Beccah, Becka, Beckah, Becki, Beckie, Beka, Bekah, Beki, Bekie, Beky

Beda (Old English) warrior.
Bedah

Bedelia (French) possesses strength.
Bedeliah, Bedelya, Bedelyah

Bedriska (Bohemian) queen of peace. The feminine form of Frederick.
Bedriskah, Bedryska, Bedryskah

Beela (Australian Aboriginal) black cockatoo (parrot).
Beala, Bealah, Beelah

Beeree (Australian Aboriginal) lagoon.
Beree

Begga (Gaelic) tiny. (Swedish) strength. The short form of Bridget.
Bega, Begah, Beggah

Bel (Hindi) apple tree in the sacred wood. (Fren) beautiful. The short form of names starting with 'Bel' e.g. Belinda.
Bell

Bela (Slavic) white. (Hung) bright one.
Bel, Belah, Bell, Bella, Bellah, Belle

Belda (French) beautiful.
Beldah

Belicia (Spanish) dedicated to God.
Beliciah, Belicya, Belicyah, Belysia, Belysiah, Belysya, Belysyah

Belilanca (Italian) fair-haired.
Belanca, Belancah, Belancka, Belanckah, Belanka, Belankah

Belina/Belinda (Spanish) beautiful woman. (O/Ger) bringer of wisdom.
Balina, Balinah, Baline, Balind, Balinda, Balindah, Balinde, Ballind, Ballinda, Ballindah, Ballinde, Belinah, Belindah, Belinde, Bellind, Bellinda, Bellindah, Bellynd,

Bellynda, Bellynde, Belva, Belynda,
Beneta, Benita, Benyt, Benyta,
Benytah, Benyte

Bella/Belle (Italian) beautiful. The
short form of Isabella, dedicated
to God.
Bela, Belah, Belau, Belia, Beliah,
Belita, Belitah, Belite, Bella, Bellau,
Belle (Fren), Belva, Belvia, Belviah,
Belvya, Belvyah

Bellanca (Greek/Italian) beautiful;
fair-haired.
Belanca, Belancah, Belancka,
Belanckah, Belanka, Belankah,
Bellancah, Bellancka, Bellanckah,
Bellanka, Bellankah, Bianca
(Span), Byanca, Byancah, Byancka,
Byanckah, Byanka, Byankah

Belphoebe (Latin/Greek) beautiful;
bright.
Belaphoebe, Belphoebea,
Belphoebee

Beltana (Australian Aboriginal)
running water.
Belltan, Belltana, Belltanah,
Belltane, Beltan, Beltane, Beltania,
Beltanja, Beltanya

Belva (Latin) beautiful view.
Belvah

Bena (Native American) pheasant.
Benah, Benna, Bennah

Benah (Hebrew) wisdom.
Bena, Benna, Bennah

Benecia/Benedicta/Benita (Latin)
blessed. The feminine form of
Benedict.
Bendite, Beneciah, Benecya,
Benecyah, Benedetta (Ital),
Benedettah, Benedette, Benedictina
(Ger), Benedictine, Benedikta
(Ger), Benedycta, Benedykta,
Beneisha, Benish, Benisha,
Benishia, Benita, Benitah, Benite,

Bennicia, Benniciah, Bennicie,
Bennicya, Bennycia, Bennyciah,
Bennycya, Bennycyah, Benoite
(Fren), Bent, Benta, Bentah, Bente,
Benwenuta, Benyta, Benytah,
Benyte, Betina, Betinah, Betine,
Bettina, Bettinah, Bettine, Bettyna,
Bettynah, Bettyne, Betyna, Betynah,
Betyne

Benigna (Latin) gracious; kind;
gentle.
Benignah, Benigne, Benygna,
Benygne

Benton (English) from the moor
town.
Bentan, Bentin, Bentun, Bentyn

Berdine (German) glorious one
who brightly shines from within.
Berdina, Berdinah, Berdyn,
Berdyna, Berdynah, Berdyne

Berenice/Bernice (Greek) strong
like a bear; warrior. The feminine
form of Bernie.
Bernece, Berneece, Berneese,
Bernese, Berneta, Bernetah,
Bernete, Bernetta, Bernettah,
Bernette, Bernica, Bernicah,
Bernicka, Bernickah, Bernika,
Bernikah, Bernyc, Bernyce, Bernyse,
Vernice, Vernise

Berit (German) glorious.
Beret, Bereta, Berete, Berett, Beretta,
Berette, Biret, Bireta, Birete, Birett,
Biretta, Birette, Byret, Byreta,
Byrete, Byrett, Byretta, Byrette

Bernadette/Bernadine
(French/English) strong and
brave little bear; little warrior.
The feminine form of Bernard.
Bernadeen, Bernadeena,
Bernadeenah, Bernadeene,
Bernaden, Bernadena, Bernadenah,
Bernadene, Bernadet, Bernadeta,
Bernadetah, Bernadete, Bernadett,

Bernadette/Bernadine cont.
Bernadetta, Bernadettah, Bernadina
(Span/Ital), Bernadinah,
Bernadine, Bernadit, Bernadita,
Bernadytah, Bernadyte, Bernadyn,
Bernadyna (Pol), Bernadynah,
Bernadyne, Bernit, Bernita,
Bernitah, Bernite, Bernyt, Bernyta,
Bernytah, Bernyte

Bernia (Latin) warrior.
Berniah, Bernya, Bernyah

Bernice (Greek) strong and brave
like a bear; warrior. The feminine
form of Bernie.
Berenice (Fren), Bernece, Berneece,
Berneese, Bernese, Berneta,
Bernetah, Bernete, Bernetta,
Bernettah, Bernette, Bernica,
Bernicah, Bernicka, Bernickah,
Bernika, Bernikah, Bernyc, Bernyce,
Bernyse, Vernice, Vernise, Veronica,
Veronika, Veronique (Fren),
Veronik (Ger)

Berontha (Australian Aboriginal)
crow.
Beronthah

Berry (Australian Aboriginal) white
box tree. (O/Eng) berry. The short
form of Bernice, strong and brave
like a bear.
Beree, Berey, Beri, Berie, Berree,
Berrey, Berri, Berrie, Bery

Bertha (Old English/Teutonic)
bright; shining; illustrious. The
feminine form of Bert.
Bercta, Berta (Ger/Span), Berte,
Berth, Berthah, Berthe (Fren/Ger),
Berthel, Bertolda, Bertilla, Bertille,
Bertina, Bertle, Birth, Birtha, Birthe,
Byrth, Byrtha, Byrthah, Holda,
Holla, Huldr

Berthilda/Bertilde/Bertina (Old
English/Teutonic) bright; shining;
illustrious. The feminine form of
Bert.
Berteana, Berteanah, Berteena,
Berteenah, Berteene, Berthildah,
Berthilde, Bertinah, Bertine,
Berthylda, Berthyldah, Berthylde,
Bertilda, Bertildah, Bertilde,
Bertylda, Bertyldah, Bertylde,
Bertyna, Bertynah, Bertyne,
Birteana, Birteanah, Birteane,
Birteena, Birteenah, Birteene,
Birtina, Birtinah, Birtine, Birtyna,
Birtynah, Birtyne, Byrteana,
Byrteanah, Byrteane, Byrteena,
Byrtina, Byrtinah, Byrtine, Byrtyna,
Byrtynah, Byrtyne

Bertrade (Old English/Teutonic)
shining counsel.
Bertrada, Bertradah

Berwyn (Old English/Teutonic)
little, bright, shining, illustrious
friend.
Berwin, Berwina, Berwinah,
Berwine, Berwyna, Berwynah,
Berwyne, Berwynn, Berwynna,
Berwynnah, Berwynne

Beryl (Greek) sea-green jewel.
Beral, Beril, Berila, Berile, Berill,
Berille, Beryle, Berylee, Berylla,
Rylla

Bessie (Hebrew) holy and sacred to
God. The short form of Elizabeth.
Besee, Besey, Besi, Besie, Bess,
Bessee, Bessey, Bessi, Bessy, Besy

Beth (Hebrew) from the house of
God; holy and sacred to God. The
short form of names starting with
or containing 'Beth' e.g.
Elizabeth/Bethany.
Bethal, Bethel, Bethil, Bethol,
Bethyl

Betha (Celtic) life. The Swiss form
of Betty, from the house of God.
Bethah, Bethal, Bethel, Bethil,
Bethol, Bethyl

Bethan/Bethanny (Aramaic) from
the house of God's grace. A
combination of Beth/Annie.
Bethan, Bethana, Bethanah,
Bathane, Bethanee, Bethaney,
Bethani, Bethania, Bethaniah,
Bethanie, Bethann, Bethanna,
Bethannah, Bethany, Bethena,
Bethenee, Betheney, Bethina,
Bethinah, Bethine, Bethyn,
Bethyna, Bethynah, Bethyne

Bethel (Hebrew) from the house of
God.
Bethal, Bethall, Bethell, Bethil,
Bethill, Bethol, Betholl, Bethyl,
Bethyll

Bethesda (Hebrew) from the house
of Mercy.
Bethesdah

Bethia (Hebrew) daughter.
(Gae) life.
Bethiah, Bethya, Bethyah

Betsy (Hebrew/American) holy and
sacred to God. A short form of
Elizabeth.
Betsee, Betsey, Betsi, Betsia, Betsiah,
Betsie, Betsya, Betsyah, Betsye

Bette/Betty (French/Hebrew) from
the house of God. A short form
of Bethel/Elizabeth, holy and
sacred to God.
Bet, Beta, Betah, Bete, Betea, Betee,
Betey, Beti, Betia, Betie, Betha,
Betje (Dut), Betka (Boh), Bett,
Betta, Bettah, Bette, Bettee, Bettey,
Bettja, Bettje, Bettys (Wel), Betuska
(Boh), Bety

Betulah (Hebrew) woman.
Betula, Betulla, Betullah

Beulah (Hebrew) married woman.
Buela

Beverly (Old English) from the
beaver stream in the meadow.
Beverie, Beverlea, Beverleah,
Beverlee, Berelei, Beverleigh,
Beverley, Beverlie, Beverly, Bevlea,
Bevlea, Bevlee, Bevlei, Bevleigh,
Bevley, Bevli, Bevlia, Bevliah, Bevly

Bevin (Irish) sweet-singing woman.
Bevina, Bevinah, Bevine, Bevyn,
Bevyna, Bevynah, Bevyne

Bian (Vietnamese) secret.
Biana, Bianah, Biane, Biann,
Bianna, Biannah, Bianne, Byan,
Byana, Byanah, Byane, Byann,
Byanna, Byannah, Byanne

Bianca (Italian) white.
Biancha, Bianka, Biankah, Biannca,
Biannka, Biannqua, Biannquah,
Bianqua, Bianquah, Blannca,
Blannka, Byanca, Byancah, Byanka,
Byankah, Byanqua, Byanquah

Bibi (Arabic) lady.
Bebe, BeBe, Bea, Beabea, Bea Bea,
Bee, Beebee, Bee Bee, Byby

Bibiana (Latin) lively.
Bibi, Bibianah, Bibiane, Bibiann,
Bibianna, Bibiannah, Bibianne,
Bibyan, Bibyana, Bibyanah,
Bibyann, Bibyanna, Bibyannah,
Bibyanne, Bybian, Bybiana,
Bybianah, Bybiane, Bybiann,
Bybianna, Bybiannah, Bybianne,
Bybyan, Bybyana, Bybyanah,
Bybyane, Bybyann, Bybyanna,
Bybyannah, Bybyanne, Vibiana

Bilhah (Hebrew) tender.
Bilha, Bylha, Bylhah

Billie (Old English) wilful. The
feminine form of Billy.
Bilea, Bileah, Bilee, Bilei, Bileigh,
Biley, Bili, Bilie, Billea, Billee,

Billie cont.
Billena, Billeenah, Billey, Billi,
Billie, Billy, Billyana, Bilyana,
Billyanna, Billyannah, Bily,
Bilyana, Bilyanah, Bylea, Byleah,
Bylee, Bylei, Byleigh, Byley, Byli,
Bylie, Byll, Byllea, Bylleah, Byllee,
Byllei, Bylleigh, Bylli, Byllie, Bylly,
Byly

Bimbeen (Australian Aboriginal)
woodpecker.
Binbeena

Bina (Swahili) dancer. (Heb) wise
and understanding.
Binah, Byna, Bynah

Binda (Australian Aboriginal) deep
water.
Bindah, Bynda, Byndah

Binga (Teutonic) from the kettle-
shaped hollow.
Bingah, Bynga, Byngah

Birdie (English) bird.
Birde, Birdea, Birdee, Birdeen,
Birdeena, Birdeenah, Birdeene,
Birdel, Birdela, Birdelah, Birdele,
Birdella, Birdellah, Birdena,
Birdenah, Birdene, Birdenia,
Berdeniah, Berdenie, Birdet,
Birdeta, Birdetah, Birdete, Birdett,
Birdetta, Birdettah, Birdette,
Birdina, Birdinah, Byrd, Byrda,
Byrde, Byrdeena, Byrdeenah,
Byrdeene, Byrdett, Byrdetta,
Byrdette, Byrdina, Byrdinah,
Byrdine, Byrdyna, Byrdynah,
Byrdyne

Birdita (English) little bird.
Birditta, Birditte, Byrditta, Byrditte

Bjorg (Scandinavian) salvation; help.
Bjorga, Bjorgah

Bladina (Latin) warm and friendly.
Bladean, Bladeana, Bladeanah,
Bladeane, Bladeen, Bladeena,
Bladeene, Bladene, Bladine,
Bladyn, Bladyna, Bladyne

Blaine (Irish) slender. (O/Eng)
flame.
Blain, Blaire, Blayn, Blayne

Blair (Latin) from the marsh on the
plain. (Scot) field of battle.
Blaire, Blayr, Blayre

Blaise (English) burning flames.
Blais, Blaisia, Blaiz, Blazia, Blaize,
Blasia, Blayse, Blayz, Blayza, Blayze,
Blaze, Blazia, Blazya

Blake (Old English) dark
hair/complexion.
Blaik, Blaike, Blaiklea, Blaikleah,
Blaiklee, Blaiklei, Blaikleigh,
Blaikley, Blaikli, Blaiklie, Blaikly,
Blakelea, Blakeleah, Blakelee,
Blakelei, Blakeleigh, Blakeley,
Blakeli, Blakelie, Blakely, Blayk,
Blayklea, Blaykleah, Blayklee,
Blayklei, Blaykleigh, Blaykli,
Blayklie, Blaykly

Blanca (Spanish) white.
Bijanka, Blancah, Blanka
(Ger/Dut/Nor), Blankah, Blannca,
Blanncah, Blannka, Blannkah,
Blannqua, Blannquah, Blanqua,
Blanquah, Blinnie (Ir)

Blanche (French) white; fair-haired.
Blanch, Blanchardina,
Blanchardine, Blinnie, Bluinse (Ir),
Blanka (Ger/Dut/Nor), Branca
(Port), Branka

Blanda (Hebrew) compliment giver.
Blandah, Blandia, Blandiah,
Blandya, Blandyah

Bleniki (Hawaiian) white.
Blanikee, Blanikey, Blanikie,
Blaniky

Blessing (Old English) one who is a blessing.
Bless, Blessa, Blessi, Blessie, Blessin, Blessinga, Blessy

Bliss (Old English) bringer of happiness.
Blis, Blisa, Blissa, Blisse, Blys, Blysa, Blyss, Blyssa

Blodwen (Old Welsh) white flower.
Blodwin, Blodwina, Blodwinah, Blodwine, Blodwyn, Blodwyna, Blodwynah, Blodwyne, Blodwynn, Blodwynna, Blodwynnah, Blodwynne

Blondelle (French/Old English) she is fair-haired.
Blondel, Blondele, Blondell, Blondella, Blondelia, Blondeliah, Blondelya, Blondelyah

Blondie (English) fair-haired.
Blondea, Blondee, Blondi, Blondia, Blondiah, Blondy, Blondya, Blondyah

Blossom (Old English) blooming like a flower.
Blossoma

Blum (Yiddish) flower.
Bluma, Blumah

Bly (Native American) high.
Bligh, Blygh

Blythe (Old English) cheerful; gentle.
Bliss, Blyss, Blithe, Blyth, Blythe

Bo (Chinese) precious.
Beau, Bow

Boann (Irish) white cow.
Bo-Ann, Boana, Boanah, Boane, Boanna, Boannah, Boanne, Bo-Ann, Bo-Anna, Bo-Annah, Bo-Anne

Bobbi (Teutonic) bright; famous. The short form of Roberta. The feminine form of Bobby/Robert.
Bobbea, Bobbee, Bobbey, Bobby, Bobea, Bobee, Bobey, Bobi, Bobie, Boby

Bodil (Norse) warrior.
Bodila, Bodilah, Bodyl, Bodyla, Bodylah

Bombala (Australian Aboriginal) where the waters meet.
Bombalah

Bona (Latin) good. The feminine form of Bono.
Bonah, Bono

Bonal (Australian Aboriginal) place with lots of grass.
Bonala, Bonalah, Bonale,Bonall, Bonalla, Bonallah, Bonalle, Bonel, Bonela, Bonelah, Bonell, Bonella, Bonellah, Bonelle

Bondi (Australian Aboriginal) sound of tumbling water.
Bondie, Bondy, Bondye

Bonita (Spanish) pretty; little.
Bonitah, Bonitta, Bonittah, Bonnita, Bonnitta, Bonnyta, Bonnitta, Bonyta, Bonytta

Bonne/Bonnie/Bonny (Scottish) pretty; good. (Ir) pretty; charming.
Bonea, Bonee, Boney, Boni, Bonia, Boniah, Bonie, Bonnea, Bonnee, Bonney, Bonni, Bonnia, Bonniah, Bonnibela, Bonnibelah, Bonnibele, Bonnibella, Bonnibellah, Bonnibell, Bonnibelle, Bonie, Bunee, Buney, Buni, Bunia, Buniah, Bunie, Bunnea, Bunnee, Bunney, Bunni, Bunnia, Bunniah, Bunnie, Bunny, Buny

Boronia (Australian Aboriginal) boronia flower.
Boronee, Boroney, Boroni, Boroniah, Boronie, Borony, Boronya, Boronyah

Bowral (Australian Aboriginal) large; high.
Bowrall, Bowralle, Bowrel, Bowrela, Bowrelah, Bowrele, Bowrell, Bowrella, Bowrellah, Bowrelle

Bozenka (Slavic) God will favour; born at Christmas time.
Bozena, Bozenah

Bracken (English) fern.
Brackin, Brackyn, Braken, Brakin, Brakyn

Bradlee (Old English) from the broad meadow. (Scott) clearing in the woods. The feminine form of Bradley.
Bradlea, Bradleah, Bradlei, Bradleigh, Bradley, Bradli, Bradlia, Bradliah, Bradlie, Bradly, Bradlya, Bradlyah

Branda (Hebrew) blessing.
Brandah

Brandy/Brandyce (Dutch) brandy; wine.
Brandais, Brande, Brandea, Brandeace, Brandease, Brandeece, Brandeese, Brandee, Brandi, Brandia, Brandice, Brandie, Brandina, Brandine, Brandis, Brandisa, Brandise, Brandiss, Brandissa, Bradisse, Brandyn, Brandyna, Brandys, Brandysa, Brandyse, Brandyss, Brandyssa, Brandysse

Brangane (Welsh) white raven.
Brangan, Brangana, Branganah

Breana (Celtic/Old English) strong, gracious victory.
Brana, Breanah, Breane, Breanna, Breannah, Breanne, Breeana, Breeanah, Breeane, Breeann, Breeanna, Breeannah, Breeanne, Breeannie, Briana, Brianah, Briane, Briannah, Brianne, Briel, Briela, Brielah, Briele, Briell, Briella, Brielle, Brina, Brina, Brinna, Brinnah, Bryana, Bryanna, Bryannah, Bryanne, Bryel, Bryela, Bryele, Bryell, Bryella, Bryelle

Breck (Irish) freckled.
Brec, Breca, Brecah, Breckah, Brek, Breka, Brekah

Bree (Irish) strong victory. The short form of names staring with 'Bree' e.g. Breena.
Brea, Breah, Beay, Breea, Breeah, Brei, Breigh, Brey, Bri, Bria, Briah, Brie (Fren), Bry, Brya, Bryah, Brye

Breen (Irish) from the fairy palace.
Brea, Breana, Breanah, Breane, Bree, Breenah, Breene, Breenia, Breeniah, Breina, Breinah, Brena, Brenah, Brina, Brinah, Bryna, Brynah

Breeze (Old English) windy; carefree.
Brease, Breaz, Breaza, Breazah, Breaze, Brees, Breese, Breez, Breeza, Briez, Brieza, Brieze, Bryez, Bryeza, Bryeze

Brenda (Old English) fire stoker.
Branda, Brandah, Brandea, Brendah, Brennda, Brenndah, Briennah, Brienne, Brinda, Brindah, Brinnda, Brinndah, Brynda, Bryndah, Brynnda, Brynndah

Brieena (Irish/Gaelic) little raven; raven-haired.
Breanna, Breanne, Brennah,

Briana, Brianna, Briannah,
Briannka, Brieann, Brieanna,
Brieannah, Brieannan, Brieannkah,
Briearne, Bryan, Bryana, Bryanah,
Bryann, Bryanna, Bryannah,
Bryanne

Bretta (Irish/Gaelic) from Britain.
The feminine form of Brett.
Bret, Breta, Brett, Bretta, Brettah,
Brette, Brettea, Brettee, Brettia,
Britnee, Britney, Britt, Brittania,
Brittani, Brittannie, Brittany,
Brittanny, Britten, Britteny, Bryta,
Brytah, Brytia, Brytiah, Brytta,
Bryttah, Bryttnea, Bryttnee,
Bryttney, Bryttni, Bryttnia, Bryttnie,
Bryttny

Bria (Irish/Gaelic) hill.
(Celt) strong; honourable.
A feminine form of Brian.
Brea, Breah, Breea, Breeah, Briah,
Briea, Brya, Bryah

Brianna/Brianne (Celtic/Old
English) strong; graceful victory;
hill. (Celt) strong; honourable.
A feminine form of Brian.
Brana, Breana, Breanah, Breanna,
Breannah, Breanne, Breeana,
Breeanah, Breeane, Breeann,
Breeanna, Breeannah, Breeanne,
Breeannie, Breian, Breiana,
Breianah, Breiane, Breiann,
Breianna, Breiannah, Breianne,
Briana, Brianah, Briane, Briannah,
Brianne, Briel, Briela, Brielah,
Briele, Briell, Briella, Brielle, Brina,
Brina, Brinna, Brinnah, Bryana,
Bryanna, Bryannah, Bryanne, Bryel,
Bryela, Bryele, Bryell, Bryella,
Bryelle

Briar (French) heather.
Brear, Brier, Briet, Brieta, Brietah,
Brietta, Briettah, Brya, Bryah, Bryar

Bridey (Irish) strength. A form of
Bridget.
Bridea, Brideah, Bridee, Bridi,
Bridie, Bridy, Brydea, Brydee,
Brydey, Brydi, Brydie, Brydy

Bridget (Irish) strength.
Beret, Bereta, Berget, Bergeta,
Birgit, Birgita, Birgitt, Birgitta,
Birgitte, Bridey, Bridger, Bridgeta,
Bridgetah, Bridgete, Bridgett,
Bridgetta, Bridgettah, Bridgette,
Bridgit, Bridgita, Bridgitah,
Bridgite, Bridgett, Bridgitta,
Bridgittah, Bridgitte, Brydget,
Brydgeta, Brydgetah, Brydgete,
Brydgett, Brydgetta, Brydgettah,
Brydgette

Brie (French) from Brie in France.
Brea, Breah, Bree, Brei, Brey, Briel,
Briela, Briele, Briell, Briella, Brielle,
Briena, Brienah, Briene, Brion,
Briona, Brione, Briet, Brieta, Briete,
Briett, Brietta, Briette, Bry, Bryel,
Bryela, Bryelah, Bryele, Bryell,
Bryella, Bryelle

Brielle (French) she is from Brie in
France. A short form of Gabrielle,
God is my strength; she of God.
Breael, Breaele, Breaell, Breaelle,
Breel, Breele, Breell, Breelle, Briel,
Briela, Brielah, Briele, Briell,
Briella, Briellah, Bryel, Bryela,
Bryelah, Bryele, Bryell, Bryella,
Bryellah, Bryelle, Gabrielle

Brina (Latin) boundary. (Ir) strong;
virtuous; honourable. (Eng)
princess. The short form of
Sabrina. (Heb) seventh daughter;
promise. A form of Bathsheba/
Sheba.
Breana, Breanah, Breena, Breenah,
Breina, Breinah, Breyna, Breynah,
Brinah, Bryna, Brynah

Briona (Irish) hill. (Celt) strong;
honourable. A feminine form of
Brian.
Breaona, Breaonah, Breeona,
Breeonah, Breiona, Breionah,
Breona, Breonah, Breyona,
Breyonah, Brionah, Brione,
Brionna, Brionnah, Brionne,
Briony, Bryona, Bryonah, Bryone,
Bryony

Brisa (Spanish) beloved.
Brisah, Brisha, Brishia, Brissa,
Brysa, Brysah, Bryssa, Bryssah

Brita/Britin/Britt/Britta
(Irish/English/Swedish) strong
spirit. (Eng) from Britain.
Breat, Breata, Breatah, Breatin,
Breatina, Breatinah, Breatine,
Breatta, Breatta, Breatte, Breattin,
Breattina, Breattinah, Breattine,
Bret, Breta, Bretah, Brett, Bretta,
Brettah, Brette, Bretin, Bretina,
Bretinah, Bretine, Bretyn, Bretyna,
Bretynah, Bretyne, Britin, Brintina,
Britinah, Britine, Britt (Swed),
Britta (Swed), Brittah, Britte,
Brittin, Brittina, Brittine, Brittinee,
Brittiney, Britini, Britinie, Brittiny,
Bryt, Bryta, Brytah, Bryte, Brytta,
Bryttah, Brytte, Bryttin, Brittina,
Brittinah, Brittine, Bryttin, Bryttina,
Bryttine, Bryttnee, Bryttney, Bryttni,
Bryttnie, Bryytny

Brittany (Irish) from Britain.
Brita, Britah, Britan, Britana,
Britanah, Britane, Britanee,
Britaney, Britani, Britanie, Britann,
Britanna, Britannah, Britanne,
Britanee, Britaney, Britenee,
Briteney, Britenie, Britenie, Briteny,
Britnee, Britney, Britni, Britnie,
Britt, Britta, Brittan, Brittana,
Brittanah, Brittainnee, Brittainney,
Brittainni, Brittainnie, Brittainny,
Brittenee, Britteney, Britteni,

Brittenie, Britteny, Brytanee,
Brytaney, Brytani, Brytania,
Brytanie, Brytany, Bryttanee,
Bryttaney, Bryttani, Bryttania,
Bryttanie, Bryttany

Bronwyn (Welsh) white friend.
Bronia, Broniah, Bronie, Bronnee,
Broney, Bronwin, Broonwina,
Bronwinah, Bronwine, Bronwyn,
Bronwyna, Bronwynah, Bronwyne,
Bronwynn, Bronwynna,
Bronwynnah, Bronwynne

Brooke (English) from the stream.
Brook, Brookee, Brookey,
Brookelina, Brookeline, Brookelyn,
Brookelyna, Brookelyne, Brookel,
Brookela, Brookele, Brookelle,
Brookellin, Brookellina,
Brookelline, Brookellyn,
Brookellyna, Brookellyne, Brookia,
Brookiah, Brookie, Brooklin,
Brooklina, Brookline, Brooklyn,
Brooklyna, Brooklyne

Brooklyn (English) from the pool
by the stream.
Brook, Brookelina, Brookeline,
Brookelyn, Brookelyna,
Brookelyne, Brookel, Brookela,
Brookelah, Brookele, Brookella,
Brookellah, Brookelle, Brookellin,
Brookellina, Brookelline,
Brookellyn, Brookellyna,
Brookellyne, Brooklin, Brooklina,
Brookline, Brooklyn, Brooklyna,
Brooklyne

Brosina (Greek) divine immortal.
The short form of Ambrosia. The
feminine form of Ambrose.
Ambrosina, Ambrosinah,
Ambrosine, Ambrosyn,
Ambrosyna, Ambrosynah,
Ambrosyne, Brosin, Brosinah,
Brosine, Brosyn, Brosyna,
Brosynah, Brosyne

Bruna/Brunhilda (German) armoured warrior.
Brinhild, Brinhilda, Brinhilde, Brunhild, Brunhildah, Brunhilde, Brunnhild, Brunnhilda, Brunnhildah, Brunnhilde, Brynhild, Brynhilda, Brynhildah, Brynhilde, Brynhyld, Bryndylda, Brynhyldah, Brynhylde

Bryga (Polish/Irish) strength. A form of Bridget.
Brygid, Brygida, Brygitka

Bryn/Bryna (Latin) boundary. (Wel) from the mountain.
Brin, Brina, Brinah, Brinan, Brinn, Brinna, Brinnah, Brinnan, Bryna, Brynah, Brynan, Brynee, Bynne

Bryony (English) twisting vine; bear. The feminine form of Bryon. (Ger) cottage.
Brionee, Brioney, Brinoni, Brinonie, Briony, Bryonee, Bryoney, Bryoni, Bryonie, Bryony

Buffy (English) one who shines or polishes. (Amer) buffalo of the plains.
Bufee, Bufey, Buffee, Buffey, Buffi, Buffie, Bufi, Bufie, Bufy

Bunny (English) little rabbit.
Bunee, Buney, Buni, Bunie, Bunnee, Bunney, Bunni, Bunnie, Buny

Burgundy (French) from Burgundy, a wine-making area in France. A red/brown colour.
Burgandee, Burgandey, Burgandi, Burgandie, Burgandy, Burgundee, Burgundey, Burgundi, Burgundy

Byanna (Irish) hill. (Celt) strong; honourable. (Eng) near the graceful one. A feminine form of Brian.
Bian, Biana, Bianah, Biane, Biann, Biannah, Bianne, Breana, Breanah, Breane, Breann, Breanna, Breannah, Breanne, Breean, Breenah, Breeane, Breeann, Breeanna, Breeannah, Breeanne, Breian, Breianah, Breiane, Breiann, Breianna, Breiannah, Breianne, Breyan, Breyanah, Breyane, Breyann, Breyanna, Breyannah, Breyanne, Briana, Brianah, Briane, Briann, Brianna, Briannah, Brianne, Bryana, Bryanah, Bryane, Bryann, Bryannah, Bryanne, Byan, Byana, Byanah, Byane, Byann, Byanna, Byannah, Byanne, Briann, Brianna, Briannah, Brianne, Bryana, Bryanah, Bryane, Bryann, Bryannah, Bryanne

Byhalia (Choctaw) white oak.
Bihalia, Bihaliah, Byhaliah, Byhalya, Byhalyah

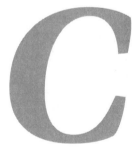

Cachet (French) desired.
Cache, Cachea, Cachee

Cadence (Latin) to beat a rhythm.
Cadena, Cadenah, Cadenza, Cadenzah, Kadena, Kadenah, Kadenza, Kadenzah

Cady (Latin) to beat a rhythm. The short form of Cadence.
Cadea, Cadee, Cadey, Cadi, Cadia, Cadiah, Cadie, Cadya, Cadyah

Caeley (Arabic/Hebrew/Old English) crown of laurel leaves in the meadow. (O/Eng) from the pure meadow.
Calea, Caeleah, Caelee, Caelei, Caeleigh, Caeli, Caelia, Caelie, Caely, Cailea, Caileah, Cailee, Cailei, Caileigh, Caili, Cailia, Cailie, Caily, Caylea, Cayleah, Caylee, Caylei, Cayleigh, Cayley, Cayli, Caylia, Caylie, Cayly, Kaela, Kaelah, Kaelea, Kaeleah, Kaelee, Kaelei, Kaeleigh, Kaeley, Kaeli, Kaelia, Kaeliah, Kaelie, Kaely, Kahla, Kahlah, Kahlea, Kahleah, Kahlee, Kahlei, Kahleigh, Kahley, Kahlei, Kahlie, Kahly, Kaila, Kailah, Kailea, Kaileah, Kailee, Kailei, Kaileigh, Kailey, Kaili, Kailia, Kailiah, Kailie, Kaily, Kalea, Kaleah, Kalee, Kalei, Kaleigh, Kaley, Kali, Kalia, Kaliah, Kalie, Kaly, Kalya, Kayla, Kaylah, Kaylea, Kayleah, Kaylee, Kaylei, Kayleigh, Kayley, Kayli, Kaylia, Kayliah, Kaylie, Kayly, Kaylya, Kealea, Kealeah, Kealee, Kealei, Kealeigh, Keali, Kealia, Kealiah, Kealie, Kealy

Caera (Irish) brown/red complexioned.
Caerah

Cai (Vietnamese) woman. (Ir) purity.
Cae, Cay, Caye

Cailida/Cailidora (Spanish) adorable.
Caelida, Caelidah, Cailidah, Cailidorah, Callidora (Grk), Callidorah, Caylida, Caylidah, Kailida, Kailidah, Kaylida, Kaylidah

Cailin (Welsh/Irish) from the pure pool.
Caelean, Caeleana, Caeleanah, Caeleane, Caeleen, Caeleena, Caeleenah, Caeleene, Caelen,

Caelena, Caelenah, Caelene, Caelin, Caelina, Caelinah, Caeline, Caelyn, Caelyna, Caelynah, Caelyne, Caileen, Caileena, Caileenah, Caileene, Cailena, Cailenah, Cailene, Cailina, Cailine, Cailyn, Cailyna, Cailyne, Caylean, Cayleana, Cayleanah, Cayleane, Cayleen, Cayleena, Cayleenah, Caylen, Caylena, Caylenah, Caylene, Caylin, Caylina, Cayline, Caylyn, Caylyna, Caylyne

Caimilw (African) life continues.
Caymile

Cainwen (Welsh) fair-haired one who is blessed.
Cainwin, Caynwin, Caynwyn

Caitlin (Irish/Latin) from the pure pool. The Irish form of Catherine.
Caetlan, Caetlana, Caetlane, Caetlen, Caetlena, Caetlene, Caetlin, Caetlina, Caetline, Caetlyn, Caetlyna, Caetlyne, Caitlan, Caitlana, Caitlane, Caitlen, Caitlena, Caitlene, Caitlyn, Caitlyna, Caitlyne, Catlin, Catlina, Catline, Catlyn, Catlyna, Catlyne, Kaitlan, Kaitlen, Kaitlin, Kaitlina, Kaitline, Katlin, Katlina, Katline, Katlyn, Katlyna, Katlyne

Cakusola (African) loving.
Cakusolah

Cala (Arabic) castle.
Calah, Calan, Calana, Calia, Caliah, Calla, Callah

Calamity (Latin/English/American) misfortune.
Calamitea, Calamitee, Calamitey, Calamiti, Calamitia, Calamitie, Kalamitea, Kalamitee, Kalamitey, Kalamiti, Kalamitia, Kalamitie, Kalamity

Calandra (Greek) carefree; the lark bird.
Caelan, Caelana, Cailan, Cailana, Calan, Calana, Calanah, Calandrea, Calandria, Calandriah, Caleida, Calendra, Calendrah, Calandre, Caylan, Caylana, Caylanah, Caylandra, Caylandrea, Caylandria, Caylandriah, Caylana, Caylanah

Calantha (Greek) flower.
Calanthah, Calanthia, Calanthiah, Calanthya, Calanthyah

Calca (Australian Aboriginal) star.
Calcah

Caledonia (Latin) from Scotland.
Caledona, Caledoniah, Caledonya, Caledonyah, Caldona, Caldonah, Caldonia, Caldoniah, Caldonya, Caldonyah

Caley (Irish/Old English) slender one from the meadow.
Calea, Caleah, Calee, Calei, Caleigh, Cali, Calia, Caliah, Callea, Calleah, Callee, Callei, Calleigh, Calley, Calli, Callia, Calliah, Callie, Cally, Caly

Calida (Spanish) warm; ardent.
Calina, Calinda, Callida, Callinda, Callyda, Callydah, Calyda, Calydah, Kalida, Kalidah, Kallida, Kallidah, Kallyda, Kallydah, Kalyda, Kalydah

Calla (Greek) beautiful.
Callah, Kalla, Kallah

Callan (German) talker; chatterer. (O/Nrs) to cry out.
Callen, Callin, Callon, Callun, Callyn, Kallan, Kallen, Kallin, Kallon, Kallun, Kallyn

Callie (Arabic) fortress.
Calea, Caleah, Calee, Calei, Caleigh, Caley, Cali, Calia, Caliah, Callea, Calleah, Callee, Callei, Calleigh, Calley, Calli, Callia, Calliah, Cally, Caly

Calliope (Greek) muse.
Calliopee, Kalliope, Kalliopee

Callista (Greek) beautiful.
Calesta, Calestah, Calista, Calistah, Callesta, Callestah, Callysta, Callistah, Callystah, Calysta

Callula (Latin) beautiful light.
Calula, Calulah, Callulah, Kallula, Kallulah, Kalula, Kalulah

Calumina (Scottish) little dove.
Caluminah, Calumyna, Calumynah

Calvina (Latin) bald one. The feminine form of Calvin.
Calveana, Calveanah, Calveane, Calveania, Calveaniah, Calveane, Calveena, Calveenah, Calveenia, Calveeniah, Calvinah, Calvine, Calvinetta, Calvinette, Calvyna, Calvynah, Calvyne

Calypso (Greek) hidden.
Calipso

Cam (Vietnamese) sweet citrus.
Kam

Cambria (Latin) from Wales.
Camalia, Camallia, Camber, Cambriah, Cambrya, Cambryah, Camela, Camelia, Camelita, Camella, Camellita, Kamelia, Kamellia

Camelia (Latin) beautiful flower.
Cameliah, Camelya, Camelyah, Kamelia, Kameliah, Kamylia, Kamyliah

Cameo (Latin) portrait carved onto a shell or gem.
Camio, Camyo, Kameo, Kamio, Kamyo

C

Cameron (Scottish) crooked nose. (Kurd) happy.
Cameran, Camerana, Cameren, Cameri, Cameria, Cameriah, Camerie, Camerin, Camerya, Cameryah, Cameryn, Camesha, Cameshia, Kameron, Kamerona, Kameronia, Kamesha, Kameshia

Cami (French) young ceremonial attendant; messenger. The short form of Camille.
Camee, Camey, Camia, Camiah, Camie, Camy, Camya, Camyah

Camilla/Camille (Latin/French) young ceremonial attendant; messenger.
Camil, Camila (Span), Camilia, Camilla (Ital), Camillah, Cammila, Cammilah, Cammile, Cammill, Cammilla, Cammille, Cammyl, Cammyla, Cammylah, Cammyle, Cammyll, Cammylla, Cammyllah, Cammylle, Chamelea, Chameleah, Chamelee, Chamelei, Chameley, Chamelia, Chameliah, Chamellia, Chameliah, Chamely, Chamelya, Chamelyah

Canace (Greek) daughter of the wind God.
Kanace

Candice (Greek) pure white; glowing.
Candace, Candida, Candide (Fren), Candis, Candra, Candrah, Candyce, Kandace, Kandice, Kandise, Kandyce, Kandyse

Candra (Latin) glowing.
Crandrah, Candrea, Candria, Candriah, Candrya, Candryah, Kandra, Kandrah, Kandria, Kandriah, Kandrya, Kandryah

Candy (Latin) pure, white glow. (Amer) sweet lolly. The short form of Candace.
Candea, Candee, Candi, Candia, Candiah, Candie, Candya, Candyah, Kandea, Kandee, Kandey, Kandi, Kandia, Kandiah, Kandy, Kandya, Kandyah

Caneadea (Iroquois) horizon.
Caneadee

Cantara (Arabic) small crossing.
Cantarah

Cantrelle (French) she is like a song.
Cantrel, Cantrela, Cantrelah, Cantrele, Cantrella, Cantrellah, Kantrel, Kantrella, Kantrelle

Capri/Caprice (Italian) fanciful. The short form of Caprice.
Capree, Caprey, Capria, Capriah, Caprie, Capry, Caprya, Capryah

Cara (Italian) beloved.
Carah, Carra, Carrah, Kara, Karah, Karra, Karrah

Caress (French) tender, soft touch.
Carass, Carassa, Carassar, Caressa, Caresse, Caris, Carisa, Carisah, Carise, Cariss, Carissa, Carissah, Carisse, Caryss, Caryssa, Caryssah, Carysse, Charice, Charis, Charisah, Chariss, Charissa, Charissah, Charisse, Charys, Charysa, Charysah, Charyss, Charyssa, Charyssah, Charysse, Karisa, Karisah, Karissa, Karissah, Karysa, Karysah, Karyssa, Karyssah

Carey (Welsh) castle on the rocky island. (O/Eng) carer.
Caree, Cari (Wel), Caria, Cariah, Carie (Wel), Cary, Carya, Caryah

Cari (Turkish) gentle flowing stream.
Caree, Carey, Carie, Cary

C

Carina (Spanish) little darling.
Caran, Carana, Caranah, Carane,
Caren, Carena, Carenah, Carene,
Carin, Carinah, Carine, Carrin,
Carrina, Carrinah, Carrine, Carryn,
Carryna, Carrynah, Carryne, Caryn,
Caryna, Carynah, Caryne

Carissa (Greek) beloved.
Carass, Carassa, Carassar, Caress,
Caressa, Caresse, Caris, Carisa,
Carisah, Carise, Cariss, Carissah,
Carisse, Caryss, Caryssa, Caryssah,
Carysse, Charice, Charis, Charisah,
Chariss, Charissa, Charissah,
Charisse, Charys, Charysa,
Charysah, Charyss, Charyssa,
Charyssah, Charysse, Karisa,
Karisah, Karissa, Karissah, Karysa,
Karysah, Karyssa, Karyssah

Carita (Latin) charity.
Caritah, Caritta, Carittah, Caryta,
Carytah, Carytta, Caryttah, Charita,
Charity, Karita, Karitah, Karitta,
Karittah

Carla (German) farmer.
(Eng) strong woman.
Carila, Carilah, Carilla, Carillah,
Carlah, Carlan, Carlana, Carlanah,
Carlane, Carlea, Carleah, Carlee,
Carlei, Carleigh, Carleta, Carletha,
Carlethe, Carli, Carlia, Carliah,
Carlicia, Carlie, Carliqua,
Carliquah, Carlique, Carlisa,
Carlisah, Carlissa, Carlisssah,
Carlisse, Carlita, Carlitah, Carlite,
Carlonda, Carlondra, Carlondrea,
Carlreca, Carlondria, Carlyle,
Carlyjo, Carlyle, Carlyse, Carlysle,
Karla, Karlea, Karleah, Karlee, Karlei,
Karleigh, Karley, Karli, Karlia,
Karliah, Karly, Karlya, Karlyah
Carlyjo, Carlyle, Carlyse, Carlysle,
Karla, Karlea, Karlee, Karleigh,
Karley, Karli, Karlia, Karly

Carlene (Irish/English) little
woman. The feminine form of
Charles, strong; courageous.
Carla, Carlah, Carlan, Carlana,
Carlanah, Carlandra, Carlandrah,
Carlane, Carlean, Carleana,
Carleanah, Carleane, Carleen,
Carleena, Carleenah, Carleene,
Carlen, Carlena, Carlenah, Carlin,
Carlina, Carlinah, Carlinda,
Carlindah, Carline, Carling,
Carllan, Carllin, Carllyn, Carllyna,
Carllynah, Carllyne, Carlyn,
Carlyna, Carlynah, Carlyne

Carlin/Carling (Gaelic) little
champion. (O/Eng) strong,
courageous one from the pool.
The feminine form of Carlin.
Carla, Carlah, Carlan, Carlana,
Carlanah, Carlandra, Carlandrah,
Carlane, Carlean, Carleana,
Carleanah, Carleane, Carleen,
Carleena, Carleenah, Carleene,
Carlen, Carlena, Carlenah, Carlene,
Carlina, Carlinah, Carlinda,
Carlindah, Carline, Carling,
Carllan, Carllin, Carllyn, Carllyna,
Carllynah, Carllyne, Carlyn,
Carlyna, Carlynah, Carlyne

Carlissa (Hebrew) little woman who
is holy and sacred to God.
Carleasha, Carleashah, Carleesha,
Carleesia, Carleesiah, Carleeza,
Carlesia, Carlesiah, Carlis, Carlisa,
Carlisah, Carlise, Carlisha, Carlisia,
Carlisiah, Carliss, Carlissah,
Carlisse, Carlissia, Carlissiah,
Carlista, Carlysa, Carlysah,
Carlyssa, Carlyssah, Carlysta,
Carlystah

Carlotta (Italian/French) little
woman. The feminine form of
Charles, strong; courageous.
Carleta, Carletah, Carlete, Carletta,

Carlotta cont.
Carlettah, Carlette, Carlota,
Carlotah, Carlote, Carlotte

Carly (Teutonic) little and woman.
A short form of Caroline. The
feminine form of Carl/Charles,
strong; courageous.
Carlea, Carleah, Carlee, Carlei,
Carleigh, Carley, Carli, Carlia,
Carliah, Carlie, Carly, Carlya,
Carlyah

Carma (Sanskrit) destiny.
(Arab) fruit field.
Carmah, Carmal, Carmala,
Carmalah, Carmalina, Carmalinah,
Carmaline, Carmalyn, Carmalyna,
Carmalynah, Carmalyne,
Carmania, Carmaniah, Carmanya,
Carmanyah, Karma, Karmah,
Karmal, Karmala, Karmale

Carmela (Hebrew) vineyard; garden.
Carmelah, Carmelia, Carmeliah,
Carmelie, Carmell, Carmella,
Carmelle, Carmely, Carmelya,
Carmil, Carmila, Carmile, Carmill,
Carmilla, Carmille, Carmillia,
Carmilliah, Carmillya, Carmillyah,
Carmyllia, Carmylliah, Carmyllya,
Carmyllyah, Carmyla, Carmylah,
Carmyle, Carmylla, Carmylle

Carmen (Latin) song.
Carma, Carmah, Carmainm,
Carmaina, Carmaine, Carman,
Carmana, Carmanah, Carmelina,
Carmeline, Carmelita, Carmencita,
Carmena, Carmene, Carmia,
Carmiah, Carmin, Carmina,
Carmine, Carmita, Carmon,
Carmona, Carmone, Carmyn,
Carmyna, Carmynta

Carmine (Latin) scarlet red.
Carmina, Carminah, Carmine,
Carmyn, Carmuna, Carmynah,
Carmyne, Karmina, Karminah,

Karmine, Karmyn, Karmyna,
Karmynah, Karmyne

Carna (Latin) flesh colour.
(Heb) horn of God.
Carnah, Carniel, Carniela,
Carnielah, Carniell, Carniella,
Carnielle, Carnit, Carnita, Carnite,
Carnyta, Carnytah, Carnyte, Karna,
Karnah, Karniel, Karniela,
Karnielah, Karniell, Karniella,
Karnielle, Karnit, Karnyt, Karnyta,
Karnytah, Karnyte

Carnelian (Latin) red/yellow
translucent stone.
Carnelia, Carneliah, Carnelya,
Carnelyah, Carnelyan

Caroi (Latin) strong, courageous
woman. The feminine form of
Carl.
Caroy

Carol (German) farmer; strong;
courageous. (Eng) joyful
Christmas song.
Caral, Carala, Caralah, Carall,
Carel, Carela, Carele, Carell,
Carella, Carelle, Caril, Carila,
Carilah, Carile, Carill, Carole,
Caroll, Carral, Carrala, Carralah,
Carrall, Carralla, Carrallah, Carrel,
Carrell, Carrella, Carrellah,
Carrelle, Carril, Carrill, Carrilla,
Carrillah, Carrol, Carroll, Carryl,
Carryll, Caryl, Caryla. Carylah,
Caryle, Caryll, Carylla, Caryllah,
Carylle

Carolann (German/Hebrew)
graceful farmer. (O/Eng) graceful;
strong; courageous.
Carolan, Carolana, Carolanah,
Carolane, Carolanna, Carolanne

C

Carolina/Caroline (Italian/French) little woman. (Ger) farmer; strong; courageous. (Eng) joyful line from a Christmas song.
Caralan, Caralana, Caralanah, Caralane, Caralin, Caralina, Caralinah, Caraline, Carilean, Carileana, Carileanah, Carileane, Carileen, Carileena, Carolean, Caroleana, Caroleanah, Caroleane, Caroleen, Caroleena, Caroleenah, Caroleene, Carolin, Carolinah, Caroline, Carolyn, Carolyna, Carolynah, Carolyne, Carralean, Carraleana, Carraleanah, Carraleane, Carraleen, Carraleena, Carraleenah, Carraleene, Carrallin, Carralina, Carralinah, Carraline, Carralyn, Carralyna, Carralynah, Carralyne, Carrelean, Carreleana, Carreleanah, Carreleane, Carreleen, Carreleena, Carreleenah, Carreleene, Carrelin, Carrelina, Carrelinah, Carreline, Carrelyn, Carrelyna, Carrelynah, Carrelyne, Carrileen, Carrileena, Carrileenah, Carrileene, Carrilin, Carrilina, Carrilinah, Carriline, Carroleen, Carroleena, Carroleenah, Caroleene, Carrolin, Carrolina, Carrolinah, Carroline, Carrolyn, Carrolyna, Carrolynah, Carrolyne, Carrolynn, Carrolynna, Carrolynah, Carrolynne

Caron (Welsh) loving; kind-hearted.
Caaran, Caaren, Caarin, Caaron, Caaryn, Caran, Caren, Carin, Carran, Carren, Carrin, Carron, Carrun, Carryn, Carun, Caryn, Kaaran, Kaaren, Kaarin, Kaaron, Kaaryn, Karan, Karen, Karin, Karon, Karran, Karren, karrin, Karron, Karrun, Karryn, Karun, Karyn

Carpathia (Greek) fruit.
Carpathiah, Carpathya, Carpathyah

Carra (Irish) friend.
Cara, Carah, Carrah, Kara, Karah, Karra, Karrah

Carrie (French/English) little, strong, courageous woman. The short form of names starting with 'Car' e.g. Caroline.
Caree, Carey, Cari, Carie, Carree, Carrey, Carri, Carry, Cary, Karee, Karey, Kari, Karie, Karree, Karrey, Karri, Karrie, Karry, Kary

Caryl (Welsh) beloved.
Caril, Carila, Carilah, Carile, Carol, Carola, Carolah, Caroll, Carolla, Carollah, Carolle, Carryl, Carryla, Carrylah, Carryle, Caryla, Carylah, Caryle, Caryll, Carylla, Caryllah, Carylle, Karyl, Karyla, Karylah, Karyle, Karyll, Karylla, Karyllah, Karylle

Caryn (Greek/Danish) purity. A form of Karen.
Caaran, Caaren, Caarin, Caaron, Caaryn, Caran, Caren, Carin, Caron, Carran, Carren, Carrin, Carron, Carrun, Carryn, Carun, Kaaran, Kaaren, Kaarin, Kaaron, Kaaryn, Karan, Karen, Karin, Karon, Karran, Karren, karrin, Karron, Karrun, Karryn, Karun, Karyn

Carys (Welsh) love.
Carass, Carassa, Carassar, Caress, Caressa, Caresse, Caris, Carisa, Carisah, Carise, Cariss, Carissah, Carisse, Caryss, Caryssa, Caryssah, Carysse, Charice, Charis, Charisah, Chariss, Charissa, Charissah, Charisse, Charys, Charysa, Charysah, Charyss, Charyssa, Charyssah, Charysse, Karisa, Karisah, Karissa, Karissah, Karysa, Karysah, Karyssa, Karyssah

Casey (Irish) brave.
Cacee, Cacey, Caci, Cacia, Cacie,

Casey cont.

Cacy, Caecee, Caecey, Caeci,
Caecie, Caecy, Caicee, Caicey, Caici,
Caicie, Caicy, Caisee, Caisey, Caisi,
Caisie, Caisy, Casee, Casi, Casia,
Casie, Casy, Caycee, Caycey, Cayci,
Caycie, Caysee, Caysey, Caysi,
Caysie, Caysy, Kacee, Kacey, Kaci,
Kacie, Kacy, Kaicee, Kaicey, Kaici,
Kaicie, Kaicy, Kaycee, Kaycey, Kayci,
Kaycie, Kaycy

Cass/Cassie (Greek) prophet. The
short form of names starting with
'Cass' e.g. Cassandra.
Cas, Casi, Casie, Cassa, Cassi, Cassie,
Cassy, Casy, Caz, Cazi, Cazie, Cazy,
Cazzi, Cazzie, Cazzy, Kas, Kasi,
Kasie, Kass, Kassee, Kassey, Kassi,
Kassie, Kassy, Kasy, Kaz, Kazi, Kazie,
Kazy, Kazz, Kazzi, Kazzie, Kazzy

Cassandra (Greek) prophet.
Casandera, Casandra, Casandre,
Casancrey, Casandri, Casandria,
Casandrina, Casandrine,
Casaundra, Casaundre, Casondra,
Casondre, Casondria, Casondriah,
Cassander, Cassandera, Cassandre
(Fren), Cassondra, Cassondre,
Cassundra, Cassundre, Cassundria,
Cassundrina, Cazzandra,
Cazzandre, Cazzandria, Cazzondra,
Cazzondre, Cazzondria, Kasandra,
Kasandrah, Kasandre, Kasandria,
Kasandrina, Kasandrine, Kassandra,
Kassandrah, Kassandre (Fren),
Kassundra, Kassundre, Kassundria,
Kassundriah, Kazzandra,
Kazzandre, Kazzandria,
Kazzandriah, Kazzandrya,
Kazzandryah

Cassia (Latin) flowering.
Casia, Casiah, Cassiah, Casya,
Cassyah, Cazia, Caziah, Cazya,
Cazyah, Cazzia, Cazziah, Cazzya,
Cazzyah, Kasia, Kasiah, Kassia,

Kassiah, Kassya, Kassyah, Kasya,
Kasyah, Kazia, Kaziah, Kazya,
Kazyah, Kazzia, Kazziah, Kazzya,
Kazzyah

Cassidy (Irish) clever; curly-haired.
Casadee, Casadey, Casadi, Casadia,
Casadiah, Casadie, Casady,
Casidee, Casidey, Casidi, Casidia,
Casidiah, Casidie, Casidy,
Cassadee, Cassadey, Cassadi,
Cassadia, Cassadie, Cassady,
Cassidee, Cassidey, Cassidi,
Cassidia, Cassidie, Cassydi,
Cassydie, Cassydy, Casydi, Casydie,
Casydy, Cazidy, Cazzidy, Kasadee,
Kasadey, Kasadi, Kasadia, Kasadie,
Kasady, Kasidee, Kasidey, Kasidi,
Kasidia, Kasidie, Kasidy, Kassidee,
Kassidey, Kassidi, Kassidia,
Kassidie, Kassidy, Kasidy, Kassidee,
Kassidey, Kassidi, Kassidia,
Kassidie, Kassidy, Kasydee, Kasydey,
Kassydi, Kassydie, Kassydy, Kasydy,
Kazidy, Kazydy

Catava (African) sleeping.
Catavah

Cathal (Irish) eye of the battle.
Cathall, Cathalla, Cathalle, Cathel,
Cathell, Cathella, Cathelle, Kathal,
Kathall, Kathalla, Kathalle, Kathel,
Kathell, Kathella, Kathelle

Catherine (Greek) purity.
Cairena, Cairene, Cairina,
Cairinah, Cairine, Caitlin (Ir),
Caitrin, Catalina, Catalinah,
Cataline, Catana (Span), Catania,
Cataniah, Catanya, Catanyah,
Cataut (O/Fren), Catelini, Cateret,
Caterina (Ital), Caterinah, Caterine,
Catha, Catharin, Catharina (Port),
Catharinah, Catharine, Catheau,
Catherina, Catherinah, Cathlean,
Cathleana, Cathleanah, Cathleane,
Cathleen, Cathleena, Cathleenah,
Cathleene, Cathrina, Cathrinah,

Cathrine, Cathryn, Cathryna,
Cathrynah, Cathryne, Cathwyg,
Cathy, Catlin, Caton, Catrion,
Catriona (Gae), Catrionah,
Catrione, Cattarin, Cattarina (Ital),
Cattarineh, Cattarine, Catuja
(Span), Catya, Catyah, Cawth (Ir),
Ekatrina Kaatje (Dut), Kaddo (Est),
Kaferin, Kaferina, Kaferinah,
Kaferine, Kaferyn, Kaferyna,
Kaferynah, Kaferyne, Kafferin,
Kafferina, Kafferinah, Kafferine,
Kafferyn, Kafferyna, Kafferynah,
Kafferyne, Kardreinl, Kajsa (Swed),
Kalina (Swed), Kalinah, Kaline,
Karan (Grk), Karean, Kareana,
Kareanah, Kareane, Kareen,
Kareena, Kareenah, Kareene, Karen
(Grk/Austr), Karena, Karenah,
Karene, Karin, Karina (Scan),
Karinah, Karine, Karlinka (Slav),
Karlinkah, Karolin, Karolina (Lith),
Karolinah, Karoline (Ger), Karolyn,
Karolyna, Karolynah, Karolyne,
Karstin (Dan), Karstina, Karstinah,
Karstine, Kashe (Dan), Kasen
(Dan), Kasena, Kasenah, Kasene,
Kasia, Kasiah, Kasie, Kata, Katal,
Katalin (Hun), Katalina, Katalinah,
Kataline, Katarin, Katarina
(Lith/Swed), Katarina, Katarinah,
Katarine, Kataryn, Kataryna,
Katarynah, Kataryne, Katarzyna
(Pol), Kate, Katey, Kateren,
Katharin, Katharina, Katharinah,
Katharine, Katharyn, Katharyna,
Katharynah, Katharyne, Katherin,
Katherina, Katherinah, Katherine,
Katheryn, Katheryna, Katherynah,
Katheryne, Kathran, Kathren,
Kathrin, Kathron, Kathrun,
Kathryn, Kathy, Kati, Katie, Katja,
Katreen (Eng), Katreena,
Katreenah, Katreene, Katren (Eng),
Katrena, Katrenah, Katrene, Katri
(Est), Katria, Katriah, Katrian,
Katriana, Katrianah, Katriane,

Katriann, Katrianna, Katriannah,
Katrianne, Katrien (Ger), Katriena,
Katrienah, Katrienja, Katrijin,
Katrina (Aust), Katrinah (Aust),
Katrinka, Katrinna (Aust),
Katrinnah, Katrinne, Katryn,
Katryna, Katrynah, Katryne, Kattel,
Katterie (Slav), Katterle, Katushka,
Katya (Russ), Keri, Kerie, Kerri,
Kerrie, Kerry, Kery

Cathleen (Irish/Greek) purity.
Cathalean, Cathaleana,
Cathaleanah, Cathaleane,
Cathaleen, Cathaleena,
Cathaleena, Cathaleenah,
Cathaleene, Cathalen, Cathalena,
Cathalenah, Cathalene, Cathalin,
Cathalina, Cathalinah, Cathaline,
Cathalyn, Cathalyna, Cathalynah,
Cathalyne, Catheleen, Catheleena,
Catheleenah, Catheleene,
Cathelen, Cathelena, Cathelenah,
Cathelene, Cathelin, Cathelina,
Cathelinah, Catheline, Cathelyn,
Cathelyna, Cathelynah, Cathelyne,
Cathlean, Cathleana, Cathleanah,
Cathleane, Cathleena, Cathleena,
Cathleenah, Cathleene, Cathlen,
Cathlena, Cathlenah, Cathlene,
Cathlin, Cathlina, Cathlinah,
Cathline, Cathlyn, Cathlyna,
Cathlynah, Cathlyne, Kafflean,
Kaffleana, Kaffleanah, Kaffleane,
Kaffleen, Kaffleena, Kaffleenah,
Kaffleene, Kaffleen, Kaffleena,
Kaffleenah, Kaffleene, Kafflein,
Kaffleina, Kaffleinah, Kaffleine,
Kafflin, Kafflina, Kafflinah,
Kaffline, Kafflyn, Kafflyna,
Kafflynah, Kafflyne, Kaflean,
Kafleana, Kafleanah, Kafleane,
Kafleen, Kafleena, Kafleena,
Kafleenah, Kafleene, Kaflein,
Kafleina, Kafleinah, Kafleine,
Kaflin, Kaflina, Kaflinah, Kafline,
Kaflyn, Kaflyna, Kaflynah, Kaflyne,

C

Cathleen cont.
Kathleena, Kathleenah, Kathleene,
Kathlein, Kathleina, Kathleinah,
Kathleine, Kathlin, Kathlina,
Kathlinah, Kathline, Kathlyn,
Kathlyna, Kathlynah, Kathlyne

Cathy (Greek) purity. The short
form of Catherine.
Caffee, Caffey, Caffi, Caffie, Caffy,
Cath, Cathea, Cathee, Cathey,
Cathi, Cathie, Kaffee, Kaffey, Kaffi,
Kaffie, Kaffy, Kath, Kathea, Kathee,
Kathey, Kathi, Kathie, Kathy

Catrina (Slavic/Greek) purity. A
form of Katrina.
Catereana, Catereanah, Catereane,
Catereena, Catereenah, Catereene,
Caterina, Caterinah, Caterine,
Cateryna, Caterynah, Cateryne,
Catina, Catinah, Catreana,
Catreanah, Catreen, Catreena,
Catreenah, Catreene, Catren,
Catrena, Catrenah, Catrene,
Catrenia, Catrinah, Catrine,
Catrinia, Catriona, Catrionah,
Catrione, Catryn, Catryna, Catryne,
Catrynia, Catrynya, Katereana,
Katereanah, Katereane, Katereena,
Katereena, Katereenah, Katereene,
Katerina, Katerinah, Katerine,
Kateryna, Katerynah, Kateryne,
Katreana, Katreanah, Katreane,
Katreen, Katreena, Katreenah,
Katreene, Katrina, Katrinah,
Katrine, Katryna, Katrynah, Katryne

Cayla (Hebrew) crown of laurel.
Caela, Caelah, Caelea, Caeleah,
Caelee, Caelei, Caeleigh, Caeley,
Caeli, Caelia, Caeliah, Caelie,
Caely, Cahla, Cahlah, Cahlea,
Cahleah, Cahlee, Cahlei, Cahleigh,
Cahley, Cahli, Cahlie, Cahly, Caila,
Cailah, Cailea, Caileah, Cailee,
Cailei, Caileigh, Caili, Cailia,
Cailiah, Cailie, Caily, Cala, Calah,

Calea, Caleah, Calee, Calei,
Caleigh, Caley, Cali, Caliah, Calie,
Caly, Caylah, Caylea, Cayleah,
Caylee, Caylei, Cayleigh, Cayley,
Cayli, Caylia, Cayliah, Caylie,
Cayly, Kaela, Kaelah, Kaelea,
Kaeleah, Kaelee, Kaelei, Kaeleigh,
Kaeley, Kaeli, Kaelia, Kaeliah,
Kaelie, Kaely, Kahla, Kahlah,
Kahlea, Kahleah, Kahlee, Kahlei,
Kahleigh, Kahley, Kahlei, Kahlie,
Kahly, Kaila, Kailah, Kailea,
Kaileah, Kailee, Kailei, Kaileigh,
Kailey, Kaili, Kailia, Kailiah, Kailie,
Kaily, Kalea, Kaleah, Kalee, Kalei,
Kaleigh, Kaley, Kali, Kalia, Kaliah,
Kalie, Kaly, Kalya, Kayla, Kaylah,
Kaylea, Kayleah, Kaylee, Kaylei,
Kayleigh, Kayley, Kayli, Kaylia,
Kayliah, Kaylie, Kayly, Kayla

Ceara (Irish/Gaelic) spear.
Cearah, Seara, Searah

Cecania (German) freedom.
Cecanie, Cecaniah, cecanya,
Cecanyah, Secania, Sesaniah,
Secanie, Sesanya, Sesanyah

Cecilia (Latin) unseeing. The
feminine form of Cecil.
Cacelea, Caceleah, Cacelee,
Cacelei, Caceleigh, Caceley, Caceli,
Cacilia (Ger), Caciliah, Cacilie
(Ger), Caecil, Caecilia, Caeciliah,
Caecilie, Cecile, Ceciliah
(Span/Ital), Cecilie (Ger), Cecily
(O/Eng), Cecilya (Illy), Cecylia,
Cecyliah, Cecylya, Cecylyah,
Cecylja (Pol), Celia (Swed/Ital),
Celiah, Celie (Fren), Celina,
Celinah, Celine (Fren), Celeka,
Celine (Fren), Cicely, Cilina,
Cilinah, Cylina, Cylinah, Cylyne,
Hiria, Leola, Sheelagh (Ir/Gae),
Sheelah (Ir/Gae), Sheila (Ir/Gae),
Sile (Ir), Sileas (Scot), Sissel (Ir),
Zezilya, Zilia (Ven), Ziliola

C

Cedrica (Welsh) gift; splendour.
(O/Eng) war chief. The feminine
form of Cedric.
Cedricah, Cedryca, Cedrycah

Ceinlys (Welsh) gem.
Ceinlis, Ceynlis, Ceynlys, Seinlis,
Seinlys, Seynlys, Seynlys

Ceinwen (Welsh) beautiful, precious
stone.
Ceinwin, Ceinwyn, Ceinwynn,
Ceinwynne, Ceynwin, Ceynwyn,
Ceynwynn, Ceynwynne

Celandine (Greek/French) little
swallow; yellow flowering plant.
Celandina, Celandinah,
Celandrina, Celandrinah,
Celandrine, Celandryna,
Celandrynah, Celandryne

Celena (Greek/French) moon;
heavenly.
Caleena, Caleene, Calina, Caline,
Calyn, Calyna, Calyne, Celean,
Celeana, Celeanah, Celeane,
Celeen, Celeena, Celeenah,
Celeene, Celin, Celina, Celinah,
Celinda, Celinka, Celine, Celka,
Celyn, Celyna, Celynah, Celyne,
Celyne, Seleena, Seleene, Selina,
Seline, Selyn, Selyna, Selyne

Celeste (Greek/French) moon;
heavenly.
Celesta, Celestah, Celestar,
Celestelle, Celestia, Celestial,
Celestiar, Celestina, Celestine,
Celestyn, Celestyna (Pol),
Celestyne, Celina, Celinda, Celine,
Celinka, Selest, Selesta, Selestah,
Seleste, Selestin, Selestina,
Selestinah, Selestine, Selestyna,
Selestynah, Selestyne

Celestina (Greek/French/Latin) little
moon; little heavenly one.
Celeste, Celesteana, Celesteanah,
Celesteane, Celesteen, Celesteena,

Celesteenah, Celesteene, Celestin,
Celestinah, Celestine, Celestyn,
Celestyna, Celestynah, Celestyne,
Selest, Selestina, Selestinah,
Selestine, Seleseana, Seleseanah,
Seleseane, Seleseena, Seleseenah,
Seleseene, Selestina, Selestinah,
Selestine, Selestyna, Selestynah,
Selestyne

Celie (Greek/French) moon;
heavenly.
Celea, Celeah, Celee, Celei,
Celeigh, Celey, Celi, Cely, Selea,
Seleah, Selee, Selei, Seleigh, Seley,
Seli, Selie, Sely

Celine (Greek/French) moon;
heavenly.
Celeana, Celeanah, Celeane,
Celeena, Celeenah, Celeene,
Celina, Celinah, Celinia, Celiniah,
Celyna, Celynah, Celyne, Selina,
Selinah, Seline, Selinia, Seliniah,
Selyna, Selynah, Selyne

Cella (Italian/French) she is
freedom.
Cellah, Cellia, Celliah, Cellya,
Cellyah, Sella, Sellah, Sellia,
Selliah, Sellya, Sellyah

Celosia (Greek) flaming.
Celosiah, Celosya, Celosyah,
Selosia, Selosiah, Selosya, Selosyah

Celyren (Welsh) holly.
Celeeren, Celeighren, Celiren

Cera (Irish/Welsh) red/brown
complexioned; belt.
Ceara, Cearah, Ciar, Ciara, Ciarah,
Ciora, Ciorah, Cyra, Cyrah, Sera,
Serah, Sira, Sirah, Syra, Syrah

Cerelia (Latin) from the spring in
the meadow.
Cereliah, Cerelya, Cerelyah, Serelia,
Sereliah, Serelya, Serelyah

Cerella (Latin) spring time.
Cerela, Cerelah, Cerelisa, Cerelise,
Cerellah, Cerelle, Ceres, Ceress,
Ceressa

Ceres (Roman) goddess of the
harvest. (Lat) candle.
Cerelia, Cereliah, Cerelya, Cerelyah

Ceridwen (Welsh) poetry; white.
The Welsh goddess of poetry.
Ceridwyn, Ceridwen, Cerydwen,
Cerydwin, Cerydwyn, Cerydwynn,
Cerydwynne, Seridwen, Seridwyn,
Seridwynn, Seridwynne

Cerise (French) cherry.
Carice, Carise, Caryce, Caryse,
Cariss, Cerice, Ceryce, Ceryse,
Charise, Charriss, Charrissa,
Charrissee, Sherise, Sheriss,
Sherissa, Sherisse

Cerys (Welsh) love.
Ceris, Serys

Chaanach (Hebrew) graceful.
Chanach

Chablis (French) dry, white wine.
Chablea, Chableah, Chablee,
Chabley, Chabli, Chablia, Chablie,
Chabliss, Chably, Chablys,
Chablyss

Chadee (French) from Chad in
Africa. The feminine form of
Chad, from the warrior's estate.
Chadae, Chadai, Chadey, Chaddae,
Chaddai, Chadday, Chade, Chadea,
Chadee, Chadey, Chadi, Chadia,
Chadiah, Chadie, Chady

Chahna (Hindi) loving.
Chahnah

Chai (Hebrew) life.
Chae, Chaela, Chaeli, Chaelia,
Chaella, Chaelle, Chaena, Chay

Chaka/Chakia/Chakra (Sanskrit)
energy circle. A form of Chakra.
Chakra, Chakrah, Chakiah,
Chakira, Chakria, Chakriya,
Chakya, Chakyah, Chakyra,
Chakyrah, Shakra, Shakrah,
Shakeeia, Shakeeiah, Shakeeya,
Shakeeyah, Shakeia, Shakeiah,
Shakeya, Shakiya, Shakiyah,
Shakya, Shakyah, Shekela, Shekia,
Shekiah, Shekya, Shekyah

Chalice (French) goblet.
Chalace, Chalcia, Chalcie, Chalece,
Chaliece, Chaliese, Chalisa,
Chalise, Chalisk, Chalissa, Challa,
Challain, Challaina, Challaine,
Challis, Challisa, Challise, Challiss,
Challissa, Challisse, Chalyce,
Chalyse, Challyce, Challysa,
Challyse, Chalyce, Chalyse

Chalina (Spanish) rose.
Chalin, Chalinah, Chaline, Chalyn,
Chalyna, Chalynah, Chalyne,
Shalina, Shalinah, Shaline, Shalyn,
Shalyna, Shalynah, Shalyne

Chalonna (Latin) solitary.
Chalona, Chalonah, Chalone,
Chalonee, Chalonnah, Chalonne,
Chalonnee

Chamania (Hebrew) sunflower.
Chamaniah, Chamanya,
Chamanyah

Chambray (French) light fabric.
Chambrae, Chambrai, Chambre,
Chambree, Chambrey, Chambri,
Chambria, Chambrie, Chambry,
Shamrae, Shambrai, Shambre,
Shambree, Shambrey, Shambri,
Shambria, Shambry

Chameli (Hindi) jasmine flower.
Chamelia, Chameliah, Chamelie,
Chamely

C

Chan (Cambodian) tree which is
sweet smelling.
Chana, Chanae, Chanah, Shana,
Shanae, Shanah

Chana (Hebrew) God is gracious.
A form Hannah.
Chanah, Channa, Channah, Shana,
Shanah, Shanna, Shannah

Chanda (Sanskrit) goddess.
Chandah, Chandea, Chandee,
Chandey, Chandi, Chandia,
Chandiah, Chandie, Chandy,
Chandya, Shanda, Shandea,
Shandee, Shandey, Shandi,
Shandie, Shandy

Chandani (Hindi) moonlight.
Chandanee, Chandaney, Chandania,
Chandaniah, Chandany,
Chandanya, Chandanyah

Chandella (French) candle.
Chandal, Chandala, Chandalah,
Chandale, Chandel, Chandela,
Chandelah, Chandele, Chandell,
Chandella, Chandellah, Shandel,
Shandela, Shandelah, Shandele,
Shandell, Shandella, Shandellah,
Shandelle

Chandra/Chandria (Sanskrit)
moon.
Chandra, Chandrah, Chandriah,
Chandrya, Chandryah, Shandria,
Shandriah, Shandrya, Shandryah

Chanel (French) from the strait.
Chanal, Chanall, Chanalla,
Chanalle, Chanell, Chanella,
Chanelle, Channel, Channell,
Chanelle

Chanina (Hebrew) graceful.
Chaninah, Chanyna, Chanynah

**Chantal/Chantelle/Chontal/
Chontelle** (French) song.
Chantal, Chantala, Chantalah,
Chantale, Chantel, Chantela,

Chantelah, Chantele, Chantell,
Chantella, Chantellah, Chantelle,
Chantila, Chantile, Chantill,
Chantilla, Chantille, Chantoia,
Chantoya, Chantril, Chantrill,
Chantrille, Chaunta, Chontel,
Chontela, Chontelah, Chontele,
Chontell, Chontella, Chontellah,
Chontelle, Shantal, Shantel,
Shantela, Shantelah, Shantele,
Shantell, Shantella, Shantellah,
Shontel, Shontela, Shontelah,
Shontele, Shontell, Shontella,
Shontellah, Shontelle

Chantara (American/French) song.
A form of Chantal.
Chantarah, Chantia, Chantiah,
Chantarra, Chantarrah, Chantarria,
Chantarriah, Chantarrya,
Chantarryah, Chantya, Chantyah,
Shantara, Shantarah, Shantaria,
Shantariah, Shantarra, Shantarrah,
Shantarria, Shanntarriah,
Shanntarya, Shanntaryah

Chantilly (French) fine lace.
Chantilea, Chantileah, Chantilee,
Chantilei, Chantileigh, Chantili,
Chantilia, Chantilie, Chantilla,
Chantillea, Chantilleah, Chantillee,
Chantillei, Chantilleigh,
Chantilley, Chantilli, Chantillia,
Chantillie, Chantily, Chantyly,
Shantilea, Shantileah, Shantilee,
Shantiley, Shantili, Shantilie,
Shantillea, Shantilleah, Shantillee,
Shantillei, Shantilleigh, Shantilli,
Shantillie, Shantilly, Shantylea,
Shantyleah, Shantylee, Shantylei,
Shantyleigh, Shantyley, Shantylli,
Shantyllie, Shantylly, Shantyly

Chapa (Sioux) beaver.
Chapah

Chapawee (Sioux) busy beaver.

C

Chara (Greek) joy.
Charah, Shara, Sharah

Chardonnay (French) dry, white wine.
Chardae, Chardai, Chadon, Chardona, Chardonay, Chardonee, Chardonnae, Chardonnee, Shardonae, Shardonai, Shardonay, Shardonaye

Charis/Charissa/Charisse (French) tender touch. (Grk) graceful.
Charisa, Charidah, Charise, Chariss, Charissa, Charissah, Charisse, Charys, Charysa, Charysah, Charyse, Charyss, Charyssa, Charyssah, Charysse

Charity (Latin) charitable; caring.
Charissa, Carita, Caritaa, Caritah, Caritas, Charita, Charitah, Charitas, Charitea, Charitee, Charitey, Chariti, Charitia, Charitiah, Charitie, Charitina, Charatinah, Charitine, Charitiyna, Charityne, Charyty, Charytia, Charytiah, Charyty, Charytya, Charytyah

Charla (English) strong; courageous. The feminine form of Charles. A short form of Charlene.
Charlah

Charleen (German) strong, courageous one from the meadow.
Charlean, Charleana, Charleane, Charleena, Charleene, Charlein, Charleina, Charleine, Charleyn, Charleyna, Charleyne, Charlin, Charlina, Charline, Charlyn, Charlyna, Charlyne, Sharlean, Sharleana, Sharleane, Sharleen, Sharleena, Sharleene, Sharlein, Sharleina, Sharleine, Sharleyn, Sharleyna, Sharleyne, Sharlin, Sharlina, Sharline, Sharlyn, Sharlyna, Sharlyne

Charlie (German/English) strong, courageous one from the meadow. The feminine form of Charles. A short form of Charlene.
Charla, Charlae, Charlai, Chalah, Charlea, Charleah, Charlee, Charlei, Charleigh, Charley, Charlia, Charliah, Charly, Charlya

Charlotte (French) little, strong, courageous woman.
Carla, Carlean, Carleana, Carleane, Carleen, Carleena, Carleene, Carlein, Carleina, Carleine, Carleyn, Carleyna, Carleyne, Carlot, Carlota, Carlotah, Carlote, Carlott, Carlotta, Carlottah, Carlotte, Carolet, Caroleta, Caroletah, Carolete, Carolett, Caroletta, Carolettah, Carolette, Charla, Charlah, Charlean, Charleana, Charleane, Charleen, Charleena, Charleene, Charlein, Charleina, Charleine, Charlena, Charlenah, Charlene, Charlet, Charleta, Charletah, Charlete, Charlett, Charletta, Charlettah, Charlette, Chalin, Chalina, Charlinah, Charline, Charlot, Charlota, Charlotah, Charlote, Charlott, Charlotta, Charlottah, Linuscha, Lolotte, Lotje, Sharlet, Sharleta, Sharletah, Sharlete, Sharlett, Sharletta, Sharlettah, Sharlette, Sharlot, Sharlota, Sharlotah, Sharlote, Sharlott, Sharlotta, Sharlottah, Sharlotte

Charmaine (German) strong; courageous. A femimine form of Charles.
Charmain, Charmaina, Charmainah, Charmayn,

Charmayna, Charmaynah,
Charmayne, Karmain, Karmaina,
Karmaine, Karmayn, Karmayna,
Karmayne, Karmein, Karmeina,
Karmeine, Karmeyn, Karmeyna,
Karmeyne, Kharmain, Kharmaina,
Kharmaine, Kharmayn, Kharmayna,
Kharmayne, Kharmein, Kharmeina,
Kharmeine, Kharmeyn, Kharmeyna,
Kharmeyne

Charmane (Latin) singer.
Charmain, Charmaina,
Charmainah, Charmayn,
Charmayna, Charmaynah,
Charmayne, Karmain, Karmaina,
Karmaine, Karmayn, Karmayna,
Karmayne, Karmein, Karmeina,
Karmeine, Karmeyn, Karmeyna,
Karmeyne, Kharmain, Kharmaina,
Kharmaine, Kharmayn, Kharmayna,
Kharmayne, Kharmein, Kharmeina,
Kharmeine, Kharmeyn, Kharmeyna,
Kharmeyne

Charo (Spanish) little Rosa; little rose.
Charoe, Charow

Charrissee (French) cherry.
Charisa, Charidah, Charise,
Charrisa, Charrisah, Charrise,
Charriss, Charrissa, Charrissah,
Charrisse, Charrys, Charrysa,
Charrysah, Charryse, Charryss,
Charryssa, Charryssah, Charrysse,
Charysa, Charysah, Charyse,
Charyss, Charyssa, Charyssah,
Charysse

Chasca (Incan) goddess of the dawn.
Chaska

Chastity (Latin) purity.
Chastitea, Chastitee, Chastitey,
Chastiti, Chastitie

Chava (Hebrew/Yiddish) bird.
Chavah, Chavala, Chavalah,

Chavarra, Chavarria, Chave,
Chaveli, Chavelia, Chavelie,
Chavetta, Chavette, Chaviva,
Chavonna, Chavonne, Chavvis,
Chavvisa, Chavvissa

Chavella (Spanish) holy and sacred to God. A form of Elizabeth.
Chavel, Chavela, Chavelah,
Chavele, Chavell, Chavella,
Charvellah, Charvelle

Chavi (Gypsy) little girl.
Chavee, Chavey, Chavia, Chaviah,
Chavie, Chavy, Chavya, Chavyah

Chavon (Hebrew) God is gracious. A form of Siobhain.
Chavona, Chavonah, Chavone,
Chavonda, Chavondah,
Chavondria, Chavondriah,
Chavone, Chavonn, Chavonna,
Chavonnah, Chavonne,
Chavaughn, Chavaughna,
Chavaughne, Chavawn,
Chavawnah, Chavawne, Chevon,
Chevona, Chevonn, Chevonna,
Chevonnah, Chevonne,
Chevaughn, Chevaughna,
Chevaughne, Chevawn, Chevawna,
Chevawnah, Chevawne

Chaya (Hebrew) life.
Chaia, Chaiah, Chaike, Chailea,
Chaileah, Chailee, Chailei,
Chayleigh, Chailey, Chaili, Chalia,
Chailiah, Chailie, Chaily, Chayah,
Chayka, Chayla, Chaylea,
Chayleah, Chaylee, Chayleena,
Chayleene, Chaylei, Chayleigh,
Chaylena, Chaylene, Chayley,
Chayli, Chaylie, Chayly

Chaylea (Hebrew/Old English) life meadow.
Chaia, Chaiah, Chaike, Chailea,
Chaileah, Chailee, Chailei,
Chayleigh, Chailey, Chaili, Chalia,
Chailiah, Chailie, Chaily, Chayah,

Chaylea cont.
Chayka, Chayla, Chaylea,
Chayleah, Chaylee, Chayleena,
Chayleene, Chaylei, Chayleigh,
Chaylena, Chaylene, Chayley,
Chayli, Chaylie, Chayly

Chechoter (Seminole) dawn.

Cheera (Greek) happy.
Cheerah, Cheeria, Cheeriah,
Cheery, Cheerya, Cheeryah

Chelsea (Old English) from the port of ships; from the chalk sea.
Chelcea, Chelcee, Chelcey, Chelci,
Chelcia, Chelciah, Chelcie, Chelcy,
Chelsee, Chelsi, Chelsie, Chelsy

Chemarin (Hebrew) girl who wears black.
Chemarina, Chemarine,
Chermaryn, Chermaryna,
Chermaryne

Chemosh (Hebrew) peace.

Chen (Chinese) precious.

Chenetta (Greek) goose.
(O/Fren) oak tree.
Chenet, Cheneta, Chenetah,
Chenete, Chenett, Chenettah,
Chenette

Chenia (Hebrew) God is gracious.
Cheniah, Chenya, Chenyah

Chenoa (Native American) white dove.
Chenoah

Cher (French) beloved. A form of Cherily/Cherie.
Chere, Cheree, Cherey, Cheri,
Cherie, Cherlan, Cherlana,
Cherlane, Cherree, Cherrey, Cherri,
Cherrie, Cherry, Chery, Sher, Shere,
Sheree, Sherey, Sheri, Sherie, Sherr,
Sherree, Sherrey, Sherri, Sherrie,
Sherry

Cherelle (French) she is the beloved. A form of Cheryl.
Charel, Charela, Charleah, Charele,
Charell, Charella, Charellah

Cherie (French) beloved cherry tree.
Cheree, Cherey, Cheri, Cherree,
Cherrey, Cherri, Cherrie, Cherry,
Chery, Sheree, Sherey, Sheri, Sherie,
Sherree, Sherrey, Sherri, Sherrie,
Sherry, Shery

Cherilyn (French/Welsh) from the cherry tree near the pool.
(O/Eng) beloved from the pool.
Cherilin, Cherilina, Cherilinah,
Cheriline, Cherilyna, Cherilynah,
Cherilyne, Sherilin, Sherilina,
Sherilinah, Sheriline, Sherilyn,
Sherylyna, Sherylynah, Sherylyne

Cherise (French) cherished.
Charisa, Charisah, Charise, Charys,
Charysa, Charysah, Charyse,
Cherece, Chereece, Chereese,
Cheresa, Cherese, Cherice, Cherys,
Cherysa, Cherysah, Cheryse

Cherish (English) cherished.
Charish, Charisha, Charishe,
Charysha, Charyshah, Cheerish,
Cheerisha, Cherisa, Cherisah,
Cherise, Cherishe, Cherrish,
Cherrisha, Cherrishe, Cherysh,
Cherysha, Cheryshe

Cherokee (Choctaw) people of the cave country; people with a different speech. A tribal name.
Cherika, Cherikia, Cherita,
Cherokei, Cherokey, Cheroki,
Cherokia, Cherokie, Cheroky,
Sherokee

Cherry (Old English) cherry tree.
(Fren) beloved.
Chere, Cheree, Cherey, Cherida,
Cherise, Cherita, Cherree, Cherrey,
Cherri, Cherrie, Cherrye, Chery

Cheryl (Welsh) love.
Cheral, Cherel, Cherell, Cherella,
Cherelle, Cheril, Cherila, Cherille,
Cherrel, Cherrela, Cherrelle,
Cherril, Cherrila, Cherrile, Sheril,
Sherill, Sherille, Sheryl, Sheryll,
Sherylle

Cheyenne (Native American) a
tribal name. (O/Fren/Hebrew)
graceful oak tree.
Cheian, Cheiann, Cheianne,
Cheyan, Cheyana, Cheyane,
Cheyann, Cheyanna, Cheyanne,
Cheyena, Cheyene, Cheyenn,
Cheyenna, Chyan, Chyann,
Chyanna, Chyanne, Chyen,
Chyena, Chyene, Chyenn,
Chyenna, Chyenne

Chezna (Slavic) peace.
Chesna, Chesnah, Chessna,
Chessnah, Cheznah, Cheznia,
Chezniah, Cheznya, Cheznyah

Chiara (Italian) clear; bright.
Cheara, Chyara

Chika (Japanese) one who is near
and dear; beloved.
Chikah, Chyka, Chykah

Chiku (Swahili) one who chatters.

Chilali (Native American) snow
bird.
Chilalea, Chilaleah, Chilalee,
Chilalei, Chilaleigh, Chilalie,
Chilaly

Chimalis (Native American) blue
bird.
Chymalis

Chimene (French) hospitable.

China (Chinese) fine porcelain.
(Geographical) the country.
Chinaetta, Chinah, Chinasa,
Chinda, Chine (Fren), Chinea,
Chinesia, Chinita, Chinna,

Chinwa, Chyna, Chynah, Chynna,
Chynnah

Chinira (Swahili) God will receive.
Chinara, Chinarah, Chinirah,
Chynira, Chynirah

Chinue (Ibo) with God's own
blessing.

Chiquita (Spanish) little girl.
Chaqueta, Chaquita, Chica,
Chikata, Chikita, Chiqueta,
Chiquila, Chiquite, Chiquitha,
Chiquithe, Chiquitia, Chiquitta

Chita (Middle English) kitten.

Chitsa (Native American) fair-
haired.
Chitsah

Chiyo (Japanese) eternal.
Chiya

Chizu (Japanese) a thousand storks.

Chloe/Chloris (Greek) flowering;
goddess of agriculture.
Chloea, Chloee, Chloey, Chloris,
Chlorisa, Chlorise, Chlorys,
Chlorysa, Cholryse, Cloe, Cloea,
Cloee, Cloey, Cloi, Cloie, Cloris,
Clorisa, Clorise, Clorys, Clorysa,
Cloryse, Clowee, Clowey, Clowi,
Clowie, Khloe, Khloea, Khloee,
Khloey, Khloi, Khloie, Khloris,
Khlorisa, Khlorise, Khlorys,
Khlorysa, Khloryse, Khloy, Kloe,
Kloea, Kloee, Kloey, Kloi, Kloie,
Klowee, Klowey, Klowi, Klowie,
Klowy

Cho (Japanese) butterfly; born at
dawn. (Kor) beautiful.

Cholena (Native American) bird.
Choleana, Choleanah, Choleane,
Choleena, Choleenah, Choleene,
Choleina, Choleinah, Choleyna,
Choleynah, Choleyne, Cholenah,
Cholene, Cholina, Cholinah,

Cholena cont.
Choline, Cholyna, Cholynah,
Cholyne

Chooli (Navajo) mountain.
Choolea, Chooleah, Choolee,
Choolei, Chooleigh, Choolie,
Chooly

Choomia (Gypsy) kiss.
Choomiah, Choomya, Choomyah

Chriki (Swahili) blessed.

Chrissanth (French) golden flower.
Chrisanth, Chrisantha,
Chrisanthia, Chrisanthiah,
Chrisanthya, Chrisanthyah,
Chrysantha, Chrysanthe,
Chrysanthia, Chrysanthiah,
Chryzanta, Chryxzanta, Chryzante,
Chryzanthia, Chryzanthiah,
Chryzanthya, Chryzanthyah

Chrissy (German/Greek/English)
Christian. The short form of
names stating with 'Chris' e.g.
Christine.
Chrisea, Chrisee, Chrisi, Chrisie,
Chrissea, Chrissee, Chrissey,
Chrissi, Chrissie, Chrissy, Chrisy,
Chrys, Chrysi, Chrysie, Chryss,
Chryssi, Chryssie, Chryssy, Chrysy

Christa (German/Greek) Christian.
A short form of Christabel.
Christah, Christar, Christara,
Christarah, Chrysta, Chrystah,
Chrystar, Chrystara, Crysta,
Crystah, Chrystar, Crystara,
Crystarah

Christabel (Latin/French) beautiful
Christian.
Christabeel, Christabela,
Christabelah, Christabele,
Christabell, Christabella,
Christabellah, Christabelle,
Christobel, Christobell,
Christobella, Christobelle,

Cristabel, Cristabelah, Cristabele,
Cristabell, Cristabella, Cristabellah,
Cristabelle, Chrystabel,
Chrystabela, Chrystabelah,
Chrystabele, Chrystabell,
Chrystabella, Chrystabellah,
Chrystabelle, Chrystobel,
Chrystobela, Chrystobelah,
Chrystobele, Chrystobell,
Chrystobella, Chrystobellah,
Chrystobelle

Christen (Greek) Christian. A form
of Christina.
Christan, Christen, Christin,
Christon, Christyn, Chrystan,
Chrysten, Chrystin, Chryston,
Chrystyn, Crestian, Crestiana,
Crestianah, Crestiane, Crestiann,
Crestianna, Crestiannah,
Crestianne, Crstyan, Crestyana,
Crestyanah, Crestyane, Crestyann,
Crestyanna, Crestyannah,
Crestyanne, Cristan, Cristen,
Cristia, Cristian, Cristiana,
Cristianah, Cristiane, Cristiann,
Cristianna, Cristiannah, Cristianne,
Cristin, Criston, Cristyn, Kristan,
Kristen, Kristia, Kristian, Kristiana,
Kristianah, Kristiane, Kristiann,
Kristianna, Kristiannah, Kristianne,
Kristin, Kriston, Kristyn, Krystan,
Krysten, Krystin, Kryston, Krystyn

Christian (Greek) Christian. A form
of Christina.
Christiana, Christianah, Christiane,
Christiann, Christianna,
Christiannah, Christianne,
Christianni, Christiannia,
Christianniah, Christianne,
Christien, Christeina, Christeinah,
Christeine, Christeinn, Christeinna,
Christeinnah, Christeinne,
Chrystian, Chrystian, Chrystiana,
Chrystianah, Chrystiane,
Chrystiann, Chrystiannah,
Chrystianne, Chrystyan,

Chrystyana, Chrystyanah,
Chrystyane, Chrystyann,
Chrystyanna, Chrystyannah,
Chrystyanne, Khristian, Khristien,
Khristyn, Kristian, Kristiana,
Kristianah, Kristiane, Kristiann,
Kristianna, Kristiannah, Kristianne,
Kristien, Kriston, Kristyn

Christie (Latin) little Christian.
Christee, Christey, Christi, Christie,
Christy, Chrystee, Chrystey, Chrysti,
Chrystie, Chrysty, Khristee,
Khristey, Khristi, Khristie, Khristy,
Khrystee, Khrystey, Khrysti,
Khrystie, Khrysty

Christina/Christine (Greek/Latin)
little Christian.
Christain, Christaina, Christainah,
Christaine, Christayn, Christayna,
Christaynah, Christayne, Christan,
Christana, Christanah, Christane,
Christean, Christeana, Christeanah,
Christeane, Christeen, Christeena,
Christeenah, Christeene, Christein,
Christeina, Christeinah, Christeine,
Christia, Christian, Christiana
(Ger), Christianah, Christiane,
Christin, Christinah, Christine,
Christyn, Christyna, Christynah,
Christyne, Chrystyn, Chrystyna,
Chrystynah, Chrystyne, Cristabel,
Cristabela, Cristabelah, Cristabele,
Crisabell, Cristabella, Cristabellah,
Cristabelle, Cristain, Cristaina,
Cristainah, Cristaine, Cristan,
Cristana, Cristanah, Cristane,
Cristean, Cristeana, Cristeanah,
Cristeane, Cristeen, Cristeena,
Cristeenah, Cristeene, Cristein,
Cristeina, Cristeinah, Cristeine,
Cristen, Cristena, Cristenah,
Cristene, Cristin, Cristina,
Cristinah, Cristinah, Cristine,
Crystyn, Crystyna, Crystynah,
Crystyne, Khristean, Khristeana,
Khristeanah, Khristeane, Khristeen,

Khristeena, Khristeenah,
Khristeene, Khristein, Khristeina,
Khristeinah, Khristeine, Khristin,
Khristina, Khristinah, Khristine,
Khristyn, Khristyna, Khristynah,
Khristyne, Khrystyn, Khrystyna,
Khrystynah, Khrystyne, Krista,
Kristabel, Kristabela, Kristabelah,
Kristabele, Kristabell, Kristabella,
Kristabellah, Kristabelle, Kristain,
Kristaina, Kristainah, Kristaine,
Kristan, Kristana, Kristanah,
Kristane, Kristayn, Kristayna,
Kristaynah, Kiystayne, Kristeen,
Kristeena, Kristeenah, Kristeene,
Kristein, Kristeina, Kristeinah,
Kristeine, Kristin, Kristina,
Kristinah, Kriston, Kristyn,
Kristyna, Kristynah, Kristyne,
Kristynn, Kristynna, Kristynnah,
Kristynne, Krysta, Krystal, Krystan,
Krystana, Krystanah, Krystane,
Krystean, Krysteana, Krysteanah,
Krysteane, Krysteen, Krysteena,
Krysteenah, Krysteene, Krystein,
Krysteina, Krysteinah, Krysteine,
Krysten, Krystena, Krystenah,
Krystene, Krystenia, Krystenina,
Krystin, Krystina, Krystinah,
Krystine, Kryston, Krystyn,
Krystyna, Krystynah, Krystyne,
Krystynn, Krystynna, Krystynnah,
Krystynne

Christmas (English) born at
Christmas time.
Chrystmas

Christy (Greek) Christian. The short
form of names starting with
'Christ' e.g. Christine.
Christee, Christey, Christi, Christia,
Christie, Cristee, Cristey, Cristi,
Cristia, Cristie, Cristy, Crystee,
Crystey, Crysti, Crystia, Crystie,
Crysty, Khristee, Khristey, Khristi,
Khristie, Khristy, Khrystee,
Khrystey, Khrysti, Khrystie, Khrysty

C

Chrys (English/Greek) Christian. A form of names starting with 'Chris' e.g. Christine. The feminine form of Chris.
Chris, Chriss, Chryss, Cris, Criss, Cryss, Khris, Khriss, Khrys, Khryss, Kris, Kriss, Krys, Kryss

Chrysanthe (Greek) golden flower.
Chrisanth, Chrisantha, Chrisanthia, Chrisanthiah, Chrisanthya, Chrisanthyah, Chrysantha, Chrysanthia, Chrysanthiah, Chryzanta, Chryxzanta, Chryzante, Chryzanthia, Chryzanthiah, Chryzanthya, Chryzanthyah

Chryseis (Greek/Latin) golden; daughter of the gold.
Chryseys, Chryzanta (Pol), Chryzanthe

Chu (Chinese) pearl.

Chu (Native American) rattle-snake girl.
Chumanah, Chumanna, Chumannah

Chumani (Sioux) dew drop.
Chumanee

Chun (Burmese) the renewal of nature.

Ciana (Italian) God is gracious. A form of Jane. (Chin) China.
Cianah, Ciandra

Ciannait (Irish) ancient.
Cianait

Ciara (Irish) black.
Ciarah, Ciarra, Ciarrah, Ciera, Cierah, Cierra, Cierrah, Cyarah, Cyarra, Cyarrah, Cyera, Cyerah, Cyerra, Cyerrah

Cicely (Latin) unseeing.
Cicelea, Ciceleah, Cicelee, Cicelei, Ciceleigh, Ciceley, Ciceli, Cicelie, Siselea, Siseleah, Siselee, Siselei, Siseleigh, Siseli, Siselie, Sisely

Cien (Irish) ancient.
Cian, Ciana, Cianah, Ciena, Ciena, Cienah

Cinderella (French) little one from the ashes.
Cinderel, Cinderela, Cinderelah, Cinderele, Cinderellah, Cinderelle, Cynderel, Cynderela, Cynderelah, Cynderell, Cynderella, Cynderellah, Cynderelle, Sinderel, Sinderela, Sinderele, Sinderell, Sinderella, Sinderelle, Synderell, Synderella, Synderelle

Cindy (French) little ashes. The short form of Cinderella or Cynthia, moon.
Cindea, Cindeah, Cindee, Cindey, Cindi, Cindie, Cyndea, Cyndeah, Cyndee, Cyndey, Cyndi, Cyndie, Cyndy, Sindea, Sindeah, Sindee, Sindey, Sindi, Sindie, Sindy, Syndea, Syndeah, Syndee, Syndey, Syndi, Syndie, Syndy

Cinnamon (Old French) fragrant.
Cinamon, Cynamon, Cynnamon, Sinamon, Sinnamon, Synamon, Synnamon

Cinnia (Latin) curly-haired.
Cinia, Ciniah, Cinniah, Sinia, Siniah, Sinnia, Sinniah

Cipriana (Italian) lady from Cyprus.
Cipriann, Ciprianna, Ciprianne, Cyprian, Cypriana, Cyriane, Cyprienne

Cirilla (Greek) lordly.
Cirila, Cirilah, Cyrila, Cyrilla, Cyrille, Cyryll, Cyrylla, Cyrylle

C

Cissy (Latin/American/English) sister; unseeing. The short form of names starting with 'Ces' e.g. Cecilia.
Cissi, Cissie, Sissi, Sissie, Sissy

Claire/Clara/Clare (Latin) brilliant.
Chiara (Ital), Claara, Claarah, Claare, Claira, Clairah, Claire (Fren), Clar, Clarah, Clare, Claret, Clareta (Span), Claretah, Clarete, Clarett, Claretta, Clarettah, Clarette, Clarinda, Clarina, Clarinah, Clarine, Clarita (Span), Claritah, Clarite, Claryt, Claryta, Clarytah, Claryte, Clarytt, Clarytta, Claryttah, Clarytte, Klaara, Klaarah, Klaare, Klara (Ger), Klarah, Klaret, Klareta, Klaretah, Klarete, Klarett, Klaretta, Klarettah, Klarette, Sorcha (Scott)

Clarenza (Latin) famous one. The feminine form of Clarence, illustrious, shining and famous one.
Clarensia, Clarensiah, Clarensya, Clarensyah, Clarenzia, Clarenziah, Clarenzya, Clarenzyah

Clarest (French) most brilliant.
Claresta, Clarestah, Clarestar, Clarestarr

Claribell (Latin) bright; clear; beautiful.
Clarabel, Clarabela, Clarabelah, Clarabele, Clarabell, Clarabella, Clarabellah, Clarabelle, Claribel, Claribela, Claribelah, Claribele, Claribella, Claribellah, Claribelle, Clarobel, Clarobela, Clarolbelah, Clarobele, Clarobell, Clarobella, Clarobelle, Clarybel, Clarybela, Clarybelah, Clarybele, Clarybell, Clarybella, Clarybelle

Clarice (French) brilliant; bright; clear. The French form of Clara.
Clareace, Clarease, Clareece,

Clareese, Claric, Claris, Clarise, Clariss, Clarisse, Claryc, Claryce, Clarys, Claryse

Clarimond (Old French) light from the new world. (O/Ger) brilliant protector.
Clarimon, Clarimund, Clarymon, Clarymond, Clarymund

Clarinda (Latin/Teutonic) bright; wise. (Span) brilliant; beautiful.
Clairinda, Clairynda, Clarinda, Clarindah, Clarynda, Claryndah

Clarissa (Greek) bright; clear.
Claris, Clarisa, Clarisah, Clarise, Clariss, Clarissah, Clarisse, Clarys, Clarysa, Clarysah, Claryse, Claryss, Claryssa, Claryssah, Clarysse, Klarisa, Klarisah, Klarise, Klarissa, Klarissah, Klarisse, Klarysa, Klarysah, Klaryse, Klaryss, Klaryssah, Klarysse

Clarita (Spanish/Latin) clear; bright. A form of Clara, brilliant.
Clareata, Clareatah, Clareate, Clareeta, Clareetah, Clareete, Clareta, Claretah, Clarete, Claretta, Clarettah, Clarette, Clarita, Claritah, Clarite, Claritta, Claritte, Claryta, Clarytah, Claryte, Clarytta, Claryttah, Clarytte, Klareata, Klareatah, Klareate, Klareeta, Klareetah, Klareete, Klareta, Klaretah, Klarete, Klaretta, Klarettah, Klarette, Klarita, Klaritah, Klarite, Klaritta, Klaritte, Klaryta, Klarytah, Klaryte, Klarytta, Klaryttah, Klarytte

Claudette (French) little weak one. The feminine form of Claude.
Claudet, Claudeta, Claudetah, Claudete, Claudett, Claudetta, Claudettah, Clawdet, Clawdeta, Clawdetah, Clawdete, Clawdett, Clawdetta, Clawdettah, Clawdette

Claudia (French) weak. The feminine form of Claude.
Claud, Clauda, Claudah, Claude, Claudea, Claudee, Claudet, Claudeta, Claudete, Claudett, Claudetta, Claudettah, Claudette (Fren), Claudiah, Claudin, Claudina, Claudinah, Claudine (Fren), Clause (Fren), Claudyn, Claudyna, Claudynah, Claudyne, Klaudia, Klaudiah, Klaudja (Lith), Klaudya (Lith), Klaudyah

Cleantha (Greek) flower of glory.
Cliantha, Clyantha

Clematis (Greek) brushwood; vine. The name of a flower.
Clematisa, Clematise, Clematiss, Clematissa, Clematisse, Clematys, Clematysa, Clematyse, Clematyss, Clematyssa, Clematysse

Clementia (Latin) mild; gentle.
Clemence (Fren), Clemency (Eng), Clemente (Fren), Clementia, Clemntiah, Clementina (Ger), Clementinah, Clementine (Eng), Clemenza (Pol), Klemence, Klemency, Klemenina, Klemente, Klementia, Klementiah, Klementina, Klementinah, Klementine, Klementyna, Klementynah, Klementyne

Clementine (Greek) merciful.
Clemence, Clemency, Clementia, Clementiah, Clementina, Clementinah, Clementine, Clementyn, Clementyna, Clementynah, Clementyne, Clemenza, Klementin, Klementina, Klementinah, Klementine, Klementyn, Klementyna, Klementynah, Klementyne

Cleo (Greek) little fame.
Clea, Clio, Kleo, Klio

Cleone (Greek) famous.
Cleaona, Cleaonee, Cleoney, Cleoni, Cleonie, Cleony

Cleopatra (Greek) famous; her father's pride and joy.
Kleopatra

Cleta (Greek) famous.
Cletah

Cleva (Middle English) from the cliff. The feminine form of Cleve/Clive.
Clevah, Clevara, Clevarah

Clio (Greek) the proclaimer.
Cleo, Kleo, Klio

Clorinda (Persian) famous beauty.
Clorind, Clorynd, Clorynda

Clotilda (Teutonic) famous in the loud battle.
Chlotilda, Chlotilde, Clotilde, Klothida, Klothilde

Clove (Latin) nail; aromatic spice.

Clover (Old English) luck; the clover plant (finding a four leaf clover is believed to bring luck).
Claver (O/Eng), Clova, Clovar, Clovah

Clymene (Greek) famous.
Climen, Climena, Clymen, Clymena, Clymene

Coahoma (Choctaw) red panther.
Coahomah

Cocheta (Native American) foreigner.
Cochetah

Coco (Spanish) coconut.
Koko

Cody (Old English) cushion; pillow. (Ir/Gae) helpful.
Codea, Codee, Codey, Codi, Codie,

Kodea, Kodee, Kodey, Kodi, Kodie,
Kody

Colby (English) by the coal town;
dark-haired.
Colbea, Colbee, Colbey, Colbi,
Colbie

Colette (Greek/French) little
victorious army.
Colet, Coleta, Coletah, Colete,
Colett, Coletta, Colettah, Kolet,
Koleta, Koletah, Kolete, Kolett,
Koletta, Kolettah, Kolette

Colina (Irish) young child.
(Ir) peaceful dove.
(O/Eng) from the coal pool.
The femine form of Colin.
Colean, Coleana, Coleane, Coleen,
Coleena, Coleenah, Coleene,
Colinah, Coline, Colyn, Colyna,
Colynah, Colyne

Colleen (Irish) girl.
Colean, Coleana, Coleane, Coleen,
Coleena, Coleenah, Coleene,
Colinah, Colinah, Coline, Collean,
Colleana, Colleane, Colleen,
Colleena, Colleenah, Colleene,
Collinah, Collinah, Colline,
Collyn, Collyna, Collynah, Collyne,
Colyn, Colyna, Colynah, Colyne

Columba (Latin) dove.
Colina, Colinah, Coline, Colombe
(Fren), Coulumbe (Fren), Columbia,
Columbina, Columbinah,
Columbine, Columbyna,
Columbynah, Columbyne

Combara (Australian Aboriginal)
tomorrow.
Combarah

Comfort (Latin) one who brings
comfort or solace.
Comforta

Conception (Latin) the beginning.
Concepcion, Concepta, Concetta
(Ital), Conchita (Span)

Concha (Spanish) shell.
Conchata

Conchetta (Italian) purity.
Concettina

Conchita (Spanish) the beginning.
Chita, Concepta, Conceptia,
Concha, Concian, Conciana,
Concianah, Conciann, Concianna,
Conciannah, Concianne

Concordia (Latin) harmony; peace.
Concorda, Concrodah, Concordia,
Concordiah, Concordya,
Concordyah

Connie (Latin) constant; steadfast.
The short form of Constance.
Conee, Coney, Coni, Conie,
Connee, Conney, Conni, Conny,
Cony

Conradine (German) bold, wise
counsel. The feminine form of
Conrad.
Conradina, Conradyna, Conradyne

Consolata (Italian) consolation.

Constance (Latin) constant;
steadfast.
Congalie, Constancia (Span),
Constancy, Constanta, Constantina
(Eng), Constantine, Constanza,
Constanze (Ger), Custance,
Gostanza, Konstance, Konstancia
(Boh/Lith), Konstancja, Konstancy,
Konstancyna (Pol), Kotika (Rus),
Kotka (Rus)

Consuela (Spanish) consolation.
Consolata, Consuelo (Ital/Span)

Content (Latin) satisfaction.
Contenta

Coolalie (Australian Aboriginal) south wind.
Coolali, Coolalia, Coolaliah, Coolalya, Coolalyah

Cora (Greek) girl.
Corah, Kora, Korah

Corabelle (Greek/French) beautiful girl.
Corabel, Corabela, Corabelah, Corabele, Corabell, Corabella, Corabellah, Korabel, Korabela, Korabelah, Korabele, Korabell, Korabella, Korabellah

Coral (Latin) from the sea.
Coralea, Coraleah, Coralee, Coralei, Coraleigh, Coralia, Coraliah, Coralie (Fren), Coralin, Coralina, Coralinah, Coraline, Corel, Corela, Corelah, Corele, Corell, Corella, Corellah, Corelle, Coril, Corila, Corilah, Corile, Corill, Corilla, Corillah, Corille, Coryl, Coryla, Corylah, Coryle, Coryll, Corylla, Coryllah, Corylle

Coralee (Greek/English) girl from the meadow.
Coralea, Coraleah, Coralei, Coraleigh, Corali, Coralie, Coraly, Koralea, Koraleah, Koralei, Koraleigh, Korali, Koralie, Koraly

Corazon (Spanish) heart.
Corazona

Cordelia (Celtic) jewel from the sea.
Cordelie (Fren), Cordellia, Cordellya, Cordula, Cordulia, Kordel, Kordelia, Kordellia, Kordellya, Kordellyah, Kordelya, Kordelyah, Kordula (Ger)

Cordella (Latin) warm-hearted.
Cordel, Cordela, Cordelah, Cordele, Cordella, Cordellah, Cordelle

Coreita (Greek) girl.
Coreta, Coretah, Corettah

Corey (Irish) from the hollow.
Coree, Cori, Corie, Cory, Koree, Korey, Kori, Korie, Kory

Cori (Greek) girl.
Coree, Corey, Corie, Cory, Koree, Korey, Kori, Korie, Kory

Corina (Greek) girl.
Corean, Coreana, Coreanah, Coreane, Coreen, Coreena, Coreenah, Coreene, Corin, Corinah, Corinda, Corine, Corrin, Corrina, Corrinah, Corrine, Corrinn, Corrinna, Corrinnah, Corrinne, Correan, Correana, Correanah, Correane, Correen, Correena, Correenah, Correene, Corren, Correna, Correnah, Correne, Corryn, Corryna, Corrynah, Corryne, Coryn, Coryna, Corynah, Coryne

Corinne (French) from the hollow.
Corin, Corinn, Coryn, Corynn, Corynne

Corisande (Greek) girl.
Corysande

Corissa (Latin/Greek) girl.
Corisa, Corisah, Corissah, Corysa, Corysah, Coryssa, Coryssah

Corliss (Old English) cheerful.
Corlis, Corlisa, Corlisah, Corlise, Corlissa, Corlissah, Corlisse, Corlys, Corlysa, Corlysah, Corlyse, Corlyss, Corlyssa, Corlyssah, Corlysse

Cornelia (Latin) horn-coloured; horn blower; the cornell tree. A feminine form of Cornelius.
Cornelie (Fren), Cornella, Cornelle, Cornelya, Kornelia, Korneliah, Kornelya, Kornelyah

Corona (Latin) crowned.
Coronah, Coronna, Coronnah,

Korona, Koronah, Koronna,
Koronnah

Corra (Irish) from the mountain
valley.
Cora, Corah, Corrah, Kora, Korah,
Korra, Korrah

Corvina (Latin) raven.
Corvinah, Corvyna, Corvynah

Cory (Irish) head protection; helmet
used for battle. (Ir) from the
hollow.
Coree, Corey, Cori, Corie, Koree,
Korey, Kori, Korie, Kory

Cosette (Teutonic) lamb.
Coset, Coseta, Cosetah, Cosete,
Cosett, Cosetta, Cosettah

Cosima (Greek) universal harmony.
The feminine form of Cosmo.
Cosimah, Cosyma, Cosymah

Courtney (Old French) short-nosed.
(O/Eng) of the court.
Cortnae, Cortnai, Cortnay,
Cortnea, Cortnee, Cortney,
Cortneia, Cortni, Cortnie, Cortny,
Corttney, Courtena, Courtenay,
Courtene, Courtlin, Courtlina,
Courtlinah, Courtline, Courtlyn,
Courtlyna, Courtlynah, Courtlyne,
Courtlynn, Courtnae, Courtnai,
Courtnay, Courtnee, Courtnei,
Courtni, Courtnie, Courtny,
Courtoni, Courtonie, Courtony

Creola (French) home raised.
Creolah

Cressida (Greek) golden.
Cresida, Cressyda, Cresyda

Crisiant (Welsh) crystal.
Crisianta, Crisiante, Crysiant,
Crysianta, Crysiante, Crysyant

Crispina (Latin) curly-haired.
Crispin, Crispine, Crispyn,
Crispyna, Cryspyne

Crystal (Greek) gem; ice. (Lat) clear.
Christal, Chrystal, Chrystalina,
Chrystaline, Chrystel, Cristal,
Cristalie, Cristalina, Cristaline,
Cristalle, Cristel, Cristela, Cristelia,
Cristalina, Cristell, Cristella,
Cristelle, Crystal, Crystala, Crystale,
Crystell, Crystella, Crystelle, Krista,
Kristabel, Kristabele, Kristabell,
Kristabella, Kristabelle, Kristal,
Kristale, Kristall, Kristalle, Kristel,
Kristele, Kristell, Kristella, Kristelle,
Krystal (USA), Krystalbel,
Krystalbele, Krystalbell,
Krystalbella, Krystabelle, Krystel,
Krystele, Krystell, Krystella,
Krystelle, Krystelina, Krysteline,
Krystell, Krystella, Krystelle, Krystle
(USA), Krystyl, Krystyle, Krystyll,
Krystylle

Crystalin (Latin/Welsh) from the
crystal pool.
Christalin, Christalina, Christaline,
Chrystalin, Chrystalina,
Chrystaline, Cristalin, Cristalina,
Cristaline, Cristalyn, Cristalyna,
Cristalyne, Crystalina, Crystaline,
Crystalyn, Crystalyna, Crystalyne,
Khristalin, Khristalina, Khristaline,
Khrystalin, Khrystalina,
Khrystaline, Kristalin, Kristalina,
Kristaline, Kristalyn, Kristalyna,
Kristalyne, Krystalina, Krystaline,
Krystalyn, Krystalyna, Krystalyne

Curra (Australian Aboriginal) water
spring.
Currah

Cushla (Irish) dear.

Cuthberta (Old English) brilliant.
The feminine form of Cuthbert.
Cuthbertina, Cuthbirta,
Cuthbirtina, Cuthburga,
Cuthburta, Cuthburtine,
Cuthbyrta, Cuthbyrtina

Cveta (Slavic) flower.

Cybil (Greek) prophet. A form of Sybil.
Cebel, Cebela, Cebele, Cibel, Cibela, Cibele, Cibell, Cibella, Cibelle, Cybel, Cybela, Cybele, Cybell, Cybella, Cybelle, Cybyl, Cybyla, Cybyle, Cybyll, Cybylla, Cybylle

Cyma (Greek) flowering.
Cima, Cimah, Cymah

Cymbaline (Celtic) lord of the sea.
Cimbalina, Cymbalina

Cynara (Greek) artichoke; thistle.
Cinara, Cinarah, Cynarah, Sinara, Sinarah, Synara, Synarah

Cynthia (Greek) moon.
Cinthea, Cinthia, Cinthiah, Cinthya, Cinthyah, Cynthea, Cynthiah, Cynthya, Cynthyah, Sinthea, Sinthia, Sinthiah, Sinthya, Sinthyah, Synthea, Synthia, Synthiah, Synthya, Synthyah

Cypris (Greek) from the island of Cyprus.
Cipres, Cipress, Cypriana, Cypriane

Cyra (Persian) sun.
Cira, Cirah, Cyrah, Kira, Kirah, Kyra, Kyrah

Cyrena (Greek) alluring one; Siren.
Ciren, Cirena, Cirenah, Cirene, Cyren, Cyrenah, Cyrene, Cyrenia, Cyreniah, Siren, Sirena, Sirenah, Sirene, Syren, Syrena, Syrenah, Syrenia, Syreniah, Syrenya, Syrenyah

Cyria (Greek) lordly ruler. The feminine form of Cyril.
Ciria, Ciriah, Cyriah, Cyrya, Cyryah, Siria, Siriah, Syria, Syriah, Syrya, Syryah

Cyriaca (Greek) child born on a Sunday.
Ciriaca, Ciriacah, Cyriacah

Cyrilla (Latin) lordly ruler. The feminine form of Cyril.
Cerella, Cirilla, Cirylla, Cyrella, Cyrelle

Cytherea (Greek) from the island of Cythera.
Citherea, Sitherea, Sytherea

Czenzi (Hungarian) to increase.
Czenzee, Czenzey, Czenzie, Czenzy

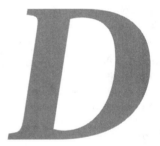

Dacia (Greek) pure white; glowing.
Dacea, Dacee, Dacey, Daciah, Dacie, Dacy, Dacya, Dacyah

Dae (English) born during the day.
Dai, Daia, Daiah, Day, Daya, Dayah

Daffodil (French) (Botanical) the daffodil flower.

Dagmar (German) glorious.
Dagmara, Dagmarah, Dagmaria, Dagmariah, Dagmarya, Dagmaryah

Dagny (Scandinavian) day.
Dagna, Dagnah, Dagnana, Dagnia, Dagniah, Dagnanna, Dagne, Dagnee, Dagney, Dalia, Daliah (Heb), Dalialah, Daliyah

Dahila (Scandinavian) from the valley.
Dahiliah, Dahyla, Dahylah

Dahlia (English) (Botanical) the dahlia flower.
Dahliah, Dahlya, Dahlyah

Dai (Japanese) great. (Eng) day.
Dae, Daija, Daijon, Day, Daye

Daila (Latvian) beautiful.
Daela, Daelah, Dailah, Dayla, Daylah

Daisy (English) (Botanical) the day's eye; yellow or white flower.
Daisee, Daisey, Daisi, Daisia, Daisie, Dasee, Dasey, Dasi, Dasie, Dasy, Daysee, Daysey, Daysi, Daysia, Daysie, Daysy

Daiya (Polish) gift.
Daia, Daiah, Daiyah, Daya, Dayah

Dakota (Sioux) friend.
Dakotah, Dakotha, Dekoda, Dekodah, Dekota, Dekotah, Dekotha, Takota, Takotah

Dale (English) from the valley.
Dael, Daela, Dahli, Dahlia, Dahlie, Dail, Daila, Daile, Dalelean, Daleleana, Dalena, Dalenah, Dalene (Ger), Dalina, Dalinah, Daline, Dalyn, Dalyna, Dalyne, Dayl, Dayla, Dayle

Dalit (Hebrew) flowing water.
Dalyt

Dallas (Irish) wisdom. (Geographical) city in Texas.
Dalishia, Dalishya, Dalisia, Dalissia, Dalissiah, Dallys, Dalyss, Dalyssa, Dalysse, Dalyce, Dalys, Dalyss, Dalyssa, Dalysse

Dalya (Hebrew) tree branch.
Dalia, Daliah, Dalyah

Dama (Latin) gentle; noble.
Damah, Damara, Damaris, Dame, Damita, Damitah, Damyta, Damytah

Damaris (Greek) gentle.
Damara, Damara, Damarius, Damary, Damarys, Damaryss, Damaryssa, Dameress, Dameressa, Dameris, Damiris, Dammaris, Dammeris, Damris, Damriss, Damrissa, Damarys, Damarysa, Damaryss, Damaryssa, Damarysse, Demara, Demaras, Demaris, Demariss, Demarissa, Demarys, Demarysa, Demarysah, Demaryse, Demaryss, Demaryssa, Demaryssah, Demarysse

Damia (Greek) goddess of the forces of nature.
Damiah, Damya, Damiah, Damya, Damyah

Damiana (Greek) tamed. The feminine form of Damian.
Damianah, Damiane, Damianna, Damiannah, Damiannae, Damyana, Damyanah, Damyann, Damyanna, Damyannah, Damyanne

Damica (French) friendly.
Dameeca, Dameecah, Dameeka, Dameka, Damekah, Damicah, Damicka, Damika, Damikah, Demeeca, Demeecah, Demeeka, Demica, Demicah, Demicka, Demika, Demikah, Demyca, Demycah, Demycka, Demyka, Demykah

Damita (Spanish) noble.
Dameesha, Dameeta, Dameetah, Damesia, Damesiah, Dametia, Dametiah, Dametra, Dametrah, Damyta, Damytah

D

Damzel (Old Devon) plum.
Damzela, Damzele, Damzell,
Damzella, Damzellah, Damzelle

Dana (English) bright day; from
Denmark. (Ir) fire.
Daena, Daenah, Daina, Dainah,
Danae (Grk), Danah, Danala,
Danale, Danalee, Danarra, Danean,
Daneana, Dania, Daniah, Danja,
Danjah, Danna, Dayna, Daynah

Danessa (Hebrew/French/Greek)
God is my judge; butterfly. A
form of Vanessa.
Danesa, Danesah, Danessah,
Danisa, Danisah, Danissa,
Danissah, Danissia, Danissiah,
Danysa, Danysah, Danyssa,
Danyssya

Daniah (Hebrew) God is my judge.
Dania, Danya, Danyah

Danica (Slavic) morning star.
Daneeca, Daneecah, Daneeka,
Daneekah, Danikah, Danikia,
Danikiah, Daniqua, Daniquah,
Danique, Danyca, Danycah,
Danycka, Danyka, Danykah,
Danyqua, Danyquah, Danyque

Danice (Hebrew) God is my
gracious judge; combination of
Danielle/Janice.
Dania, Daniah, Danica, Danicah,
Danice, Danis, Danisa, Danisah,
Danise, Daniss, Danissa, Danissah,
Danisse, Danyce, Danys, Danysa,
Danysah, Danyse

Danielle (Hebrew) God is my judge.
A feminine form of Daniel.
Danae (Grk), Danal (Austl),
Daneen, Daneena, Daneil (Heb),
Daneille, Danial, Danialla,
Danialle, Danica (Slav), Danielan,
Daniele, Danielka, Daniell,
Daniella, Daniellah, Danika,

Danikah, Danille, Danit (Heb),
Danniele, Danniella, Dannielle
(Austr), Danyela, Danyele,
Danyella, Danyelle, Doniel,
Doniela, Doniele, Doniell,
Doniella, Donielle, Donniel,
Donniela, Donniele, Donniell,
Donniella, Donnielle, Donnyel,
Donnyela, Donnyele, Donnyell,
Donnyella, Donnyelle, Donyel,
Donyela, Donyela, Donyelah,
Donyele, Donyell, Donyella,
Donyellah, Donyelle

Danna (Hebrew) God is my judge.
Danah, Dannah

Dannal (Hebrew) God is my judge.
A form of Danielle.
Danal, Danala, Danalah, Dannala,
Dannalah

Dani (Hebrew) God is my judge. A
short form of Danielle.
Danee, Daney, Danie, Dannee,
Danney, Danni, Dannie, Dannii,
Danniie, Danny, Dany

Daphne (Greek/Botanical) plant
with bell-shaped flowers.
Dafnee, Dafney, Dafni, Dafnie,
Dafny, Daphnee, Daphney,
Daphni, Daphnie, Daphny

Dara (Hebrew) compassionate.
Dahra, Dahrah, Darah, Darka,
Daralea, Daralee, Daraleigh,
Daraley, Darda, Dardah, Darice,
Darilyn, Darilyna, Darisa, Darissa,
Darra, Darrah

Darah (African American/Greek)
wealthy princess. A combination
of Daria/Sarah.
Dara

Daralis (Old English) beloved.
Daralisa, Daralisah, Daralise,
Daralysa, Daralyse

Darby (Irish) freedom; (Scand) from the estate by the deer.
Darbea, Darbee, Darbi, Darbia, Darbiah, Darbie

Darcelle (French) she is from the fortress; she has dark hair/complexion.
Darcee, Darcel, Darcela, Darcelah, Darcele, Darcell, Darcella, Darcellah

Darcy (Irish) dark-haired/complexioned one. (Fren) fortress.
Darcea, Darcee, Darci, Darcia, Darciah, Darcie, Darsea, Darsee, Darsey, Darsi, Darsie, Darsy

Daria (Greek) wealthy. The feminine form of Darius, ruler.
Dariah, Darian, Dariana, Dariane, Dariann, Darianna, Darianne, Darria, Darriah, Darrya, Darryah, Darya, Daryah

Darice (Persian) queen.
Dareece, Darees, Daricia, Dariciah, Daryca, Darycah, Darycia, Darys, Darysa, Darysah, Darysia, Darysiah, Darysya, Darysyah

Darielle (French/Greek) she is a gift.
Dariel, Dariela, Darielah, Dariele, Dariella, Dariellah, Daryel, Daryela, Daryelah, Daryele, Daryell, Daryella, Daryellah, Daryelle

Darilyn (Old English) little darling one from the pool.
Daralin, Daralina, Daralinah, Daraline, Daralyna, Daralyne, Darileana, Darileanah, Darileen, Darileena, Darileenah, Darilin, Darilina, Darilinah, Darline, Darilyn, Darilyna, Darilynah, Darilyne, Darylin, Darylina, Darylinah, Daryline, Darylyn, Darylyna, Darylynah, Darylyne

Darla (English) little darling.
Darlah

Darlene (French) little darling.
Darilean, Darileana, Darileanah, Darileane, Darileen, Darileena, Darileenah, Darileene, Darleen, Darleena, Darleenah, Darleene, Darlen, Darlena, Darlenah, Darlenee, Darlin, Darlina, Darlinah, Darline, Darlyn, Darlyna, Darlynah, Darlyne

Darnelle (Irish/French) she is darling.
Darnel, Darnela, Darnelah, Darnele, Darnell, Darnella, Darnellah, Darnetta, Darnette, Darnice, Darnise, Darnita, Darnyel, Darnyela, Darnyelah, Darnyell, Darnyella, Darnyelle

Daron (Irish) great.
Daronica, Daronicah, Daronicka, Daronickah, Daronik, Daronika, Daronikah, Daroniqua, Daroniquah, Daronique, Daronyca, Daronycah, Daronycka, Daronyckah, Daronyka, Daronykah, Daronyqua, Daronyquah

Darrelyn (English) beloved from the pool; combination of Darryl/Lyn.
Darelin, Darylin, Darylyn

Daru (Hindi) pine tree.
Darua, Darue, Daroo

Daryl (French) little darling from the oak tree grave; gift. The feminine form of Darryl.
Darel, Darela, Darelah, Darell, Darella, Darellah, Darelle, Daril, Darila, Darile, Darill, Darilla, Darillah, Darille, Darril, Darrila,

Daryl cont.
Darrilah, Darrile, Darrill, Darrill,
Darrilla, Darrille, Darryl, Darryla,
Darryle, Darryll, Darrylla, Darrylle,
Daryl, Daryla, Darylah, Daryle,
Daryll, Darylla, Daryllah, Darylle

Daryn (Greek) gift. The feminine
form of Darren.
Darin, Darina, Darinah, Daron,
Darona, Daronah, Daryn, Daryna,
Darynah

Dasha (Russian) gift of God.
Darsha, Darshah, Dash, Dashah

Dashawna (Irish/African American)
God is gracious. The feminine
form of Shawn.
Dasean, Daseana, Daseanah,
Dashaughn, Dashaugna,
Dashaughnah, Dashaun,
Dashauna, Dashaunah, Dashawn,
Dashawnah, Daiseana, Daiseanah,
Daishaughna, Daishaughnah,
Daishaun, Daishauna,
Daishaunah, Daishawn,
Daishawna, Daishawnah,
Daishawn, Daishawna,
Daishawnah, Daysean, Dayseana,
Dayseanha, Dayshaughna,
Dayshaughnah, Dayshaun,
Dayshauna, Dayshawn, Dayshawna

Dashiki (Swahili) African skirt.
Dashi, Dashia, Dashika, Dashka,
Desheka, Deshiki

Davalinda (Hebrew/Spanish) pretty
beloved.
Davalindah, Davalinde, Davelinda,
Davelynda, Davilinda, Davilynda,
Davylinda, Davylindah, Davyllynda

Davida/Davita (Hebrew) beloved.
The feminine form of David.
Daveda, Daveen, Davene, Davina,
Davinna, Davita, Devina, Devinna,
Veda, Vida, Vidah, Vyda, Vydah

Davonna (Scottish/English/Hebrew)
beloved.
Davon, Davona, Davonah,
Davonda, Davondah, Davonnah

Dawatha (Swahili) the last born
one.
Dawath, Dawathah

Dawn (English) sunrise.
Dawana, Dawanah, Dawandra,
Dawandrea, Dawanna, Dawannah,
Dawin, Dawina, Dawna, Dawnah,
Dawne, Dawnee, Dawnell,
Dawnella, Dawnelle, Dawnet,
Dawneta, Dawnete, Dawnett,
Dawnetta, Dawnette, Dawnisha,
Dawnishia, Dawnlin, Dawnlina,
Dawnline, Dawnlyna, Dawnlyne,
Dawnn, Dawnna, Dawnnah,
Dawnrae, Dawnyell, Dawnyella,
Dawnyelle

Daya (Hebrew) bird. (Sans) one
with compassion.
Daea, Daeah, Daia, Daiah, Dayah

Dayna (English) bright day.
Daena, Daenah, Daina, Dainah,
Dana, Danah, Daynah

Dea (Latin) goddess.
Deah, Deana, Deanah, Deane,
Deann, Deanna, Deannah, Deanne

Deana (Latin) divine. (Eng) one
who lives in the valley. The
feminine form of Dean.
Deanah, Deaniel, Deaniela,
Deanielah, Deaniele, Deaniell,
Deaniella, Deaniellah, Deanielle,
Deanisha, Deanna, Deannah,
Deena, Deenah, Deenna, Deennah,
Dina, Dinah, Dinna, Dinnah,
Dyna, Dynah, Dynna, Dynnah

Deandra (French/Greek) strong, brave, courageous one from the valley. The feminine combination of Dean/Andre. (Lat) divine.
Deandrah, Deandre, Deandria, Deandriah, Deandrya, Deandryah

Deanna (Latin/Hebrew) divine; gracious. (Eng) one who lives in the valley. The feminine form of Dean.
Deahana, Deahanah, Deahanna, Deahannah, Deahanne, Deana, Deanah, Deannah

Debbie (Hebrew) bee. The short form of Deborah.
Debbea, Debbee, Debbey, Debbi, Debbie, Debby, Debea, Debee, Debey, Debi, Debie, Deby

Deborah/Debra (Hebrew) bee.
Debbora, Debborah, Debbera, Debberah, Debbora, Debborah, Debbra, Debbrah, Debera, Deberah, Debora, Debra (Austr/Amer), Debrah

Dede (African) first-born daughter.

Dedra (Irish) sorrowful wanderer. A form of Deirdre.
Deadra, Deadrah, Deedra, Deedrah, Deedri, Deedrie, Dedrah

Dee-Dee (Hebrew) cherished. A short form of names starting with 'De' e.g. Deirdre.

Degula (Hebrew) excellent.
Degulah

Deianeira (Greek) the wife of Hercules.
Daeanaira, Daeanirah, Daeianeira, Daeianeirah, Daianaira, Daianairah, Dayanaira, Dayanairah, Deianaira, Deianairah, Deianeirah

Deirdre (Irish) sorrowful wanderer.
Dedra, Dedrah, Deerdra, Deerdrah, Deerdre, Deidra, Deidrah, Deirdree, Didi, Dierdra, Dierdre, Dierdrie, Dyerdre, Dydree, Dydri, Dydrie, Dydry

Deita (Greek) covering the earth. A form of Demetria, goddess of fertility.
Deatra, Deatrah, Deetra, Deetrah, Deitra, Deitrah, Deytra, Deytrah

Deja (French) before
Daija, Daisia, Daja, Dasha, Deejai, Dejanel, Dejanela, Dejanelah, Dejanele, Dejanell, Dejanella, Dejanellah, Dejanelle, Dejay, Dejaya, Dejon

Deka (Somalian) pleasing.
Dekah

Delana (German) noble protector.
Dalana, Dalanah, Dalanna, Dalannah, Dalaina, Dalainah, Dalaine, Dalayna, Dalaynah, Daleena, Dalena, Dalenah, Dalenna, Dalennah, Dalina, Dalinah, Dalinda, Dalinna, Dalena, Dalenah, Dalenna, Delana, Delanah, Delanna, Delannah, Delaina, Delainah, Delayna, Delaynah

Delany (Irish) the challenger's descendant.
Dalanee, Dalaney, Dalania, Dalena, Dalene, Dalaney, Delainee, Delainey, Delana, Delanee, Delaney, Delani, Delanie, Dellanee, Dellaney, Dellani, Dellanie, Dellany

Deleena (French) little darling.
Deleana, Deleanah, Deleane, Deleenah, Deleene, Deleina, Deleinah, Deleine, Deleyna, Deleynah, Deleyne, Delina, Delinah, Deline, Delyna, Delynah, Delyne

D

Delia (Greek) visible.
Dehlia, Delea, Deleah, Delinda, Delina, Deline, Dellia, Delliah, Dellya, Dellyah, Delya, Delyah

Delicia (English) delightful.
Delesha, Delica, Delice, Delight, Delighta, Delisa, Delisah, Delise, Dellisha, Delisia, Delisiah, Deliz, Deliza, Delizah, Delize, Delizia, Delya, Delys, Delyse, Delysia, Delysia, Delysya, Delysyah

Delija (Polish) sea daughter.
Delijah

Delilah (Hebrew) one who broods.
Dalia, Daliah, Dalialah, Dalila, Dalilah, Delila, Delilla, Delyla, Delylla

Delma (Spanish) from the sea.
(Ger) noble protector.
Delmah, Delmar, Delmara, Delmarah, Delmare, Delmaria, Delmariah, Delmarya, Delmaryah

Delores (Spanish) sorrowful.
Delora, Delorah, Delore, Deloree, Delorey, Deloria, Deloriah, Delories, Deloris, Deloriss, Delorissa, Deloriessah, Delorisse, Delorita, Deloritta, Deloritte, Delorys, Deloryse, Deloryss, Deloryta, Delorytta, Deloryttah

Delpha (Greek) dolphin.
Delfi, Delfie, Delfin, Delfina, Delfine, Delfyn, Delfyna, Delfynah, Delfyne, Delphi, Delphina, Delphinah, Delphine, Delphinie, Delphinium, Delphy, Delphyna, Delphynah, Delphyne

Delphine (Greek) from Delphi.
Delfina, Delfinah, Delfine, Delfyna, Delfynah, Delfyne, Delpha, Delphe, Delphi, Delphia, Delphiah, Delphie, Delphina, Delphinia, Delphiniah, Delvina,

Delvinah, Delvine, Delvinia, Delviniah, Delvyna, Delvynah, Delvyne, Delvynia, Delvyniah, Delvynya, Delvynyah

Delsie (English/Spanish) sorrow.
Delcea, Delcee, Delsea, Delsee, Delsi, Delsia, Delsy

Delta (Greek) fourth-born daughter.
Deltah, Deltar, Deltara, Deltarah, Deltare, Deltaria, Deltariah, Deltarya, Delatyah

Delwyn (Welsh) attractive, blessed friend.
Delwin, Delwyn

Delyth (Welsh) attractive; neat.
Delith, Delitha, Delithah, Delytha, Delythia, Delythiah, Delythya, Delythyah

Demelda (Greek) to proclaim.
Demeldah, Demelde, Demilda, Demildah, Demilde, Demylda, Demyldah, Demylde

Demetria (Greek) covering of earth; of Demeter, goddess of fertility.
Deitra, Demeetra, Demeetrah, Demetra, Demetrah, Demetrice, Demetris, Demetrish, Demetrius, Demita, Demitah, Demitra, Demitrah, Dymeetra, Dymeetrah, Dymetra, Dymetrah, Dymitria, Dymitriah, Dymytria, Dymytriah, Dymytrya, Dymytryah

Demi (Greek) covering of earth; of Demeter, goddess of fertility. The short form of Demetria.
Demee, Demey, Demie, Demmee, Demmey, Demmi, Demmie, Demmy, Demy

Dena (Native American) valley.
Deana, Deanah, Deena, Deenah, Denae, Denah, Deney, Dina, Dinah, Dyna, Dynah

Denae (Hebrew) innocent.
Denai, Denay

Deni (French/Australian) follower
of Dionysus, the god of wine;
celebration. A short form of
Denise. The feminine form of
Dennis.
Denee, Deney, Denie, Dennee,
Denney, Denni, Dennie, Denny,
Deny

Denise (French) follower of
Dionysus, the god of wine;
celebration. The feminine form of
Dennis.
Danice, Danise, Denece, Denese,
Denica, Denicah, Denice, Deniece,
Deniese, Denisha, Denishia,
Deniss, Denissa, Denisse, Dennyce,
Dennyse, Denys, Denyse, Denyss,
Dineece, Dineese, Dinice, Dinise,
Dinyce, Dinyse, Dynice, Dynise,
Dynyce, Dynyse

Denna (Anglo Saxon) from the
valley.
Deana, Deanah, Deanna,
Deannah, Dena, Dene, Dennah,
Deene, Dina, Dinah, Dinna,
Dinnah, Dyna, Dynah, Dynna,
Dynnah

Deodata (Greek) God has given.
Deodatah

Derede (Greek) gift of God.
Dered

Derika (German) gifted ruler of the
people. The feminine form of
Derek.
Dereka, Derekah, Derekia,
Derekiah, Derekya, Derekyah,
Derica, Dericah, Dericka, Derikah,
Deriqua, Deriquah, Derique,
Derrica, Derricah, Derricka,
Derrika, Derrikah, Derriqua,
Derryca, Derycah, Derycka, Deryka,
Deryqua, Deryquah, Deryque

Derora (Hebrew) stream.
Derorah, Derore

Derry (Irish) red-haired one.
Deree, Derey, Deri, Derie, Derree,
Derrey, Derri, Derrie, Dery

Deryn (Welsh) bird.
Deran, Derana, Deranah, Derane,
Deren, Derena, Derenah, Derene,
Derin, Derina, Derinah, Derine,
Deron, Derona, Deronah, Derone,
Derran, Derrana, Derranah,
Derrane, Derrin, Derrina, Derrinah,
Derrine, Derryn, Derryna,
Derrynah, Derryne, Deryna,
Derynah, Deryne

Desi (French) desired. A short form
of Desiree.
Desea, Desee, Desey, Desie, Desir,
Desira, Desirah, Desy

Desire/Desiree (French) desired.
Desara, Desarah, Desarae, Desaral,
Desarai, Desaray, Desare, Desarea,
Desaree, Desarey, Desaria, Desarie,
Desary, Deserae, Deserah, Deserai,
Deseraia, Deseraie, Desere,
Deseree, Deserey, Deseri, Deseria,
Deserie, Deserrae, Desserrai,
Deserray, Desira, Desirah, Desirai,
Desirae, Desirea, Desirey, Desiri,
Desrai, Desray, Dessirae, Dessire,
Dessiree, Desyrae, Desyrai, Desyray,
Dezarae, Dezerai, Dezeray, Dezere,
Dezerea, Dezeree, Dezerie, Dezirae,
Deziree, Dezorae, Dezorai,
Dezoray, Dezrae, Dezrai, Dezray,
Dezzirae, Dezzrae, Dezzrai,
Dezzray

Dessa (Greek) wandering.
Desa, Desah, Dessah

Destiny (French) fate.
Desnina, Desnine, Desta, Destah,
Destanee, Destaney, Destani,
Destania, Destanie, Destannee,
Destanney, Destanni, Destannia,

Destiny cont.
Destannie, Destanny, Destany,
Destenee, Desteney, Desteni,
Destenia, Destenie, Desteny,
Destinee, Destiney, Destini,
Destinia, Destiniah, Destinie,
Destinnee, Destinnia, Destinnie,
Destinny, Destyni, Destynia,
Destyniah, Destynya, Destynyah

Deva (Hindi) divine; goddess of the moon.
Deava, Deavah, Deeva, Deevah,
Devah, Diva, Divah, Dyva, Dyvah

Deveney (Irish) poet. (Scott) loved. The feminine form of Devon.
Devan, Devana, Devane, Devania,
Devanie, Devany, Deven, Devena,
Devene (Scott), Devenja, Devenje,
Deveny, Deveyn, Deveyna,
Deveyne, Devina, Devine, Devinna,
Devinne, Devon, Devyn, Devyna,
Devyne, Devynee, Devyney,
Devyni, Devynia, Devyniah,
Devyny, Devynya, Devynyah

Devi (Hindi) goddess of power and destruction.
Devee, Devey, Devie, Devy

Devon (Irish) poet. (Lat) perfection. (O/Eng) feminine form of Devon, from Devonshire; people of the deep valley.
Devona, Devonah, Devonn,
Devonna, Devonnah, Divona,
Divonah, Divonna, Divonnah,
Dyvona, Dyvonah, Dyvonna,
Dyvonnah

Devora (Hebrew) speaking kindly.
Devorah, Divona, Divonah,
Dyvon, Dyvonah, Dyvora, Dyvorah

Dextra (Latin) dexterous; skilful, right-handed.
Dextrah

Dezba (Navajo) war.
Dezbah

Dhara (Hindi) from the earth.
Dharah

Di (Latin) divine; short form of names starting with 'Di' e.g. Diana.
Dy

Diamond (Greek/English) diamond; precious.
Diamonda, Diamondah,
Diamonde, Dimantra (Fren),
Dimond, Dimonda, Dimondah,
Dimonde, Dyamond, Dyamonda,
Dyamondah, Dyamonde,
Dymond, Dymonda, Dymondah,
Dymonde, Dymont, Dymonte

Diana/Diane (Latin) goddess of the hunt, the moon, fertility. (Eng) divine; graceful.
Dalana, Dalanna, Dayana,
Dayanna, Diaan, Diaana, Diaanah,
Diaane, Dianah, Dianalyn,
Dianalyna, Dianalyne, Dianarose,
Dianatris, Dianca, Diandra, Diane,
Dianelis, Diania, Dianiah,
Dianiella, Dianielle, Dianita,
Dianna, Diannah, Dianne, Dianya,
Dianyah, Dihan, Dihana, Dihanah,
Dihane, Dihann, Dihanna,
Dihanne, Dyaan, Dyaana,
Dyaanah, Dyaane, Dyan, Dyana,
Dyanah, Dyhan, Dyhana,
Dyhanah, Dyhane, Dyhann,
Dyhanna, Dyhannah, Dyhanne

Diantha (Greek) divine flower.
Diandra, Diandre, Dianthah,
Dianthe, Dyantha, Dyanthah,
Dyanthe, Dyanthia, Dyanthiah,
Dyanthya, Dyanthyah

Didi (Hebrew) beloved.
Dydy

Dido (Greek) teacher.
Dydo

Dillian (Latin) object of love and devotion.
Dilliana, Dillianna, Dilliannah, Dilliane, Dillianne, Dylian, Dyliana, Dylianah, Dyliane, Dyllian, Dylliana, Dylliane, Dylliann, Dyllianna, Dylliannah, Dyllianne, Dylyan, Dylyana, Dylyanah, Dylyane, Dylyann, Dylyanna, Dylyannah, Dylyannah, Dylyanne

Dilys (Welsh) truth.
Dilis, Dilisa, Dilisah, Dillis, Dillisa, Dillisah, Dillys, Dillysa, Dillysah, Dilys, Dilysa, Dilysah, Dyllys, Dyllysa, Dyllysah, Dylys, Dylysa, Dylysah

Dima (Hebrew) raining.
Dimah, Dyma, Dymah

Dinah (Hebrew) freedom.
Deana, Deanah, Deena, Deenah, Dina, Dyna, Dynah

Dinka (Swahili) people.
Dinkah, Dynka, Dynkah

Dione (Greek) daughter of heaven and earth; mother of Aphrodite, the goddess of love.
Dion, Diona, Dionah, Dionee, Dioney, Dioni, Dionie, Diony, Dyon, Dyona, Dyonah, Dyone, Dyonee, Dyoney, Dyoni, Dyonie, Dyony

Dior (French) golden.
Diora, Diorah, Diore, Diorra, Diorrah, Diorre, Dyor, Dyora, Dyorah, Dyorra, Dyorrah, Dyorre

Dita (Slavic) wealthy gift.
Ditah, Dyta, Dytah

Ditzah (Israeli) coy.
Ditza, Diza, Dytza, Dytzah

Divinia (Latin) divine. (Ir) ox.
Deveena, Devina, Devinah, Devinia, Deviniah, Diveena, Divina, Divinah, Diviniah, Dyveena, Dyvina, Dyvinah, Dyvinia, Dyviniah, Dyvyna, Dyvynah, Dyvynia, Dyvyniah, Dyvynya

Divya (Hindi) heavenly; divine.
Divia, Diviah, Dyvia, Dyviah, Dyvya, Dyvyah

Dixie (French) tenth-born child. (Eng) wall.
Dixee, Dixey, Dixi, Dixy, Dyxee, Dyxey, Dyxi, Dyxie, Dyxy

Diza (Hebrew) joy.
Ditza, Ditzah, Diza, Dizah, Dyza, Dyzah

Doanne (Irish) poem. (O/Eng) from down the hill. (Eng/Heb) graceful doe.
Doan, Doana, Doanah, Doann, Doanna, Doannah, Doanne, Doean, Doeana, Doeanah, Doeane, Doeann, Doeanna, Doeannah, Doeanne.

Docila (Latin) gentle.
Docilah, Docile, Docilla, Docillah, Docille, Docyl, Docyla, Docylah, Docyle, Docyll, Docylla, Docyllah, Docylle

Doda (Hebrew) friend; aunt.
Dodah, Dodee, Dodey, Dodi, Dodie, Dody

Dodie (Hebrew) beloved. A short form of Dorothy, gift.
Doda, Dodah, Dode, Dodea, Dodee, Dodi, Dodia, Dodiah, Dody, Dodya, Dodyah

Doli (Navajo) blue bird.
Dolee, Doley, Dolie, Doly

Dolly (English) beautiful; doll-like.
Dolea, Doleah, Dolee, Dolei, Doleigh, Doley, Doli, Dolia,

Dolly cont.
Doliah, Dolie, Dollea, Dolleah, Dollee, Dollei, Dolleigh, Dolley, Dolli, Dollie, Doly

Dolores (Spanish) sorrowful.
Delores

Dolphina (English/Latin) dolphin.
Dolphina, Dolphinah, Dolphine, Dolphyn, Dolphyna, Dolphynah, Dolphyne

Domencia (Italian) born on a Sunday.
Domenca, Domenciah, Domencya, Domencyah

Domina (Latin) noble birth.
Dominah, Domyna, Domynah

Dominica (Latin) of the Lord. A feminine form of Dominic.
Domeneka, Domenica, Domenicah, Domenicka, Domenika, Domeniqua, Domeniquah, Domenique, Dominica, Dominicah, Dominicka, Dominika, Dominga, Domini, Dominia, Dominiah, Dominiqua, Dominquah, Dominique, Dominixa, Dominixe, Domino, Dominyika, Domka, Domnica, Domnicah, Domnicka, Domnika, Domoniqua, Domoniquah, Domonique

Domino (English/Latin) of the Lord. A feminine form of Dominic.
Domina, Domyna, Domyno

Donata (Latin) gift.
Donatha, Donathia, Donathiah, Donathya, Donathyah, Donatta

Donna (Italian) lady.
Dona, Donah, Donnah, Donnae, Donnai, Donnay, Donnaya, Donnica, Donnicka, Donnika,

Donnike, Donnisa, Donnise, Donniss, Donnissa, Donnisse, Donnita, Donnite, Donnyta, Donnytta, Donnytte, Dontia, Dontiah, Dontya, Dontyah

Dora (Greek) gift.
Dorah, Doralia, Doraliah, Doralie, Doralisa, Doralise, Doralin, Doralina, Doraline, Doralyn, Doralyna, Doralynah, Doralyne, Doran, Dorana, Doranah, Dorchen, Dorece, Doree, Doreece, Doreen, Doreena, Doreese, Doressa, Doresse, Doretta, Dorette, Dorika, Dorinda, Dorita, Doritah, Doritta, Doritte, Dorytt, Dorytta, Dorytte

Dorabella (Greek) beautiful gift.
Dorabel, Dorabela, Dorabelah, Dorabele, Dorabell, Dorabellah, Dorabelle

Dore (French) golden.
Dorea, Doreah, Doree, Dorey, Dori, Doria, Doriah, Dorie, Dory, Dorya, Doryah, Dorye

Doreen (Irish) moody. (Fren) golden.
Dorean, Doreana, Doreanah, Doreane, Doreena, Doreenah, Doreene, Dorena, Dorenah, Dorene, Dorin, Dorina, Dorinah, Dorinda, Dorine, Doryn, Doryna, Dorynah, Dorynda, Doryne

Dorena (French) golden girl.
Dorean, Doreana, Doreanah, Doreane, Doreen, Doreena, Doreenah, Doreene, Dorenah, Dorene, Dorin, Dorina, Dorinah, Dorinda, Dorine, Doryn, Doryna, Dorynah, Dorynda, Doryne

Doretta (Greek) little gift.
Doret, Doreta, Doretah, Dorete, Doretha, Dorett, Dorettah, Dorette, Dorit, Dorita, Doritah, Dorite,

Doritt, Doritta, Dorittah, Doritte,
Doryt, Doryta, Dorytah, Doryte,
Dorytt, Dorytta, Doryttah, Dorytte

Doria (Greek) sea. A form of Doris.
Dora, Dorah, Dore, Doree, Dorey,
Dori, Doriah, Dorie, Dorinda,
Dorinde, Dorra, Dorrah, Dorre,
Dorrey, Dorri, Dorria, Dorrie,
Dorry, Dorrya, Dorryah, Dory,
Dorya, Doryah

Dorinda (Greek/Spanish) beautiful
gift. A form of Dorothy.
Dorindah, Dorynda, Doryndah

Doris (Greek) sea.
Doreece, Doreese, Dorice, Dorise,
Dorreece, Dorreese, Dorris, Dorrys,
Dorryse, Dorys

Dorita (Hebrew) generation.
Doret, Doreta, Doretah, Dorete,
Doretha, Dorett, Doretta, Dorettah,
Dorette, Dorit, Doritah, Dorite,
Doritt, Doritta, Dorittah, Doritte,
Doryt, Doryta, Dorytah, Doryte,
Dorytt, Dorytta, Doryttah, Dorytte

Dorma (Latin) sleeping.
Dormah, Dormara, Dormarah,
Dormare, Dormaria, Dormariah,
Doramary, Dormaryah

Dorothy/Dorothea (Greek) gift.
Dasha, Dasya, Doortje (Dut),
Dorafee, Dorathy, Dorathya,
Dorafey, Dorathee, Dorathey,
Dorathi, Dorathia, Dorathie,
Dorathy, Dordei, Dordi, Dorefee,
Dorefey, Dorefi, Dorefia, Dorethie,
Doretta, Dorette, Dorifee, Dorifey,
Dorifi, Dorifia, Dorifie, Dorka,
Dorle, Dorlisa, Dorlise, Dorofee,
Dorofey, Dorofi, Dorofia, Dorofie,
Dorofy, Dorofye, Dorolice,
Dorolise, Dorolisia, Dorota,
Dorothea, Dorothee, Dorothey,
Dorothi, Dorothia, Dorothie,
Dorottia, Dorottya, Doryfee,

Doryfey, Doryfi, Doryfia, Doryfie,
Doryfya, Doryfye

Dorrit (Greek) dwelling. (Heb)
generation.
Dorit, Dorita, Doritah, Dorite,
Doritta, Dorittah, Dorrite, Doryta,
Dorytah, Dorytta, Doryttah

Dottie (Greek) gift. A short form of
Dorothy.
Dotea, Dotee, Dotey, Doti, Dotie,
Dott, Dottea, Dottee, Dottey, Dotti,
Dotty, Doty

Douna (Slavic) from the valley.
Dounah

Dove (English) bird of peace.
Dova, Dovah, Dovee, Dovia,
Doviah, Dovya, Dovyah, Duv,
Duva, Duvah, Duvia, Duviah,
Duvya, Duvyah

Dowsabel (English) pretty; sweet.
Dowsabela, Dowsabelah,
Dowsabele, Dowsabell,
Dowsabella, Dowsabellah,
Dowsabelle

Dreama (Old English) one who
dreams.
Dreamah, Dreamar, Dreamara,
Dreamare, Dreamaria, Dreamariah,
Dreamarya, Dreamaryah, Dreema,
Dreemah, Dreemar, Dreemara,
Dreemarah, Dreemare, Dreemaria,
Dreemariah, Dreemarya,
Dreemaryah

Drew (Greek) strong, brave,
courageous one. A feminine short
form of Andrew.
Drewa, Drewah, Drewee, Drewia,
Drewiah, Drewie, Drewy, Dru,
Drue

Drina (Spanish) helper of
humankind.
Drinah, Dryna, Drynah

Druella (Latin) fast; level-headed.
Drewila, Drewilah, Drewile,
Drewill, Drewilla, Drewillah,
Drewille, Druila, Druilla, Druillah,
Druille, Druyl, Druyla, Druylah,
Druyle, Druylla, Druyllah, Druylle

Drusilla (Latin) strength.
Drewcela, Drewcella, Drewcila,
Drewcilla, Drewcyla, Drewcylah,
Drewcylla, Drewcyllah, Drewsila,
Drewsilah, Drewsilla, Drewsillah,
Drewsyla, Drewsylah, Drewsylla,
Drewsyllah, Drucela, Drucella,
Drucilla, Drucillah, Drucyla,
Drucylah, Drucyle, Drucylla,
Drucyllah, Drucylle, Druscila,
Druscille, Drusila, Drusilah,
Drusillah, Drusille, Drusyla,
Drusylah, Drusyle, Drusylla,
Drusyllah, Drusylle

Dudee (Gypsy) star; bright light.
Dudea, Dudey, Dudi, Dudie, Dudy

Duena (Spanish) chaperon;
companion.
Duenah, Duenna, Duennah

Dulcie (Latin) sweetnees.
Delcea, Delcee, Delcina, Delcinah,
Delcine, Delsea, Delsee, Delsey,
Delsi, Delsie, Delsy, Douce, Douci,
Doucie, Dulce, Dulcea, Dulcee,
Dulcey, Dulci, Dulcia, Dulciana,
Dulciana, Dulciann, Dulcianna,
Dulcianne, Dulibel, Dulcibela,
Dulcibell, Dulcibella, Dulcibelle,
Dulcina, Dulcine, Dulcinea, Dulcy,
Dulsea, Dulsee, Dulsey, Dulsi,
Dulsie, Dulsy

Durene (Latin) enduring.
Durean, Dureana, Dureanah,
Dureane, Dureen, Dureena,
Dureenah, Dureene, Durena,
Durenah, Durga, Durgah, Durin,
Durina, Durinah, Durine, Duryn,
Duryna, Durynah, Duryne

Dustine (German) warrior. The
feminine form of Dustin.
Dustean, Dusteana, Dusteanah,
Dusteane, Dusteena, Dusteenah,
Dusteene, Dustina, Dustinah,
Dustyna, Dustynah, Dustyne

Dusty (English) covered in dust.
A short form of Dustin, warrior.
Dustea, Dustee, Dustey, Dusti,
Dustie

Dyani (Native American) deer.
Dianee, Dianey, Diani, Dianie,
Diany, Dyami, Dyanee, Dyaney,
Dyanie, Dyany

Dyllis (Welsh) sincere; true.
Dilis, Dilisa, Dilisah, Dillis, Dillisa,
Dillisah, Dylis, Dylisa, Dylisah,
Dyliss, Dylissa, Dylissah, Dylysa,
Dylisah, Dylyss, Dylyssa, Dylyssah

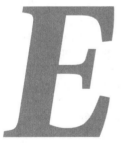

Eadda (Old English) prosperous.
Eada, Eadah, Eaddah

Eadoin (Irish) one with many
friends.
Eadiyn

Ealga (Irish) noble one.
Ealgah

Earlene (English) promise. (Eng)
noble. The feminine form of Earl.
Earleen, Earleena, Earlina,

Earlinah, Earline, Earlyn, Earlyna, Earlynah, Earlyne

Eartha (English) child of the earth.
Earthah, Earthia, Earthiah, Earthya, Earthyah, Ertha, Erthah, Heartha, Hertha, Herta, Hertah

Easter (English) born at Easter time. A form of Esther, star.
Eastera, Easterina, Easterine, Easteryn, Easteryna, Easteryne

Eavan (Irish) fair-haired.
Eavana, Eavanah, Eavane

Ebba (English) flowing tide.
Eba, Ebah, Ebbah

Eberta (Teutonic) bright.
Ebertah, Eberte, Ebirt, Eburt, Ebyrt

Ebony (English) black.
Ebonee, Eboney, Eboni, Ebonie

Ebun (Nigerian) gift.
Ebuna, Ebunah

Eca (Nigerian) bird.
Ecah

Echo (Greek) repeated sound.
Echoe, Eco

Eda (Old English) happy.
Edah, Edda, Eddah

Edana (Celtic) desired. (Ir) little fiery one.
Dana, Edanah, Edna, Ednah

Edborough (Old English) prosperous; happy fortress.
Bedbury, Edburgh, Edina, Edinburgh, Edyn, Edyna, Edynburgh

Edda (Old Norse) poetry.
Eda, Edah, Eddah

Eddi (English) property guardian.
Eddee, Eddey, Eddie, Eddy, Edee, Edey, Edi, Edie, Edy

Ede (Greek) generation.
Edee

Edeline (German) noble.
Edelin, Edelina, Edelinah, Edelyn, Edelyna, Edelynah, Edelyne

Eden (Hebrew) pleasure.
Edan, Edana, Edena, Edene, Edin, Edina, Edinah, Edine, Edon, Edona, Edonah, Edone, Edyn, Edyna, Edynah, Edyne

Edeva (Old English) expensive gift.
Eddeva, Eddevah, Eddeve, Edevah

Edian (Hebrew) God's decoration.
Edia, Edya, Edyah

Edina (Old English) prosperous, happy fortress; from Edborough.
Edena, Edena, Edenah, Edinah, Edine, Edyna, Edynah, Edyne

Edith (Old English) prosperous; happy.
Edgith, Edgyth, Edie, Edit, Edita (Ital), Editha, Edithe, Edyth, Edytha, Edythe

Ediva (English) wonderful gift.
Edith, Editha, Edivah, Edyva, Edyvah

Edlyn (Old English) little noble; prosperous.
Edlin, Edlina, Edline, Edlyna, Edlyne

Edmee (Old English) wealthy protector. A feminine form of Edmond.
Eddme, Eddmee, Edmey

Edmonda (Old English) wealthy protector. A feminine form of Edmond.
Edmona, Edmonah, Edmondea, Edmondee, Edmondey, Edmuna, Edmunah, Edmunda, Edmundea, Edmundey

Edna (Celtic) desired.
(Heb) rejuvenation.
Ednah

Edon (Irish) little fiery one. The
feminine form of Aidan.
Edan, Eden, Edin, Edona, Edonah,
Edone

Edrea (Old English) wealthy ruler.
The feminine form of Edric.
Edreah, Edria, Edriah, Edra, Edrah,
Edrya, Edryah

Edrice (English) strong property
owner.
Edrica, Edricah, Edrecia, Edriciah,
Edryca, Edrycah, Edrycia, Edryciah,
Edrycya, Edrycyah

Edris (Old English) wealthy ruler.
Edrea, Edree, Edren, Edrena,
Edrene, Edrina, Edrine, Edriss,
Edrissa, Edrisse, Edrys, Edryss,
Edryssa, Edrysse

Edwardina (Old English) wealthy
ruling guardian. The feminine
form of Edward.
Edwardinah, Edwardine,
Edwardyna, Edwardynah,
Edwardyne, Edwyna, Edwyne

Edwige (French) war; joy.
Edwig

Edwina (Old English) wealthy friend.
The feminine form of Edwin.
Edween, Edweena, Edweenah,
Edweene, Edwinah, Edwine,
Edwinna, Edwinnah, Edwinne,
Edwyna, Edwynah, Edwyne

Eepa (Hawaiian) one with
supernatural powers.
Eepah

Effie (Old Scottish) pleasant; good
reputation. (Grk) singer; speaker.
The short form of Euphemia.
Efea, Efee, Effea, Effee, Effi, Effy,
Efi, Efie, Efy

Efia (African) born on a Friday.
Efiah, Efya, Efyah

Efrata (Hebrew) respectable.
Efratah

Efrona (Hebrew) sweet-singing
bird.
Efronah, Efronna, Efronnah

Ega (Nigerian) bird.
Egah

Egberta (Old English) bright sword.
The feminine form of Egbert.
Egbertah, Egberte, Egbirt, Egbirte,
Egburt, Egburte, Egbyrt, Egbyrte

Egypt (Egyptian) from Egypt.
Egype

Ehani (Hindi) desired.
Ehanee, Ehaney, Ehanie, Ehany

Ehawee (Sioux) laughter.
Ehawey, Ehawi, Ehawie, Ehawy

Eiddwen (Welsh) fair; faithful.
Eiddwin, Eddwina, Eddwinah,
Eddwine, Eddwyn, Eddwyna,
Eddwynah, Eddwyne, Edwina,
Edwinah, Edwine, Edwyn, Edwyna,
Edwynah, Edwyne, Eiddwena,
Eiddwenah, Eiddwene, Eiddwyn,
Eiddwyna, Eiddwynah, Eiddwyne,
Eyddwin, Eyddwina, Eyddwinah,
Eyddwine, Eyddwyn, Eyddwyna,
Eyddwynah, Eyddwyne

Eifiona (Welsh) from Wales.
Eifionah

Eilah (Hebrew) oak.
Eilia, Eilya, Eilyah

Eileen (Greek) shining light. The Irish form of Helen.
Ailean, Aileana, Aileen, Aileena, Ailein, Aileina, Aileyn, Aileynah, Ailin, Ailina, Ailyn, Ailyna, Aylean, Ayleana, Ayleen, Ayleena, Aylein, Ayleina, Ayleyn, Ayleyna, Aylin, Aylina, Aylyn, Aylyna, Eilean, Eilean, Eileena, Eileenah, Eileene, Eleen, Eleena, Eleenah, Eleene, Elin, Elina, Elyn, Elyna, Eylean, Eyleana, Eyleen, Eyleena, Eylein, Eyleina, Eyleyn, Eyleyna, Eylin, Eylina, Eylyn, Eylyna

Eilwen (Welsh) fair friend.
Eilwena, Eilwenah, Eylwen, Elywena, Elywenah

Eir (Old Norse) peaceful healer.
Eira, Eirah, Eyr, Eyra, Eyrah

Eira (Welsh) snow.
Eir, Eirah, Eyr, Eyra, Eyrah

Eiralys (Welsh) snowdrop.
Eyralys

Eirene (Greek) peaceful.
Eirena, Eyren, Eyrena, Eyrene, Irene

Eirian (Welsh) silver.
Eyrian, Eyryan, Irian, Iryan

Eiriol (Welsh) snowdrop.
Iriol

Eirpne (Greek) peaceful.
Eyrpne

Eirwen (Welsh) white snow.
Eirwena, Eirwenah, Eirwene, Eyrwen, Irwen, Irwena, Irwenah, Irwene

Eithne (Celtic) fiery.
Aine, Ethne

Ekala (Australian Aboriginal) lake.
Ekalah

Ekua (Ghanian) born on a Wednesday.
Ekuah

Ela (Polish/German) noble; serene.
Elah, Ella, Ellah

Elaine (Greek) light.
Elain, Elainah, Elaine, Elana, Elane, Elani, Elayna, Elaynah, Elayne

Elama (Hebrew) people of God.
Elamah

Elana (Slavic) spirited. (Heb) oak tree.
Elanah, Elane, Elanna, Elannah, Elanne, Ellana, Ellanah, Ellann, Ellanna, Ellannah

Elanora (Australian Aboriginal) from the sea side.
Elanorah, Elanore, Ellanora, Ellanorah, Ellanore, Ellanorra, Ellanorrah, Ellanorre

Elata (Latin) praised; elevated.
Elatah, Ellata, Ellatah

Elberta (Teutonic) noble; bright.
Elbertah, Elberte, Elbirta, Elbirtah, Elburta, Elburtah, Elbyrta, Elbyrtah, Ellberta, Ellbertah, Ellberte, Ellbirta, Ellbirtah, Ellburta, Ellburtah, Ellbyrta, Ellbyrtah

Eldora (Spanish) gilded; covered with gold. The feminine form of Eldorado. (O/Ger) wise one.
Eldorah, Elldora, Elldorah

Eldrida (Old English) wise.
Eldridah, Eldryda, Eldrydah, Eldryde

Eleanor (Greek) light.
Alienor, Alienora, Annora, Annore, Eleanora, Eleanore, Elenora (Ital), Elenore (Ger/Dan), Eleonore (Fren), Elinor, Elinora, Elinore,

Eleanor cont.
Elleanor, Elleanora, Elleanore,
Ellynor, Ellynoa, Ellynore, Elna,
Elnora, Elora, Elorah, Elyenora,
Elynor, Elynora, Elynorah, Elynore,
Leanor (Span), Lenor, Lenora,
Lenore, Leonor, Leonora, Leonore

Electra (Greek) electric.
Electrah, Elektra, Elektrah

Eleebana (Australian Aboriginal)
beautiful.
Elebana, Ellebanah, Elebanna,
Elebannah, Eleebanna, Eleebannah

Eleele (Hawaiian) eyes of black.

Elena/Eleni (Greek/Scottish) shining
light. The Italian form of Helen.
Elenah, Elenee, Elenie, Eleny

Elenola (Hawaiian) bright.
Elenolah

Eleora (Hebrew) the Lord is my
bright light.
Eleorah

Eletta (English) elf.
Eleta, Eletah, Elete, Elett, Elettah,
Elette

Elfreda (Old English) powerful elf.
Elfreda, Elfredah, Elfrede, Elfrida,
Elfrydah, Elfride, Elfieda, Elfriede

Elga (Gothic/Slavic) holy.
Elgah, Elgar, Elgara

Elgiva (Old English) noble elf;
giver.
Elgivah, Elgivar, Elgyva, Elgyvah

Eli (Scandinavian) light.
Elee, Eley, Elie, Ely

Eliana (Hebrew) God has answered.
Elianah, Elianna, Eliannah,
Elianne, Elliana, Ellianah, Ellianna,
Ellilannah, Ellilanne, Ellyana,
Ellyannah, Ellyanne, Elyana,

Elyanah, Elyanna, Elyannah,
Elylanne

Elicia (Hebrew) holy and sacred to
God. A form of Elisha, truthful.
(Ger) noble.
Elicea, Eliceah, Eliciah, Ellicia,
Elliciah, Ellysia, Ellysiah, Elysia,
Elysiah, Elysya, Elysyah

Elidi (Greek) sun gift.
Elidee

Elika (Hawaiian) eternal ruler.
Elikah, Elyka, Elykah

Eliora (Hebrew) light of God.
Elilorah, Eliloria, Eliloriah,
Elilorya, Eliloryah

Elisa (Spanish/Hebrew/English)
holy and sacred to God. A form
of Elizabeth.
Elecea, Eleesa, Elesa, Elesia, Ellisia,
Ellsya, Ellisa, Ellsia, Ellissa, Elysa,
Elysia, Elysiah, Elyssia, Elyssya,
Elysya

Elise (French/English) holy and
sacred to God. A form of
Elizabeth.
Eleece, Eleesa, Elis, Elisa, Elisah,
Elissa, Elisse, Elleece, Elleesa,
Elleese, Ellisa, Ellise, Ellyce, Ellysa,
Ellyse

Elisha (Greek) truthful.
(Ger) noble.
Eleacia, Eleecia, Eleesia, Eleesha,
Eleeshia, Elesha, Eleshia, Elishiah,
Elleecia, Elleeciah, Elleesia, Ellisa,
Ellishah, Ellishia, Ellishiah,
Ellysha, Ellyshah, Ellyshia,
Ellyshiah, Ellyshya, Ellyshyah

Elissa (Greek/Hebrew) holy and
sacred to God. A short form of
Elizabeth.
Elisah, Elissah, Eliza, Elizah, Elizza,
Elizzah, Elysa, Elysah, Elyssa,

Elyssah, Elyza, Elyzah, Elyzza,
Elyzzah

Elita (Latin/French) special; chosen.
Eleata, Eleatah, Eleeta, Eleetah,
Eleita, Eleitah, Elida, Elidah, Elitia,
Elitie, Elita, Elitah, Ellitia, Ellitie,
Ellyt, Ellyta, Ellytah, Ellyte, Elyt,
Elyta, Elytah, Elyte, Lee, Leet, Leeta,
Leetah, Lei, Leit, Leita, Leitah, Lida,
Lidah, Lita, Litah, Litia, Litiah,
Lyta, Lytah, Lytia, Lytya

Eliza (Hebrew) holy and sacred to
God. A short form of Elizabeth.
Elizaida, Elizalina, Elizaline,
Elizah, Elize, Elizea, Elizeah,
Elizza, Elizzah, Elliza, Ellizah,
Ellizza, Ellizzah, Ellysa, Ellysah,
Elysa, Elysah, Elyssa, Elyssah,
Elyza, Elyzah, Ellyza, Ellyzah

Elizabeth (Hebrew) holy and sacred
to God.
Elibet, Eliabeth, Elisa (Ger), Elisabet
(Fren), Elisabeta, Elisabete,
Elisabeth, Elisabethe, Elisabetta
(Ital), Elisabette, Elisah, Elise,
Elisebet, Elisebeta, Elisebete,
Elisebeth, Elisebett, Elisebetta,
Elisebette, Elisheba, Elishebah,
Elisheva, Elishevah, Elisa, Elisah,
Elise, Elissa, Elissah, Elisse, Eliska
(Boh), Elissa (Pho), Eliza, Elizabea,
Elizabee, Elizabet, Elizabeta,
Elizabete, Elizabett, Elizabetta,
Elizabette, Elizaveta (Pol), Elizavetta
(Rus), Elizebet, Elizebeta, Elizebete,
Elizabett, Elka (Pol), Ellisa,
Ellisabeth, Ellisah, Ellise, Ellizabeth,
Ellizebet, Ellizebeta, Ellizebete,
Ellizebeth, Ellysabet, Ellysabeta,
Ellysabete, Ellysabett, Ellysabetta,
Ellysabette, Ellysebet, Ellysebeta,
Ellysebete, Ellysebett, Ellysebetta,
Ellysebette, Elsa (Swed/Ger), Elsah,
Elsabet (Ger), Elsabete, Elsabeth,
Elsabett, Elsbet (Ger), Elsbeth,

Elsbietka, Elschen, Else, Elsebin
(Dan), Elsje (Dut), Elspet, Elspeth
(Scot), Elspia, Elspie, Elsy, Elysa,
Elysabet, Elysabeta, Elysabete,
Elysabeth, Elysabett, Elyssa, Elysse,
Elzbieta (Lith), Elzinha (Span/Port),
Erzsebet, Erihapeti (NZMaori),
Erzsebet, Helsa (Dan), Ilizzabet,
Lisabeth, Lisenka (Rus), Liserli
(Swis), Lisettina (Ital), Liso (Est),
Lisset (Ger), Lizbeta (Slav), Lizette
(Fren), Lyzabeth, Lyzebeth, Lusa
(Finn)

Elk (Hawaiian) black.
(Nat/Amer) deer.
Elka, Elkah, Elke, Elkee, Elkey

Elka (Polish/Hebrew) holy and
sacred to God. A short form of
Elizabeth.
Elkah, Ilka, Ilkah

Elke (German) noble.
Elkee, Elkey, Elki, Elkie, Elky

Ella (Teutonic) little fairy girl.
Ellamae, Ella-mae, Ella-Mai,
Ellamai, Ella-mai, Ella-Mai,
Ellamay, Ella-may, Ella-May,
Ellimay, Elli-may, Elly-May

Elle (French) she.
El, Ela, Elah, Ele, Ell, Ella, Ellah

Ellen (Scottish/Greek) shining light.
The Scottish form of Helen.
Elan, Elen, Elena, Elenah, Elene,
Eleni, Elenie, Elin, Elina, Elinah,
Eline, Elinud, Ellena, Ellenah,
Ellene, Ellyn, Ellyna, Ellynah,
Ellyne

Elli (Norse) old soul.
Ele, Elea, Eleah, Elee, Elei, Eleigh,
Eley, Eli, Elia, Eliah, Elie, Ellea,
Elleah, Ellee, Ellei, Elleigh, Elley,
Ellia, Elliah, Ellie, Elly, Ellya, Ely

Ellice (Greek) noble.
Elice, Elise, Ellyce, Ellyse, Elyce, Elyse

Elma (Turkish) fruit which is sweet.
Ellma, Ellmah, Ellmar, Ellmara, Ellmarah, Elmah, Elmar, Elmara, Elmarah

Elmina (Old English) noble; famous. The feminine form of Elmer.
Alminah, Almira, Almirah, Almiria, Almiriah, Almyna, Almynah, Almyra, Almyrah, Elminah, Elmira, Elmirah, Elmiria, Elmiriah, Elmyna, Elmynah, Elmyra, Elmyrah, Elmyria, Elmyriah, Elmyrya, Elmyryah

Elmira (Arabic/Spanish) princess. A form of Almira. The feminine form of Elmer, noble; famous.
Elmear, Elmearah, Elmeera, Elmeerah, Elmeira, Elmeirah, Elmera, Elmerah, Elmiria, Elmiriah, Elmyra, Elmyrah

Elodie (Latin/German) wealthy; flower.
Alodea, Alodee, Alodey, Alodi, Alodia, Alodiah, Alodie, Alody, Alodya, Alodyah, Alodye, Elodea, Elodee, Elodey, Elodi, Elodia, Elodiah, Elody, Elodya, Elodyah, Elodye

Eloisa/Eloise (Italian/Teutonic) famous in war; healthy.
Aloisa, Aloysa, Elouisa, Elouisah, Elousie, Eloysa

Elsa/Elsie (German) noble. The Hebrew form of Elizabeth, holy and sacred to God.
Ellcea, Ellcee, Ellcey, Ellci, Ellcia, Ellcie, Ellcy, Ellsah, Ellsea, Ellsee, Ellsey, Ellsi, Ellsia, Ellsie, Ellsy, Elcea, Elcee, Elcey, Elsah, Ellsee, Ellsey, Ellsi, Ellsia, Ellsy

Elva (English) elf.
Elvah, Elvara, Elvarah, Elvena, Elvenea, Elvia, Elviah, Elvie, Elvina, Elvinah, Elvine, Elvinea, Elvinia, Elvinna, Elvinnia, Elvyna, Elvynah, Elvyne, Elvynia, Elvyniah, Elvynie, Elvyny, Elvynya, Elvynyah, Elvynye, Elvynye

Elvina (English) little elf.
Elvinah, Elvinia, Elviniah, Elvyna, Elvynah, Elvyne

Elvira (Latin) blond-haired. (Ger) closed. (Span) elf.
Elvera, Elverah, Elvina, Elvinah, Elvirah, Elvyra, Elvyrah, Elwira, Elwirah, Elwyra, Elwyrah

Elvie/Elvy (English) elf.
Elvea, Elvee, Elvey, Elvi, Elvia, Elviah, Elvira, Elvirah, Elvya, Elvyah, Elvyra, Elvyrah

Elysia (Latin) blissful; sweet.
Elisa, Elisah, Elise, Elysha, Elishia, Elysya, Elysyah, Ilisha, Ilishia, Ilysha, Ilysia

Emanuela/Emmanuelle (Hebrew) God is with us. The feminine form of Emmanuel.
Emanuel, Emanuele, Emanuell, Emanuella, Emanuellah, Emanuelle, Emmanuel, Emmanuele, Emmanuell, Emmanuella, Emmanuellah, Emmanuelle

Eme (Hawaiian) loved.
Emee, Emey

Emeni (Tongan) amen.
Emenee, Emeney, Emenie, Emenia, Emeniah, Emeny

Emerald (French) precious green gem stone.
Emelda, Emeldah, Emmarald, Emmerald, Esmaralda, Esme, Esmeralda, Esmerelda

Emere (New Zealand Maori) hard-working. A form of Emily, one who flatters.
Emera, Emerah, Emerra, Emerrah, Emerre

Emily (French/Latin) one who flatters. (Ger) hard-working. The short form of Emmaline.
Emilea, Emileah, Emilee, Emilei, Emileigh, Emiley, Emili, Emilia, Emiliah, Emilie, Emilya, Emilyah, Emilye, Emmalea, Emmaleah, Emmalee, Emmalei, Emmaleigh, Emmaley, Emmali, Emmalia, Emmaliah, Emmalie, Emmaly, Emmalya, Emmalye, Emmilea, Emmileah, Emmilee, Emmilei, Emmileigh, Emmiley, Emmili, Emmilia, Emmilie, Emmily, Emmilya, Emmilye

Emma (French/Latin) one who flatters. (Ger) hard-working. The short form of Emmaline.
Ema, Emah, Emalin, Emalina, Emaline, Emalyn, Emalyna, Emalyne, Emelin, Emelina, Emeline, Emelyn, Emelyna, Emillin, Emillina, Emilline, Emmah, Emmalin, Emmalina, Emmelin, Emmelina, Emmeline, Emmylin, Emmylina, Emmyline, Emylin, Emylina, Emyline, Emylyn, Emylyna, Emylyne

Emmaline (French/Latin) one who flatters. (Ger) hard-working.
Emalin, Emalina, Emaline, Emalyn, Emalyna, Emalyne, Emelin, Emelina, Emeline, Emelyn, Emelyna, Emillin, Emillina, Emilline, Emmalin, Emmalina, Emmelin, Emmelina, Emmeline, Emmylin, Emmylina, Emmyline, Emylin, Emylina, Emyline, Emylyn, Emylyna, Emylyne

Emmylou (German) famous, hard-working warrior.
Emiloo, Emilou, Emilu, Emmiloo, Emmilou, Emmilu, Emmyloo, Emmylu, Emylou, Emylu

Ena (Irish) shining light. A form of Helen.
Enah

Enakai (Hawaiian) sea of fire.
Enakaih

Enchantra (English) spellcaster; enchanting.
Enchantrah, Enchantria, Enchantrya, Enchantryah

Endora (Hebrew) from the fountain of youth; adorable.
Endorah, Endorra, Endorrah

Endotya (Australian Aboriginal) beautiful.
Endotah

Enfys (Welsh) rainbow.

Engel/Engelina (Greek) angel; messenger of God. A form of Angel.
Engela, Engelah, Engell, Engella, Engelle, Enjel, Enjela, Enjelah, Enjele, Enjell, Enjella, Enjellah, Enjelle

Engracia (Spanish) graceful.
Engrace, Engracee, Engraciah, Engracya, Engrasia, Engrasiah, Engrasya

Enid (Welsh) spirit of life.
Enida, Ennid, Ennida, Ennyd, Ennyda, Ennyah, Enyd, Enyda, Enydah

Enrica (Spanish/German) ruler of the house. The feminine form of Henry.
Enricah, Enrick, Enricka, Enrickah, Enrieta, Enrietta, Enriette, Enrika, Enrikah, Enrikka, Enrikkah,

Enrica cont.
Enrikke, Enriqua, Enrique, Enryc, Enryca, Enrycah, Enryka, Enrykah

Enya (Scottish/Gaelic/African) jewel; fiery.
Enia, Eniah, Enyah, Kenia, Keniah, Kenya

Eos (Greek) goddess of dawn.
Eosa, Eosah

Eostafie (Slavic/Greek) healthy.
Eos, Eostafi, Eostafia, Eostafiah, Eostafie, Eostafy

Epiphany (Hebrew) born on January 6th, a Christian festival.
Befiena, Ephana, Epifanee, Epifaney, Epifani, Epifania, Epifanie, Epiphama, Epiphanee, Epiphaney, Epiphani, Epiphania, Epiphanie, Epyfanee, Epyfaney, Epyfani, Epyfania, Epyfanie, Epyfany, Epyphanee, Epyphanee, Epyphani, Epyphania, Epyphanie, Epyphany, Theophania, Thophanie, Thophano

Epona (Roman) horse goddess.
Eponah, Eponia, Eponiah, Eponya, Eponyah

Eponi (Tongan) ebony; black.
Eponee, Eponey, Eponie, Epony

Erasma (Greek) desired.
Erasmah

Erela (Hebrew) angel.
Erelah, Erell, Erella, Erellah

Erica (Scandinavian) ruler. (O/Eng) brave ruler. The feminine form of Eric.
Ericah, Ericka, Erickah, Erika, Erikah, Eriqua, Erique, Eryca, Erycah, Eryka, Erykah

Erin/Erinna (Irish) peace. (Celt) from Ireland.
Eran, Erana, Eren, Erena, Erenah, Erene, Ereni, Erenia, Eriniah, Erinan, Erine, Erineta, Erinete, Erinett, Erinetta, Erinette, Erinn, Erinna, Erinnah, Erinne, Eryn, Eryna, Eryne, Erynna, Erynnah, Erynne

Erline (Celtic) promise. (O/Eng) little elf.
Erlean, Erleana, Erleanah, Erleane, Erleen, Erleena, Erleene, Erlin, Erlina, Erlynah, Erlyn, Erlyna, Erlynah, Erlyne

Eshe (Swahili) life.
Esha, Eshah

Esi (Ghanian) born on a Sunday.
Esee, Esey, Esie, Esy

Esme (French/Greek/Spanish) precious green gem stone. A form of Emerald.
Esma, Esmae, Esmah, Esmai, Esmay, Esmee, Esmei, Esmey

Esmeralda (Spanish) precious green gem stone. A form of Emerald.

Esperance (French) hope.
Esperanza (Span)

Estee (English/Persian) star.
Esta, Estah, Estey, Esti, Estie, Esty

Estelle (French/Latin) she is a star.
Estee, Estel, Estela, Estelah, Estele, Esteleta, Estelin, Estelina, Esteline, Estelita, Estell, Estella, Estellah, Estellin, Estellina, Estelline, Estellita, Esthel, Esthela, Esthele, Esthell, Esthella, Esthelle, Estrela, Estrelah, Estrele, Estrell, Estrella, Estrelle, Estrelleta, Estrelita, Estrelyta, Estrelytah, Estrilita, Estilitah, Estrilyta, Estrilytah, Estrylita, Estrylitah, Estrylyta, Estrylytah

Esther (Persian) star.
Esta, Estah, Estar, Ester (Hung), Estera (Pol), Esterre (Fren), Eszter,

Hadassa (Heb), Hersta, Herstar, Hestar, Hester, Hestera

Etenia (Native American) wealthy.
Eteniah, Etenya, Etenyah

Ethana (Hebrew) strong, steadfast; reliable. The feminine form of Ethan.
Ethanah, Ethena, Ethenah

Ethel (English) noble.
Ethela, Ethelah, Ethelda, Ethelin, Ethelina, Etheline, Ethella, Ethelle, Ethelyn, Ethelyna, Ethelyne, Ethelynn, Ethelynna, Ethelynne

Etoile (French) star.
Etoila, Etoilah, Etoyla, Etoylah, Etoyle

Etta (German) little. The short form of names ending in 'etta' e.g. Annetta.
Etka, Etke, Ettah, Etti, Ettie, Etty, Ety, Itka, Itke, Itta

Etumu (Native American) bear in the sun's light.

Eudore (Greek) honourable gift.
Eudora, Eudorah

Eudyce (Greek) wide.
Euridice, Euridyce, Eurydyce

Eu (Greek/French/Hebrew) noble one whose God is gracious.
Eugenea, Euganee, Euganey, Eugani, Eugania, Euganiah, Eugany, Euganya, Euganyah, Eujanee, Eujaney, Eujani, Eujania, Eujaniah, Eujanie, Eujany, Eujanya, Eujanyah

Euganie/Eugenia (Greek) noble; well born. The feminine form of Eugene.
Eugeena, Eugeenah, Eugeenee, Eugeeney, Eugeeni, Eugeenia, Eugeeniah, Eugeenie, Eugenee, Eugeney, Eugeni, Euganiah,

Eugenie, Eugeniah, Eugina, Eugine, Eugyna, Eugynah, Eugynia, Eugynie, Eugyny, Eujanee, Eujaney, Eujani, Eujania, Eujaniah, Eujanie, Eujany, Eujanya, Eujanyah, Evgenia, Evgeniah, Evgenya, Evgenyah

Eulalia (Greek) well spoken.
Eula, Eulah, Eulalea, Eulalee, Eulalie, Eulalya, Eulalyah, Eulalyam Eulia, Euliah, Eulya, Eulyah

Eun (Korean) silver.
Euna, Eunah

Eunice (Greek) happy.
Euna, Eunah, Eunique, Eunise, Euniss, Euniss, Eunisse, Eunys, Eunysa, Eunysah, Eunyse

Euphemia (Greek) one with a good reputation.
Effam, Eufemia, Eufemiah, Euphan, Euphemie, Euphemy, Euphemya, Euphemyah

Eustacia (Greek) productive. (Lat) calm.
Eustaciah, Eustacya, Eustasia, Eustasiah, Eustasya, Eustasyah

Eva (Hebrew) life. A form of Eve.
Evah, Evalea, Evaleah, Evalee, Evalei, Evaleigh, Evaley, Evali, Evalia, Evalie, Evaly, Evike

Evaline (French/Hebrew) life. A form of Eve.
Evalea, Evalean, Evaleana, Evaleanah, Evaleane, Evaleen, Evaleena, Evaleenah, Evaleene, Evalin, Evalina, Evalyn, Evalyna, Evalyne, Eveleen, Eveleena, Eveleene, Evelin, Evelina, Eveline, Evelyn, Evelyna, Evelynah, Evelyne

Evangelina (Greek) good news giver; angel; messenger of God.
Evangeleana, Evangeleanah,

Evangelina cont.
Evangeleane, Evangeleena, Evangeleene, Evangelia, Evangelica, Evangeline, Evangeliqua, Evangelique, Evangelista, Evangelyn, Evangelyna, Evangelynah, Evangelyne

Evania (Irish) youthful warrior.
Evana, Evanah, Evania, Evaniah, Evanja, Evanjah, Evann, Evanna, Evannah, Evanne, Evannja, Evannjah, Evanny, Evannya, Evany, Evanya, Evanyah

Evanthe (Greek) flower.
Evana, Evanah, Evanna, Evannah, Evantha

Eve (Hebrew) life.
Eav, Eave, Evee, Evey, Evelin, Evelina, Eveline, Evelyn, Evelyna, Evelyne, Evey, Evi (Hung), Evita, Evuska, Evva (Russ), Ewa (Pol), Evvee, Evvey, Evvi, Evvia, Evvie, Evvy, Evvya, Ewa, Ewah, Ewusche (Lett), Yev, Yeva, Yeve

Eveleen (Celtic) pleasant life.
Evalean, Evaleen, Evalin, Evalyn, Evelean, Eveleana, Eveleanah, Eveleane, Eveleena, Eveleenah, Eveleene, Evelen, Evelena, Evelenah, Evelene, Evelin, Evelina, Evelinah, Eveline, Evelyn, Evelyna, Evelynah, Evelyne

Evelyn (Hebrew/Welsh) from the pool of life.
Evalean, Evaleen, Evalin, Evalyn, Evelean, Eveleana, Eveleanah, Eveleane, Eveleen, Eveleena, Eveleenah, Eveleene, Evelen, Evelena, Evelenah, Evelene, Evelin, Evelina, Evelinah, Eveline, Evelyna, Evelynah, Evelyne

Everilda (Teutonic) from the wild boar battle.
Everild, Everilde, Everyld, Everylda, Everyldah, Everylde

Evette (French) young archer. A form of Yvette.
Evet, Eveta, Evete, Evetta

Evita (Spanish/Hebrew) life. A form of Eve.
Eveta, Evetah, Evetta, Evettah, Evitta, Evyta, Evytta

Evonne (French) archer. A form of Yvonne.
Evanna, Evanne, Eveni, Evenie, Evenne, Eveny, Evetta, Evon, Evona, Evonah, Evone, Evonn, Evonna, Evonny, Evony

Eyota (Native American) greatest.
Eyotah

Ezra (Hebrew) helpful.
Ezrah, Ezria, Ezriah, Ezrya, Ezryah

Ezrela (Hebrew) reaffirming the belief in God.
Esrela, Esrelah, Esrele, Esrell, Esrella, Esrellah, Esrelle, Ezrelah, Ezrele, Ezrella, Ezrellah, Ezrelle

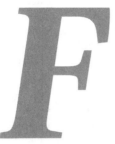

Fabayo (Nigerian) lucky birth.
Fabio

Fabia (Latin) prosperous bean
grower. The feminine form of
Fabian.
Fabiah, Fabiana, Fabianah,
Fabiann, Fabianna, Fabiannah,
Fabianne, Fabienn, Fabienna,
Fabiennah, Fabienne (Fren),
Fabiola (Span), Fabiolah, Fabya,
Fabyah, Fabyan, Fabyana,
Fabyanah, Fabyane, Fabyann,
Fabyanna, Fabyannah, Fabyanne

Fabrienne (French) little
blacksmith. The feminine form of
Fabron.
Fabrian, Fabrianah, Fabriann,
Fabrianna, Fabriannah, Fabrianne,
Fabrien, Fabriena, Fabrienah,
Fabriene, Fabrienn, Fabrienna,
Fabriennah, Fabryan, Fabryana,
Fabryanah, Fabryane, Fabryann,
Fabryanna, Fabryannah, Fabryanne,
Fabryen, Fabryena, Fabryenah,
Fabryene, Fabryenn, Fabryenna,
Fabryennah, Fabryenne

Fabrizia (Italian) worker.
Fabriziah, Fabrizya, Fabrizyah,
Fabryzia, Fabryziah, Fabryzya,
Fabryzyah

Fadila (Arabic) virtue, purity.
Fadilah, Fadyla, Fadyah

Fai (Tongan) stingray.
Fae, Faie, Faya, Fayah, Fayana,
Fayanah, Fayann, Fayanna,
Fayannah, Fayanne, Faye, Fayet,
Fayett, Fayetta, Fayettah, Fayette,
Fayin, Fayina, Fayinah, Fayine, Fei,
Fey, Feya, Feyah, Feye

Faina/Faine (Old English) joyful.
Fainah, Faine (Tuet), Fayna,
Faynah, Fayne, Feana, Feanah,
Fenna, Fennah

Fair (Old English) fair-haired.
Faira, Fairlea, Fairleah, Fairlee,
Fairlei, Fairleigh, Fairley, Fairli,
Fairlia, Fairliah, Fairlie, Fairly

Fairlee (Old English) from the
yellow meadow.
Fairlea, Fairleah, Fairlei, Fairleigh,
Fairley, Fairli, Fairlia, Fairliah,
Fairlie, Fairly, Fairlya, Fayrlea,
Fayrleah, Fayrlee, Fayrlei, Fayrleigh,
Fayrley, Fayrli, Fayrlia, Fayrliah,
Fayrlie, Fayrly, Fayrlya

Faith (Middle English) forever true.
Faeth, Faethe, Faithe, Fayeth,
Fayethe, Fayth, Faythe, Fidel,
Fidela, Fidelah, Fidele, Fidella,
Fidellah, Fidelle, Fidelia, Fidelaih,
Fidelitee, Fidelitey, Fideliti,
Fidelitie, Fidelity

Faizah (Arabic) victorious.
Faiza, Fayza, Fayzah

Falala (Tongan) trustworthy.
Falalah

Falda (Icelandic) folding wings.
Faida, Faidah, Faldah, Fayda,
Faydah

Faline (Latin) cat-like.
Falean, Faleana, Faleanah, Faleane,
Faleen, Faleena, Faleenah, Faleene,
Falina, Falinah, Falinia, Faliniah,
Falyn, Falyna, Falynah, Falyne,

F

Faline cont.
Felina, Felinah, Feline, Felinia,
Feliniah, Felyn, Felynah, Felyne

Fallon (Irish/Gaelic) the ruler's
granddaughter.
Fallan, Fallann, Fallanna,
Fallannah, Fallanne, Fallen,
Fallenn, Fallenna, Fallenna,
Fallennah, Fallenne, Fallin, Fallina,
Fallinah, Falline, Fallona, Fallonah,
Fallone, Fallonia, Falloniah,
Fallonya, Fallonyah, Fallyn,
Fallyna, Fallynah, Fallyne

Falzah (Arabic) triumph.
Falza

Fanchon (French) freedom.
Fanchona, Fanchonah, Fanchone

Fancy (French) engaged.
(Eng) decorative.
Fancee, Fanci, Fancia, Fancie

Faren (English) wandering.
Faran, Fare, Farin, Farina, Farine,
Faron, Farona, Farrahn, Farran,
Farrand, Farren, Farrin, Farron,
Farryn, Farye, Faryn, Feran, Ferin,
Feron, Ferran, Ferren, Ferrin,
Ferron, Ferryn

Farica (Teutonic) peace ruler.
Faricah, Faricka, Farika, Farikah,
Fariqua, Fariquah, Farique, Faryca,
Farycah, Farycka, Faryka, Faryqua,
Faryquah, Faryque

Farrah (Old English) beautiful;
pleasant. (Arab) happiness.
Fara, Farah, Faran, Farana, Farand,
Faranda, Farande, Farane, Faria,
Fariah, Farra, Farrand, Farranda,
Farrande, Farria, Farriah, Farrya,
Farryah, Farya, Faryah

Fatima (Arabic) daughter of the
prophet.
Fatimah, Fatma, Fatmah, Fatyma,
Fatymah

Faun (Latin) young deer.
Fauna, Faunah, Faune, Faunia,
Fauniah, Fauny, Faunya, Faunyah,
Fawn, Fawna, Fawnah, Fawne,
Fawnia, Fawniah, Fawny, Fawnya,
Fawnyah

Fausta/Faustine (Latin) lucky.
Faustah, Faustean, Fausteana,
Fausteanah, Fausteane, Fausteen,
Fausteena, Fausteenah, Fausteene,
Faustin, Faustina (Ital), Faustinah,
Faustine, Faustyn, Faustyna (Pol),
Faustynah, Faustyne

Favor (Old French) helper.
Favora, Favorah, Favore, Favour,
Favoura, Favourah, Favoure

Fawn (Old French) baby deer, fawn;
reddish/brown-haired.
Faun, Fauna, Faunah, Faune,
Faunia, Fauniah, Fauny, Faunya,
Faunyah, Fawna, Fawnah, Fawne,
Fawnia, Fawniah, Fawny, Fawnya,
Fawnyah

Faxon (German) long-haired.
Faxan, Faxana, Faxanah, Faxane,
Faxann, Faxanna, Faxannah,
Faxanne, Faxen, Faxin, Faxina,
Faxinah, Faxine, Faxyn, Faxyna,
Faxynah, Faxyne

Fay (Old French) fairy; true.
Fae, Fai, Faie, Faya, Fayah, Fayana,
Fayanah, Fayann, Fayanna,
Fayannah, Fayanne, Faye, Fayet,
Fayett, Fayetta, Fayettah, Fayette,
Fayin, Fayina, Fayinah, Fayine, Fei,
Fey, Feya, Feyah, Feye

Fayme (Old French) famous
reputation.
Faim, Faima, Faime, Fama, Fame,
Faym, Fayma

Fayola (Nigerian) lucky.
Faiola, Faiolah, Fayolah

Fayre (Old English) fair-haired.
Fair, Faira, Fairah, Faire, Fairey,
Fairy, Fare, Faree, Farey, Fari, Farie,
Fary, Fayree, Fayrey, Fayri, Fayrie,
Fary, Fear, Feara, Fearah, Fearee,
Fearey, Feari, Fearie, Feary

Fayza (Arabic) winner.
Faiza, Faizah, Fayzah

Fealty (Old French) faithful.
Fealti, Fealtie

Febe (Italian/Greek) shining; pure; bright. A form of Phoebe.
Febo (Span/Grk), Feebee, Feebe, Phoebe

Fedora (Greek) divine gift.
Fedorah, Fedorra, Fedorrah

Feeli (Tongan) fairy.
Feelie

Feena (Irish) little deer.
Feana, Feanah, Feenah

Feige (Hebrew) bird.
Feyge

Felda (Teutonic) from the field.
Feldah, Feldia, Feldiah, Feldya, Feldyah

Felice/Felicia (Greek) fortunate. The feminine form of Felix.
Falica, Felice, Feliciana (Span), Felicianna (Ital), Felicidad (Span), Felicija (Lith), Felicijanna (Pol), Felicissma (Ital), Felicitee, Felicitey, Felicitas, Felicity, Feliciza, Felicula, Felicyanna, Felicyanne, Felis, Felisa, Felise, Felisia, Felisiah, Felyc, Felyce, Felycha, Felycia, Felyciah, Felycie, Felycya, Felycyah, Felycye, Felys, Felyse, Felysha, Felysia, Felysiah, Felysie, Felysya, Felysyah, Felysye

Felicitas (Italian) fortunate; Roman goddess of good fortune.
Felicita, Felicitah, Felicyta, Felicytah, Felicytas, Felicita, Felycitah, Felycyta, Felycytah, Felycytas

Felicity (English/Latin) fortunate; Roman goddess of good fortune.
Falicitee, Falicitey, Faliciti, Falicitia, Falicitie, Falicity, Felicitee, Felicita, Felicitas, Felicite, Felicitey, Feliciti, Felicitia, Felicitie, Felycitee, Felycitey, Felyciti, Felycitie, Felycity, Felycytee, Felycytey, Felycyti, Felycytie, Felycyty

Felise (French) happy.
Felisa, Felysa, Felyse

Felora (Hawaiian) flower.
Felorah

Femi (Nigerian) love me. (Fren) woman.
Femia, Femiah, Femy, Femya, Femyah

Fenella (Irish/Gaelic) white-shouldered.
Fenel, Fenell, Fenellah, Fenelle, Fenna, Fennah, Fennal, Fennall, Fenalla, Fenallah, Fennelle, Finel, Finell, Finella, Finellah, Finelle, Finnal, Finnala, Finnall, Finallah, Finnalle, Finnghala, Finonnula, Fynela, Fynelah, Fynele, Fynell, Fynella, Fynelle, Fynnela, Fynnelah, Fynnele, Fynnell, Fynnella, Fynnellah, Fynnelle

Fenna (Norse/Irish) fair-haired.
Fena, Fenah, Fennah, Fina, Finah, Finna, Finnah, Fyna, Fynah, Fynna, Fynnah

Fern (Old English) fern; feather. The short form of names starting with 'Fern' e.g. Fernanda.
Ferna, Fernah, Ferne, Firn, Firne, Furn, Furne, Fyrn, Fyrne

Fernanda (Teutonic/Spanish)
adventurous.
Fernand, Fernandah, Fernande
(Fren), Ferdinanda, Ferdinandah,
Ferdinande, Fernand, Fernandah,
Fernande, Fernandina, Ferdandinah,
Ferdandine, Ferdandyn,
Ferdandyna, Ferdandyne

Fernley (English) from the fern
meadow.
Fernlea, Fernleah, Fernlei,
Fernleigh, Fernli, Fernlie, Fernly

Feronia (Etruscan) goddess of
flowers.
Feroniah, Feronie, Feronya,
Feronyah

Ferranta (Italian/Teutonic)
adventurer; peace maker.
(Goth) life adventure. The
feminine form of Ferdinand.
Ferrantah, Ferrante (Fren)

Fetuu (Tongan) star.

Fiala (Slavic) violet flower.
Fialah, Fyala, Fyalah

Fidelity (Latin) faithful.
Faith, Faithe, Fayth, Faythe, Fide,
Fidea, Fideah, Fidee, Fidela,
Fidelah, Fidelia, Fideliah, Fides,
Fydea, Fydee, Fydelitee, Fydelitey,
Fydeliti, Fydelitie, Fydelyty

Fidell (Latin/French) she is faithful.
Fidela, Fidelia, Fidelita, Fidelity,
Fidell, Fidellah, Fidelle, Fydel,
Fydela, Fydelah, Fydele, Fydell,
Fydella, Fydellah, Fydelle

Fidelma (Irish/Latin) faithful.
Fydelma

Fifi (French/Hebrew) God has
added a child. The French short
form of Josephine.
Fe, Fee-Fee, Fefe, Fe-Fe, Fefi, Fefie,
Fefy, Fi, Fifi, Fi-Fi, Fifina, Fifinah,

Fifine, Fiffi, Fiffie, Fiffy, Fy, Fyfy, Fy-
Fy, Phi, Phiphi, Phi-Phi, Phyphy,
Phy-Phy

Filia (Greek) friend.
Filiah, Filya, Fylia, Fyliah, Fylya,
Fylyah

Filippina (Italian) one who loves
horses.
Filipina

Filma (Teutonic) one who is veiled.
Filmah, Filmar, Filmara, Filmarah,
Filmaria, Filmariah, Filmarya,
Filmaryah, Fylma, Fylmah,
Fylmara, Fylmarah, Fylmaria,
Fylmariah, Fylmarya, Fylmaryah

Filomena (Greek) she is loved.
A form of Philomena.
Filemon, Filomenah, Fylomena,
Fylomenah

Finna (Irish/Norse) fair-haired.
Fenna, Fennah, Finnah, Fyna,
Fynah, Fynna, Fynnah

Finola (Gaelic) white-shouldered;
fair-haired.
Finella, Finellah, Finelle, Finnula,
Finnulah, Finnule, Finolah,
Fionnvale, Fynola, Fynolah, Nuala,
Nualah

Fiona (Gaelic) fair-haired; ivory-
skinned.
Feeona, Feeonah, Feeoni, Feeonie,
Feeony, Feona, Feonah, Feonia,
Feoniah, Fionah, Fionna, Fionnah,
Fionni, Fionnia, Fionniah, Fionne,
Fionnea, Fionneah, Fionnee,
Fionnuala, Fionnualah, Fyona,
Fyonah, Fyoni, Fyonia, Fyoniah,
Fyonie, Fyony, Fyonya, Fyonyah,
Nuala, Nualah, Phiona, Phionah,
Phyona, Phyonah

Fionnula (Irish/Gaelic) white-shouldered.
Fenella, Fenellah, Fenelle, Finella, Finellah, Finelle, Fionula, Fionulah, Fionnulah

Fipe (Polynesian) bright.

Fira (English) fiery.
Firah, Fyra, Fyrah

Fisi (Polynesian) flowering.

Fiusa (Tongan) the fuchsia flower.
Fuchsia, Fuchsiah, Fyusha

Flair (English) style.
Flaira, Flaire, Flare, Flayr, Flayra, Flayre

Flame (Latin/English) fiery.
Flaim, Flaima, Flaime, Flaym, Flayma, Flayme

Flanna (Irish/Gaelic) red-haired; fiery.
Flana, Flanah, Flannah

Flannery (Irish) red-haired; fiery. (O/Fren) flat metal.
Flana, Flanah, Flanna, Flannah, Flanneree, Flannerey, Flanneri, Flannerie

Flavia (Latin) golden; fair-haired.
Flaviah, Flavianna, Flavianne (Fren), Flavus, Flavya, Flavyah, Flawia (Pol), Flawiah, Flawya, Flawyah

Fleta (Teutonic) swift. (O/Eng) clean; beautiful; an inlet of water.
Fleata, Fleatah, Fleeta, Fleetah, Fletah, Flita, Flitah, Flyta, Flytah

Fleur/Fleurette (French) flower.
Fleuret, Fleurett, Fleuretta, Fleurettah, Flora, Florah, Floree, Florey, Flowa, Flowah, Flower

Flo (Latin/American/English) blooming; flowering. The short form of names starting with 'Flo' e.g. Florence.
Flow

Flora (Latin) plant. The short form of Florence, blossoming flowers.
Fiora, Fiore (Fren), Fiorella (Ital), Flaura, Flaurah, Flauria, Flauriah, Flaury, Flaurya, Flauryah, Fleur (Fren), Fliora (Lith), Fliorah, Floortje (Dut), Flouretta, Flourette, Flor (Span), Florah, Flore (Fren), Florel, Florell, Florella, Florellah, Florelle, Floretta, Florettah, Florette, Flori, Floria, Floriah, Florias, Floris, Floriss, Florissa, Florissah, Florisse, Florist, Flory, Florya, Floryah, Flow

Florence (Latin) blossoming flowers.
Fiorella, Fiorelle, Fiorenza, Fiorenze, Flarance, Flarence, Flora, Florance, Florel, Florell, Florella, Florelle, Floren, Florena, Florene, Floranc, Florance, Florancia, Floranciah, Florancie, Florenc, Florencia (Span), Florenciah, Florencija (Lith), Florencya (Pol), Florentia (Span), Florenza (Ital), Florida, Floridah, Florind, Florinda, Florindah, Florinde, Floryn, Floryna, Florynah, Florynd, Florynda, Floryndah, Florynde, Floryne, Floven, Flovena, Flovene, Floventia (Ger), Floventiah, Floventya, Floventyah

Floria (Latin/Basque) blooming; flowering. A form of Flora, plant.
Floriah, Florya, Floryah

Florida (Latin) blooming flowers. The Spanish form of Florence.
Floridah, Floridia, Floridiah, Floryda, Florydah

Florie (English/Latin) blooming;
flowering. The short form of
names starting with 'Flo' e.g.
Florence.
Floree, Florey, Floria, Floriah, Flory,
Floryah

Florimel (Greek) nectar; sweet.
Florimela, Florimele, Florimell,
Florimella, Florimelle, Florymel,
Florymela, Florymele, Florymell,
Florymella, Florymelle

Florine (Latin) blossoming flowers.
A form of Florence.
Florina, Florinah, Floryn, Floryna,
Florynah, Floryne

Floris (English/Latin) flowers.
Florisa, Florisah, Florise, Floriss,
Florissa, Florissah, Florisse, Florys,
Florysa, Florysah, Floryse, Floryss,
Floryssa, Floryssah, Florysse

Flower (French/English) blossom
flower.
Flowa

Fola (Yoruba) honour.
Folah

Folade (Nigerian) bringer of
honour.

Folami (Nigerian) respected.
Folamee, Folamie, Folamy

Foluke (Nigerian) in God's care.
Foluc, Foluck, Foluk

Fonda (Latin) foundation.
(Span) inn.
Fondah, Fondea, Fonta, Fontah

Fontane/Fontanna (French) from
the fountain.
Fontain, Fontaina, Fontainah,
Fontaine, Fontana, Fontanah,
Fontanna, Fontannah, Fontayn,
Fontayna, Fontaynah, Fontayne

Fortuna/Fortune (Latin/Italian/
Spanish) lucky; fortunate.
Faustean, Fausteana, Fausteanah,
Fausteane, Fausteen, Fausteena,
Fausteenah, Fausteene, Faustina,
Faustinah, Faustine, Faustyn,
Faustyna, Faustynah, Faustyne,
Fortunah, Fortunata, Fortunate,
Fortune (Lat), Fortunia, Fortuniah,
Fortunya, Fortunyah

Fosetta (French) dimpled.
Foset, Foseta, Fosetah, Fosete,
Fosett, Fosettah, Fosette (Fren)

Fotini (Greek) light.
Fotinia, Fotiniah, Fotinya,
Fotinyah, Fotynia, Fotyniah,
Fotynya, Fotynyah

Fran (Latin) freedom. The short
form of Frances.
Frain, Frann, Frayn

France (Latin) freedom.
(Geographical) the country.

Frances (Latin) freedom from
France. (O/Eng) honest. The
feminine form of Francis.
Cecca (Ital), Ceccarella (Ital),
Ceccina (Ital), Fanechka, Fania,
Faniah, Farruka, Franca (Ital),
Francah, Franceja, Francesca (Ital),
Francheta, Franchetah, Franchete,
Franchett, Franchetta, Franchettah,
Franchette (Fren), Franchtje (Dut),
Francillon (Fren), Francina,
Francine, Francisca (Span),
Franciska (Pol), Francoise (Fren),
Francyna, Francyne, Franis, Franisa,
Franisah, Franise, Franiss, Franissa,
Franissah, Franisse, Franka,
Frankah, Franke, Frantis, Frantisa,
Frantisah, Frantise, Frantisek
(Boh), Frantiss, Frantissa,
Frantissah, Frantisse, Franulka
(Pol), Franziska (Ger/Russ),

F

Fransquita, Frazea (Span), Pancha (Span), Paquita (Span), Phargkiske

Francesca (Italian/Latin) freedom. A form of Frances.
Franceska, Francessca, Francesta, Franchesca, Francheska, Francisca, Franciska, Franciszka, Franciszka, Frantiska, Franzet, Franzeta, Franzetah, Franzete, Franzett, Franzetta, Franzettah, Franzette, Franziska, Franzyska

Franci (Hungarian/French/Latin) freedom. A form of Frances.
Francee, Francey, Francia, Francie, Francy, Francya, Francye

Francine (French/Latin) freedom. A form of Frances.
Francin, Francina, Francyn, Francoise, Francyna, Francyne, Fransin, Fransina, Fransinah, Fransine, Fransyn, Fransyna, Fransynah, Fransyne, Franzin, Franzina, Franzinah, Franzine, Franzyn, Franzyna, Franzynah, Franzyne

Frankie (Latin/American/English) freedom. A form of Frances. The feminine form of Frank.
Frankee, Frankey, Franki, Frankia, Frankiah, Franky, Frankya

Frayda (German) joy.
Fraida, Fraidah, Frayde, Fraydina, Fraydine, Fraydyna, Fraydyne, Freida, Freidah, Freide, Freyda, Freydah

Frazea (Spanish/Latin) freedom. A form of Frances.
Franzeah, Franzia, Franziah, Franzya, Franzyah

Freda (Teutonic) old counsellor; wise judge. A feminine form of Alfred/Fred.
Freeda, Freedah, Fredah, Fredel,

Fredela, Fredelah, Fredele, Fredell, Fredella, Fredellah, Fredelle, Fredia, Frediah, Fredya, Fredyah, Freida, Friedah, Freyda, Freydah

Freddie (German/English) old counsellor; wise judge. A short form of Frederica. A feminine form of Alfred/Fred.
Fredee, Freddee, Freddey, Freddi, Freddia, Freddy, Fredee, Fredey, Fredi, Fredia, Fredie, Fredy, Fredya, Fredyah

Fredella (Teutonic/English) old counsellor; wise judge. A feminine form of Alfred/Fred.
Fredel, Fredela, Fredalah, Fredele, Fredell, Fredellah, Fredelle

Frederica/Frederique (Teutonic) old counsellor; wise judge. A feminine form of Alfred/Fred.
Farica, Faricah, Federica (Ital/Span), Feriga, Freda, Fredah, Fredda, Freddah, Fredericka (Ger), Frederiqua, Frederiquah, Frederique (Fren), Frederyc, Frederyck, Frederyk, Fredia, Frediah, Fredra, Fredrah, Fredrika, Frerika, Fredriqu, Fredriqua, Fredriquah, Fredrique, Fiddy (Ir), Fridrike, Friederike (Ger), Fredrica, Fredricah, Fridrada, Frideike (Lith), Frideryqu, Frideryqua, Frideryquah, Frideryque, Fritzi, Fritzie, Fryderika, Fryderika, Fryderikah, Fryderiqu, Fryderiqua, Fryderiquah, Fryderique

Freida (German) old counsellor; wise judge. A short form of Frederica. A feminine form of Alfred/Fred and Siegfried, victorious ruler.
Frayda, Freda, Fredda, Fredela, Fredele, Fredell, Fredella, Fredelle, Fredia, Freeda, Freedah, Freeha, Freia, Freiah, Freyda, Freydah,

G

Freida cont.
Frida, Fridah, Frideborg, Frieda,
Fryda, Frydah

Freya (Scandinavian) noble lady; a
goddess of love.
Fraja, Fray, Fraya, Frayah, Freia,
Freiah, Freja, Frehah, Frey, Freyah

Fridrun (Teutonic) peaceful
wisdom.
Fredrun, Frydrun

Fritzi (Teutonic) peaceful ruler. The
feminine form of Fritz.
Fritzee, Fritzey, Fritzie, Fritzy,
Frytzee, Frytzey, Frytzi, Frytzie,
Frytzy

Frodina (German) intelligent
friend.
Frodinah, Frodine, Frodyn,
Frodyna, Frodynah, Frodyne

Fronde (Latin) leafy branch.
Fronda, Frondah

Fronia (Latin) forehead.
Froniah, Fronya, Fronyah

Fuji (Japanese) wisteria tree.
Fujee, Fujie, Fujy

Fujo (Swahili) her parents are
divorced.

Fulande (Hindi) flower.
Fuland

Fulla (German) full.
Fula, Fulah, Fullah

Fulvia (Latin) tawny; fair/brown-
haired.
Fulvi, Fulviah, Fulvie, Fulvy,
Fulvya, Fulvyah

Fusi (Polynesian) banana.
Fusee, Fusie, Fusy

Future (Latin) unknown future.
Futura, Futruah, Futuria, Futuriah,
Futurya, Futuryah

Fuyu (Japanese) winter.

Fynballa (Gaelic) fair-shouldered.
Finbala, Finbalah, Finballa,
Finballah, Fynbala, Fynbalah,
Fynballah

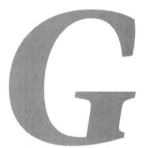

Gable (Old French) little one with
the strength of God. A form of
Gabrielle. A feminine form of
Gabriel.
Gabal, Gabala, Gabalah, Gabale,
Gaball, Gaballa, Gaballah, Gaballe,
Gabel, Gabela, Gabelah, Gabele,
Gabell, Gabella, Gabellah, Gabelle

Gabor (Hungarian/Hebrew)
strength of God. A feminine form
of Gabriel.
Gabora, Gaborah, Gabore

Gabriella/Gabrielle/Gaby (Italian)
strength of God. A feminine form
of Gabriel.
Gab, Gabb, Gabbea, Gabbee,
Gabbey, Gabbi, Gabbie, Gabby,
Gabea, Gabee, Gabell, Gabella,
Gabellah, Gabellia, Gabey, Gabi,
Gabie, Gabriel, Gabriela,
Gabrielah, Gabriell, Gabriellah,
Gabriellia, Gabriello (Ital),
Gabrila, Gabrilla, Gabriolett,
Gabrioletta, Gabriolette, Gabryel
(Pol), Gabryela (Pol), Gabryiela,

G

Gaby (Fren), Gavra (Slav),
Gavrielle, Gavrilla, Gavrille, Gavryl,
Gavryla, Gavryle, Gavryll, Gavrylla,
Gavrylle

Gada (Hebrew) lucky.
Gadah

Gady (Old English) little friend.
Gadea, Gade, Gadey, Gadi, Gadie

Gaetana (Hebrew/Greek) graceful earth.
Gaetan, Gaetanah, Gaetane,
Gaetanna, Gaetanne, Gaitana,
Gaitanah, Gaitann, Gaitanna,
Gaitanne, Gaytana, Gaytane,
Gaytanna, Gaytanne

Gage (Old French) promise.
Gaeg, Gaege, Gaig, Gaige, Gayg,
Gayge

Gai/Gay (Old French) lively.
Ga, Gae, Gaie, Gaye

Gaia (Greek) earth.
Gaea, Gaeah, Gaiah, Gaiea, Gaya,
Gayah

Gail (Old English) lively, merry singer. (Heb) born of a joyous father. A short form of Abigail.
Abigail, Gael, Gaela, Gaell, Gaella,
Gaelle, Gaile, Gailean, Gaileana,
Gaileane, Gaileen, Gaileena,
Gailina, Gailine, Gailyn, Gailyna,
Gailyne, Gale (Nrs), Galey, Galie,
Gayel, Gayell, Gayella, Gayelle,
Gayl, Gayla, Gayle (Eng), Gayleen,
Gayleena, Gaylia, Gayliah, Gaylina,
Gayline, Gaylyn, Gaylyna,
Gaylynah, Gaylyne

Gala (Norwegian) singer. (Ital) fine.
Galah, Galla, Gallah

Galatea (Greek) cream colour.
Galanth, Galanthe, Galanthea,
Galatee, Galatey, Galati, Galatia,
Galatiah, Galatie, Galaty, Galatya,
Galatyah

Galaxy (Latin) star system.
Galaxee, Galaxey, Galaxi, Galaxia,
Galaxiah

Galena (Greek) calm healer.
Galana, Galanah, Galane, Galean,
Galeana, Galeane, Galeena,
Galeenah, Galeene, Galenah,
Galene, Galina, Galinah, Galine,
Gallana, Gallanah, Gallane,
Galleena, Galleena, Galleenah,
Galleene, Galen, Galenah, Galene,
Gallin, Gallina, Gallinah, Galline,
Gallyn, Gallyna, Gallynah,
Gallyne, Galyn, Galyna, Galynah,
Galyne

Gali (Hebrew) spring; fountain on a hill.
Galea, Galeah, Galee, Galei,
Galeigh, Galey, Galia, Galiah,
Galie, Gallea, Galleah, Gallee,
Gallei, Galleigh, Galley, Galli,
Gallie, Gally, Galy

Galilani (Cherokee) friend.
Galilanee, Galilaney, Galilnie,
Galilany

Galina (Russian) white light. (Grk) calm. Russian form of Helen, shining light.
Galaina, Galainah, Galaine,
Galayna, Galaynah, Galayne,
Galean, Galeana, Galeanah,
Galeane, Galeen, Galeena,
Galeenah, Galeene, Galena,
Galenah, Galene, Galenka,
Galiana, Galianah, Galiane,
Galinah, Galine, Galinka, Galka,
Galkah, Galinka, Galochka, Galya,
Galyag, Galyn, Galyna, Galynah,
Galyne

Galla (Celtic) stranger.
Gala, Galah, Gallah

Gamel (Scandinavian) elder.
Gamala, Gamalah, Gamale,
Gamela, Gamelah, Gamele

Ganan (Australian Aboriginal) west.
Ganana, Gananah

Ganesa (Hindi) lucky.
Ganesah, Ganessa, Ganessah

Ganya (Hebrew) garden of the Lord.
Gania, Ganiah, Ganya, Ganyah

Garda (German) guardian.
Gardah

Gardenia (English) (Botanical)
sweet-smelling garden flowers.
Gardeen, Gardeena, Gardeene,
Garden, Gardena, Gardene,
Gardin, Gardina, Gardine, Gardyn,
Gardyna, Gardyne

Garland (English) from the battle
ground. (O/Fren) wreath of
flowers.
Garlan, Garlana, Garlanah,
Garlane, Garleen, Garleena,
Garleenah, Garleene, Garlena,
Garlenah, Garlene, Garlind,
Garlinda, Garlindah, Garlinde,
Garlyn, Garlynd, Garlynda,
Garlyndah, Garlynde

Garnet (Middle English) dark red;
precious gem.
Garneta, Garnetah, Garnete,
Garnett, Garnetta, Garnettah,
Garnette

Garyn (English) spear carrier.
Garan, Garana, Garane, Garin,
Garina, Garine, Garran, Garrana,
Garrane, Garrin, Garrina, Garrine,
Garyn, Garyna, Garyne, Garynna,
Garynne

Gasha (Russian/Greek) kind; good.
A form of Agatha.
Gashah, Gashka

Gasparde (French) guardian of the
treasure. A form of Casper.
Gaspard, Gasparda

Gavrella (Hebrew) hawk with the
strength of God. The
combination of Gavin/Gabrielle.
Gavila, Gavilla, Gaville, Gavrel,
Gavrela, Gavrelah, Gavrelia,
Gavreliah, Gavrell, Gavrella,
Gavrellah, Gavrelle, Gavrid,
Gavrieela, Gavriela, Gavrielle,
Gavrilla, Gavrille, Gavryl, Gavryla,
Gavryle, Gavryll, Gavrylla, Gavrylle

Gayadin (Australian Aboriginal)
platypus (Australian mammal
with fur, webbed feet and a duck-
like bill).
Gaeadin, Gaiadin, Gayadin,
Gayadyn

Gaylia (English) lively.
Gaelia, Gaeliah, Gailia, Gailiah,
Gayliah

Gayna (English/Welsh) white wave.
A form of Guinevere.
Gaena, Gaenah, Gaina, Gainah,
Gaynah

Gem/Gemma (Latin/Italian) jewel.
Gema, Gemah, Gemee, Gemey,
Gemia, Gemiah, Gemie, Gemma,
Gemmah, Gemmee, Gemmey,
Gemmi, Gemmia, Gemmiah,
Gemmy, Gemy, Jem, Jema, Jemah,
Jemee, Jemey, Jemia, Jemie, Jemm,
Jemma, Jemmah, Jemmee,
Jemmey, Jemmia, Jemmy, Jemy

Gena (French/Welsh) white wave. A
short form of Genevieve.
Geanna, Geannah, Geena, Geenah,
Genah, Gina, Ginah, Gyna, Gynah

Geneva (Old French) juniper tree.
Geneeva, Geneevah, Genevah,
Genevera, Geneva, Genevah,
Genevra (Fren), Genevrah,
Genevia, Geneviah, Genevra,
Genneeva, Genneevah, Ginevra,
Ginevrah, Ginneeva, Ginneevah,
Ginneva, Ginnevah, Gyniva,

Gynivah, Gynniva, Gynnivah,
Gynnyva, Gynnyvah, Jeneva,
Jenevah, Jenevia, Jeneviah

Genevieve (Teutonic/French) white wave.
Faik, Geneva, Geneviev, Genevion
(Fren), Genevra, Genofeva (Ger),
Genofwica (Illy), Genovefa,
Genovera, Genowefa, Genowica,
Ginette (Fren), Ginevieve,
Gynevieve, Janavive, Janeva,
Javotte, Jenevieve, Jenofeba,
Jenofeva, Vanora, Vefeli, Vevay,
Vevetta, Vevette, Zinerva, Zinervah,
Zynerva, Zynervah

Genna (Welsh) white wave.
Gena, Genah, Gennae, Gennah,
Gennai, Gennay, Genni, Gennie,
Genny, Geny

Georgeanne (Greek/English/ Hebrew) graceful farmer. The feminine form of George.
Georgeann, Georgeannah,
Georgeannah, Georgeannia,
Georget, Georgett, Georgetta,
Georgette, Georgiann, Georgianna,
Georgiannah, Georgianne,
Georgyan, Georgyana, Georgyanah,
Georgyane, Georgyann,
Georgyanna, Georgyannah,
Georgyanne

Georgene (English/Greek) farmer.
Georgeana, Georgeanah,
Georgeane, Georgeena, Georgeene,
Georgeina, Georgena, Georgenah,
Georgenia, Georgiena, Georgienna,
Georgienne, Georgina, Georginah,
Georgine, Georgyn, Georgyna,
Georgyne

Georgette (French/Greek) little farmer.
Georget, Georgeta, Georgete,
Georgett, Georgetta

Georgia (Latin/Greek) farmer.
Georgeann, Georgeanna,
Georgeannah, Georgeanne,
Georgena, Georget, Georgett,
Georgetta, Georgette, Georgiana,
Georgianah, Georgiann,
Georgianna, Georgiannah,
Georgianne, Georgina, Georgine,
Georgya, Giorgi, Giorgia (Ital),
Giraida (Ital)

Georgianna (Latin/Greek) graceful farmer.
Georgeann, Georgeannah,
Georgeanne, Georgeannia,
Georget, Georgett, Georgetta,
Georgette, Georgiann,
Georgiannah, Georgianne,
Georgyan, Georgyana, Georgyanah,
Georgyane, Georgyann,
Georgyanna, Georgyannah,
Georgyanne

Georgina/Georgine (Latin/Greek) farmer.
Georgean, Georgeana, Georgeanah,
Georgeane, Georgeen, Georgeena,
Georgeenah, Georgeenia,
Georginah, Georgine, Georgyn,
Georgyna, Georgynah, Georgyne,
Jeorgina, Jeorginah, Jeorgine,
Jeorjina, Jeorjinah, Jeorjine,
Jeorjyna, Jeorjyne

Geraldine (Teutonic) brave spear carrier. The feminine form of Gerald.
Geralda, Geraldeen, Geraldeena,
Geraldeenah, Geraldina,
Gerhardina, Gerhardine, Geriann,
Gerianna, Geriannah, Gerlina,
Gerlinda, Gerrianne, Jeraldina,
Jeraldina, Jeraldine, Jeraldyn,
Jeraldyna, Jeraldyne

Geralyn (German/Welsh) mighty woman with a spear from the pool.
Geralin, Geralina, Geraline, Geralyna, Geralyne

Gerda (German) beloved warrior. The short form of Gertrude, spear strength.
Gerdah

Geri (German/American) brave spear carrier. The short form of Geraldine.
Geree, Gerey, Gerie, Gerree, Gerrey, Gerri, Gerrie, Gerry, Gery, Jeree, Jerey, Jeri, Jerie, Jerree, Jerrey, Jerri, Jerrie, Jerry, Jery

Germaine (French) from Germany.
Germa, Germain, Germana, Germane, Germayn, Germayne, Jerma, Jermain, Jermaine, Jermane, Jermayn, Jermayne

Germina (Greek) twin.
Gemini, Geminia, Germini, Germinie, Germyn, Germyna, Germyne

Gertrude (Teutonic) spear strength.
Geede (Lett), Geertui, Geertrud, Geertruda, Geertrude, Geertrudi, Geertrudie, Geertrudy, Geitruda (Ital), Gerruda, Gerrudah, Gertraud (Ger), Gertraude, Gertruda, Gertudah, Gertrudes, Gertrudia, Gertrudis (Span), Gertruide (Dut/Pol/Lith), Gertruyd, Gertruyde, Girtrud, Girtruda, Girtrude, Gyrtrud, Gyrtruda, Gyrtrude

Gervaise (French) skilled with a spear.
Gervis, Gervayse, Jatrad, Jedert

Gessica (Italian/Hebrew) wealthy. A form of Jessica.
Gesica, Gesika, Gesikah, Gessica, Gessika, Gessikah, Gesyca, Gesyka, Gessica, Gessika, Gessyca, Gessyka, Jessica, Jessyca

Geva (Hebrew) hill.
Gevah

Ghada (Arabic) young; tender.
Gada, Gadah, Ghadah

Ghita (Italian) pearl.
Ghyta, Gita, Gyta

Gia (Italian) God is gracious.
Giah, Gya, Gyah

Giacinta (Italian) hyacinth; purple. A form of Jacinta.
Giacynta, Giacyntah, Gyacinta, Gyacynta

Giacobba (Hebrew) replacer. The feminine form of Jacob.
Giacoba, Giacobah, Giacobbah, Gyacoba, Gyacobba, Gyacobbah

Gian (Italian/Hebrew) God is gracious. A feminine form of John.
Geona, Geonna, Giana, Gianah, Gianel, Gianela, Gianele, Gianell, Gianella, Gianelle, Gianet, Gianeta, Gianete, Gianett, Gianetta, Gianette, Giannah, Gianoula, Gyan, Gyana, Gyanah, Gyann, Gyanna, Gyannah

Gidget (English/American) cute; giddy.
Gydget

Gigi (German) brilliant.
Geegee, Geygey, Gygy, Jeejee, Jeyjey, Jiji

Gila/Gilana (Hebrew) joy.
Gila, Gilah, Gilanah, Gilane, Gilania, Gilainie, Gyla, Gylah, Gylan, Gylana, Gylanah, Gylane

Gilberta/Gilberte (German) trust; promise. (Heb) joy. The feminine form of Gilbert.
Gilbert, Gilbertia, Gilbertina, Gilbertine, Gilbertyna, Gilbertyne, Gilbirt, Gilbirta, Gilbirte, Gilbirtia, Gilbirtina, Gilbirtine, Gilburta, Gilburte (Teut), Gilburtia, Gilburtina, Gilburtyna, Gilbyrta, Gilbyrte, Gilbyrtia, Gilbyrtina, Gilbyrtyna, Gylberta, Gylbertah, Gylberte, Gylbertina, Gylbertynan, Gylbirta, Gylbite, Gylbirtia, Gylbirtina, Gylbirtyna, Gylburta, Gylburte, Gylburtia, Gylburtina, Gylburtyna, Gylbyrta, Gylbyrte, Gylbyrtia, Gylbyrtina, Gylbyrtyna

Gilda (Old English) covered in gold. (Celt) God's servant.
Gildah, Gilded, Gylda, Gyldah, Gylded

Gillian (Latin) young bird. The feminine form of Julian, belonging to the youth.
Gila, Gilana, Gilena, Gilenia, Gilian, Giliana, Giliane, Gilleann, Gilleanna, Gilleanne, Gilliana, Gilliane, Gillien, Gylian, Gyliana, Gyliane, Gyllian, Gylliana, Gylliane, Gyllyan, Gyllyana, Gyllyane, Jillian, Jilliann, Jillianna, Jilliane, Jyllian, Jylliana, Jyllianah, Jylliane, Jylliann, Jyllianna, Jylliannah, Jyllianne, Jyllyan, Jyllyanah, Jyllyane, Jyllyann, Jyllyanna, Jyllyannah, Jyllyanne

Gin (Japanese) silver.
Gina, Gyn, Gyna

Gina (Japanese) silver. (Lat) queen. (Heb) garden. (Grk) farmer. A short form of Georgina.
Geena, Geenah, Gena, Genah, Ginah, Ginea, Gineah, Ginia, Gyna, Gynah, Gynia, Gynya

Ginger (Old English) red-haired; ginger spice.
Ginata, Ginatah, Ginja, Ginjah, Ginjar, Ginjer, Gynger, Gynjer

Ginia (Latin) purity. A short form of Virginia.
Ginata, Giniah, Gynia, Gyniah, Gynya, Gynyah

Ginnifer (Welsh) white wave; fair-haired. A form of Jennifer.
Genifer, Gennifer, Ginifer, Gynifer, Gyniffer

Ginny (Latin) purity. A short form of Virginia.
Ginnee, Ginni, Ginnie, Giny, Gyni, Gynie, Gynn, Gynni, Gynnie, Gynny, Gyny, Jinnee, Jinney, Jinni, Jinnie, Jinny, Jiny

Giordana (Italian/Hebrew) flowing down; descending. The feminine form of Jordan.
Giadana, Giadanah, Giadanna, Giadannah, Giodana, Giodanah, Giodanna, Giodannah, Giordanah, Giordanna, Giordannah, Gyodana, Gyodanah, Gyodanna, Gyodannah, Gyordana, Gyordanah, Gyordanna, Gyordannah

Giorsal (Scottish) graceful.
Giorsala, Giorsalah, Gyorsal, Gyorsala, Gyorsalah

Giovanna (Italian) God is gracious. A form of Jane.
Giavana, Giavanah, Giavannah, Giovana, Giovanah, Giovannah, Giovona, Giovonah, Giovonna, Giovonnah, Gyovan, Gyovana, Gyovanna, Gyovannah

Giralda (Teutonic) spear ruler.
Giraldah, Gyralda, Gyraldah

Girra (Australian Aboriginal) creek.
Gira, Girah, Girrah, Gyra, Gyrrah

Gisa (Hebrew) carved stone.
Gisah, Gysa, Gysah

Gisela (Teutonic) promise.
Ghislaine, Giselda, Gisele, Giselle,
Gysel, Gysela, Gysele, Gysell,
Gysella, Gyselle, Itisberga

Giselle (English) protector with a
sword.
Gisel, Gisela, Giselah, Gisele,
Giselia, Gisell, Gisella, Gisellah,
Gissel, Gissela, Gissele, Gissell,
Gissella, Gisselle, Gizel, Gizela,
Gizele, Gizella, Gizelle, Gysel,
Gysela, Gysele, Gysell, Gysella,
Gyzel, Gyzela, Gyzele, Gyzell,
Gyzella, Gyzelle

Gita (Sanskrit) song. (Slav) pearl.
Gitah, Gitka, Gitta, Gittah,
Gituska, Gyta, Gytah

Gitana (Spanish) gypsy.
Gitanna, Gytana, Gytanna

Githa (Greek) good.
Gitel (Heb), Gitela, Gitelah, Gitele,
Gitell (Heb), Gitella, Gitellah,
Gitelle, Githah, Gytel, Gytell,
Gytella, Gytellah, Gytelle, Gytha,
Gythah

Gladys (Celtic) princess. (Lat) small
sword.
Gladsis, Gladdys, Gladis, Gladuse
(Corn), Gladyss, Gleddis, Gleddys,
Gleddis, Gleddys, Godonne,
Godonne (Fren), Gwladys

Glenda (Irish) from the valley. A
feminine form of Glen.
Glendah, Glennda, Glenndah

Glenna (Irish) from the valley. A
feminine form of Glen.
Glen, Glenda, Glendah, Gleneesha,
Gleneisha, Glennesha, Glennis,

Glenneesha, Glennisha,
Glennishia, Glennys, Glynna,
Glynnis, Glynnys

Glennis/Glynnis (Irish) from the
valley. A feminine form of Glen.
Genda, Glenice, Glenicia, Glenis,
Glenna, Glenne, Glynis, Glynnis
(Wel), Glennys, Glenys

Gloria (Latin) glorious.
Glore, Gloree, Glorey, Glori,
Gloriah, Glorian, Gloriana,
Gloriane, Gloriann, Glorianna,
Glorianne, Glorien, Glory, Glorya,
Gloryah, Glorye

Glorien (Latin) glorious.
Glorian, Gloriana, Gloriane,
Gloriann, Glorianna, Glorianne,
Gloryan, Gloryana, Gloryane,
Gloryann, Gloryanna, Gloryanne,
Gloriena, Gloriene, Glorienn,
Glorienna, Glorienne, Gloryen,
Gloryena, Gloryene, Gloryenn,
Gloryenna, Gloryenne

Glory (Latin) glorious.
Glorea, Gloree, Glori, Gloriann,
Glorianna, Glorianne, Glorie,
Gloryann, Gloryanna, Gloryanne

Godiva (Old English) gift of God.
Godivah, Godyva, Godyvah

Golda (Old English) gold.
Goldah, Goldarina, Goldeena,
Goldeene, Goldena, Goldene,
Goldina, Goldinah, Goldine,
Goldyn, Goldyna, Goldynah,
Goldyne

Goldie (English) gold.
Goldea, Goldee, Goldey, Goldi,
Goldia, Goldiah, Goldie, Goldy,
Goldya, Goldyah

Goma (Swahili) dance of joy.
Gomah

Gopi (Sanskrit) cow herder.
Gopie, Gopy

Grace (Latin) graceful; blessed.
Engracia, Giorsal (Scott), Gracella,
Gracelia, Gracia, Graciella,
Gracielle, Graciosa (Span), Graice,
Graise, Grase, Grata, Gratia,
Gratiana, Gratiane, Grayce, Graycia,
Grazia (Ital), Graziella, Grazielle,
Grazina, Greice, Greyce, Greyse

Gracia (Latin) graceful.
Graciah, Graicia, Graiciah, Graisia,
Graisiah, Grasia, Grasiah, Graycia,
Grayciah, Graysia, Grasiah, Grazia,
Graziah, Graziel, Graziela,
Graziele, Graziell, Graziella,
Grazielle, Graziosa, Grazyna

Gratiana (Hebrew) graceful.
Gratian, Gratiane, Gratiann,
Gratianna, Gratianne, Gratyan,
Gratyana, Gratyane, Gratyann,
Gratyanna, Gratyanne

Greer (Scottish) watchful. The
Scottish feminine form of
Gregory.
Grear, Grier, Gryer

Greta (Greek) pearl. (Eng) daisy.
The Slavic/Swedish/German form
of Margaret.
Grata, Gratah, Greata, Greatah,
Greeta, Greetah, Gretah, Gretal,
Gretchen, Grete, Gretel, Gretna,
Gretta, Grettal, Gretyl, Gretyll

Gretchen (German/Greek) pearl. A
form of Margaret.
Greta, Gretah, Gretchan, Gretchin,
Gretchon, Gretchun, Gretchyn

Gretel (Greek) pearl.
Gretal, Gretall, Gretil, Gretill,
Gretell, Gretyl, Gretyll

Grischa (Russian) watchful. The
feminine form of Gregory.
Gryscha

Griselda (Teutonic) war heroine.
Griseldios, Griseldis, Grishilda,
Grishild, Grishilde, Grissel,
Grisselda, Grizel, Grizelda,,
Grizella, Grizelle, Gryselda,
Gryzelda

Guda (Scandinavian) divine; good.
Gudah

Gudrun (Old Norse) divine
wisdom; good friend.
(Scand) warrior.
Gudren, Gudrin, Gudrina,
Gudrine, Gudrinn, Gudrinna,
Guddrinne, Gudrun, Gudruna

Guilda (English/Italian) guide from
the forest. The feminine form of
Guy.
Guildah, Guylda, Guyldah

Guinevere/Genevieve (Welsh) white
wave.
Gaynor, Genevieve, Genevive,
Genivive, Gennifer, Ginevra,
Gonor, Guenevere, Guinievre,
Guinivive, Guynieve, Guyniviv,
Guynivive, Gwenivere, Gwenora,
Gwenore, Gwiniviev, Gwinivieve,
Gwynifor, Gwynivere, Gwynivive,
Janifier, Jennifer, Ona, Oona, Una,
Vannora, Vanora, Wanda, Wander,
Wannore

Gulla (Scandinavian) yellow.
(Nrs) divine sea.
Gula, Gulah, Gullah

Gunda (Norwegian) woman warrior.
Gundah

Gurit (Hebrew) innocent baby.
Gurita, Gurite, Guryta, Guryte

Gurley (Australian Aboriginal)
willow tree.
Gurlea, Gurleah, Gurlee, Gurlei,
Gurleigh, Gurli, Gurlie, Gurly

Gustee (English) windy.
Gustea, Gustey, Gusti, Gustie,
Gusty

Guyra (Australian Aboriginal)
fishing place.
Guira, Guirah, Guyrah

Gwen (Welsh) white. The short form
of names beginning with 'Gwen'
e.g. Gwendolyn.
Gwenesha, Gweness, Gwenessa,
Gweneta, Gwenetta, Gwenette,
Gwenisha, Gwenishia, Gwenita,
Gwenite, Gwenitta, Gwenitte,
Gwenn, Gwenneta, Gwenete,
Gwenetta, Gwenette, Gwin, Gwine,
Gwineta, Gwinete, Gwinisha,
Gwinita, Gwinite, Gwinitta,
Gwinitte, Gwinn, Gwinne, Gwyn,
Gwynn, Gwynne

Gwenda (Welsh) white. A form of
Gwendolyn.
Gwinda, Gwynda, Gwynedd

Gwendolyn (Welsh) white moon.
(O/Eng) fair one from the pool.
Guendolen, Gwendolen,
Gwendolin, Gwendolina,
Gwendoline, Gweneth, Gwenetta,
Gwenette, Gwindolin, Gwindolina,
Gwindoline, Gwindolyn,
Gwindolyna, Gwindolyne,
Gwynaeth, Gwyndolin,
Gwyndolina, Gwyndoline,
Gwyndolyn, Gwyndolyna,
Gwyndolyne, Gwynedd

Gwun (Native American) flute.
Gwuna

Gwyneth (Welsh) white wave.
Gweneth, Gwenneth, Gwennyth,
Gwenyth, Gwineth, Gwinneth,
Gwyneth, Gwynneth

Gypsy (Old English) wanderer.
Gipsea, Gipsee, Gipsey, Gipsi,
Gipsie, Gipsy, Gypsea, Gypsee,
Gypsey, Gypsi, Gypsie

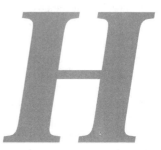

Hachi (Native American)
(Seminole) river.
Hachee, Hachie, Hachy

Hadara (Hebrew) adorned with
beauty.
Hadarah, Hadaria, Hadariah,
Hadarya, Hadaryah

Hadiya (African) (Swahili) gift.
Hadiyah

Hadley (English) from the heather
meadow.
Hadlea, Hadleah, Hadlee, Hadlei,
Hadleigh, Hadley, Hadli, Hadlie,
Hadly

Hafwen (Welsh) fair summer.
Hafwena, Hafwenah, Hafwin,
Hafwina, Hafwinah, Hafwine,
Hafwyn, Hafwyna, Hafwynah,
Hafwyne

Hagar (Hebrew) abandoned.
Hagara, Hagarah, Hagaria,
Hagariah, Hagarya, Hagaryah,
Hajar, Hajara, Hajarah, Hajaria,
Hajariah, Hajarya, Hajaryah

H

Hahau (Tongan) dew.

Haidee (Greek) modest.
Haidea, Haideah, Haidey, Haidi,
Hadia, Hady, Hadya, Hadyea,
Hadyee, Hadyey

Haido (Greek) caress.
Haydo

Hailey (Scottish) hero. (O/Eng)
from the hay meadow.
Hailea, Haileah, Hailee, Hailei,
Haileigh, Haili, Hailie, Haily, Haylea,
Hayleah, Haylee, Haylei, Hayleigh,
Hayley, Hayli, Haylie, Hayly

Haiwee (Native American)
(Shoshone) dove.
Haiwi, Haiwie, Haiwy

Hala (Latin) salty.
Halah

Haldana (Old Norse) half Danish.
The feminine form of Halden.
Haldanah, Haldania, Haldaniah,
Haldanna, Haldannah, Haldanya,
Haldanyah, Haldannya,
Haldannyah

Haley (Scandinavian) heroine.
(O/Eng) ingenious; from the hay
meadow.
Hailea, Haileah, Hailee, Hailei,
Haileigh, Hailey, Haili, Hailia,
Hailiah, Hailie, Halea, Haleah,
Halee, Halei, Haleigh, Hali, Halia,
Haliah, Halie, Haly, Halya, Halyah

Halfrida (Teutonic) peaceful
heroine. (O/Eng) peaceful home.
Halfreda, Halfredah, Halfredda,
Halfreddah, Halfrida, Halfridah,
Halfrieda, Halfryda, Halfrydah

Halia (Hawaiian) she looks like a
beloved relative.
Haleaah, Haleea, Haleeah, Haleia,
Haleiah, Haliah, Halya, Halyah

Haliaka (Hawaiian) house leader.
Haliakak, Halyaka, Halyakah

Halima (African) (Swahili) gentle.
Haleema, Haleemah, Halimah,
Halyma, Halymah

Halimeda (Greek) one who thinks
of the sea.
Halimedah, Halymeda,
Halymedah

Halina (Hawaiian) resemblance.
Halinah, Haline, Halyn, Halyna,
Halynah, Halyne

Halla (African) (Swahili)
unexpected guest; unexpected
gift.
Hala, Halah, Hallah, Hallia,
Halliah, Hallya, Hallyah, Halya,
Halyah

Hallie (Greek) one who thinks of
the sea.
Hallea, Halleah, Hallee, Hallei,
Halleigh, Halley, Halli, Hallia,
Halliah, Hally, Hallya, Hallyah

Halona (Native American) lucky.
Allona, Allonah, Alona, Alonah,
Hallona, Hallonah, Halonah

Hana (Hawaiian) work. (Jap)
blossom flower. (Heb) God is
gracious. A form of Hannah.
Hanah, Hanna, Hannah

Hanako (Japanese) flower child.

Hanele (Hebrew) merciful.
Hanal, Hanall, Hanalla, Hanalle,
Hanel, Hanela, Hanelah, Hanele,
Hanell, Hanella, Hanelle, Hannel,
Hannell, Hannella, Hannelle

Hanifah (Arabic) true believer.
Hanifa, Hanyfa, Hanyfah

Hannah (Hebrew) God is gracious.
Ann, Anna, Annah, Chana,
Chanah, Channa, Channah, Hana,

Hannah cont.
Hanah, Hanna, Hanita, Hanitah,
Henna, Hennah, Honna, Honnah,
Johana, Johanah, Johanna,
Johannah

Hanya (Australian Aboriginal)
stone.
Hania, Haniah, Hanyah

Hao (Vietnamese) tasteful; good.

Happi (English) delightful.
Happea, Happee, Happey, Happie,
Happy

Harah (Australian Aboriginal) sky.
Hara

Haralda (Old Norse) powerful army
commander. The feminine form
of Harold.
Harelda, Hareldah, Heralda,
Heraldah

Harlene (English) from the hare
meadow.
Harlean, Harleana, Harleanah,
Harleane, Harleen, Harleena,
Harleenah, Harleene, Harlena,
Harlenah, Harlin, Harlinah,
Harline, Harlyn, Harlyna,
Harlynah, Harlyne

Harley (Old English) from the hare
meadow.
Harlea, Harleah, Harlean,
Harleana, Harleanah, Harleane,
Harleen, Harleena, Harleenah,
Harlei, Harleigh, Harlein, Harleina,
Harleinah, Harleine, Harlene,
Harleyn, Harleyna, Harleynah,
Harleyne, Harlin, Harlina,
Harlinah, Harline, Harlyn,
Harlyna, Harlynah, Harlyne

Harmony (Latin) harmonious.
Harmonia, Harmoniah, Harmone,
Harmonee, Harmoney, Harmoni,
Harmonia, Harmoniah, Harmonie,
Harmony, Harmonya, Harmonyah

Harriet (Old French) powerful army
commander. The feminine form
of Harry.
Harriett, Harietta, Harriette, Hariot,
Hariott, Harriot, Harriott, Harryet,
Harryeta, Harryetah, Harryete,
Harryett, Harryetta, Harryettah,
Harryette, Haryet, Haryeta,
Haryetah, Haryete, Haryett,
Haryetta, Haryettah, Haryette

Hasia (Hebrew) protected by the
Lord.
Hasiah, Hasya, Hasyah

Hasina (African) (Swahili) good.
Hasinah, Hasyn, Hasyna, Hasynah,
Hasyne

Hateya (Native American) to push
away with the foot.
Hateia, Hateiah, Heteyah

Hathor (Egyptian) sky goddess.
Hathora, Hathorah, Hathore

Haukea (Hawaiian) snow.
Haukia, Haukiah, Haukya,
Haukyah

Hausu (Native American) bear
yawning.

Hawa (Arabic) love. (Heb) the
breath of life.
Hawah

Haya (Arabic) modest.
Haia, Haiah, Hayah

Hayat (Arabic) life.
Haiat

Hayley (Old English) high clearing.
Hailea, Haileah, Hailee, Hailei,
Haileigh, Hailey, Haili, Hailia,
Hailiah, Hailie, Halea, Haleah,
Halee, Halei, Haleigh, Hali, Halia,
Haliah, Halie, Haly, Halya, Halyah,
Haylea, Hayleah, Haylee, Haylei,
Hayleigh, Hayli, Haylia, Hayliah,
Haylie, Hayly

Hazel (Old English) hazelnut tree; a light yellow-brown colour.
Haizel, Haizelah, Haizell, Haizella, Haizellah, Haizelle, Hayzal, Hayzala, Hayzalah, Hayzale, Hayzall, Hayzalla, Hayzallah, Hayzalle, Hazal, Hazall, Hazalla, Hazallah, Hazalle, Hazell, Hazella, Hazelle, Hazzal, Hazzel, Hazzell, Hazzella, Hazzellah, Hazzelle, Heyzal, Heyzel

Heather (Middle English) from the place where heather grows.
Heathar, Hethar, Hether, Hevar, Hever

Heavenly (English) angel-like; heavenly.
Heavenlea, Heavenleah, Heavenlee, Heavenlei, Heavenleigh, Heavenley, Heavenli, Heavenlie

Hebe (Greek) young.
Heba, Hebah, Hebee, Hebey, Hebi, Hebia, Hebie, Heby

Hedda (Teutonic) one who struggles.
Heda, Hedah, Heddah, Hedvige, Hedwig, Hedwiga, Hedwyga, Hendvig, Henvyg

Hedwig (Teutonic) fighter.
Avice, Avis, Edo, Edvige, Eide, Havoise, Hawise, Heda, Hedda (Ger), Hedu (Slav), Hedvig, Hedvige (Fren), Hedwegis, Hedwyg, Heidi, Jadviga

Hedy (Greek) sweet; pleasant. The short form of names starting with 'Hed' e.g. Hedda.
Heddee, Heddey, Heddi, Heddie, Heddy, Hedee, Hedey, Hedi, Hedie

Heidi (Swiss) noble.
Heidea, Heidee, Heidey, Heidie, Heidy, Hidea, Hidee, Hidey, Hidi, Hidie, Hydea, Hydee, Hydey, Hydi, Hydie, Hydy

Helaku (Native American) sunny day.
Helakoo

Helen (Greek) shining light.
Aila, Aileen, Aileena, Ailene, Aleen, Aleena, Eileen, Eileena, Elaine, Elana, Elanah, Elane, Elayne, Eleanor, Eleanora, Eleanore, Eleen, Elena (Ital), Elene, Eleni, Elenora, Elenore, Elinor, Elinora, Elinore, Elladina, Elladine, Ellen, Ellena, Ellene, Elletta, Ellette, Ellyn, Ellynn, Elna, Elnora, Elora, Elyn, Galina, Helaina, Helan, Helana, Helanah, Helean, Heleana, Heleanah, Heleen, Heleena, Heleenah, Helena, Helenah, Helene (Ger/Fren), Helenka, Helin, Helina, Helinah, Helyn, Helyna, Helynah, Ileana, Leanora, Leanore, Lenora, Lenore, Leonora, Leonore, Leora, Lora, Nora, Norah, Valenka, Yelena, Yelenah, Yelina, Yelinah, Yelyna, Yelynah

Helena (Greek) shining light.
Halaina, Halainah, Halaine, Halayn, Halayna, Halaynah, Halayne, Helain, Helaina, Helainah, Helaine, Helana, Helanah, Helane, Helayn, Helayna, Helaynah, Helayne, Heleana, Heleena, Heleenah, Helenah, Helina, Helinah, Hellain, Hellaina, Hellaine, Hellan, Hellana, Hellanah, Helyna, Helynah, Holain, Holaina, Holainah, Holaine, Holana, Holanah, Holane, Holayn, Holayna, Holaynah, Holayne

Helga (Teutonic Religious) (Nrs) holy.
Helgah

Helice (Greek) spiral.
Helicia, Heliciah, Helyce, Helycia,
Helyciah, Helycya, Helycyah

Helki (Native American) to touch.
Helkee, Helkie, Helky

Helma (Teutonic) little determined
guardian. The short form of
Wilhelmina.
Halma, Halmah, Helmah, Hilma,
Hilmah, Hylma, Hylmah

Heloise (French) famous in war;
healthy. The French form of
Eloise.
Heloisa, Heloisah, Heloysa,
Heloysah, Heloyse

Helsa (English) swan. The Danish
form of Elizabeth, holy and
sacred to God.
Helsah, Helsia, Helsiah, Helsya,
Helsyah

Heltu (Native American) friendly
bear.
Heltoo

Henrietta (French) ruler of the
house. The feminine form of
Henry.
Eiric (Scot), Enrichetta (Ital),
Enrika, Enriquetta (Span),
Enriquette, Hendrica (Dut),
Hendrika (Dut), Hendrinka,
Hendrinkah, Henka, Henrieta
(Lith), Henriette (Fren), Henrinka
(Swed/Slav), Henriquetta,
Henriquette, Henriquieta (Port),
Henriquiette, Henryet, Henryeta,
Henryetah, Henryete, Henryett,
Henryetta, Henryettah, Henryette,
Henryetta, Henryettah, Henryette,
Henryka, Henrykah, Jendriska,
Jetje, Jette, Jindriska

Hera (Greek) queen of the heavens;
in Greek mythology, the wife of
Zeus.
Herah, Heria, Heriah, Herya,
Heryah

Herberta (German) brilliant
warrior. The feminine form of
Herbert.
Herbertah, Herbertia, Herbertiah,
Herbirta, Herbirtah, Herbirtia,
Herburta, Herburtah, Herburtia,
Herbyrta, Herbyrtah

Herma (Latin) square pillar made of
stone.
Erma, Ermah, Hermah, Hirma,
Hirmah, Hyrma, Hyrmah

Hermoine (Greek) daughter of the
earth; noble woman.
Hermia, Hermina, Herminah,
Hermine (Fren), Herminia (Pol),
Herminiah, Hermion, Hermiona,
Hermyon, Hermyona, Hermyonah,
Hermyone

Hermosa (Spanish) beautiful.
(Lat) lovely.
Hermosah

Hertha (Teutonic) mother earth.
Heartha, Hearthah, Hearthea,
Heartheah, Hearthia, Hearthiah,
Hearthya, Hearthyah, Herthah,
Herthia, Herthiah, Herthya,
Herthyah

Hester (Greek) evening star.
Hespar, Hesta, Hestar, Hestarr,
Hestia, Hestiah, Hestya, Hestyah

Hestia (Persian) myrtle tree.
(Grk) star.
Hestiah, Hestya, Hestyah

Heta (Native American) hunting
rabbits.
Hetah

Hialeah (Cherokee) beautiful meadow.
Hialea, Hialee, Hialei, Hialeigh, Hiali, Hialie, Hialy, Hyalea, Hyaleah, Hyalee, Hyalei, Hyaleigh, Hyali, Hyalie, Hyaly

Hiawasee (Cherokee) meadow.
Hyawasee

Hiawatha (Native American) river maker.
Hiawathah, Hyawatha, Hyawathah

Hibernia (Latin) from Ireland.
Hibernina, Hiberninah, Hibernine, Hibernya, Hibernyah, Hybernyna, Hybernynah, Hybernyne

Hibiscus (Latin) marshmallow flowering plant found in the moors.
Hibyscus, Hybyscus

Hika (Polynesian) daughter.
Hikah, Hyka, Hykah

Hilary (Greek) cheerful.
Hilaire, Hilarea, Hilaree, Hilarey, Hilari, Hilaria (Lat), Hilarie, Hillarea, Hilllaree, Hillarey, Hillari, Hillarie, Hillary, Hylarea, Hylaree, Hylarey, Hylari, Hylarie, Hylarie, Hylary, Hyllarea, Hyllaree, Hyllarey, Hyllari, Hyllarie, Hyllary, Ilaria, Milara

Hilda (Teutonic) battle stronghold; warrior. The short form of Hildegarde.
Hildah, Hilde, Hildee, Hildi, Hildia, Hildie, Hillda, Hilldah, Hilldee, Hilldey, Hilldi, Hilldia, Hilldie, Hilldy, Hylda, Hyldah, Hyldea, Hyldee, Hyldey, Hyldi, Hyldie, Hyldy, Hylldea, Hylldee, Hylldey, Hylldi, Hylldie, Hylldy, Hyldy

Hildegarde (Teutonic) battle stronghold; warrior.
Hildaagard, Hildaagarde, Hildagard, Hildagarde, Hildegard, Hildegaurd, Hildeguarda, Hildeguarde, Hyldaagard, Hyldaagarde, Hyldaaguard, Hyldaaguarde, Hyldagard, Hyldagarde, Hyldegard, Hyldegarde, Hyldeguard, Hyldeguarde

Hildemar (Teutonic) glorious.
Hildemara, Hildemare, Hyldemar, Hyldermara, Hyldemare

Hildreth (Teutonic) battle counsellor.
Hyldreth

Hilma (German) protected.
Hilmah, Hylma, Hylmah

Hina (Tongan) spider.
Hinah, Hyna, Hynah

Hinda (Hebrew) female deer, doe.
Hindah, Hynda, Hyndah

Hine (Polynesian) girl.
Hina, Hinah, Hyn, Hyna, Hynah, Hyne

Hinemoa (New Zealand Maori) one who swims the lake to be with her lover.
Hinemoah, Hynemoa, Hynemoah

Hiriko (Japanese) generous.
Hiryko, Hyriko, Hyryko

Hiriwa (Polynesian) silver.
Hiriwah, Hirywa, Hirywah, Hyriwa, Hyriwah, Hyrywa, Hyrywah

Hiroko (Japanese) generous.
Hyroko

Hisa (Japanese) long-lived.
Hisae, Hisah, Hisako, Hisayo, Hysa, Hysah

Hiva (Tongan) song.
Hivah, Hyvah

Hoa (Vietnamese) flower; blossom.
Hoah

Hoaka (Hawaiian) bright.
Hoakah

Holda (Teutonic) beloved. The Scandinavian form of Bertha, bright; shining; illustrious.
Holdah, Holde, Holle, Hulda (Ger), Huldah

Holla (Teutonic) the goddess of fruitfulness.
Hola, Holah, Hollah

Hollace (English) from the holly tree.
Holace, Hollice, Hollis, Hollise, Hollyce, Hollyse

Hollis (English) holly tree.
Holice, Holisa, Holisah, Holise, Holiss, Holissa, Holissah, Holisse, Holisse, Hollice, Hollyce, Hollys, Hollysa, Hollysah, Hollyse, Hollyss, Hollyssa, Hollyssah, Hollysse, Holyce, Holys, Holysa, Holysah, Holyse, Holyss, Holyssa, Holyssah, Holysse

Holly (Old English) holly tree.
Holea, Holeah, Holee, Holei, Holeigh, Holey, Holi, Holie, Holle, Hollea, Holleah, Hollee, Hollei, Holleigh, Holley, Holli, Hollie, Hollye, Holy

Hone (Tongan) honey; bee.
Honee, Honey, Honi, Honia, Honiah, Honie, Hony

Honesta (Latin) honest; trustworthy.
Honest, Honestah, Honestee, Honestey, Honesti, Honestia, Honestie, Honesty

Honey (Old English) sweet; honey.
Honea, Honeah, Honee, Honora, Honori, Honoria, Honorie, Honorina, Honorine, Honnea, Honnee, Honney, Honni, Honnie, Honny, Hunea, Hunee, Huney, Huni, Hunie, Hunnee, Hunney, Hunni, Hunni, Hunnie, Hunny

Hoong (Chinese) pink.

Honor (Latin) honourable.
Honora, Honorah, Honoria, Honoriah, Honour (Aust/Eng), Honoura, Honourah, Honouria, Honouriah, Honoury, Honourya, Honouryah

Honovi (Native American) (Hopi) powerful buck.
Honovee, Honovey, Honovie, Honovy

Hoolana (Hawaiian) happy.
Hoolanah

Hope (Old English) hope; desire.

Hopi (Native American) peace. A tribal name.
Hopee, Hopey, Hopie, Hopy

Horatia (Latin) time keeper. (Grk) promise. The feminine form of Horace.
Horacia, Horaciah, Horacya, Horacyah, Horatya, Horatyah

Hortense (Latin) farmer.
Hortensia (Ger/Dut/Dan), Hortensiah, Hortensya, Hortensyah, Ortense, Ortensia (Ital), Orazia, Oraziah, Orazya, Orazyah

Hoshi (Japanese) star.
Hoshee, Hoshey, Hoshie, Hoshy

Howi (Native American) dove.
Howee, Howey, Howie, Howy

Huata (Native American) seeds in a basket.
Huatah

Huberta (Teutonic) bright mind or heart. The feminine form of Hubert.
Hubertah, Hubertia, Hubertiah, Hubertya, Hubertyah, Hughbirta, Hughbirtah, Hughbirtia, Hughbirtiah, Hughbirtya, Hughbirtyah, Hughburta, Hughburtah, Hughburtia, Hughburtiah, Hughburtya, Hughburtyah, Hughbyrta, Hughbyrtah, Hughbyrtia, Hughbyrtiah, Hughbyrtya, Hughbyrtyah

Hue-Lan (Chinese) pink.

Huelo (Tongan) ray of light.

Huette (Old English) intelligent. (O/Ger) heart; mind. A feminine form of Hugh.
Huet, Hueta, Huetah, Huete, Huett, Huetta, Huettah, Huit, Huita, Huitah, Huitt, Huitta, Huittah, Huitte, Hughet, Hugheta, Hughetah, Hughete, Hughett, Hughetta, Hughettah, Hughette, Huyet, Huyeta, Huyetah, Huyete, Huyett, Hueyetta, Huyettah, Huyette

Huguette (French) little intelligent one. (O/Ger) heart; mind. A feminine form of Hugh.
Hugeta, Hugetah, Hughete, Hugetta

Huhulu (Tongan) one who glows.
Huhulo, Huhuloo

Hula (Hebrew) maker of music.
Hulah

Humilia (Polish) humble.
Humiliah, Humillia, Humilliah, Humylia, Humyliah, Humylya, Humylyah

Humita (Hopi) corn that has been shelled.
Humitah, Humyta, Humytah

Hunter (English) hunter.
Hunta, Huntah

Huyana (Miwok) rain falling.
Huyanah

Hyacinth (Greek) (Botanical) the hyacinth flower; purple.
Giacinta (Ital), Giacintah, Giacynta, Giacyntah, Hyacinth (Fren), Hyacintha, Hyacinthe, Hyacinthia (Span), Hyacinthie (Ger), Jacent, Jacenta, Jacentah, Jacinda, Jacindah, Jacindia, Jacinta, Jacintah, Jacinth, Jacintha, Jacinthe, Jacinthy, Jacynda, Jacyndah, Jacynta, Jacyntah, Jacynth, Jacytha, Jacynthe, Jacyntheia

Ia (Celtic) the yew tree.
Iah

Ianira (Greek) enchantress.
Ianirah, Ianyra, Ianyrah

Ianthe (Greek) violet-coloured flower.
Ianthia, Iantha, Ianthina, Ianthine, Ianthya, Ianthyah, Janthina

Ida (Old English) prosperous; hard-working; happy.
Idda, Idaia, Idal, Idaleen, Idaleena, Idaleene, Idaena, Idalene, Idalia, Idalina, Idaline, Idamae, Idania, Idarina, Idarine, Idaya, Ide, Idell, Idella, Idelle, Idetta, Idetta, Idette, Iduska, Idys, Iida (Finn), Iidda, Yda, Ydah

Idabelle (Old English) beautiful; prosperous; hard-working; happy.
Idabel, Idabela, Idabelah, Idabele, Idabell, Idabella, Idabellah

Idalia (Greek/Spanish) sun.
Idaliah, Idalya, Idalyah

Idelia (German) noble.
Ideliah, Idelya, Idelyah

Idelle (Celtic) bountiful; plenty.
Idela, Idelah, Idele, Idell, Idella, Idellah

Idola (Greek) visionary; idolised.
Idol, Idolah

Idra (Aramaic) fig tree.
Idrah

Ierne (Latin) from Ireland.
Ierna, Iernah

Iesha (Swahili) life.
Iaisha, Ieachia, Ieachya, Ieaisha, Ieasha, Ieesha, Ieeshia, Ieisha, Ieishia, Ieshia, Ieysha, Ieyshah, Leshya, Leshyah

Ignacia (Latin) fiery. A feminine form of Ignatius.
Ignaci, Ignaciah, Ignacie, Ignacya (Pol), Ignacyah, Ignasha, Ignashah, Ignashia, Ignashya, Ignashyah, Ignatia, Ignatya, Ignatyah, Ignazia, Ignazya, Ignazyah, Ignezia, Ignezya, Ignezyah, Ignia, Igniah, Inignatia, inignatiah, Inignatya, Inignatyah, Ignya, Ignyah

Ignia (Latin) fiery. A feminine form of Ignatius.
Igniah, Ignya, Ignyah

Igraine (Celtic) graceful.
Igraina, Igrainah, Igrayn, Igrayna, Igraynah, Igrayne

Ikia (Hebrew) God is my salvation. The Hawaiian feminine form of Isaiah, God is generous; God is my helper.
Ikaisha, Ikea, Ikeasha, Ikeashia, Ikeesha, Ikeeshia, Ikeisha, Ikeishi, Ikeishia, Ikesha, Ikeshia, Ikiah, Ikya, Ikyah

Ila (Hungarian/Greek) light. (O/Fren) island.
Ilah

Ilana (Hebrew) tree.
Ilanah, Ilane, Ilanee, Ilaney, Ilani, Ilainie, Ilanah, Ilane, Illana, Illanah, Illane, Illanee, Illaney, Illani, Illania, Illanie, Illanit, Illanna, Illannah, Illanne, Ileana, Ileane, Ileanee, Ileaney, Ileani, Ileanie, Ileanna, Ileannah, Ileany, Ileina, Ileinah, Ileine, Ileinee, Ileiney, Ileini, Ileinie, Ileiny, Ileyna, Ileynah, Ileynee, Ileyney, Ileyni, Ileynie, Ileyny, Ilina, Ilinah, Ilinee, Iliney, Ilini, Ilinie, Iliny, Ilyna, Ilynah, Ilynee, Ilyny, Ilyney, Ilyni, Ilynie, Ilyny

Ilene (Irish) light.
Ilean, Ileana, Ileanah, Ileane, Ileen, Ileena, Ileenah, Ileene, Ileina, Ileinah, Ileine, Ileyna, Ileynah, Ileyne, Ilina, Ilinah, Iline, Ilyna, Ilynah, Ilyne, Ilynee, Ilyney, Ilyni, Ilynie, Ilyiny

Iliana (Greek) light. (Heb) God has answered me.
Ileana, Ileane, Ileanna, Ileanah, Ileanne, Ilia, Iliah, Iliani, Iliania,

I

Illianah, Illiane, Illyana, Illyane, Illyanna, Illyanne

Ilima (Hawaiian) flower.
Ilimah, Ilyma, Ilymah

Ilise (German) noble.
Elsa, Elsah, Elsie, Ilissa, Ilissah, Ilisse, Illisa, Illisah, Illissa, Illlissah, Illysa, Illysah, Illyssa, Illyssah, Illysse, Ilysa, Ilysah, Ilyssa, Illyssah, Ilysse

Ilisha (Hebrew) life.
Aisha, Elisha, Ilishia, Ilycia, Ilysha, Ilyshia, Lisha, Lishia, Lysha, Lyshia

Ilka (Scottish/Middle English) flattering. The Slavic form of Helen, shining light.
Elka, Elke, Elki, Elkie, Elky, Ilke, Ilki, Ilkie, Ilky

Ilona (Hungarian) shining light; beautiful.
Alona, Ilka (Hung), Illona, Illonia, Illonya, Ilone, Iloni, Ilonie, Ilonka, Iluska, Ilyona, Lona, Lonka

Ilsa (Teutonic) noble woman.
Elsa, Else, Elsi, Elsie, Ilse, Ilissa, Illisa, Illissa, Illysa, Illyssa, Ilysa, Ilyssa

Iluminada (Spanish) one who shines.
Ilumina, Iluminah, Ilumine, Ilumyna, Ilumynah, Ilumyne

Ilysa (Latin) blissful. (Grk) logical.
Ilisa, Ilisah, Ilissa, Ilissah, Ilysah, Ilyssa, Ilyssah

Ima (Japanese) present. (Ger) hard-working.
Imah

Imala (Native American) strong-minded.
Imalah

Iman (Arabic) believer.
Imana, Imanah, Imanee, Imani, Imania, Imaniah, Imanie, Imany

Imber (Polish) ginger.
Imbera, Imberah, Imbere

Imelda (German) warrior.
Imalda, Imeldah, Irmhilde, Melda

Imena (African) dreamer.
Imee, Imenah, Imene

Imeria (Latin) royal.
Imperiah, Imperial

Immookalee (Cherokee) waterfall.
Immokalea, Immokaleah, Immokalei, Immokaleigh, Immokali, Immokalie, Immokaly

Imogene (Latin) image; likeness. (Ir) she is the image of her mother.
Emogen, Emogena, Emogene, Emojean, Emojeana, Imagena, Imagene, Imagina, Imajean, Imogeen, Imogeene, Imogen, Imogenia, Imogina, Imogine, Imogyn, Imogyne, Imojean, Imojeen, Innogen, Innogena, Innogene

Ina (Irish) purity.
Ena, Enya, Ianna, Ianne

Inari (Finnish) lake.
Inaree, Inarey, Inarie, Inary

Inas (Polynesian) wife of the moon.
Inasa, Inasah

Inca (Incan) Incan, an ancient race of people.
Incah, Incan, Incana, Inka, Inkah

India (Hindi) from India.
Indea, Indi, Indiah, Indiana, Indiane, Indie, Indy, Indya

**Indiana (English/American) Indian
territory.**
Indeana, Indeanna, Indeanah,
Indianna, Indiannah, Indianne,
Indyana, Indyanah, Indyann,
Indyanna, Indyannah, Indyanne

**Indigo (Latin) dark blue/violet
colour.**
Indego

Indira (Hindi) great.
Indirah, Indyra, Indyrah

**Induna (Old Norse) lover.
(O/Ger) hard-working.**
Indonia, Indunah

Inez (Spanish) purity.
Ines (Ital), Inessa (Russ), Inetta

**Inga (Scandinavian) the beautiful
daughter of the hero.**
Ingaberg, Ingaborg, Ingah, Inge,
Ingeberg, Ingeborg, Ingela

**Ingar (Australian Aboriginal)
crayfish.**
Ingara, Ingarah

**Inge (Old Norse) meadow.
(O/Eng) to extend.**
Inga, Ingaberg, Inger, Ingerith,
Ingrede, Ingrid, Inguanna, Inky

**Ingrid (Scandinavian) beautiful
daughter of the hero.**
Inga, Ingaberg, Ingaborg, Inger
(Scand), Ingeberg (Scand),
Ingeborg, Inger, Ingunna (Scand)

Iniga (Latin) fiery.
Ignatia, Inigah, Inyga, Inygah

Inoa (Hawaiian) chanting.
Inoah

**Inocencia (Spanish) innocence;
purity.**
Innocentia, Innocenciah,
Innocencya, Innocencyah,

Innocenzia, Innocenziah,
Innocenzya, Innocenzyah

Inola (Cherokee) black fox.
Inolah

Ioana (Hebrew) God is gracious.
Ioanah, Ioanna, Ioannah, Ioanne

**Iola (Greek) violet-coloured flower.
(Wel) worthy of the Lord.**
Ioanna, Ioanne, Iola, Iolah, Ione,
Ioni, Ionia, Ioniah

**Iolana (Hawaiian) soaring like a
hawk.**
Iolanah, Iolane, Iolann, Iolanna,
Iolannah, Iolanne

**Iolanda (French) hyacinth; purple.
A form of Yolanda.**
Iolande, Iolantha, Iolanthe

Ione (Greek) violet-coloured stone.
Iona, Ionee, Ioney, Ioni, Ionie, Iony

Iora (Latin) gold.
Iorah

Iphigenia (Greek) sacrifice.
Iphigena, Iphigeniah, Iphigenya,
Iphigenya, Iphigenyah

**Ira (Australian Aboriginal) camp.
(Heb) watchful. (Ara) stallion.**
Irah

**Ireland (Irish/Old English) from
Ireland.**

Irene (Greek) peaceful.
Eereen, Eereena, Eereene, Eireen,
Eireena, Eirena, Eirene, Ereen,
Ereena, Erena, Irean, Ireana,
Ireanah, Ireane, Ireen, Ireena,
Ireenah, Irena, Irenah, Irenee,
Irenka, Irina (Lith), Irinah, Irine,
Iryn, Iryna, Irynah, Iryne

Irenta (Latin) filled with rage.
Irentah, Ireta, Iretah, Irete, Iretta,
Irettah, Irette, Irete

Iriny (Greek) peace. The short form
of Irene.
Irenee, Ireney, Ireni, Irenie, Iryni,
Irynie, Iryny

Iris (Greek) rainbow. (Botanical)
the iris flower.
Irisa, Irisha, Iriss, Irissa, Irisse, Irita,
Irys, Irysa, Irysah, Iryse, Iryssa,
Iryssah, Irysse

Irma (Latin) noble; high ranking.
(Ger) honourable.
Erma, Ermina, Ermine, Irmah,
Irmina, Irmine, Irmintrude

Irmgaard (German) noble.
Irmguard

Irmina (Latin) noble.
Irmin, Irminah, Irmine, Irmyn,
Irmyna, Irmynah, Irmyne

Irva (Old English) sea farer.
Irvah, Irvettta, Irvette

Irvette (Old English) little sea
friend. The feminine form of
Irving, boar friend; green river.
Irvet, Irveta, Irvetah, Irvete, Irvett,
Irvetta, Irvettah

Isa (Greek) little. (O/Ger) lady with
the iron will. The short form of
Isabella, dedicated to God.
Isah, Issa, Issah

Isabella/Isabelle (Old Spanish)
dedicated to God.
Belica, Belita, Ezabel, Ezabell,
Ezabella, Ezabelle, Isabeal, Isabeau,
Isabel, Isabele, Isabelhina,
Isabelita, Isabella (Fren/Ital),
Isabelle (Ger/Fren), Isbel, Iseabal
(Scott), Sobel (Scott), Isobell,
Isobella, Isobelle, Isopel, Issabel,
Issabell, Issabella, Issabelle,
Issabelle, Izabel, Izabele, Izabell,
Izabella, Izabelle, Ysabel, Ysabela,
Ysabelah, Ysabele, Ysabell,

Ysabella, Ysabellah, Ysabelle,
Ysibel, Ysibela, Ysibelah, Ysibele,
Ysibell, Ysibella, Ysibellah,
Ysibelle, Ysybel, Ysybela, Ysybelah,
Ysybele, Ysybell, Ysybella, Ysybelle

Isadora (Latin/Greek) gift of Isis.
(Eng) adored. The feminine form
of Isidore.
Isadoria, Isadoriah, Isadorya,
Isadoryah, Izadora, Izadorah,
Izadore

Isatas (Native American) snow.

Isha (Hindi) woman.
Ishah

Isis (Egyptian) goddess of nature,
the moon, fertility.
Ices, Icess, Isiss, Issisa, Issise, Issys,
Isys

Isla (Celtic) island.
Islah

Ismaela (Hebrew) God listens.
Ismaila, Ismayla

Ismena (Greek) wisdom.
Ismenah, Ismenia, Ismeniah,
Ismenya, Ismenyah

Isoka (Nigerian) God's gift.
Isokah

Isola (Italian) island.
Isolah

Isolde (Welsh) fair-haired.
(O/Ger) ruler.
Isault, Isolda, Isolad, Isolt, Izot
Yseult, Ysolde, Ysolt

Ita (Gaelic) thirsting for the truth.
Itah, Itar

Italia (Latin) woman from Italy.
Italea, Italeah, Italee, Italei,
Italeigh, Italiah, Italy, Italya, Italyah

Ituha (Native American) oak tree.

Iuana (Native American) wind over a bubbling stream.
Iuanah

Iva (Russian) willow.
(O/Fren) yew tree.
Ivah

Ivah (Hebrew) God is gracious.
Iva

Ivanna (Hebrew) God is gracious. The feminine form of Ivan The Russian form of Joanna/Jane.
Ivanah, Ivania, Ivaniah, Ivanka, Ivanna, Ivannah, Ivannia, Ivanniah, Ivannka, Ivannya, Ivannyah, Ivanya, Ivanyah

Iverna (Latin) from Ireland.
Ivana, Ivanah, Ivanna, Ivannah, Ivernah

Ivory (African American) ivory; white.
Ivoree, Ivorey, Ivori, Ivorie

Ivy (Old English) (Botanical) ivy vine.
Iva, Ivalyn, Ivalynn, Ivee, Ivey, Ivi, Ivia, Iviann, Ivianna, Ivianne, Ivie, Ivye

Izusa (Native American) white stone.
Izusah

Ja (Hawaiian) fiery.
Jah

Jaamini (Hindi) evening.
Jaaminee, Jaaminey, Jaaminie, Jaaminy

Jacey (Tupi-Guarani) moon.
(Grk) beautiful. (Span) purple. The short form of Jacinda/Jacinta, hyacinth; purple.
Jacea, Jacee, Jaci, Jacia, Jaciah, Jacie, Jaciel, Jaciela, Jaciele, Jacy, Jacya, Jacyah, Jacylin, Jacylina, Jacylinah, Jacyline, Jacylyn, Jacylyna, Jacylynah, Jacylyne

Jaci (Hebrew) replacer.
Jacea, Jacee, Jacey, Jacia, Jaciah, Jacie, Jackea, Jackee, Jackey, Jacki, Jackie, Jacky, Jacqui, Jacquie, Jacquey, Jacy, Jacya, Jacyah

Jacinda (Greek) beautiful.
(Heb) replacer.
(Span/Grk) hyacinth; purple.
Jacenda, Jacenta, Jacentah, Jacindah, Jacinde, Jacindea, Jacindee, Jacindey, Jacindi, Jacindia, Jacindie, Jacindy, Jacinth, Jacintha, Jacinthe, Jacynda, Jacyndah, Jacynta, Jacynth, Jacynthe, Jakinda, Jakindah, Jakynda, Jakyndah, Jasinda, Jasindah, Jasinde, Jasindea, Jasindey, Jasindi, Jasindia, Jasindy,

J

Jaxina, Jaxine, Jaxyn, Jaxyna,
Jaxynah, Jaxyne

Jacinta (Spanish/Greek) hyacinth;
purple.
Giacinta, Hiacinth, Hiacintha,
Hiacinthe, Hyacinth, Hyacintha,
Hyacinthe, Jacanta, Jacenta,
Jacenta, Jacente, Jacinda, Jacindah,
Jacinde, Jacindea, Jacindee, Jacindi,
Jacindia, Jacindy, Jacinna, Jacinnia,
Jacintah, Jacinte, Jacinth, Jacintha,
Jacinthe (Fren), Jacinthia, Jacyn,
Jacynda, Jacyndah, Jacyndea,
Jacyndee, Jacyndi, Jacyndia,
Jacyndy, Jacyntha, Jacynthia,
Jacynthy, Jacynthe, Jasinda,
Jasindah, Jasinde, Jasinta, Jasintah,
Jasinte, Jasynda, Jasyndah,
Jasyndea, Jasyndee, Jasyndey,
Jasyndi, Jasyndia, Jasyndie, Jasyndy,
Jazinda, Jazindah, Jazindea,
Jazindee, Jazindia, Jazindie,
Jazindy, Jazinta, Jazintah, Jazynte,
Jaxinta, Jaxintah, Jaxinte

Jacki/Jacky/Jacqui (Hebrew)
replacer. The short form of
Jacqueline. The feminine form of
Jack.
Jacea, Jacee, Jacey, Jackea, Jackee,
Jackey, Jacki, Jackia, Jackiah, Jacky,
Jacquay, Jacquai, Jacquay, Jacque,
Jacquei, Jacquey, Jacqui (Fren),
Jacy, Jakea, Jakee, Jaki, Jakia,
Jakiah, Jakie, Jakkea, Jakkee, Jakki,
Jakkia, Jakkiah, Jakkie, Jakky,
Jakkya, Jakkyah, Jakquai, Jakquee,
Jakquei, Jakquey, Jakqui, Jakquie,
Jakquy, Jaky, Jaquai, Jaquee, Jaquei,
Jaquey, Jaqui, Jaquie, Jaquy, Jaky

Jacoba/Jacoby (Latin) replacer. The
feminine form of Jacob.
Jacobea, Jacobee, Jacobeell,
Jacobella (Ital), Jacobi, Jacobia,
Jacobiah, Jacobie, Jacobina,
Jacobinah, Jacobine, Jacoby,

Jacobya, Jacobyah, Jacobye,
Jacovina (Russ), Jacovinah,
Jacovine, Jocovyn, Jocovyna,
Jocovynah, Jocovyne, Jakoba,
Jakobah, Jakobea, Jakobee,
Jakobey, Jakobi, Jakobia, Jakobiah,
Jakobie, Jakoby, Jakobya, Jakuba
(Pol), Jakubah

Jacqueena (Hebrew/French/English)
replacer; replacer queen.
Jacqueen, Jacqueena, Jacqueenah,
Jacqueene, Jacqueenia,
Jacqueeniah, Jacqueenie, Jaqueen,
Jaqueena, Jaqueenah, Jaqueene,
Jaqueenia, Jaqueeniah, Jaqueenie,
Jaqueeny, Jaqueenya, Jaqueenyah

Jacqueline (French) replacer. The
feminine form of Jacques/Jack.
Jacalean, Jacaleana, Jacaleanah,
Jacaleane, Jacaleen, Jacaleena,
Jacaleenah, Jacaleene, Jacalein,
Jacaleina, Jacaleinah, Jacaleine,
Jacaleyn, Jacaleyna, Jacaleynah,
Jacaleyne, Jacalin, Jacalina,
Jacalinah, Jacaline, Jacalyna,
Jacalyna, Jacalynah, Jacalyne,
Jacelean, Jaceleana, Jaceleanah,
Jaceleane, Jaceleen, Jaceleena,
Jaceleenah, Jaceleene, Jacelein,
Jaceleina, Jaceleinah, Jaceleine,
Jaceleyn, Jaceleyna, Jaceleynah,
Jaceleyne, Jacelin, Jacelina,
Jacelinah, Jaceline, Jacelyn,
Jacelyna, Jacelynah, Jacelyne,
Jacelynn, Jacelynna, Jacelynnah,
Jacelynne, Jacilin, Jacilina,
Jacilinah, Jaciline, Jackalean,
Jackaleana, Jackaleanah,
Jackaleane, Jackaleen, Jackaleena,
Jackaleenah, Jackaleene, Jackalein,
Jackaleina, Jackaleinah, Jackaleine,
Jackaleyn, Jackaleyna, Jackaleynah,
Jackaleyne, Jackalin, Jackalina,
Jackalinah, Jackaline, Jackalyn,
Jackalyna, Jackalynah, Jackalyne,
Jackilean, Jackileana, Jackileanah,

Jacqueline cont.

Jackileane, Jackileen, Jackileena,
Jackileenah, Jackileene, Jackilein,
Jackileina, Jackileinah, Jackileine,
Jackileyn, Jackileyna, Jackileynah,
Jackileyne, Jacolean, Jacoleana,
Jacoleanah, Jacoleane, Jacoleen,
Jacoleena, Jacoleenah, Jacoleene,
Jacolein, Jacoleina, Jacoleinah,
Jacoleine, Jacolin, Jacolina,
Jacolinah, Jacoline, Jacolyn,
Jacolyna, Jacolynah, Jacolyne,
Jacolynn, Jacolynna, Jacolynnah,
Jacolynne, Jacquelean, Jacqueleana,
Jacqueleanah, Jacqueleane,
Jacqueleen, Jacqueleena,
Jacqueleenah, Jacqueleene,
Jacquelein, Jacqueleina,
Jacqueleinah, Jacqueleine,
Jacqueleyn, Jacqueleyna,
Jacqueleynah, Jacqueleyne,
Jacquelin, Jacquelina, Jacquelinah,
Jacquelyn, Jacquelyna,
Jacquelynah, Jacquelyne,
Jacquelynn, Jacquelynna,
Jacquelynnah, Jacquelynne,
Jacylean, Jacyleana, Jacyleanah,
Jacyleane, Jacyleen, Jacyleena,
Jacyleenah, Jacyleene, Jacylein,
Jacyleina, Jacyleinah, Jacyleine,
Jacyleyn, Jacyleyna, Jacyleynah,
Jacyleyne, Jacylin, Jacylina,
Jacylinah, Jacyline, Jacylyn,
Jacylyna, Jacylynah, Jacylyne,
Jacylynn, Jacylynna, Jacylynnah,
Jacylynne, Jakalean, Jakaleana,
Jakaleanah, Jakaleane, Jakaleen,
Jakaleena, Jakaleenah, Jakaleene,
Jakalein, Jakaleina, Jakaleinah,
Jakaleine, Jakaleyn, Jakaleyna,
Jakaleynah, Jakaleyne, Jakalin,
Jakalina, Jakalinah, Jakaline,
Jakalyn, Jakalyna, Jakalynah,
Jakalyne, Jakalynn, Jakalynna,
Jakalynnah, Jakalynne, Jakolean,
Jakoleana, Jakoleanah, Jakoleane,
Jakoleen, Jakoleena, Jakoleenah,

Jakoleene, Jakolein, Jakoleina,
Jakoleinah, Jakoleine, Jakoleyn,
Jakoleyna, Jakolin, Jakolina,
Jakolinah, Jakoline, Jakolyn,
Jakolyna, Jakolynah, Jakolyne,
Jakolynn, Jakolynna, Jakolynnah,
Jakolynne, Jakquelean,
Jakqueleana, Jakqueleanah,
Jakqueleane, Jakqueleen,
Jakqueleena, Jakqueleenah,
Jakqueleene, Jakquelein,
Jakqueleina, Jakqueleinah,
Jakqueleine, Jakqueleyn,
Jakqueleyna, Jakqueleynah,
Jakqueleyne, Jakquelin, Jakquelina,
Jakquelinah, Jakqueline, Jakquelyn,
Jakquelyna, Jakquelynah,
Jakquelyne, Jakquelynn,
Jakquelynna, Jakquelynnah,
Jakquelynne, Jaquelean,
Jaqueleana, Jaqueleanah,
Jaqueleane, Jaqueleen, Jaqueleena,
Jaqueleenah, Jaqueleene, Jaquelein,
Jaqueleina, Jaqueleinah,
Jaqueleine, Jaqueleyn, Jaqueleyna,
Jaqueleynah, Jaqueleyne, Jaquelin,
Jaquelina, Jaquelinah, Jaqueline,
Jaquelyn, Jaquelyna, Jaquelynah,
Jaquelyne, Jaquelynn, Jaquelynna,
Jaquelynnah, Jaquelynne,
Jaquilean, Jaquileana, Jaquileanah,
Jaquileane, Jaquileen, Jaquileena,
Jaquileenah, Jaquileene, Jaquilein,
Jaquileina, Jaquileinah, Jaquileine,
Jaquileyn, Jaquileyna, Jaquileynah,
Jaquileyne, Jaquilin, Jaquilina,
Jaquilinah, Jaquiline, Jaquilyn,
Jaquilyna, Jaquilynah, Jaquilyne,
Jaquilynn, Jaquilynna,
Jaquilynnah, Jaquilynne

Jada (Hebrew) wisdom.
Jadah, Jaed, Jaeda, Jaedah, Jaida,
Jaidah, Jayda, Jaydah

Jade (Spanish) precious green gem
stone.
Gada, Gadah, Gade, Gaid, Gaida,

Gaidah, Gaide, Gayd, Gayda,
Gaydah, Gayde, Jada, Jadah, Jadda,
Jaddah, Jadea, Jadee, Jaden, Jadena,
Jadene, Jadeen, Jadeena, Jaden,
Jadena, Jadera, Jadielin, Jadielyn,
Jadienna, Jadienne, Jaed, Jaeda,
Jaedah, Jaid, Jaida, Jaidah, Jaide,
Jayd, Jayda, Jaydah, Jayde

Jadwige (Polish) safety in a time of
war.
Jadwig

Jae (Latin) the jay bird.
Jaea, Jaele, Jaelea, Jaeleah, Jaelee,
Jaelei, Jaeleigh, Jaeley, Jaeli, Jaelia,
Jaeliah, Jaelie, Jaely, Jaelya, Jaelyah,
Jai, Jaia, Jaiah, Jailea, Jaieleah,
Jailee, Jailei, Jaileigh, Jailey, Jaili,
Jailia, Jailiah, Jailie, Jaily, Jailya,
Jailyah, Jay, Jaya, Jayla, Jaylea,
Jayleah, Jaylee, Jaylei, Jayleigh,
Jayley, Jayli, Jaylie, Jayly, Jaylyn,
Jaylyna, Jaylynah, Jaylyne

Jaehwa (Korean) beautiful.

Jael (Hebrew) wild mountain goat.
Jaela, Jaelah, Jaelea, Jaeleah, Jaelee,
Jaelei, Jaeleigh, Jaeley, Jaeli, Jaelia,
Jaeliah, Jaelie, Jaell, Jaella, Jaellah,
Jaelle, Jaely, Jaelya, Jaelyah, Jaelyn,
Jaelyna, Jaelynah, Jaelyne, Jahia,
Jahiah, Jahlea, Jahleah, Jahlee,
Jahlei, Jahleigh, Jahley, Jahli, Jahlia,
Jahliah, Jahlie, Jahly, Jahlya,
Jahlyah, Jaela, Jaelah, Jaelea,
Jaeleah, Jaelee, Jaelei, Jaeleigh,
Jaeley, Jaeli, Jaelia, Jaeliah, Jaelie,
Jaelly, Jailla, Jaillah, Jaille, Jaily,
Jailya, Jailyah, Jailyn, Jailyna,
Jailynah, Jailyne, Jaela, Jaelah,
Jaelea, Jaeleah, Jaelee, Jaelei,
Jaeleigh, Jaeley, Jaeli, Jaelia, Jaeliah,
Jaelie, Jaelly, Jaylla, Jayllah, Jaylle,
Jayly, Jaylya, Jaylyah, Jaylyn,
Jaylyna, Jaylynah, Jaylyne

Jaffa (Hebrew) beautiful.
Jaffice, Jaffit, Jafit, Jafra, Yaffa, Yaffit

Jagoda (Slavic) strawberry.
Jagodah

Jaha (Swahili) dignified; proud.
Jahaida, Jahaira, Jaharra, Jahayra,
Jahida, Jahira, Jahitza, Jai, Jaiah,
Jaya, Jayah

Jaia (Hindi) victorious.
Jaea, Jaeah, Jaha, Jahah, Jaiah, Jaya,
Jayah

Jaime/Jaimee/Jamie (Hebrew/French)
I love; replacer. The feminine
form of James.
Jaema, Jaemah, Jaemea, Jaemeah,
Jaemee, Jaemey, Jaemi, Jaemia,
Jaemiah, Jaemy, Jaemya, Jaemyah,
Jahmea, Jahmee, Jahmey, Jahmi,
Jahmie, Jahmy, Jaima, Jaimah,
J'aime, J'aimee, Jaimee, Jaimea,
Jaimeah, Jaimey, Jaimi, Jaimia,
Jaimiah, Jaimie, Jaimini, Jaiminia,
Jaiminiah, Jaimmie, Jaimy, Jaimya,
Jaimyah, Jama, Jamah, Jamea,
Jameah, Jamee, Jamei, Jameisha,
James, Jamesa, Jamesah, Jamesha,
Jamesi, Jamesia, Jamesie, Jameysha,
Jami, Jamia, Jamiah, Jamie, Jamii,
Jamiia, Jamika, Jamikah, Jamilean,
Jamileana, Jamileanah, Jamileane,
Jamileen, Jamileena, Jamileenah,
Jamileene, Jamilin, Jamilina,
Jamilinah, Jamiline, Jamilyna,
Jamilynah, Jamilyne, Jamis, Jamisa,
Jamisah, Jamise, Jammea, Jammee,
Jammey, Jammi, Jammia,
Jammiah, Jammii, Jammiia,
Jammiiah, Jammiie, Jamy, Jamya,
Jamyah, Jamye, Jamyee, Jamyka,
Jamykah, Jayma, Jaymah, Jaymea,
Jaymeah, Jaymee, Jaymey, Jaymi,
Jaymie, Jaymini, Jayminia,
Jayminie, Jaymma, Jaymmea,
Jaymmeah, Jaymmi, Jaymmia,
Jaymmiah, Jaymmie, Jaymmy,

J

Jaime/Jaimee/Jamie cont.
Jaymmya, Jaymy, Jaymya, Jaymye, Jaymyea, Jaymyee

Jaira (Hebrew/Spanish) God teaches.
Jahra, Jahrah, Jairah, Jayra, Jayrah

Jakea (Hebrew) replacer. The feminine form of Jake.
Jacea, Jacee, Jacey, Jackea, Jackee, Jackey, Jacki, Jackia, Jackiah, Jackie, Jacky, Jacquay, Jacquai, Jacquay, Jacque, Jacquei, Jacquey, Jacy, Jakee, Jaki, Jakia, Jakie, Jakkea, Jakkee, Jakki, Jakkia, Jakkiah, Jakkie, Jakky, Jakkya, Jakkyah, Jaky, Jaquai, Jaquay, Jaquea, Jaquee, Jaquei, Jaquey, Jaqui, Jaquia, Jaquiah, Jaquie, Jaquy

Jakeisha (Hebrew/Swahili) life; replacer.
Jacqueesha, Jacqueisha, Jacqueysha, Jakeesha, Jakeeshia, Jakeishia, Jakeishiah, Jakeita, Jakeitah, Jakela, Jakelah, Jakelia, Jakeliah, Jakell, Jakella, Jakellah, Jakelle, Jakena, Jakenah, Jakesha, Jakeshia, Jakeshiah, Jaket, Jaketa, Jaketah, Jakete, Jaketta, Jakettah, Jakette, Jakeva, Jakevah, Jakevia, Jakeviah, Jakeysha, Jakeyshia, Jakeyshiah, Jakia, Jakiah, Jakira, Jakirah, Jakisha, Jakishia, Jakishiah, Jakiya, Jakiyah, Jakkia, Jakkiah, Jaqueisha, Jaqueishia, Jaqueishiah, Jaqueysha, Jaquisha, Jaquysha

Jakinda (Spanish) hyacinth; purple. A form of Jacinta.
Jacinda, Jacindra, Jackinda, Jackindra, Jakindra, Jakynda, Jakyndah, Jakyndra, Jakyndrah

Jala (Arabic) clear.
Jalah

Jalena (Latin) temptress. (Heb) God is gracious. A form of Jane.
Jalana, Jalanah, Jalane, Jalaina, Jalainah, Jalaine, Jalayna, Jalaynah, Jalayne, Jalean, Jaleana, Jaleanah, Jaleane, Jaleen, Jaleena, Jaleenah, Jaleene, Jalenah, Jalene, Jalin, Jalina, Jalinah, Jaline, Jalyn, Jalyna, Jalynah, Jalyne, Jelana, Jelanah, Jelane, Jelaina, Jelainah, Jelaine, Jelayna, Jelaynah, Jelayne, Jelean, Jeleana, Jeleanah, Jeleane, Jeleen, Jeleena, Jeleenah, Jeleene, Jelenah, Jelene, Jelin, Jelina, Jelinah, Jeline, Jelyn, Jelyna, Jelynah, Jelyne

Jalila (Arabic) great.
Jalilah, Jalile, Jallila, Jallilah, Jallile, Jallyl, Jallyla, Jallyle

Jalinda (African American/Hebrew/ Spanish) pretty jay bird. A combination of Jay/Linda.
Jaelinda, Jaelindah, Jaelynda, Jaelyndah, Jailinda, Jailindah, Jailynda, Jailyndah, Jaylinda, Jaylindah, Jaylynda, Jaylyndah

Jalini (Hindi) one who lives by the ocean.
Jalinee, Jaliney, Jalinie, Jaliny

Jama (Sanskrit) daughter.
Jamah, Jamia, Jamiah, Jamya, Jamyah

Jamaica (Spanish) caribbean Island.
Jamacia, Jameca, Jameka, Jamica, Jamika, Jamoka, Jemaica, Jemika, Jemyka

Jamelia (Arabic) beautiful. The feminine form of Jamal.
Jameala, Jamealah, Jameale, Jameall, Jamealla, Jamealle, Jamilia, Jamiliah, Jamilla, Jamillah, Jamille, Jamyl, Jamylla, Jamylle

J

Jamesha (Hebrew) replacer. The feminine form of James.
Jameisha, Jamesa, Jamese, Jamesisha, Jameshya, Jameshyia, Jamesia, Jamesica, Jamesika, Jamesina, Jamesinah, Jamesine, Jamessa, Jamesse, Jameta, Jametta, Jamette, Jameysha, Jameyshia, Jameyshiah, Jameyshya, Jameyshyah, Jameysina, Jameysinah, Jameysine, Jameysyna, Jameysynah, Jameysyne, Jamisha, Jammisha, Jammysha, Jamysha

Jami/Jamie (Hebrew) replacer. The feminine form of James.
Jaema, Jaemah, Jaemea, Jaemeah, Jaemee, Jaemey, Jaemi, Jaemia, Jaemiah, Jaemy, Jaemya, Jaemyah, Jahmea, Jahmee, Jahmi, Jahmia, Jahmiah, Jahmie, Jahmy, Jaima, Jaimah, J'aime, Jaime, J'aimee, Jaimee, Jaimea, Jaimeah, Jaimee, Jaimey, Jaimi, Jaimia, Jaimiah, Jaimie, Jaimini, Jaiminia, Jaiminiah, Jaimmie, Jaimy, Jaimya, Jaimyah, Jama, Jamah, Jamea, Jameah, Jamee, Jamei, Jameisha, James, Jamesa, Jamesah, Jamesha, Jamesi, Jamesia, Jamesie, Jameysha, Jamia, Jamiah, Jamii, Jamiia, Jamika, Jamikah, Jamilean, Jamileana, Jamileanah, Jamileane, Jamileen, Jamileena, Jamileenah, Jamileene, Jamilin, Jamilina, Jamilinah, Jamiline, Jamilyna, Jamilynah, Jamilyne, Jamis, Jamisa, Jamisah, Jamise, Jammea, Jammee, Jammey, Jammi, Jammia, Jammiah, Jammii, Jammiia, Jammiiah, Jammiie, Jamy, Jamya, Jamyah, Jamye, Jamyee, Jamyka, Jamykah, Jayma, Jaymah, Jaymea, Jaymeah, Jaymee, Jaymey, Jaymi, Jaymie, Jaymini, Jayminia, Jayminie, Jaymma, Jaymmea, Jaymmeah, Jaymmi, Jaymmia, Jaymmiah, Jaymmie, Jaymmy, Jaymmya, Jaymy, Jaymya, Jaymye, Jaymyea, Jaymyee

Jamila (Arabic) beautiful. The feminine form of Jamil.
Jahmeala, Jahmealah, Jahmeale, Jahmela, Jahmelia, Jahmil, Jahmila, Jahmilah, Jahmill, Jahmilla, Jahmillah, Jahmille, Jahmyla, Jahmylah, Jahmylla, Jahmyllah, Jahmylle, Jaimeala, Jaimealah, Jaimeale, Jaimila, Jaimilah, Jaimile, Jaimilla, Jaimillah, Jaimille, Jaimyla, Jailmylah, Jaimyle, Jaimylla, Jaimyllah, Jaimylle, Jameala, Jamealah, Jameela, Jameelah, Jameele, Jameelia, Jameeliah, Jamela, Jamelah, Jamelia, Jameliah, Jamell, Jamella, Jamellah, Jamelle, Jamilah, Jamilia, Jamiliah, Jamilla, Jamillah, Jamille, Jamillia, Jamilliah, Jamilya, Jamilyah, Jemeala, Jemealah, Jemeela, Jemeelah, Jemelia, Jemeliah, Jameela, Jemeelah, Jemela, Jemelah, Jemelia, Jemeliah, Jemilla, Jemillah, Jemille, Jemyl, Jemyla, Jemylah, Jemyle, Jemyll, Jemylla, Jemyllah, Jemylle

Jamilee (Hebrew/Old English) the meadow replacer. A feminine form of James.
Jahmilea, Jahmileah, Jahmilee, Jahmilei, Jahmileigh, Jahmili, Jahmilia, Jahmiliah, Jahmilie, Jahmily, Jaimilea, Jaimileah, Jaimilee, Jaimilei, Jaimileigh, Jaimiley, Jaimili, Jaimilia, Jaimiliah, Jaimilie, Jaimily, Jamilea, Jamileah, Jaimilei, Jaimileigh, Jamiley, Jamili, Jamilia, Jamiliah, Jamilie, Jamily, Jaymilea, Jaymileah, Jaymilee, Jaymilei, Jaymileigh, Jaymili, Jaymilia, Jaymiliah, Jaymilie, Jaymyly

Jamilynn (English) replacer from the pool.
Jahmielin, Jahmielina, Jahmielinah, Jahmeiline, Jahmielyn, Jahmielyna, Jahmielyne, Jahmielynn, Jahmielynne, Jahmilin, Jahmilina, Jahmilinah, Jahmiline, Jahmilyn, Jahmilyna, Jahmilyne, Jahmilynn, Jahmilynna, Jahmilynne, Jaimielin, Jaimielina, Jaimielinah, Jaimeiline, Jaimielyn, Jaimielyna, Jaimielyne, Jaimielynn, Jaimielynne, Jaimilin, Jaimilina, Jaimilinah, Jaimiline, Jaimilyn, Jaimilyna, Jaimilyne, Jaimilynn, Jaimilynna, Jaimilynne, Jamielin, Jamielina, Jamielinah, Jameiline, Jamielyn, Jamielyna, Jamielyne, Jamielynn, Jamielynne, Jamilin, Jamilina, Jamilinah, Jamiline, Jamilyn, Jamilyna, Jamilyne, Jamilynn, Jamilynna, Jamilynne, Jaymielin, Jaymielina, Jaymielinah, Jaymeiline, Jaymielyn, Jaymielyna, Jaymielyne, Jaymielynn, Jaymielynne, Jaymilin, Jaymilina, Jaymilinah, Jaymiline, Jaymilyn, Jaymilyna, Jaymilyne, Jaymilynn, Jaymilynna, Jaymilynne

Jan (English) God is gracious. The short form of names starting with 'Jan' e.g. Janelle.
Jana, Janah, Jani, Jania, Janiah, Janie, Jandi, Jandia, Jandiah, Jandie, Jandy, Jann, Janni, Jannia, Jannniah, Jannie, Janny, Jannya, Jannyah, Jany, Janya, Janyah

Jana (Slavic/Hebrew) God is gracious. A form of Jane.
Janaca, Janah, Janalea, Janalee, Janaleigh, Janaley, Janali, Janalie, Janalin, Janalina, Janaline, Janalis, Janalisa, Janalise, Janaly, Janalyn, Janalyna, Janalyne, Janalynn, Janalynna, Janalynne, Jania, Janiah, Janika, Janike, Janka, Janna,

Jannah, Janne, Jannia, Janniah, Jannya, Jannyah, Janya, Janyah, Yana, Yanah, Yania, Yaniah, Yanie, Yanna, Yannah, Yannia, Yanniah, Yannie, Yannya, Yannyah

Janae (Hebrew) God is gracious. A form of Jane.
Janaea, Janaeh, Janah, Janai, Janaia, Janay, Janaya, Janaye, Janea, Janee, Jannae, Jannai, Jannay, Jenae, Jenai, Jenaia, Jenay, Jenaya, Jenna, Jennae, Jennai, Jennay, Jennaya, Jennaye

Janaia (Arabic) fruit harvest. A form of Janna.
Janaiah, Janaya, Janaye, Janna, Jannah, Jannaia, Jannaya, Yana (Slav), Yanah, Yanna, Yannah

Janaki (Hindi) mother.
Janakee, Janakey, Janakie, Janaky

Janan (Arabic) she has heart and soul.
Jananee, Jananey, Janani, Janania, Jananiah, Jananie, Janany, Jananya, Jananyah

Jane/Janie/Jayne (Hebrew) God is gracious. The feminine form of John.
Hanneli, Jahn, Jahne, Jain, Jaine, Jana, Janaki, Janecza, Janee, Janel, Janell, Janella, Janelle, Janet, Janetje, Janett, Janetta, Janette, Janey, Jani, Jania, Janice, Janie, Janina, Janine (Fren), Janis, Janith, Janithe, Janithia, Janka, Janna, Jannah, Janne, Jannel, Jannell, Jannella, Jannelle, Jany, Janytha, Janythia, Janythiah, Jayne, Jaynee, Jenda, Jenica, Jinana, Vanya, Zaneta (Heb)

Janel/Janelle (Hebrew) God is gracious.
Jaenel, Jaenela, Jaenelah, Jaenele, Jaenell, Jaenella, Jaenellah,

J

Jaenelle, Jainel, Jainela, Jainelah,
Jainele, Jainell, Jainella, Jainelle,
Janela, Janelah, Janell, Janella,
Janellah, Jannel, Jannell, Jannella,
Jannellah, Jannelle, Janyll, Jaynel,
Jaynela, Jaynelah, Jaynele, Jaynell,
Jaynella, Jaynelle

Janessa (Hebrew/Greek) God's
gracious butterfly. A combination
of Jane/Vanessa.
Janesha, Janeska, Janiesa, Janiesha,
Janisha, Janissa, Janisse, Jannesa,
Jannesha, Jannessa, Jannisa,
Jannise, Jannissa, Jannisse, Jannys,
Jannysa, Jannysah, Jannyse, Janys,
Janysa, Janysah, Janyss, Janyssa,
Janyssah, Janysse

Janet (Hebrew) God is gracious.
Janata, Janesha, Janeta, Janete,
Janetje (Dut), Janett, Janetta,
Janette, Janita, Janith, Janitza,
Jannet, Janneta, Jannetta, Jannette,
Jannita, Jannitah, Jannite, Jannitta,
Jannittah, Jannitte, Janot, Janota,
Janote, Janta, Jante, Janyt, Janyta,
Janyte, Janytta, Janyttah, Janytte

Jania (Hebrew) God's gracious gift.
A form of Jane.
Jainia, Jainiah, Janiah, Janina,
Janine, Janna, Jannah, Jaynia,
Jayniah, Jaynee

Janice (Hebrew) God is gracious.
Janeace, Janease, Janeece, Janeese,
Janece, Janecia, Janeciah, Janeice,
Janeise, Janese, Janiece, Janiese,
Janika, Janike, Janis, Janisa,
Janisah, Janise, Janitz, Janitza,
Janizzetta, Janizzette, Janneece,
Janneice, Janniece Jannice, Jannik,
Jannika, Jannike, Jannique, Jannis,
Jannisa, Jannisah, Jannise, Jannyc,
Jannyca, Jannyce, Jannys, Jannysa,
Jannysah, Jannyse, Janyce, Janys,
Janysa, Janysah, Janyse, Jynice

Janika (Slavic/Hebrew) God is
gracious. A form of Jane.
Janeca, Janecka, Janeeca, Janeeka,
Janeica, Janeika, Jeneka, Janica,
Janick, Janicka, Janieka, Janikka,
Janikke, Janiqua, Janiquah,
Janique, Janka, Janyca, Janycah,
Janyck, Janycka, Janyk, Janyka,
Janyqua, Janyquah, Janyque,
Jenica, Jenicah, Jenicka, Jenika,
Jeniqua, Jeniquah, Jenique,
Jennica, Jennika, Jennyca,
Jennycah, Jennycka, Jennyka,
Jenyca, Jenycah, Jenyka, Jenyqua,
Jenyquah, Jenyque

Janine (French) God is gracious.
Janean, Janeana, Janeane, Janeen,
Janeena, Janeene, Janenan, Janene,
Janeva, Janina (Pol), Janinah,
Janne, Jannene, Jannina, Jannine,
Jannyna, Jannyne, Janyna, Janynah,
Janyne, Jenina, Jeninah, Jenine,
Jenyna, Jenynah, Jenyne

Janique (Hebrew) God is gracious.
A form of Jane.
Janic, Janica, Janicah, Janick,
Janicka, Janickah, Janicqua,
Janicquah, Janicque, Janik, Janika,
Janikah, Janike, Janiqua, Janiquah,
Janyc, Janyca, Janycah, Janycka,
Janyk, Janyka, Janykah, Janyke,
Janyqua, Janyquah, Janyque

Janita (Spanish/Hebrew) God is
gracious. A form of Jane/Juanita.
Janeata, Janeatah, Janeeta,
Janeetah, Janeita, Janeitah, Janitah,
Janitra, Janitza, Janyta, Janytah,
Jeneata, Jeneatah, Jeneeta,
Jeneetah, Jenita, Jenitah, Jennita,
Jennitah, Jennyta, Jenyta, Jenytah,
Juanita

Janna (Arabic) fruit harvest.
Janaia, Janaiah, Janaya, Janaye,
Jannah, Jannaia, Jannaya, Yana
(Slav), Yanah, Yanna, Yannah

Jannali (Australian Aboriginal) moon.
Janalea, Janaleah, Janalee, Janalei, Janaleigh, Janaley, Janali, Janalia, Janaliah, Janalie, Janaly, Jannalea, Jannaleah, Jannalee, Jannalei, Jannaleigh, Jannaley, Jannalia, Jannaliah, Jannalie, Jannaly, Jannalya, Jannalyah

Jany (Hindi) fire.
Janee, Janey, Jani, Janie

Japera (Zimbabwean) complete.
Japerah, Japira, Japirah, Japyra, Japyrah

Japonica (Latin) from Japan; a plant that bears fruit and has red flowers.
Japonicah, Japonicka, Japonika, Japonikah, Japonyca, Japonycah, Japonycka, Japonyka, Japonykah

Jardena (Hebrew) flowing down; descending. A form of Jordan.
Jardan, Jardana, Jardanah, Jardane, Jardania, Jaden, Jardena, Jardene, Jardenia, Jardin, Jardina, Jardinah, Jardine, Jardyn, Jardyna, Jardyne, Jardynia

Jarita (Hindi) legendary bird. (Arab) water jug.
Jareata, Jareatah, Jareet, Jareeta, Jareetah, Jareita, Jareitah, Jaria, Jariah, Jarica, Jarida, Jarietta, Jariette, Jarika, Jarina, Jarinah, Jaritta, Jaritte, Jaritza, Jarixa, Jarnita, Jarnite, Jarrika, Jarrike, Jarrina, Jarrine, Jaryta, Jarytah, Jaryte, Jarytta, Jarytte

Jarka (Czech) spring time.
Jarkah

Jarmilla (Slavic) spring.
Jarmila, Jarmilah, Jarmile, Jarmill, Jarmille, Jarmyla, Jarmylah, Jarmyle, Jarmyll, Jarmylla, Jarmyllah, Jarmylle

Jarnila (Arabic) beautiful.
Jarnilah, Jarnile, Jarnill, Jarnilla, Jarnillah, Jarnille, Jarnyl, Jarnyla, Jarnylah, Jarnyle, Jarnyll, Jarnylla, Jarnyllah, Jarnylle

Jarvia (Teutonic) keen like a spear.
Jarviah, Jarvya, Jarvyah

Jarvinia (German) intelligent; keen.
Jarviniah, Jarvinya, Jarvinyah, Jarvynya, Jarvynyah

Jasia (Hebrew/Polish) God is gracious. A form of Jane.
Jasha, Jashae, Jashala, Jashale, Jashona, Jashone, Jashonta, Jashonte, Jasya, Jasyah, Jazia, Jaziah, Jazya, Jazyah, Jazzia, Jazziah, Jazzya, Jazzyah

Jasmina/Jasmine (Persian) fragrant flower; the jasmine flower. A form of Jasmine.
Jasminah, Jasmine, Jasmyn, Jasmyna, Jasmynah, Jasmyne, Jazmin, Jazmina, Jazminah, Jazmine, Jazmyn, Jazmyna, Jazmynah, Jazmyne, Jazzmin, Jazzmin, Jazzmina, Jazzminah, Jazzmine, Jazzmyn, Jazzmyna, Jazzmynah, Jazzmyne, Jesmin, Jesmina, Jesminah, Jesmine, Jesmyn, Jesmyna, Jesmynah, Jesmyne, Jessmin, Jessmina, Jessminah, Jessmine, Jessmyn, Jessmyna, Jessmynah, Jessmyne, Jezmin, Jezmina, Jezminah, Jezmine, Jezzmin, Jezzmina, Jezzminah, Jezzmine, Jezzmyn, Jezzmyna, Jezzmynah, Jezzmyne

Jasper (English) gem stone. (Pers) guardian of the treasure.
Jaspa, Jaspah, Jaspera, Jaspere

Jaspreet (Punjabi) virtue.
Jasparit, Jasparita, Jasparite, Jasprit, Jasprita, Jasprite, Jaspryta, Jasprytah, Jaspryte

Jassi (Persian) jasmine flower. The short form of Jasmine.
Jas, Jasee, Jasey, Jasi, Jasie, Jassee, Jassey, Jassie, Jassy, Jasy, Jazee, Jazey, Jazi, Jazie, Jazy, Jazzee, Jazzey, Jazzi, Jazzie, Jazzy

Jatara (Hebrew) God is gracious. (Ir) from the rocky hill.
Jatarah, Jataria, Jatariah, Jatarra, Jatarrah, Jattaria, Jatori, Jatoria, Jatoriah, Jatorie, Jatory, Jatorya, Jatoryah

Javana (Malayan/Old English) graceful one from Java.
Javanah, Javanna, Javannah, Javanne, Javvania, Javon, Javona, Javonah, Javonia, Javonn, Javonna, Javonnah, Javonne, Javonnia, Javonniah, Javonya, Javonyah, Jawana, Jawanna, Jawn

Javiera (Spanish) new house owner.
Javeera, Javeerah, Javierah, Javyra, Javyrah

Jay (French) jaybird; one who chatters.
Jae, Jah, Jaha, Jai, Jaia, Jaiah, Jaya, Jayah, Jaye

Jaya (Hindi) victorious.
Jaea, Jaha, Jaia, Jaiah, Jayah

Jaylene (English) the blue jay bird.
Jaeleen, Jaeleena, Jaeleenah, Jaeleene, Jaelen, Jaelena, Jaelenah, Jaelene, Jaileen, Jaileena, Jaileenah, Jaileene, Jailen, Jailena, Jailenah, Jaillene, Jayleen, Jayleena, Jayleenah, Jayleene, Jaylena, Jaylenah

Jayna (Hebrew) God is gracious.
Jaena, Jaenah, Jaina, Jainah, Jaynae, Jaynah, Jaynay

Jayne (Sanskrit) victorious. (Heb) God is gracious.
Jaan, Jaana, Jaanah, Jaane, Jaen, Jaena, Jaene, Jaeen, Jaeena, Jaeene, Jain, Jaina, Jainah, Jaine, Jayn, Jayna, Jaynee, Jayni, Jaynie, Jaynita, Jaynite, Jaynitta, Jaynitte, Jaynn, Jaynna, Jaynnah, Jaynne

Jazlyn (Persian/Welsh) from the jasmine flowers near the pool.
Jazlean, Jazleana, Jazleanah, Jazleane, Jazleen, Jazleena, Jazleenah, Jazleene, Jazlin, Jazlina, Jazlinah, Jazline, Jazlyna, Jazlynah, Jazlyne, Jazlynn, Jazlynna, Jazlynnah, Jazlynne, Jazzleen, Jazzleena, Jazzleene, Jazzlin, Jazzlina, Jazzlinah, Jazzline, Jazzlyn, Jazzlyna, Jazzlynah, Jazzlyne, Jazzlynn, Jazzlynna, Jazzlynne

Jazz (English) lover of jazz music.
Jaz, Jazee, Jazey, Jazi, Jazie, Jazy, Jazzee, Jazzey, Jazzi, Jazzie, Jazzy

Jean (French) God is gracious. The feminine form of John.
Gean, Geana, Geanah, Geane, Geen, Geena, Geenee, Geenia, Genni, Gennie, Genny, Gina, Ginah, Gyn, Gyna, Gynah, Jeana, Jeancie, Jeane, Jeanee, Jeaneen, Jeanetta, Jeanette, Jeani, Jeanie, Jeanina, Jeanine, Jeanetta, Jeanette, Jeanetton (Fren), Jeann, Jeanna, Jeannah, Jeanne (Fren), Jeannine, Jeano, Jeany, Jeen, Jeena, Jeene, Jeenia, Jehan, Jenela, Jenelah, Jenele, Jenell, Jenella, Jenellah, Jenelle

Jeanette (French) God is gracious.
Janeat, Janeata, Janeatah, Janeate, Janeatt, Janeatta, Janeattah, Janeatte, Janeet, Janeeta, Janeetah, Janeete, Janet, Janeta, Janetah, Janete, Janett, Janetta, Janettah, Janette, Jeanet, Jeaneta, Jeanetah, Jeanete, Jeanett, Jeanetta, Jeanettah, Jenet, Jeneta, Jenetah, Jenete,

Jeanette cont.
Jenett, Jenetta, Jenettah, Jenette,
Jinet, Jineta, Jinetah, Jinete, Jinett,
Jinetta, Jinettah, Jinette, Jonet,
Joneta, Jonetah, Jonete, Jonett,
Jonetta, Jonettah, jonette, Jynet,
Jyneta, Jynetah, Jynete, Jynett,
Jynetta, Jynettah, Jynette

Jedda (Australian Aboriginal)
beautiful girl.
Jeda, Jedah, Jeddah

Jelena (Russian) shining light. A
form of Helen.
Jalaina, Jalaine, Jalana, Jalane,
Jalanna, Jalanne, Jalayna, Jalayne,
Jalean, Jaleana, Jaleanah, Jaleane,
Jaleen, Jaleena, Jaleenah, Jaleene,
Jalenah, Jalene, Jalaina, Jalainah,
Jalaine, Jalin, Jalina, Jalinah, Jaline,
Jalyn, Jalyna, Jalynah, Jalyne,
Jelana, Jelanah, Jelane, Jelean,
Jeleana, Jeleanah, Jeleane, Jeleen,
Jeleena, Jeleenah, Jeleene, Jelenah,
Jelene, Jelyn, Jelyna, Jelynah, Jelyne

Jem/Jemma (English) little gem.
Gem, Gema, Gemah, Gemia,
Gemiah, Gemma, Gemmah,
Gemmia, Gemmiah, Gemmya,
Gemmyah, Jem, Jema, Jemah,
Jemia, Jemm, Jemmah, Jemmia,
Jemmya, Jemmyah

Jemima (Hebrew) dove of peace.
Gemima, Gemma, Gemimah,
Jamim, Jamima, Jemimah, Jemma,
Jemmah, Jemmia, Jemmiah,
Jemyma, Jemymah, Yemina,
Yeminah, Yemyna, Yemynah

Jemina (Hebrew/Czech) gem child
of the earth.
Jeminah, Jemyna, Jemynah

Jena (Arabic) small bird.
Jenae, Jenah, Jenai, Jenal, Jenay,
Jenia, Jeniah, Jenya, Jenyah

Jendan (Zimbabwean) to give
thanks.
Jenden, Jendin, Jendon, Jendyn

Jendaya (Zimbabwean) thankful.
Jenda, Jendaia, Jendaiah, Jendaya,
Jendayah

Jenelia (Welsh/Old English) from
the white meadow.
Jenalea, Jenaleah, Jenalee, Jenalei,
Jenaleigh, Jenaley, Jenali, Jenalia,
Jenaliah, Jenalie, Jenelea, Jeneleah,
Jenelee, Jenelei, Jeneleigh, Jeneli,
Jeneliah, Jenelie, Jenelly, Jenely,
Jenilea, Jenileah, Jenilee, Jenilei,
Jenileigh, Jenili, Jenilia, Jeniliah,
Jennelea, Jenneleah, Jennelei,
Jenneleigh, Jennilea, Jennileah,
Jennileigh, Jenniley, Jennili,
Jennilia, jenniliah, Jennilie, Jennily,
Jennylea, Jennyleah, Jennylee,
Jennylei, Jennyleigh, Jennyley,
Jennyli, Jennylia, Jennyliah,
Jennylie, Jennyly, Jenylea, Jenyleah,
Jenylee, Jenylei, Jennyleigh, Jenyley,
Jenyli, Jenylia, Jenyliah, Jenylie,
Jenyly

Jenelle (English) to give in.
(Fren) she is the white wave.
Jenel, Jenele, Jenell, Jennel,
Jennele, Jennell, Jennelle

Jenice (Hebrew) God is gracious.
Jenice, Jenicee, Jenicy, Jenika,
Jenikah, Jeniqua, Jeniquah,
Jenique, Jenise, Jennica, Jennika,
Jenniqua, Jenniquah, Jennique,
Jennise, Jennyca, Jennyce, Jennyka,
Jenniqua, Jenniquah, Jennyque,
Jennyse

Jenilee (Welsh) white wave from the
meadow.
Jenalea, Jenaleah, Jenalee, Jenalei,
Jenaleigh, Jenaley, Jenali, Jenalia,
Jenaliah, Jenalie, Jenelea, Jeneleah,
Jenelee, Jenelei, Jeneleigh, Jeneli,

J

Jenelia, Jeneliah, Jenelie, Jenelly, Jenely, Jenilea, Jenileah, Jenilee, Jenilei, Jenileigh, Jenili, Jenilia, Jeniliah, Jennelea, Jenneleah, Jennelei, Jenneleigh, Jennilea, Jennileah, Jennileigh, Jenniley, Jennili, Jennilia, Jenniliah, Jennilie, Jennily, Jennylea, Jennyleah, Jennylee, Jennylei, Jennyleigh, Jennyley, Jennyli, Jennylia, Jennyliah, Jennylie, Jennyly, Jenylea, Jenyleah, Jenylee, Jenylei, Jennyleigh, Jenyley, Jenyli, Jenylia, Jenyliah, Jenylie, Jenyly

Jenna (Welsh) fair; white-haired.
Gena, Genah, Genna, Gennah, Jena, Jenah, Jennah

Jennalyn (English) white wave in the pool; fair one from the pool.
Jenalin, Jenalyn, Jennalin

Jennica (English) God is gracious.
Jenica, Jenicah, Jenicka, Jenickah, Jennicah, Jennicka, Jennickah, Jennika, Jennikah, Jennyca, Jennycah, Jennycka, Jennyckah, Jennyka, Jennykah, Jenyca, Jenycah

Jennifer (Cornish) white wave; fair-haired.
Ganor, Gaynor, Gennifer, Ginevra, Guenevere, Gwyneth, Jenafar, Jenafer, Jeneffar, Jenaffer, Jenava, Jenavah, Jenefar, Jenefer, Jenifar, Jenifer, Jennafar, Jennafer, Jennefar, Jennefer, Jennelle, Jennifar, Jenniful, Jennilea, Jennileah, Jennilee, Jennileigh, Jenniva, Jennivah, Jennyfar, Jennyfer, Jenyfar, Jenyfer

Jenny (Welsh) white. The short form of Jennifer.
Genee, Geni, Genie, Gennee, Genney, Genni, Gennie, Genny, Geny, Jenee, Jeni, Jenia, Jeniah, Jenie, Jennee, Jenney, Jenni, Jennia,
Jenniah, Jennie, Jennya, Jennyah, Jeny, Jenya, Jenyah

Jeraldine (German) brave spear carrier. The feminine form of Jerald/Gerald.
Geraldina, Geraldinah, Geraldine, Geraldeen, Geraldeena, Geraldeene, Geraldyn, Gealdyna, Geraldyne, Jeraldeen, Jeraldeena, Jeraldeene, Jeraldena, Jeraldene, Jeraldin, Jeraldina, Jeraldinah, Jeraldine, Jeraldyna, Jeraldynah, Jeraldyne

Jeremia (Hebrew) chosen by God. The feminine form of Jeremiah.
Jeramia, Jeramiah, Jeramya, Jeramyah, Jeremiah, Jeremya, Jeremyah

Jereni (Russian/Greek) peaceful.
Jerenee, Jerenia, Jereniah, Jerenie, Jereny, Jerenya, Jerenyah

Jeri (German) brave spear carrier. The short form of Jeraldine.
Geree, Gerey, Geri, Gerie, Gerree, Gerrey, Gerri, Gerrie, Gerry, Jeree, Jerey, Jerie, Jerree, Jerrey, Jerri, Jerrie, Jerry, Jery

Jerica (German/Scandinavian) mighty warrior ruler.
Jericah, Jericka, Jerika, Jerikah, Jeriqua, Jeriquah, Jeryca, Jerycah, Jerycka, Jeryka, Jerykah, Jeryqua, Jeryquah

Jerilyn (German/Welsh) brave spear carrier from the pool.
Jeralin, Jeralina, Jeralinah, Jeraline, Jeralyn, Jeralyna, Jeralynah, Jeralyne, Jerilina, Jerilinah, Jeriline, Jerilyn, Jerilyna, Jerilynah, Jerilyne, Jerilynn, Jerilynna, Jerilynnah, Jerilynne, Jerylin, Jerylina, Jerylinah, Jeryline, Jerylyn, Jerylyna, Jerylynah, Jerylyne

Jermaine (French) from Germany.
Germain, Germaina, Germainah,
Germaine, Germayn, Germayna,
Germaynah, Germayne, Jermain,
Jermaina, Jermainah, Jermayn,
Jermayna, Jermaynah, Jermayne

Jeroma (Latin) sacred name, of
God. The feminine form Jerome.
Geroma, Geromah, Jeromah,
Jerometta, Jeromette, Jeronima,
Jeronyma

Jerusha (Hebrew) marriage;
inheritance.
Jerushah, Yerusha

Jessalin (Hebrew/English) wealthy
one from the pool.
Jessalina, Jessalinah, Jessaline,
Jessalyn, Jessalyna, Jessalynah,
Jessalyne, Jessamin, Jessamina,
Jessaminah, Jassamine, Jessamyn,
Jessamyna, Jessamynah, Jessamyne

Jessamine (French/Persian) wealthy;
jasmine flower. A form of
Jasmine.
Jesamin, Jesamina, Jesaminah,
Jesamon, Jesamona, Jesamone,
Jesamyn, Jesamyna, Jesamynah,
Jesamyne, Jessamin, Jessamina,
Jessaminah, Jessamon, Jessamona,
Jessamonah, Jessamone, Jessamy,
Jessamya, Jessamyah, Jessamyn,
Jessamyna, Jessamyne, Jessemin,
Jessemina, Jesseminah, Jessemine,
Jessmin, Jessmina, Jessminah,
Jessmine, Jessmon, Jessmona,
Jessmonah, Jessmone, Jesmy,
Jessmyn, Jessmyna, Jessmynah,
Jessmyne

Jesse (Hebrew) wealthy. The short
form of names starting with 'Jess'
e.g. Jessica.
Jesea, Jese, Jesee, Jesey, Jesi, Jesie,
Jessea, Jessee, Jessey, Jessi, Jessie,
Jessy, Jesy

Jessenia (Arabic) flower.
Jescenia, Jesceniah, Jescenya,
Jescenyah, Jesenia, Jeseniah,
Jesenya, Jesenyah

Jessica (Hebrew) wealthy.
Jesica, Jesicah, Jesicka, Jesika,
Jesikah, Jessaca, Jessah, Jessalin,
Jessalina, Jessaline, Jessalyn,
Jessalynn, Jessca, Jessia, Jessiah,
Jesseca, Jessecah, Jesseka, Jessekah,
Jessia, Jessiah, Jessicah, Jessicca,
Jessicia, Jessicka, Jessieka, Jessika,
Jessikah, Jessiqua, Jessiquah,
Jessique, Jessiya, Jessyca, Jessycka,
Jessyka, Jessyqua, Jessyquah,
Jezeca, Jezecah, Jezecka, Jezeka,
Jezekah, Jezica, Jezicah, Jezicka,
Jezika, Jezikah, Jeziqua, Jeziquah,
Jezyca, Jezycah, Jezycka, Jisica,
Jisicah, Jisicka, Jisika, Jisikah,
Jisiqua, Jisiquah, Jyssica, Jyssicah,
Jyssika, Jyssikah, Jyssica, Jyssicah,
Jyssicka, Jyssika, Jyssikah, Jyssiqua,
Jyssiquah, Jyssyca, Jyssycka, Jyssyka,
Jyssykah, Jysica, Jysicah, Jysicka,
Jysyka, Jysykah, Jysyqua, Jysyquah

Jessie (Hebrew) wealthy. A short
form of Jessica.
Jesea, Jese, Jesey, Jesi, Jesie, Jesse,
Jessea, Jessee, Jessey, Jessi, Jessy,
Jesy

Jesusa (Hebrew) God will help. The
Spanish feminine form of Jesus.
Chuca, Chuchita (Span), Jesusita,
Jesusyta

Jet (English) black-coloured gem
stone.
Jeta, Jetah, Jetia, Jetiah, Jetje, Jett,
Jettah, Jette (Dan), Jetti, Jettia,
Jettiah, Jettie, Jetty, Jettya, Jettyah

Jewel (Old French) precious gem
stone.
Jewal, Jewele, Jewele (Lith), Jewell,
Jewella, Jewelle, Jewellea,

Jewelleah, Jewellee, Jewelei,
Jeweleigh, Jeweli, Jewelia, Jeweliah,
Jewelie, Jewely, Juel, Juela, Juele,
Juelea, Jueleah, Juelee, Juelei,
Jueleigh, Jueli, Juelie, Juely, Julea,
Juleah, Julee, Julei, Juleigh, Juli,
Julie, July

Jewelana (English/Hebrew)
precious, graceful gem stone.
Jewelanah, Juelana, Juelanah,
Julana, Julanah

Jezebel (Hebrew) wicked.
(Heb/Span) wealthy; beautiful.
Jesabel, Jesabelah, Jesabele,
Jesabell, Jesabella, Jessabellah,
Jessabelle, Jessabel, Jessabela,
Jessabelah, Jessabele, Jessabell,
Jessabella, Jessabellah, Jessabelle,
Jessebel, Jessebela, Jessebelah,
Jessebele, Jessebell, Jessebella,
Jessebellah, Jessebelle, Jezabel,
Jezabela, Jezabelah, Jezabele,
Jezabell, Jezabella, Jezabellah,
Jezabelle, Jezebel, Jezebela,
Jezebelah, Jezebele, Jezebell,
Jezebella, Jezebellah, Jezebelle,
Jezel, Jezela, Jezelah, Jezele, Jezell,
Jezella, Jezellah, Jezelle

Jiana (American/English) graceful.
Jianah, Jianna, Jiannah, Jyana,
Jyanah, Jyanna, Jyannah

Jiba (Australian Aboriginal) moon.
Jibah, Jibba, Jibbah, Jyba, Jybah,
Jybba, Jybbah

Jibon (Hebrew) life.
Jibona, Jibonah, Jibone, Jybon,
Jybona, Jybonah, Jybone

Jill (English/Latin) youthful.
Gill, Gillian, Gyl, Gyll, Jilietta,
Jiliette, Jillana, Jillann, Jillanna,
Jillanne, Jilliana, Jilliann, Jillianna,
Jillianah, Jyl, Jyll, Jyllana, Jyllanah,
Jyllane, Jyllann, Jyllanna,
Jyllannah, Jyllanne

Jillaine (Latin) youthful.
Jilain, Jilaina, Jilaine, Jilan, Jilana,
Jilane, Jillain, Jillaina, Jillann,
Jillanna, Jillanne, Jillayn, Jillayna,
Jillayne, Jylain, Jylaina, Jylaine,
Jylan, Jylana, Jylane, Jyllain,
Jyllaina, Jyllann, Jyllanna, Jyllanne,
Jyllayn, Jyllayna, Jyllayne

Jilli (Australian Aboriginal) today.
Jilea, Jilea, Jileah, Jilee, Jilei, Jileigh,
Jili, Jilie, Jillea, Jilleah, Jillee, Jillei,
Jilleigh, Jilley, Jillie, Jilly, Jily, Jylea,
Jyleah, Jylee, Jylei, Jyleigh, Jyli,
Jylie, Jyllea, Jylleah, Jyllee, Jyllei,
Jylleigh, Jylli, Jyllie, Jylly, Jyly

Jillian (Latin) youthful.
Gilian, Giliana, Gilianah, Giliane,
Gillian, Gilliana, Gillianah,
Gilliane, Gillyan, Gillyana,
Gillyanah, Gillyane, Gillyann,
Gillyanna, Gillyannah, Gillyanne,
Gylian, Gyliana, Gylianah,
Gyliane, Gyliann, Gylianna,
Gyliannah, Gylianne, Gyllian,
Gylliana, Gylliannah, Gyllianne,
Gyllyan, Gyllyana, Gyllyanah,
Gyllyane, Jilian, Jiliana, Jilianah,
Jiliane, Jiliann, Jilianna, Jiliannah,
Jilianne, Jilliana, Jilianah, Jilliane,
Jilliann, Jillianna, Jilliannah,
Jillianne, Jillyann, Jillyanna,
Jillyannah, Jillyanne, Jilyan,
Jilyana, Jilyana, Jilyanah, Jilyane,
Jilyann, Jilyanna, Jilyannah,
Jilyanne, Julian, Juliana, Julianah,
Juliane, Juliann, Julianna,
Juliannah, Julianne, Jylian, Jyliana,
Jylianah, Jyliane, Jyliann, Jylianna,
Jyliannah, Jylianne, Jyllian,
Jylliana, Jyllianah, Jylliane,
Jylliann, Jyllianna, Jylliannah,
Jyllianne, Jyllyan, Jyllyana,
Jyllyanah, Jyllyane, Jyllyann,
Jyllyanna, Jyllyannah, Jyllyanne

J

Jimena (Spanish) hearing.
(Heb/Ger/Dut) the strong, little
replacer. The combination of
Jim/Mena.
Jimenah, Jymena, Jymenah

Jimi (Hebrew) replacer. The
feminine form of Jimmy.
Jimee, Jimey, Jimie, Jimmee,
Jimmey, Jimmi, Jimmie, Jimmy,
Jimy, Jymee, Jymey, Jymi, Jymie,
Jymmee, Jymey, Jymi, Jymie,
Jymmee, Jymmey, Jymmi, Jymmie,
Jymmy, Jymy

Jin (Japanese) tender.
Jina, Jinah, Jinee, Jinie, Jinna,
Jinnah, Jinni, Jinnie, Jinny, Jiny,
Jyn, Jyna, Jynah, Jynee, Jynie,
Jynna, Jynnah, Jynni, Jynnie, Jynny,
Jyny

Jina (Greek) farmer. A short form of
Georgina.
Geana, Geanah, Geena, Geenah,
Gina, Ginae, Ginah, Gini, Ginie,
Ginna, Ginnah, Ginni, Ginnie,
Ginny, Giny, Gyna, Gynah, Jeana,
Jeanah, Jeena, Jeenah, Jinae, Jinah,
Jini, Jinie, Jinna, Jinnae, Jinnah,
Jinni, Jinnie, Jinny, Jiny, Jyna,
Jynah

Jinchilla (Australian Aboriginal)
cypress pine tree.
Jinchila, Jinchilah, Jinchillah,
Jinchyla, Jinchylah, Jinchylla,
Jinchyllah, Jynchila, Jynchilah,
Jynchilla, Jynchillah, Jynchyla,
Jynchylah, Jynchylla, Jynchyllah

Jingle (English) to ring lightly.
Gingle, Gyngle, Jyngle

Jinny (Welsh) white wave. A form of
Jenny.
Ginee, Giney, Gini, Ginie, Ginnee,
Ginney, Ginni, Ginnie, Ginny,
Giny, Jinee, Jiney, Jini, Jinie, Jinnee,
Jinney, Jinni, Jinnie, Jynee, Jyney,

Jyni, Jynie, Jynnee, Jynney, Jynni,
Jynnie, Jynny, Jyny

Jinx (Latin) spell.
Ginnx, Ginx, Gynx, Jinnx, Jinnxx,
Jynx, Jynnx, Jynnxx

Jirakee (Australian Aboriginal)
cascade; series of waterfalls over
rocks.
Jirakei, Jirakey, Jiraki, Jirakie, Jiriky,
Jyrakee, Jyrakei, Jyrakey, Jyraki,
Jyrakie, Jyraky

Jirina (Slavic/Greek) farmer. A form
of Georgina.
Jireana, Jireanah, Jireena, Jireenah,
Jirinah, Jiryna, Jirynah, Jyreana,
Jyreanah, Jyreena, Jyreenah, Jyrina,
Jyrinah, Jyryna, Jyrynah

Jivanta (Hindi) creating.
Jivantah, Jyvanta, Jyvantah

Jizelle (German) promise.
Gisel, Gisela, Gisele, Gisella,
Giselle, Gizel, Gizela, Gizele,
Gizell, Gizella, Gizelle, Gyzel,
Gyzela, Gyzelah, Gyzele, Gyzell,
Gyzella, Gyzelle, Jisel, Jisela, Jisele,
Jisell, Jisella, Jizel, Jizela, Jizele,
Jizella, Jyzel, Jyzela, Jyzele, Jyzell,
Jyzella, Jyzelle

Jo (Hebrew) God is gracious. The
short form of names starting with
'Jo' e.g. Joanna.
Jho, Joe, Joee, Joey, Joh

Joakima (Hebrew) God will
establish. The feminine form of
Joachim.
Joakimah

Joan (Hebrew) God is gracious. The
feminine form of John.
Joana, Joanah, Joane, Joanee,
Joaneil, Joanel, Joanela, Joanele,
Joaney, Joani, Joanie, Joann,
Joanna, Joanne, Johanna (Ger),

Jone, Jonella, Jonelle, Jonilla, Jonilee, Jhone, Shona, Shonah

Joanna (Hebrew) God is gracious and graceful.
Janetje, Janka, Jankesika, Joana, Joanah, Joananna, Joananne, Joanka, Jo-ann, Jo-anna, Jo-annah, Jo-anne, Joann, Joannah, Joanne, Joanney, Joayn, Joayna, Joayne, Joenn, Joenna, Joennah, Joenne, Johanina, Johann, Johanna, Johannah, Jovana, Jovanah, Jovanna, Jovannah, Jovanne

Joanne (Hebrew) God is gracious and graceful.
Joan, Joana, Joanah, Joane, Johana, Johanah, Johane, Johann, Johanna, Johannah, Johanne, Joann, Joanna, Joannah, Joeana, Joeanah, Joeane, Joeann, Joeanna, Joeanna, Joeannah, Joeanne, Joen, Joena, Joena, Joenah, Joenn, Joenna, Joennah, Joenne, Johan, Johana, Johanah, Johane, Johann, Johanna, Johannah, Johanne

Joaquina (Hebrew) God establishes.
Joaquinah, Joaquine, Joaquyn, Joaquyna, Joaquynah, Joaquyne

Jobeth (Hebrew) from the house of the gracious God. A combination of Jo/Beth.
Jobetha, Jobethe, Joebeth, Joebetha, Jobethe, Johbeth, Johbetha, Johbethe

Jobina (Hebrew) distressed; afflicted. A feminine form of Job.
Jobeana, Jobeanah, Jobeena, Jobeenah, Jobin, Jobinah, Jobine, Jobyna, Jobynah, Jobyne

Joby (Hebrew) distressed; afflicted. A feminine form of Job.
Jobea, Jobee, Jobey, Jobi, Jobie, Jobin, Jobina, Jobine, Jobit, Jobita, Jobite, Jobitt, Jobitta, Jobitte, Jobrina, Jobrine, Jobya, Jobye, Jobyna, Jobyne

Jocasta (Greek) shining moon. (Ital) light-hearted.
Jocastah

Joccoaa (Latin) witty.
Jocca, Jocoa, Jocoaa

Jocelyn (Latin) joyful. (O/Eng) just.
Jocalin, Jocalina, Jocaline, Jocalyn, Jocelin, Jocelina, Jocalinah, Jocaline, Josalin, Josalina, Josalinah, Josaline, Josalyn, Joselin, Joselina, Joselinah, Joselina, Joseline, Joselyn, Jossalin, Jossalina, Jossalinah, Jossaline, Jossalyn, Joslina, Joslinah, Josline, Joslyn, Joycalin, Joycalina, Jocalinah, Joycaline, Joycalyn, Joysalin, Joysalina, Joysalinah, Joysaline, Joysalyn, Jukundra, Jununda

Jodi/Jodie/Jody (Hebrew) praised; admired. (Lat) playful.
Jode, Jodea, Jodee, Jodett, Jodetta, Jodette, Jodey, Jodia, Jodie, Jodis, Jody, Joedee, Joedey, Joedi, Joedie, Joedy, Johdea, Johdee, Johdey, Johdi, Johdie, Johdy, Jowdea, Jowdee, Jowdey, Jowdi, Jowdie, Jowdy

Johanna (Hebrew) God is gracious. The feminine form of Johann.
Johana, Johanah, Johanna

Joelle (Hebrew) God is willing. The feminine form of Joel.
Joel, Jo-el, Joela, Joelah, Joele, Joelean, Joeleana, Joeleanah, Joeleane, Joeleen, Joeleena, Joeleenah, Joeleene, Joelena, Joelenah, Joelene, Joelin, Joelina, Joelinah, Joeline, Joell, Joella, Joellah, Joellen, Joellena,

Joelle cont.
Joellenah, Joellene, Jowel, Jowela,
Jowelah, Jowele, Jowell, Jowella,
Jowellah, Jowelle

Johnna (Hebrew) God is gracious. A
feminine form of John.
Jahna, Jahnaia, Jahnaya, Jhona,
Jhonna, Jianna, Jianni, Jiannini,
Johna, Johnda, Johneatha,
Johnetta, Johnette, Johni, Johnica,
Johnie, Johnika, Johnique, Johnita,
Johnitta, Johnittia, Johnnessa,
Johnni, Johnnie, Johnnielynn,
Johnnqua, Johnnquia, Johnnquiah

Joia (French) happy.
Joiah, Joya, Joyah

Jokia (Swahili) beautiful robe.
Jokia, Jokya, Jokyah

Jolan (Hungarian) the violet flower;
violet colour.
Jolana, Jolanah, Joalane, Jolanee,
Jolaney, Jolani, Jolania, Jolaniah,
Jolanie, Jolany, Jolanya, Jolanyah

Jolanda (Greek) hyacinth; purple. A
form of Yolanda.
Jolan, Jolana, Jolanah, Jolanca,
Joland, Jolande, Jolander, Jolania,
Jolanka, Jolankia, Jolanta, Jolante,
Jolantha, Jolanthe, Yoland,
Yolanda, Yolande

Jolena (French) pretty.
Jolean, Joleana, Joleanah, Joleane,
Joleen, Joleena, Joleenah, Joleene,
Jolin, Jolina, Jolinah, Joline, Jolyn,
Jolyna, Jolynah, Jolyne

Jolene (Hebrew) God increases.
Jolaina, Jolaine, Jolana, Jolane,
Jolanna, Jolanne, Jolanta, Jolante,
Jolean, Joleana, Joleane, Joleen,
Joleena, Joleene, Jolena, Jolenna,
Jolenne, Jolin, Jolina, Joline,
Jolleen, Jolleena, Jolleene, Jollin,
Jollina, Jolline, Jollyn, Jollyna,

Jollynah, Jollyne, Jolyn, Jolyna,
Jolynah, Jolyane, Jolyann,
Jolyanna, Jolyannah, Jolyanne

Jolie (Middle English) high-spirited.
(Fren) pretty.
Jole, Jolea, Joleah, Jolee, Jolei,
Joleigh, Jolena, Jolenah, Jolene,
Joley, Jolina, Jolinah, Jolinda,
Joline, Jolli, Jollea, Jolleah, Jollei,
Jolleigh, Jollie, Jollina, Jollinah,
Jollinda, Jolline, Jolly, Joly, Jolye

Joline (Hebrew) God has added a
child. A feminine form of Joseph.
Jolaina, Jolainah, Jolaine, Jolana,
Jolane, Jolanna, Jolannah, Jolanne,
Jolanta, Jolantah, Jolante, Jolean,
Joleana, Joleanah, Joleane, Joleen,
Joleena, Joleenah, Joleene, Jolena,
Jolenah, Jolene, Jolenna, Jolennah,
Jolenne, Jolin, Jolina, Jolinah,
Joline, Jollean, Jolleana, Jolleanah,
Jolleane, Jolleen, Jolleena, Jolleene,
Jollin, Jollina, Jollinah, Jollyn,
Jollyna, Jollynah, Jollyne, Jolyn,
Jolyna, Jolynah, Jolyane, Jolyann,
Jolyanna, Jolyannah, Jolyanne

Jonelle (Hebrew/French) she is
gracious to God. A combination
of Jon/Elle.
Johnel, Johnela, Johnele, Johnell,
Johnella, Johnelle, Jonel, Jonela,
Jonelah, Jonele, Jonell, Jonella

Joni (Hebrew) God is gracious.
Jona, Jonae, Jonah, Jonae, Jonai,
Jonati, Jonatie, Jonaty, Joncee,
Jonci, Joncie, Jonee, Joneeka,
Joneen, Joneena, Joneika, Joneisha,
Jonella, Jonelle, Jonessa, Jonetia,
Jonetta, Jonette, Joney, Jonie, Jonia,
Joniah, Jonica, Jonicah, Jonika,
Jonilee, Jonina, Joninah, Jonine,
Joniqua, Jonique, Jonis, Jonisa,
Jonise, Jonisha, Jonishah, Jonit,
Jonita, Jonite, Jony

J

Jonina (Hebrew) dove.
Jona, Jonah, Jonae, Jonai, Joneen, Joneena, Joneene, Jonika, Joniqua, Jonique, Jonit, Jonita, Jonite, Jonyna, Jonynah, Yoneena, Yoneene, Yonina, Yoninah, Yonine, Yonyna, Yonynah

Jonita (Latin) happy. (Heb) peace.
Jonatee, Jonatey, Jonati, Jonatie, Joneata, Joneatah, Joneeta, Joneetah, Jonit, Jonita, Jonitae, Jonitah, Jontai, Jontaia, Jontaya, Jontaye, Jonita, Jonite, Jonyta, Jonytah

Jonna (English) God is gracious. The feminine form of Jon.
Jonnah

Jonquil (Latin/English) fragrant yellow flower; the colour yellow.
Jonquila, Jonquile, Jonquill, Jonquilla, Jonquille, Jonquyl, Jonquyla, Jonquylah, Jonquyle, Jonquyll, Jonquylla, Jonquyllah, Jonquylle

Jontel (Hebrew) God is gracious. A feminine form of John.
Jontaia, Jontaya, Jontel, Jontela, Jontele, Jontell, Jontella, Jontelle, Jontia, Jontiah, Jontila, Jontricia, Jontrice

Jora (Hebrew) child born at the time of the autumn/fall rains.
Jorah, Joree, Jorey, Jori, Joria, Joriah, Joriana, Jorianah, Joriane, Joriann, Jorianna, Joriannah, Jorianne, Jorie, Jory, Joryana, Joryanah, Joryane, Joryann, Joryanna, Joryanne

Jordan (Hebrew) flowing down; descending. A feminine form of Jordan.
Jorda, Jordah, Jordain, Jordaina, Jordaine, Jordana, Jordane, Jordann, Jordanna, Jordanne, Jordayn, Jordayna, Jordayne, Jorden, Jordena, Jordene, Jordenn, Jordenna, Jordenne, Jordin, Jordina, Jordine, jordinn, Jordinna, Jordinne, Jordon, Jordona, Jordone, Jordonn, Jordonna, Jordonne, Jordyn, Jordyna, Jordyne, Jordynn, Jordynna, Jordynne

Jorja (Greek) farmer. A form of Georgia.
Georga, Georgah, Georgan, Georgana, Georgane, Georgia, Georgina, Jorga, Jorgah, Jorgan, Jorgana, Jorgane, Jorgi, Jorgia, Jorjiah, Jorgie, Jorgina, Jorgine, Jorjan, Jorjana, Jorjanah, Jorjane, Jorjia, Jorjiah, Jorjina, Jorjya, Jorjyah

Josea/Josee (French) God will increase; God has added a little child. A feminine form of Joseph.
Joesee, Joesell, Joesella, Joeselle, Joesetta, Joesette, Joesey, Josee, Josel, Josela, Josele, Josell, Josella, Joselle, Joset, Joseta, Josete, Josett, Josetta, Josette, Josey, Josi, Josia, Josiah, Josian, Josiana, Josiane, Josiann, Josianna, Josianne, Josie, Josielin, Joelina, Joseline, Josina, Josinah, Josine, Josinee, Josy, Josyn, Josyna, Josyne, Jozan, Jozana, Jozane, Joze, Jozee, Jozey, Jozi, Jozian, Joziana, Joziane, Joziann, Jozie, Jozy, Jozyn, Jozyna, Jozyne, Jozze, Jozzee, Jozzey, Jozzi, Jozzie, Jozzy

Josephine (Hebrew) God will increase; God had added a child. A feminine form of Joseph.
Fifine (Fren), Giuseppina (Ital), Josaffina, Josaffine, Josaphina, Josaphine, Josefa (Span), Josefena, Josepha (Ger), Josepha, Josephe, Josephena, Josephene, Josephin,

Josephine cont.
Josephina, Josephiney, Josephyn,
Josephyna, Josett, Josetta, Josette,
Jozafin, Jozafina, Jozafine,
Jozapata, Jozaphin, Jozaphina,
Jozaphinah, Jozaphine, Jozaphyn,
Jozaphyna, Jozaphynah,
Jozaphyne, Jozefa, Jozefin,
Jozefina, Jozefinah, Jozefine,
Jozephin, Jozephina, Jozephinah,
Jozephine, Jozephyn, Jozephyna,
Jozephynah, Jozephyne

Josette (French) God has added a
little child.
Joset, Joseta, Josetah, Josete, Josett,
Josetta, Josettah, Josit, Josita, Jositah,
Josite, Jositt, Jositta, Josittah, Jositte,
Josyt, Josyta, Josytah, Josyte, Josytt,
Josytta, Josyttah, Josytte, Jozet,
Jozeta, Jozetah, Jozete, Jozett,
Jozetta, Jozettah, Jozette

Joshalin (Hebrew) God is my
salvation. (Eng) from Josh's pool;
from the pool of salvation. The
feminine form of Joshua.
Jesua, Jesuah, Joshalin, Joshalina,
Joshlinah, Joshaline, Joshan,
Joshana, Joshanah, Joshann,
Joshanna, Joshannah, Joshanne,
Joshel, Joshela, Joshelah, Joshele,
Joshell, Joshella, Joshellah, Joshelle,
Joshet, Josheta, Joshetah, Joshete,
Joshett, Joshetta, Joshettah,
Joshette, Joshlean, Joshleana,
Joshleanah, Joshleane, Joshleen,
Joshleena, Joshleenah, Joshleene,
Joshlin, Joshlina, Joshlinah,
Joshline, Joshlyna, Joshlynah,
Joshlyne, Joshlynn, Joshlynna,
Joshlynnah, Joshlynne

Josie (French) God will increase;
God has added a little child.
Joesee, Joesell, Joesella, Joeselle,
Joesetta, Joesette, Joesey, Josea,
Josee, Josel, Josela, Josele, Josell,

Josella, Joselle, Joset, Joseta, Josete,
Josett, Josetta, Josette, Josey, Josi,
Josia, Josiah, Josian, Josiana,
Josiane, Josiann, Josianna,
Josianne, Josielin, Joelina, Joseline,
Josina, Josinah, Josine, Josinee,
Josy, Josyn, Josyna, Josyne, Jozan,
Jozana, Jozane, Joze, Jozee, Jozey,
Jozi, Jozian, Joziana, Joziane,
Joziann, Jozie, Jozy, Jozyn, Jozyna,
Jozyne, Jozze, Jozzee, Jozzey, Jozzi,
Jozzie, Jozzy

Jovanna (Latin) love; majestic. The
Slavic/English feminine form of
John, God is gracious.
Jovan, Jovana, Jovanah, Jovane,
Jovanee, Jovaney, Jovani, Jovania,
Jovaniah, Jovanie, Jovann,
Jovannah, Jovanne, Jovannee,
Jovanney, Jovanni, Jovannia,
Jovanniah, Jovannie, Jovanny,
Jovany, Jovian, Joviana, Jovianah,
Joviane, Joviann, Jovianna,
Joviannah, Jovianne, Jovon,
Jovona, Jovonah, Jovone, Jovonn,
Jovonna, Jovonne, Jovyan, Jovyana,
Jovyanah, Jovyane, Jovyann,
Jovyanna, Jovyannah, Jovyanne

Jovi (Latin) joyful.
Jovee, Jovey, Jovia, Joviah, Jovian,
Joviana, Jovianah, Joviane, Joviann,
Jovianna, Joviannah, Jovianne,
Jovie, Jovy, Jovya, Jovyah

Jovita (Latin) joyful.
Jovena, Jovenah, Jovenia, Joveniah,
Jovet, Joveta, Jovete, Jovett, Jovetta,
Jovette, Jovida, Jovidah, Jovina,
Jovinah, Jovine, Jovit, Jovita,
Jovitah, Jovite, Jovitt, Jovitta,
Jovitte, Jovyn, Jovyna, Jovynah,
Jovyne, Jovyta, Jovytah, Jovyte,
Jovytt, Jovytta, Jovyttah, Jovytte

Joy (Latin) joyful.
Joi, Joia, Joiah, Joya, Joyah

J

Joyanna (English) joyful grace.
Joian, Joiana, Joianah, Joiane, Joiann, Joianna, Joiannah, Joianne, Joyan, Joyana, Joyanah, Joyane, Joyann, Joyannah, Joyanne

Joyce (French) joyful.
Jocea, Joia, Joiah, Joice, Joise, Joya, Joycee, Joycelin, Joycelina, Joycelinah, Joyceline, Joycelyn, Joycelyna, Joycelynah, Joycelyne, Joycey, Joycia, Joyciah, Joyse, Joyous, Joyse

Joyita (Spanish) jewel.
Joyitah

Joylyn (English) archer from the pool.
Joialin, Joialina, Joialinah, Joialine, Joialyn, Joialyna, Joialyne, Joilin, Joilina, Joilinah, Joiline, Joilyn, Joilyna, Joilyne, Joylin, Joylina, Joylinah, Joyline, Joylyna, Joylyna, Joylynah, Joylyne

Joyous (Latin) bringer of joy and happiness.
Joious

Juana (Spanish) God is gracious.
Juanah, Juanna, Juannah

Juanita (Spanish) God is gracious. A feminine form of Juan/John.
Anita, Juana, Juanah, Juandalin, Juandalina, Juandalyn, Juandalyna, Juandalyne, Juaneice, Juanequa, Juaneque, Juanesha, Juanice, Juanicia, Juaniqua, Juanique, Juanisha, Juanishia, Juanna

Jubilee (Latin) celebration of joy in the meadow; child born on an anniversary.
Jubilea, Julbileah, Jubilei, Jubileigh, Jubilia, Jubiliah, Jubilie, Jubily, Jubilya, Jubilyah, Jubylea, Jubyleah, Jubylee, Jubylei, Jubyleigh, Jubyley, Jubyli, Jubylia, Jubyliah, Jubylie, Jubyly

Juci (Hungarian/Hebrew) praised. A form of Judy.
Jucee, Jucey, Jucia, Juciah, Jucie, Jucy, Jucya, Jucyah

Jucosa (Latin) playful.
Jucosah

Judith (Hebrew) praised.
Gluditta, Jita, Juczi, Judal, Judana, Judane, Jude, Judeen, Judeena, Judena, Judene, Judett, Judetta, Judette, Judina, Judine, Judit, Judith, Juditha, Judithe, Juditt, Juditta, Juditte, Judyta, Judytt, Judytta, Jujube, Jutka, Jutha, Jytte (Dan)

Judy (Hebrew) praised. The short form of Judith.
Juci (Hung), Jude, Judea, Judee, Judeen, Judeena, Judeenah, Judeene, Judey, Judi, Judian, Judiana, Judiane, Judiann, Judianna, Judiannah, Judianne, Judie, Judin, Judina, Judinah, Judine, Judyn, Judyna, Judynah, Judyne

Juh (Hindi) flower.
Ju

Juju (African) superstition; spell.

Jula (Polish/Latin) youthful. A form of Julia.
Jewpla, Jewlah, Juela, Juelah, Julah, Julca, Julcia, Julia, Juliah, Julie, Juliska, Julka, July, Julya, Julyah

Julene (Basque/Latin) youthful. A form of Julia.
Julean, Juleana, Juleanah, Juleane, Juleen, Juleena, Juleenah, Juleene, Julena, Julenah, Julenia, Juleniah, Juline, Julinca, Julinka, Juliska, Jullean, Julleana, Julleanah, Julleane, Julleen, Julleena,

J

Julene cont.
Julleenah, Julleene, Jullin, Jullina, Jullinah, Julline, Jullyna, Jullynah, Jullyne, Julyna, Julynah, Julyne

Julia/Julie (Latin) youthful. The feminine form of Julius.
Gillot, Giula, Giulia, Giuliana, Giulietta (Ital), Giuliette, Huriana, Iliska, Jewelea, Jeweleah, Jewelee, Jewelei, Jeweleigh, Jewli, Jewelia, Jeweliah, Jewlie, Jewlya, Jewlyah, Jolet, Joleta, Joletah, Jolete, Juelet, Jueleta, Jueletah, Juelete, Juelett, Jueletta, Juelettah, Juelette, Juet, Jueta, Juetah, Juete, Juett, Juetta, Juettah, Juette, Juliah, Juliana, Julianah, Juliane, Juliann, Julianna, Juliannah, Julianne, Julij, Julijana, Julijanah, Julijanna, Julijannah, Julijanne, Julian, Juliana, Julianah, Juliane, Juliann, Julianna, Juliannah, Julianne, Julienn, Julienna, Juliennah, Julienne, Juliet, Julieta (Span), Julietah, Juliete, Juliett, Julietta, Juliettah, Juliette (Fren), Julina, Julinah, Julinda, Julindah, Juline, Julita, Julitah, Julite, Julitta, Julittah, Julitte, Julka, Julya, Julyan, Yuliana, Yulia, Sheila, Sile (Ir), Sileas (Scott), Utili

Juliana (Slavic/Hungarian/Spanish/Latin/Hebrew) youthful grace.
Jewelian, Jeweliana, Jewelianah, Jeweliane, Jewelinann, Jewelianna, Jewelianne, Jewliana, Jewlianah, Jewliane, Jewliann, Jewlianna, Jewlianne, Julian, Juliana (Slav/Hung), Julianah, Juliane, Juliann, Juliannah, Julianne, Juliean, Julieana, Julieanah, Julieane, Julieann, Julieanna, Julieanne, Julyan, Julyana, Julyanah, Julyane, Julyann, Julyanna, Julyannah, Julyanne

Juliet (French/Latin) little youth.
Dawlita, Eliidan, Guilietta, Jewelett, Jeweletta, Jewelette, Jewelit, Jewelieta, Jewliett, Jewelietta, Jeweliette, Jewelyet, Jewelyeta, Jewelyett, Jewelyetta, Jewelyette, Juleata, Juleatah, Juleate, Juleet, Juleeta, Juleetah, Julette, Julet, Juleta, Juletah, Julett, Juletta, Julette, Juliett, Julietta, Juliettah, Juliette, Julit, Julitt, Julitta, Julitte, Julliet, Jullieta, Jullietah, Julliete, Julliett, Jullietta, Julliette, Julyet, Julyeta, Julyetah, Julyete, Julyett, Julyetta, Julyette

July (Latin/English) born in the month of July.
Juli, Julli, Jully

Jumana (Arabic) pearl.
Jumanah

Jun (Chinese) truthful.

Jundah (Australian Aboriginal) woman.
Junda

June (Latin) born in the month of June.
Juin, Juine, Junell, Junella, Junelle, Junett, Junetta, Junette, Juni, Junia, Junie, Juniet, Juniett, Junietta, Juniette, Junill, Junilla, Junille, Junina, Junine, Junn, Junula

Junee (Australian Aboriginal) speaking.
June, Juney, Juni, Junia, Juniah, Junie, Juny

Juniper (Latin/English) the juniper shrub.
Junyper

Juno (Latin) queen of the heavens.

Jupiter (Greek) the planet.
Jupita, Jupitah, Jupitor, Jupyta, Jupytah, Jupyter, Jupytor

Jurisa (Slavic) storm; tempest.
Jurisah, Jurissa, Jurissah, Jurysa,
Jurysah, Juryssa, Juryssah

Justa (Latin) just.
Giustina, Giustine, Justah, Juste,
Justea, Justean, Justeana, Justeane,
Justee, Justeen, Justeena, Justeene,
Justill, Justilla, Justille, Justina,
Justine, Justyn, Justyna, Justynah,
Justyne

Justice (Old French) judge; justice.
Justise, Justyce, Justyse

Justine/Justine (Latin) righteous;
just. The feminine form of Justin.
Giustina, Giustine, Gustina,
Gustinah, Gustine, Gustyn,
Gustyna, Gustynah, Gustyne,
Justah, Juste, Justea, Justean,
Justeana, Justeanah, Justeane,
Justee, Justeen, Justeena, Justeenah,
Justeene, Justein, Justeina,
Justeinah, Justeine, Justeyn,
Justeyna, Justeynah, Justeyne,
Justill, Justilla, Justille, Justinah,
Justine, Justyn, Justyna, Justynah,
Justyne

Jute (Latin) tropical yellow plant.
Jutee

Jutta (Latin) close by.
Juta, Jutah, Juttah

Jyoti (Hindi) light.
Jioti, Jyoty

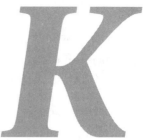

Kaanan (Hindi) forest.
Kanan

Kachine (Native American) sacred
dancer.
Kachin, Kachina, Kachinah,
Kachinee, Kachiney, Kachyn,
Kachyna, Kachynah, Kachyne

Kacie (Irish) vigorous; alert.
Caecea, Caecee, Caecey, Caeci,
Caecia, Caeciah, Caecie, Caecy,
Caesea, Caesee, Caesey, Caesi,
Caesie, Caesy, Caicea, Caicee,
Caicey, Caici, Caicia, Caiciah,
Caicie, Caicy, Caisea, Caisee,
Caisey, Caisi, Caisia, Caisiah,
Caisie, Caisy, Casea, Casee, Casey,
Casi, Casie, Casy, Caycea, Caycee,
Caycey, Cayci, Caycia, Cayciah,
Caycie, Caycy, Caysea, Caysee,
Caysey, Caysi, Caysia, Caysiah,
Caysie, Caysy, Kacey, Kacee,
Kacy, Kacya, Kaecea, Kaecee,
Kaecey, Kaeci, Kaecia, Kaeciah,
Kaecie, Kaecy, Kaesea, Kaesee,
Kaesey, Kaesha, Kaesi, Kaesia,
Kaesiah, Kaesie, Kaesy, Kaicea,
Kaicee, Kaicey, Kaici, Kaicia,
Kaiciah, Kaicie, Kaicy, Kaisea,
Kaisee, Kaisey, Kaisi, Kaisia,
Kaisiah, Kaisie, Kaisy, Kasea, Kasee,
Kasey, Kasi, Kasia, Kasiah, Kasie,
Kasy, Kayce, Kaycea, Kaycee, Kayci,
Kaycia, Kayciah, K.C.

Kadla (Australian Aboriginal) sweet.
Kadlah

Kafu (Tongan) covering.

Kagami (Japanese) mirror;
reflection; looks like her mother.
Kagamee

Kahi (Tongan) shellfish.

Kahoa (Tongan) necklace.
Kahoah

Kahoko (Hawaiian) star.

Kai (Navajo) willow tree. (Haw) sea.
(Jap) to forgive. (Wel) keeper of
keys.
Kia, Kiah, Kya, Kyah

Kaila (Tongan) to call out.
(Isr) victory.
Kaela, Kaelah, Kaelea, Kaeleah,
Kaelee, Kaelei, Kaeleigh, Kaeley,
Kaeli, Kaelia, Kaeliah, Kaelie, Kaely,
Kaila, Kailah, Kailea, Kaileah, Kailee,
Kailei, Kaileigh, Kailey, Kaili, Kailia,
Kailiah, Kailie, Kaily, Kayla, Kaylah,
Kaylea, Kayleah, Kaylee, Kaylei,
Kayleigh, Kayley, Kayli, Kaylia,
Kayliah, Kaylie, Kayly, Kaylya

Kailani (Hawaiian) sky; sea.
Kaelana, Kaelanah, Kaelanea,
Kaelanee, Kaelaney, Kaelani,
Kaelania, Kaelaniah, Kaelanie,
Kaelany, Kaelanya, Kailana,
Kailanah, Kailanea, Kailanee,
Kailaney, Kailania, Kailaniah,
Kailnie, Kailany, Kailanya, Kaylana,
Kaylanah, Kaylanea, Kaylanee,
Kaylaney, Kaylani, Kaylania,
Kaylaniah, Kaylanie, Kaylany,
Kaylanya

Kailmana (Hawaiian) diamond.
Kaemana, Kaemanah, Kaemane,
Kaiman, Kaimanah, Kaimane,
Kayman, Kaymana, Kaymanah,
Kaymane

Kaina (Welsh) beautiful.
(Ir) tribute. (Haw) eastern sky.
The feminine form of Kaine.
Kainah, Kayna, Kaynah

Kainga (Tongan) relative.
Kaingah, Kaynga, Kayngah

Kaisa (Swedish) purity.
Kaisah, Kaysa, Kaysah

Kaitlin (English) from the pure
pool.
Caitlin, Caitlyn, Caytlin, Caytlyn,
Kaitlyn, Kaytlin, Kaytlyn

Kaiyo (Japanese) one who is
forgiven.

Kakaha (Tongan) glowing with
heat.

Kakai (Tongan) people.

Kakala (Tongan) sweet-smelling
flower.
Kakalah

Kakalina (Hawaiian) purity.
Kakalinah, Kakalyna, Kakalynah

Kakalu (Tongan) cicada noise;
whistle.

Kakamika (Tongan) shrub.
Kakamikah

Kakapu (Tongan) misty.

Kakata (Tongan) laughing.
Kakatah

Kakra (Ghanian) second-born twin.
Kakrah

Kal (English) yellow flower.
Kala, Kalah

Kala (Hawaiian) sun. (Hin) black;
time.
Cala, Calah, Calla, Callah, Kalah,
Kalla, Kallah

Kalala (Hawaiian) bright.

Kalama (Hawaiian) flame.

Kalameli (Tongan) caramel.
Kalamelie, Kalamely

Kalana (Hawaiian) flat land.

Kalani (Hawaiian) sky.
Kalan, Kalana, Kalanah, Kalanea,
Kalanee, Kalaney, Kalania,
Kalaniah, Kalanie, Kalona,
Kalonah, Kalonea, Kalonee,
Kaloney, Kaloni, Kalonia,
Kaloniah, Kalonie, Kalony

Kalanit (Hebrew) flower.
Kalan, Kalanyt

Kalasia (Tongan) grace.
Kalasiah, Kalasya, Kalasyah

Kalauka (Hawaiian) famous.

Kalauni (Tongan) crown.
Kalaunea, Kalaunee, Kalauney,
Kalaunia, Kalauniah, Kalaunie,
Kalauny, Kalaunya

Kalavite (Tongan) gravity.
Kalavit, Kalavita, Kalavitah,
Kalavyta, Kalavytah

Kalea (Hawaiian) bright.
Kaleah, Kalee, Kalei, Kaleigh, Kaley,
Kali, Kalie, Kaly

Kalei (Hawaiian) pure one with a
wreath of flowers. (Eng) from the
pure meadow.
Caelea, Caeleah, Caelee, Caelei,
Caeleigh, Caeley, Caeli, Caelia,
Caeliah, Caelie, Caely, Caila,
Cailah, Cailea, Caileah, Cailee,
Cailei, Caileigh, Caili, Cailia,
Cailiah, Cailie, Caily, Cala, Calah,
Calea, Caleah, Calee, Calei,
Caleigh, Caley, Cali, Caliah, Calie,
Caly, Cayla, Caylah, Caylea,
Cayleah, Caylee, Caylei, Cayleigh,
Cayley, Cayli, Caylia, Cayliah,
Caylie, Cayly, Kaela, Kaelah,
Kaelea, Kaeleah, Kaelee, Kaelei,

Kaeleigh, Kaeley, Kaeli, Kaelia,
Kaeliah, Kaelie, Kaely, Kaila,
Kailah, Kailea, Kaileah, Kailee,
Kailei, Kaileigh, Kailey, Kaili, Kailia,
Kailiah, Kailie, Kaily, Kalea, Kaleah,
Kalee, Kaleigh, Kaley, Kali, Kalia,
Kaliah, Kalie, Kaly, Kalya, Kayla,
Kaylah, Kaylea, Kayleah, Kaylee,
Kaylei, Kayleigh, Kayley, Kayli,
Kaylia, Kayliah, Kaylie, Kayly,
Kaylya

Kalepi (Tongan) grape vine.

Kali (Sanskrit) energy. (Haw) one
who hesitates.
Caelea, Caeleah, Caelee, Caelei,
Caeleigh, Caeley, Caeli, Caelia,
Caeliah, Caelie, Caely, Caila,
Cailah, Cailea, Caileah, Cailee,
Cailei, Caileigh, Caili, Cailia,
Cailiah, Cailie, Caily, Cala, Calah,
Calea, Caleah, Calee, Calei,
Caleigh, Caley, Cali, Caliah, Calie,
Caly, Cayla, Caylah, Caylea,
Cayleah, Caylee, Caylei, Cayleigh,
Cayley, Cayli, Caylia, Cayliah,
Caylie, Cayly, Kaela, Kaelah, Kaelea,
Kaeleah, Kaelee, Kaelei, Kaeleigh,
Kaeley, Kaeli, Kaelia, Kaeliah,
Kaelie, Kaely, Kaila, Kailah, Kailea,
Kaileah, Kailee, Kailei, Kaileigh,
Kailey, Kaili, Kailia, Kailiah, Kailie,
Kaily, Kalea, Kaleah, Kalee, Kalei,
Kaleigh, Kaley, Kali, Kalia, Kaliah,
Kalie, Kaly, Kalya, Kayla, Kaylah,
Kaylea, Kayleah, Kaylee, Kaylei,
Kayleigh, Kayley, Kayli, Kaylia,
Kayliah, Kaylie, Kayly, Kaylya

Kalia (Tongan) double canoe.
Kaliah, Kalya, Kalyah

Kalifa (Somalian) holy; sacred.
Califa, Califah, Kalifah

Kalika (Greek) rosebud.
Calica, Calicah, Calicka, Calickah,
Calika, Calikah, Caly, Calyca,

Kalika cont.
Kalica, Kalicah, Kaly, Kalyca, Kalycah, Kalyka, Kalykah

Kalila (Arabic) beloved.
Calila, Calilah, Kalilla, Kalli, Kallila, Kally, Kaylil, Kylila

Kalilinoe (Hawaiian) rain.

Kalina (Polish) flower.
Kalinah, Kalyna, Kalynah

Kalinda (Australian Aboriginal) view. (Sans) sun.
Calinda, Calindah, Calinde, Calynd, Calynda, Calyndah, Calynde, Kaleena, Kalina, Kalinah, Kalindah, Kalindi, Kalindie, Kalindy, Kalynd, Kalynda, Kalynde

Kalinn (Scandinavian) river.
Kalin, Kalyn, Kalynn

Kaliope (Greek) beautiful.
Caliope, Calliope, Kalliope

Kalisitala (Tongan) crystal.
Kalisital, Kalisitalah

Kaliska (Native American) coyote chasing a deer.
Kaliskah, Kalyska, Kalyskah

Kalla (Australian Aboriginal) fiery.
Cala, Calah, Calla, Callah, Kala, Kalah, Kallah

Kallan (Scandinavian) flowing water.
Callan, Callen, Callin, Callon, Callyn, Kallen, Kallin, Kallon, Kallyn

Kallirroe (Greek) beautiful river.

Kallista (Greek) beautiful.
Calista, Calistah, Callista, Callistah, Callistar, Callistarr, Kalista, Kalistah, Kallistar, Kallistara, Kallistarah, Kallistarr, Kallistarra, Kallistarrah

Kallolee (Hindi) happy.
Kallolea, Kalloleah, Kallolei, Kalloleigh, Kalloley, Kalloli, Kallolie, Kalloly

Kaloni (Tongan) perfume.
Kalona, Kalonah, Kalonee, Kaloney, Kalonia, Kaloniah, Kalonie, Kalony, Kalonya, Kalonyah

Kaloti (Tongan) carrot.
Kalot, Kalott, Kalotti

Kalou (Tongan) crow.
Kalu

Kalyan (Australian Aboriginal) to stay near.
Calyan, Calyana, Calyanah, Kalyanah

Kama (Sanskrit) love.
Cama, Camah, Kamah, Kamia, Kamiah, Kamie, Kamlean, Kamleana, Kamleanah, Kamleane, Kamleen, Kamleena, Kamleenah, Kamleene, Kamlin, Kamlina, Kamlinah, Kamline, Kamlyn, Kamlyna, Kamlynah, Kamlyne, Kamma, Kammah, Kammalean, Kammaleana, Kammaleanah, Kammaleane, Kammaleen, Kamaleena, Kammaleenah, Kammaleene, Kammalin, Kammalina, Kammalinah, Kammaline, Kammalyn, Kammalyna, Kammalynah, Kammalyne, Kammalynn, Kammi, Kammia, Kammiah, Kammie, Kammy, Kamy

Kamala (Sanskrit) lotus flower.
Kamalah

Kamali (Zimbabwean) angel of newborn babies.
Kamalea, Kamaleah, Kamalei, Kamaleigh, Kamaley, Kamalie, Kamaly

Kamaria (African) moon.
Kamariah, Kamarya, Kamaryah

Kamata (Native American) throwing bones; fortune; fate.

Kamballa (Australian Aboriginal) young woman.
Kambala, Kambalah, Kamballah

Kame (Japanese) turtle.

Kamea (Hawaiian) only child.
Camea, Cameah, Camee, Camey, Cami, Camia, Camiah, Camie, Camy, Kameah, Kamee, Kamey, Kami, Kamia, Kamiah, Kamie, Kamy, Kamya, Kamyah

Kameko (Japanese) child of the tortoise; child who lives long.
Kameeko, Kamiko, Kamyko

Kameli (Hawaiian) honey.
Kamelia, Kameliah, Kamely, Kamelya, Kamelyah

Kami (Japanese) lord.
Camee, Camia, Camiah, Camie, Camy, Camya, Camyah, Kamee, Kamia, Kamiah, Kamie, Kamy, Kamya, Kamyah

Kamilah (Arabic) perfection.
Camia, Camiah, Camila, Camilah, Camillia, Camillah, Chamelea, Chameleah, Chamelia, Chameliah, Chamika, Chamila, Chamilla, Chamylia, Chamyliah, Chamylla, Chamyllah, Kamila, Kamilia, Kamilla, Kamillah, Kamillia, Kamilliah, Kamillya, Kamilya, Kamyla, Kamylah, Kamylla, Kamyllah

Kamilia (Slavic) sweet flower.
Camia, Camiah, Camila, Camilah, Camillia, Camillah, Chamelea, Chameleah, Chamelia, Chameliah, Chamika, Chamila, Chamilla,

Chamylia, Chamyliah, Chamylla, Chamyllah, Kamila, Kamilah, Kamiliah, Kamilla, Kamillah, Kamillia, Kamilliah, Kamillya, Kamilya, Kamyla, Kamylah, Kamylla, Kamyllah

Kamille (Arabic) perfection.
Camil, Camila (Span), Camilia, Camilla (Ital), Camillah, Cammila, Cammilah, Cammile, Cammill, Cammilla, Cammille, Cammyl, Cammyla, Cammylah, Cammyle, Cammyll, Cammylla, Cammyllah, Cammylle, Kamia, Kamilah, Kamil, Kamile, Kamilla, Kamillah, Kamyl, Kamyle, Kamyll, Kamylle

Kamoana (Hawaiian) ocean.
Kamoanah

Kanali (Tongan) canal.
Kanalia, Kanalie, Kanaly

Kanani (Hawaiian) beautiful.
Kanana, Kananah, Kananea, Kananee, Kanania, Kananiah, Kananie, Kanany, Kananya, Kananyah

Kanda (Kurdish) smile.

Kandelka (Australian Aboriginal) good.
Kandel, Kandelkah

Kaneli (Tongan) canary; yellow.
Kanelea, Kaneleah, Kanelee, Kanelei, Kaneleigh, Kanelia, Kaneliah, Kanelie, Kanely, Kanelya

Kanestie (Seneca) guide; helper.

Kani (Hawaiian) sound.
Canee, Caney, Cani, Canie, Cany, Kanee, Kaney, Kanie, Kany

Kaniva (Tongan) the Milky Way; galaxy.
Kanivah, Kanyva, Kanyvah

Kannitha (Cambodian) angel;
messenger of God.
Kanitha

Kanya (Sanskrit) young girl.
(Hindi) purity.
Kania, Kaniah, Kanja, Kanjah,
Kanya, Kanyah, Kenja, Kenjah,
Kenya, Kenyah

Kaoru (Japanese) strength; perfume.
Kaori

Kapika (Hawaiian) gazelle.

Kara (Australian Aboriginal)
possum. (Turk) black.
Cara, Carah, Carra, Carrah, Kara,
Karah, Karalea, Karaleah, Karalee,
Karalei, Karaleigh, Karaley, Karali,
Karalia, Karaliah, Karalie, Karaly,
Karra, Karrah, Karralea, Karraleah,
Karralee, Karralei, Karraleigh,
Karraley, Karrali, Karralie, Karraly

Karalana (Australian Aboriginal/
English/Greek) possum; light.
Karalain, Karalaina, Karalainah,
Karalaine, Karalanah, Karalane,
Karalayn, Karalayna, Karalaynah,
Karalayne

Karan/Karen (Greek/Australian)
purity.
Caaran, Caran, Caren, Carin,
Caron, Carran, Carren, Carrian,
Carrin, Carrina, Carrine, Carryn,
Carryna, Carrynah, Caryn, Caryna,
Carynah, Kaaran, Kaaren, Kaarin,
Kaaron, Kaarun, Kaaryn, Kara,
Karah, Karean, Kareana, Kareane,
Kareen, Kareena, Kareenah,
Kareene, Karen, Karena, Karenah,
Karene, Karensa, Karensah,
Karensia, Karensiah, Karenza,
Karenzah, Karenzia, Karenziah,
Kari, Karia, Kariah, Karin, Karina,
Karinah, Karine, Karna, Karnah,
Karon, Karona, Karonah, Karone,
Karonia, Karoniah, Karonie,

Karony, Karonya, Karra, Karrah,
Karran, Karrana, Karranah, Karrane,
Karren, Karrena, Karrenah, Karrin,
Karrina, Karrinah, Karrine, Karryn,
Karryna, Karrynah, Karryne, Karyn,
Karyna, Karynah, Karyne

Kareela (Australian Aboriginal)
wind of the south.
Kareala, Karealah, Karealla,
Kareallah, Karela, Karelah, Karella,
Karellah

Karenza (Cornish) affectionate;
loving.
Caranzah, Caranzia, Caranziah,
Carenza, Caranzya, Caranzyah,
Carenzah, Carenzia, Carenziah,
Carenzya, Carenzyah, Karansa,
Karansah, Karansia, Karansiah,
Karanza, Karanzah, Karanzia,
Karanziah, Karanzya, Karanzyah,
Karensa, Karensah, Karensia,
Karensiah, Karenzah, Karenzia,
Karenziah, Karenzya, Karenzyah

Karida (Arabic) purity.
Karidah, Karindah, Karynda,
Karyndah, Karyda, Karydah

Karima (Arabic) generous; noble.
Karim, Karimah, Karyma, Karymah

Karis (Greek) graceful.
Charis, Charisa, Charisah, Chariss,
Charissa, Charissah, Charisse,
Charys, Charysa, Charysah,
Charyss, Charyssa, Charyssah,
Charysse, Karisa, Karisah, Karise,
Kariss, Karissa, Karissah, Karisse,
Karys, Karysa, Karysah, Karyse,
Karyss, Karyssa, Karyssah, Karryse

Karisma (Greek) favourite gift.
Carisma, Carismah, Carismara,
Carismarah, Carismaria,
Carismariah, Carysma, Carysmah,
Carysmara, Carysmarah,
Carysmaria, Carysmariah,
Carysmarya, Karismah, Karismara,

K

Karismarah, Karismaria, Karismaria, Karismariah, Karysma, Karysmah, Karysmara, Karysmarah, Karysmaria, Karysmariah, Karysmarya

Kariss/Karissa (Greek) favourite.
Cares, Caresa, Caresah, Carese, Caress, Caressa, Caressah, Caresse, Cariss, Carissa, Carissah, Carisse, Carys, Carysa, Carysah, Caryss, Caryssa, Caryssah, Carysse, Kares, Karesa, Karesah, Karese, Karess, Karessa, Karessah, Karesse, Karis, Karisa, Karisah, Karise, Karissa, Karissah, Karisse, Karys, Karysa, Karysah, Karyse, Karyss, Karyssa, Karyssah, Karysse

Karla (German) farmer; strong; courageous. The feminine form of Karl.
Carla, Carlah, Carlea, Carleah, Carlee, Carlei, Carleigh, Carli, Carlie, Karlea, Karleah, Karlean, Karleana, Karleanah, Karleane, Karlee, Karleen, Karleena, Karleenah, Karleene, Karlei, Karleigh, Karlein, Karleina, Karleinah, Karleine, Karlen, Karlena, Karlenah, Karlene, Karlesha, Karley, Karleyn, Karleyna, Karleynah, Karleyne, Karlin, Karlina, Karlinah, Karline, Karlyn, Karlyna, Karlynah, Karlyne

Karli (Turkish) covered in snow.
Carlea, Carleah, Carlee, Carlei, Carleigh, Carley, Carli, Carlia, Carliah, Carlie, Carly, Karlea, Karleah, Karlee, Karlei, Karleigh, Karley, Karlia, Karliah, Karlie, Karly

Karma (Sanskrit) destiny; fate.
Carma, Carmah, Carmana, Carmane, Carmarnia, Carmarniah, Karmah, Karmana, Karmane, Karmania, Karmaniah, Karmanya, Karmanyah

Karmel (Hebrew) God's garden; fruitful vineyard.
Carmel, Carmela, Carmelah, Carmele, Carmell, Carmella, Camellah, Carmelle, Carmellia, Camelliah, Karmela, Karmelah, Karmele, Karmell, Karmella, Karmellah, Karmelle, Karmellia, Karmelliah, Karmellya, Karmellyah

Karmiti (Banti) tree.
Karmitee, Karmitey, Karmitie, Karmity, Karmytee, Karmytey, Karmyti, Karmytie, Karmyty

Karniela (Hebrew) horn-coloured; horn blower; cornell tree. A feminine form of Cornelius.
Carneiela, Carniela, Carnielah, Carniele, Carniell, Carniella, Carnielle, Carnyel, Carnyela, Carnyella, Carnyelle, Karniel, Karniela, Karnielah, Karniele, Karniella, Karnielle, Karnyel, Karnyela, Karniell, Karnyella, Karnyelle

Karol (German/Hungarian) farmer; strong; courageous.
Carol, Carola, Carole, Carolin, Carolina, Carolinah, Caroline, Carolyn, Carolyna, Carolynah, Carolyne, Karola, Karole, Karolin, Karolina (Czech), Karolinah, Karoline, Karolyn, Karolyna, Karolynah, Karolyne

Karolina (Hawaiian/French) little woman. A form of Carolina.
Karolainah, Karolayna, Karolaynah

Karri (Australian Aboriginal) eucalyptus tree.
Caree, Carey, Cari, Carie, Carree, Carrey, Carri, Carrie, Carro, Carry, Cary, Karee, Karey, Kari, Karie, Karree, Karrey, Karrie, Karry, Kary

K

Karrin (Australian Aboriginal) evening time.
Caaran, Caran, Caren, Carin, Caron, Carran, Carren, Carrian, Carrin, Carrina, Carrine, Carryn, Carryna, Carrynah, Caryn, Caryna, Carynah, Kaaran, Kaaren, Kaarin, Kaaron, Kaarun, Kaaryn, Kara, Karah, Karan, Karean, Kareana, Kareane, Kareen, Kareena, Kareenah, Kareene, Karen, Karena, Karenah, Karene, Karensa, Karensah, Karensia, Karensiah, Karenza, Karenzah, Karenzia, Karenziah, Kari, Karia, Kariah, Karin, Karina, Karinah, Karine, Karna, Karnah, Karon, Karona, Karonah, Karone, Karonia, Karoniah, Karonie, Karony, Karonya, Karra, Karrah, Karran, Karrana, Karranah, Karrane, Karren, Karrena, Karrenah, Karrina, Karrinah, Karrine, Karryn, Karryna, Karrynah, Karryne, Karyn, Karyna, Karynah, Karyne

Kasimira (Slavic) peace is announced. The feminine form of Casimir.
Casimiera, Casimira, Casimirah, Casmira, Casmirah, Casmyra, Casmyrah, Cazmira, Cazmirah, Cazmyra, Cazmyrah, Kasimiera, Kasimirah, Kasmira, Kasmirah, Kazatimru, Kazmira, Kazmirah, Kazmyra, Kazmyrah

Kasota (Native American) clear sky.
Kasotah

Kassandra (Greek) prophet.
Casandra, Casandrah, Casandria, Casandriah, Casondra, Casondrah, Cassandra, Cassandrah, Cassandria, Cassandriah, Cassondra, Cassondrah, Cazzandra, Kasandra (Span), Kasandrah, Kasondra, Kasondrah, Kassandrah, Kassandria, Kassandriah, Kassondra, Kassondrah, Kasundra, Kasundrah, Kazandra, Kazandrah, Kazandria, Kazandriah, Kazzandra, Kazzandrah, Kazzandria, Kazzandriah, Kazzandrya, Kazzandryah

Kassia (Greek) purity. (Heb) cassia tree.
Casia, Casiah, Cassia, Cassiah, Cassya, Cassyah, Casya, Casyah, Cazia, Caziah, Cazzia, Cazziah, Cazzya, Kasia, Kasiah, Kassiah, Kassya, Kassyah, Kazia, Kaziah, Kazya, Kazyah, Kazzia, Kazziah, Kazzya, Kazzyah

Kassidy (Irish/Gaelic) clever; curly-haired.
Casadea, Casadee, Casadey, Casadi, Casadia, Casadiah, Casadie, Casady, Cassadea, Cassadee, Cassadey, Cassadi, Cassadia, Cassadiah, Cassadie, Cassady, Cassidea, Cassidee, Cassidey, Cassidy, Kassadea, Kassadee, Kassadey, Kassadi, Kassadia, Kassadiah, Kassadie, Kassady, Kassadya, Kassidea, Kassidee, Kassidey, Kassidi, Kassidia, Kassidiah, Kassidie, Kazadea, Kazadee, Kazadey, Kazadi, Kazadia, Kazadiah, Kazadie, Kazady, Kazadya, Kazzadea, Kazzadee, Kazzadi, Kazzadia, Kazzadiah, Kazzadie, Kazzady

Kate (Greek) purity. A short form of Katherine.
Caet, Caete, Cait, Caite, Cate, Kadea, Kadee, Kaddia, Kaddiah, Kaddie, Kaddy, Kadi, Kadia, Kadiah, Kadie, Kait, Kaitea, Kaitee, Kaitey, Kaitie, Kaitlin, Kaitlina, Kaitlinah, Kaitline, Kaitlyn, Kaitlyna, Kaitlynah, Kaitlyne,

K

Katelea, Kateleah, Katelee, Katelei, Kateleigh, Kateley, Kateli, Katelia, Kateliah, Katelie, Kately, Katelyn, Katelyna, Katelynah, Katelyn, Katewin, Katewina, Katewinah, Katewine, Katewyn, Katewyna, Katewynah, Katewyne, Katia, Katiah, Katie, Katina, Katinah, Katinka, Katinkah, Katja (Russ), Katreena, Katrin, Katrina (Scand/Swed/Lith/Slav/Austr), Katrinah, Katrinna, Katrine, Katrinka, Katryn, Katryna, Katrynah, Katryne, Kattie (Ir), Katty, Katy, Katya (Russ), Kay, Kaye, Kayt

Kateri (Native American) purity. The first Native American saint.
Katerie, Katery

Kath (Greek) purity. A short form of Katherine.
Caf, Caff, Cath, Catha, Cathe, Cathee, Cathey, Cathia, Cathiah, Cathie, Cathy, Cathye, Katha, Kathe (Ger), Kathee, Kathey, Kathia, Kathiah, Kathie, Kathy, Kathya, Kathye

Katherine (Greek) purity.
Caferin, Caferina, Caferinah, Caferine, Cafferin, Cafferina, Cafferinah, Cafferine, Catherine, Catheryn, Catheryne, Cathleen, Ekaterina, Gaton, Kaatje (Dut), Kaddo (Est), Kaferin, Kaferina, Kaferinah, Kaferine, Kaferyn, Kaferyna, Kaferynah, Kaferyne, Kafferin, Kafferina, Kafferinah, Kafferine, Kafferyn, Kafferyna, Kafferynah, Kafferyne, Kardreinl, Kajsa (Swed), Kalina (Swed), Kalinah, Kaline, Karan (Grk), Karean, Kareana, Kareanah, Kareane, Kareen, Kareena, Kareenah, Kareene, Karen (Grk/Austr), Karena, Karenah,

Karene, Karin, Karina (Scan), Karinah, Karine, Karlinka (Slav), Karlinkah, Karolin, Karolina (Lith), Karolinah, Karoline (Ger), Karolyn, Karolyna, Karolynah, Karolyne, Karstin (Dan), Karstina, Karstinah, Karstine, Kashe (Dan), Kasen (Dan), Kasena, Kasenah, Kasene, Kasia, Kasiah, Kasie, Kata, Katal, Katalin (Hun), Katalina, Katalinah, Kataline, Katarin, Katarina (Lith/Swed), Katarina, Katarinah, Katarine, Kataryn, Kataryna, Katarynah, Kataryne, Katarzyna (Pol), Kate, Katey, Kateren, Katharin, Katharina, Katharinah, Katharine, Katharyn, Katharyna, Katharynah, Katharyne, Katherin, Katherina, Katherinah, Katheryn, Katheryna, Katherynah, Katheryne, Kathran, Kathren, Kathrin, Kathron, Kathrun, Kathryn, Kathy, Kati, Katie, Katja, Katreen (Eng), Katreena, Katreenah, Katreene, Katren (Eng), Katrena, Katrenah, Katrene, Katri (Est), Katria, Katriah, Katrian, Katriana, Katrianah, Katriane, Katriann, Katrianna, Katriannah, Katrianne, Katrien (Ger), Katriena, Katrienah, Katrienja, Katrijin (Dut), Katrijn, Katrina (Austr), Katrinah (Austr), Katrinka, Katrinna (Austr), Katrinnah, Katrinne, Katryn, Katryna, Katrynah, Katryne, Kattel, Katterie (Slav), Katterle, Katushka, Katya (Russ), Keri, Kerie, Kerri, Kerrie, Kerry, Kery

Kathleen (Greek) purity. The Irish short form of Katherine.
Cafflean, Caffleana, Caffleanah, Caffleane, Caffleen, Caffleena, Caffleenah, Caffleene, Cafflein, Caffleina, Caffleinah, Caffleine, Cafflin, Cafflina, Cafflinah, Caffline, Cafflyn, Cafflyna,

K

Kathleen cont.
Cafflynah, Cafflyne, Caflean,
Cafleana, Cafleanah, Cafleane,
Cafleen, Cafleena, Cafleenah,
Cafleene, Caflein, Cafleina,
Cafleinah, Cafleine, Caflin,
Caflina, Caflinah, Cafline, Caflyn,
Caflyna, Caflynah, Caflyne,
Cathlean, Cathleana, Cathleanah,
Cathleane, Cathleen, Cathleena,
Cathleenah, Cathleene, Cathlein,
Cathleina, Cathleinah, Cathleine,
Cathlin, Cathlina, Cathlinah,
Cathline, Cathlyn, Cathlyna,
Cathlynah, Cathlyne, Kafflean,
Kaffleana, Kaffleanah, Kaffleane,
Kaffleen, Kaffleena, Kaffleenah,
Kaffleene, Kaffleen, Kaffleena,
Kaffleenah, Kaffleene, Kafflein,
Kaffleina, Kaffleinah, Kaffleine,
Kafflin, Kafflina, Kafflinah,
Kaffline, Kafflyn, Kafflyna,
Kafflynah, Kafflyne, Kaflean,
Kafleana, Kafleanah, Kafleane,
Kafleen, Kafleena, Kafleena,
Kafleenah, Kafleene, Kaflein,
Kafleina, Kafleinah, Kafleine,
Kaflin, Kaflina, Kaflinah, Kafline,
Kaflyn, Kaflyna, Kaflynah, Kaflyne,
Kathleena, Kathleenah, Kathleene,
Kathlein, Kathleina, Kathleinah,
Kathleine, Kathlin, Kathlina,
Kathlinah, Kathline, Kathlyn,
Kathlyna, Kathlynah, Kathlyne

Katina (Australian Aboriginal) first
born child. (Grk/O/Eng) little
pure one.
Cateana, Cateanah, Cateena,
Cateenah, Cateina, Cateinah,
Cateyna, Cateynah, Catina,
Catinah, Catine, Catyn, Catyna,
Catynah, Catyne, Catynka,
Catynkah, Kateana, Kateanah,
Kateena, Kateenah, Kateina,
Kateinah, Kateyna, Kateynah,
Katinah, Katine, Katinka, Katinkah,

Katyn, Katyna, Katynah, Katyne,
Katynka, Katynkah

Katriel (Hebrew) God is my crown.
Catriel, Catriela, Catrielah,
Catriele, Catriell, Catriella,
Catriellah, Catrielle, Katriela,
Katrielah, Katriele, Katriell,
Kartriella, Katriellah, Kartrielle,
Katryel, Katryela, Katryelah,
Katriele, Katryell, Katryella,
Katryellah, Katryelle

Katrina (Scandinavian/Australian/
Swedish/Slavic/Lithuanian)
purity. A form of Katherine.
Caetreana, Caetreanah, Caetreena,
Caetreenah, Caetreina, Caetreinah,
Caetreyna, Caetreynah, Caetrina,
Caetrinah, Caetryna, Caetrynah,
Caitreana, Caitreanah, Caitreena,
Caitreenah, Caitreina, Caitreinah,
Caitreyna, Caitreynah, Caitrina,
Caitrinah, Caitryna, Caitrynah,
Catalina (Span), Catalinah,
Caterina (Ital), Caterinah,
Catriona, Catrionah, Cattarina,
Cattarinah, Caytreana, Caytreanah,
Caytreena, Caytreenah, Cayreina,
Caytreinah, Cayreyna, Caytreynah,
Caytrina, Caytrinah, Caytryna,
Caytrynah, Ekaterina, Kaetreana,
Kaetreanah, Kaetreena, Kaetreenah,
Kaetreina, Kaetreinah, Kaetreyna,
Kaetreynah, Kaetina, Kaetrinah,
Kaetryna, Kaetrynah, Kaitreana,
Kaitreanah, Kaitreena, Kaitreenah,
Kaitein, Kaitreinah, Kaitreyna,
Kaitreynah, Kaitrina, Kaitrinah,
Kaitryna, Kaitrynah, Karlinka,
Katarain, Kataraina (NZMaori),
Katarainah, Kataraine, Katarina
(Swed/Lith/Illy), Katarinah,
Katarine, Kataryn, Kataryna,
Katarynah, Katarynza (Pol),
Katchena, Katchen (Ger),
Katchena, Katereans, Katereanah,
Katereena, Katereenah, Katerina,

Katerinah, Katerini, Katerinia, Kateriniah, Kateriny (Slav), Katharina, Katharinah, Katherina (Eng), Katherinah, Kathrina-Dan), Kathrinah, Kathryna, Kathrynah, Katreana, Katreanah, Katreena, Katreenah, Katreina, Katreinah, Katreyna, Katreynah, Katryna, Katrynah, Kayreana, Kayreanah, Kaytreena, Kaytreenah, Kaytreina, Kaytreinah, Kaytreyna, Kaytreynah, Kayrina, Kaytrinah, Kaytryna, Kaytrynah

Katrinelle (Greek/French) she is purity.
Katrin, Katrina, Katrinah, Katrinal, Katriel, Katriela, Katriele, Katriell, Katriella, Katrielle, Katrinel, Katrinela, Katrinele, Katrinell, Katrinella, Katrynel, Katrynela, Katrynele, Katrynell, Katrynella, Katrynelle

Kauser (Arabic) plenty.
Kausera

Kawana (Australian Aboriginal) wild flower.
Kawanah

Kay (Greek) purity. The short form of Kate/Katherine.
Cae, Caea, Caeh, Caelea, Caelean, Caeleana, Caeleane, Caelee, Caeleen, Caeleena, Caeleene, Caelei, Caelein, Caeleina, Caeleine, Caeli, Caelin, Caelina, Caeline, Caely, Caelyn, Caelyna, Caelyne, Cah, Cai, Caia, Caiah, Cailea, Cailean, Caileana, Caileane, Cailee, Caileen, Caileena, Caileene, Cailei, Cailein, Caileina, Caileine, Caileyn, Caileyna, Caileyne, Caili, Cailin, Cailina, Cailine, Caily, Cailyn, Cailyna, Cayline, Cayly, Caylyn, Caylyna, Caylyne, Cay, Caye, Kae, Kaelea, Kaelean, Kaeleana, Kaeleane, Kaelee,

Kaeleen, Kaeleena, Kaeleene, Kaelei, Kaelein, Kaeleina, Kaeleine, Kaeleyn, Kaeleyna, Kaeleyne, Kaeli, Kaelin, Kaelina, Kaeline, Kaely, Kaelyn, Kaelyna, Kaelyne, Kah, Kai, Kaia, Kaiah, Kailea, Kailean, Kailean, Kaileane, Kailee, Kaileena, Kaileene, Kailei, Kailein, Kaileina, Kaileine, Kaili, Kailin, Kailina, Kailine, Kaily, Kailyn, Kailyna, Kayline, Kayly, Kaylyn, Kaylyna, Kaylyne, Kaja, Kaya, Kaye, Kaylea, Kaylean, Kayleana, Kayleane, Kaylee, Kayleen, Kayleena, Kayleene, Kaylei, Kaylein, Kayleina, Kayleine, Kaylena, Kaylene, Kayli, Kaylin, Kaylina, Kayline, Kaylyn, Kaylyna, Kaylyne

Kaya (Japanese) place of rest.
Caea, Caia, Caiah, Caya, Cayah, Kaea, Kaia, Kaiah, Kaya, Kayah

Kayalana (Greek/English) pure light.
Kaialana

Kayla (English) purity. (Heb) crown.
Caela, Caelah, Caelea, Caeleah, Caelee, Caelei, Caeleigh, Caeley, Caeli, Caelia, Caeliah, Caelie, Caely, Cahla, Cahlah, Cahlea, Cahleah, Cahlee, Cahlei, Cahleigh, Cahley, Cahli, Cahlie, Cahly, Caila, Cailah, Cailea, Caileah, Cailee, Cailei, Caileigh, Caili, Cailia, Cailiah, Cailie, Caily, Cala, Calah, Calea, Caleah, Calee, Calei, Caleigh, Caley, Cali, Caliah, Calie, Caly, Cayla, Caylah, Caylea, Cayleah, Caylee, Caylei, Cayleigh, Cayley, Cayli, Caylia, Cayliah, Caylie, Cayly, Kaela, Kaelah, Kaelea, Kaeleah, Kaelee, Kaelei, Kaeleigh, Kaeley, Kaeli, Kaelia, Kaeliah, Kaelie, Kaely, Kahla, Kahlah, Kahlea, Kahleah, Kahlee,

Kayla cont.
Kahlei, Kahleigh, Kahley, Kahlei, Kahlie, Kahly, Kaila, Kailah, Kailea, Kaileah, Kailee, Kailei, Kaileigh, Kailey, Kaili, Kailia, Kailiah, Kailie, Kaily, Kalea, Kaleah, Kalee, Kalei, Kaleigh, Kaley, Kali, Kalia, Kaliah, Kalie, Kaly, Kalya, Kayla, Kaylah, Kaylea, Kayleah, Kaylee, Kaylei, Kayleigh, Kayley, Kayli, Kaylia, Kayliah, Kaylie, Kayly, Kaylya

Kaylee (Old English/Greek) from the pure meadow.
Caela, Caelah, Caelea, Caeleah, Caelee, Caelei, Caeleigh, Caeley, Caeli, Caelia, Caeliah, Caelie, Caely, Cahla, Cahlah, Cahlea, Cahleah, Cahlee, Cahlei, Cahleigh, Cahley, Cahli, Cahlie, Cahly, Caila, Cailah, Cailea, Caileah, Cailee, Cailei, Caileigh, Caili, Cailia, Cailiah, Cailie, Caily, Cala, Calah, Calea, Caleah, Calee, Calei, Caleigh, Caley, Cali, Caliah, Calie, Caly, Cayla, Caylah, Caylea, Cayleah, Caylee, Caylei, Cayleigh, Cayley, Cayli, Caylia, Cayliah, Caylie, Cayly, Kaela, Kaelah, Kaelea, Kaeleah, Kaelee, Kaelei, Kaeleigh, Kaeley, Kaeli, Kaelia, Kaeliah, Kaelie, Kaely, Kahla, Kahlah, Kahlea, Kahleah, Kahlee, Kahlei, Kahleigh, Kahley, Kahlei, Kahlie, Kahly, Kaila, Kailah, Kailea, Kaileah, Kailee, Kailei, Kaileigh, Kailey, Kaili, Kailia, Kailiah, Kailie, Kaily, Kalea, Kaleah, Kalee, Kalei, Kaleigh, Kaley, Kali, Kalia, Kaliah, Kalie, Kaly, Kalya, Kayla, Kaylah, Kaylea, Kayleah, Kaylee, Kaylei, Kayleigh, Kayley, Kayli, Kaylia, Kayliah, Kaylie, Kayly, Kaylya, Kealea, Kealeah, Kealee, Kealei, Kealeigh, Keali, Kealia, Kealiah, Kealie, Kealy

Kaz (Australian/Greek) purity. A short form of Karen.
Kazz

Kazimiera (Polish) peace is proclaimed.
Kasimerah, Kasimiera, Kasimira, Kasimirah, Kasmira, Kasmirah, Kasmiria, Kasmiriah, Kasmirya, Kasmiryah, Kasmyra, Kasmyrah, Kazmira, Kazmirah, Kazmiria, Kazmiriah, Kazmyra, Kazmyrah, Kazmyria, Kazmyriah, Kazmyrya, Kazmyryah, Kazzmira, Kazzmirah, Kazzmiria, Kazzmiriah, Kazzmirya, Kazzmiryah, Kazzmyrya, Kazzmyryah

Keala (Hawaiian) pathway.
Kealah, Keela, Keelah, Keila, Keilah, Keyla, Keylah

Kedma (Hebrew) towards the east.
Kedmah

Keely (Irish/Gaelic) beautiful.
Kealea, Kealeah, Kealee, Kealei, Kealeigh, Kealey, Keali, Kealia, Kealiah, Kealie, Kealy, Kealya, Keelea, Keeleah, Keelee, Keelei, Keeleigh, Keeley, Keeli, Keelia, Keeliah, Keelya, Keighlea, Keighleah, Keighlee, Keighlei, Keighleigh, Keighley, Keighli, Keighlia, Keighliah, Keighlie, Keighly, Keilea, Keileah, Keilei, Keileigh, Keiley, Keili, Keilia, Keiliah, Keilie, Keily, Keilya, Kelee, Kelei, Keleigh, Keley, Keli, Kelia, Keliah, Kelie, Kely, Kely, Keylea, Keyleah, Keylee, Keylei, Keyleigh, Keyley, Keyli, Keylia, Keyliah, Keylie, Keyly

Keena (Irish) fast; brave.
Keana, Keanah, Keenah, Keina, Keinah, Keyna, Keynah

K

Kefira (Hebrew) young lioness.
Kefirah, Kefire, Kefyra, Kefyrah,
Kefyre

Kei (Hawaiian) glorious.
Kee, Key

Keighlea (Irish/Old English) pure
one from the meadow.
Keelea, Keeleah, Keelee, Keelei,
Keeleigh, Keeley, Keeli, Keelia,
Keeliah, Keelie, Keely, Keighlea,
Keighlee, Keighlei, Keighleigh,
Keighley, Keighli, Keighlia,
Keighliah, Keighly, Keilea, Keileah,
Keilee, Keilei, Keileigh, Keiley,
Keili, Keilia, Keiliah, Keilie, Keily,
Kelea, Keleah, Kelee, Kelei, Keleigh,
Keley, Keli, Kelia, Keliah, Kelie,
Kellea, Kelleah, Kellee, Kellei,
Kelleigh, Kelley, Kelli, Kellia,
Kelliah, Kellie, Kellina, Kellinah,
Kelline, Kelton, Kelula, Kelulah,
Kielea, Kieleah, Kielee, Kielei,
Kieleigh, Kieley, Kieli, Kielia,
Kieliah, Kielie, Kiely, Kyle (Ir),
Kylea, Kyleah, Kylee, Kylei, Kyleigh,
Kyli, Kylie (Aust/AustKoor), Kyly

Keija (Swedish/Greek) purity. A
form of Katherine.
Kei, Ki, Ky

Keiki (Hawaiian) child.
Keyki, Kiki

Keiko (Japanese) pretty; adored.
Keyko

Keilana (Hawaiian) glorious calm.
Kealana, Kealanah, Kealane,
Kealaina, Kealainah, Kealaine,
Kealanah, Kealanna, Kealannah,
Kealanne, Keelana, Keelanah,
Keelaina, Keelainah, Keelane,
Keelayn, Keelayna, Keelaynah,
Keelayne, Keilanah, Keilane,
Keilaina, Keilanah, Keilaine,
Keilanna, Keilannah, Keilanne,
Keilayn, Keilayna, Keilaynah,
Keilayne, Keylana, Keylanah,
Keylane, Keylaina, Keylainah,
Keylaine, Keylayn, Keylayna,
Keylaynah, Keylayne

Keilani (Hawaiian) glorious chief.
Kealana, Kealanah, Kealane,
Kealanee, Kealaina, Kealainah,
Kealaine, Kealainee, Kealanah,
Kealanna, Kealannah, Kealanne,
Kealannee, Keelana, Keelanah,
Keelane, Keelanee, Keelaina,
Keelainah, Keelane, Keelanee,
Keelayn, Keelayna, Keelaynah,
Keelayne, Keelaynee, Keilana,
Keilanah, Keilane, Keilanee,
Keilaina, Keilanah, Keilaine,
Keilainee, Keilanna, Keilannah,
Keilanne, Keilannee, Keilayn,
Keilayna, Keilaynah, Keilayne,
Keilaynee, Keylana, Keylanah,
Keylane, Keylanee, Keylaina,
Keylainah, Keylaine, Keylainee,
Keylayn, Keylayna, Keylaynah,
Keylayne, Keylaynee

Keina (Australian Aboriginal)
moon.
Keinah, Keyna, Keynah

Keisha (Swahili) favourite.
Aisha, Aishah, Eisha, Eishah,
Eysha, Eyshah, Iesha, Ieshah, Isha,
Keasha, Keesham Keeshia,
Keeshiah, Keeshy, Keeshya,
Keeshyah, Keishah, Keishia,
Keishiah, Keishya, Keishyah,
Keysha, Keyshah, Keyshia,
Keyshiah, Keyshya, Keyshyah,
Lakeasha, Lakeashia, Lakeashiah,
Lakeashya, Lakeashyah, Lakeesha,
Lakeeshia, Lakeeshiah, Lakeeshya,
Lakeeshyah, Lakeisha, Lakeishia,
Lakeishiah, Lakeshia, Lakeshiah,
Lakeshya, Lakeshyah, Lakeysha,
Lakeyshah

Kelby (Scandinavian) dweller by the place near the fountain spring.
Kelbea, Kelbee, Kelbey, Kelbi, Kelbie

Kelda (Scandinavian) clear mountain; spring of life.
Keldah, Keldra, Keldrah

Kele (Tongan) clay.
Kelea, Keleah, Kelee, Kelei, Keleigh, Keli, Kelie, Kely

Kelesi (Tongan) grace.
Kelesia, Kelesiah, Kelesie, Kelesy, Kelesya, Kelesyah

Keletina (Hawaiian) heavenly.
Keletinah, Keletyna, Keletynah

Keli (Tongan) mine.
Kelea, Keleah, Kelee, Kelei, Keleigh, Keley, Kelia, Keliah, Kelie, Kely, Kelya, Kelyah

Kelila (Hebrew) victory; crown of laurels.
Kaile, Kalila, Kalilah, Kayle, Kelilah, Kelula, Kelulah, Kyla, Kyle, Kyleen, Kylene, Lila, Lilah, Lylia, Lyliah, Lylya, Lylyah

Kelly (Irish/Gaelic) warrior; dweller from the farm near the woods.
Kalea, Kaleah, Kalee, Kalei, Kaleigh, Kaley, Kali, Kalia, Kaliah, Kalie, Kaly, Keelea, Keeleah, Keelee, Keelei, Keeleigh, Keeley, Keeli, Keelia, Keeliah, Keelie, Keely, Keighlea, Keighleah, Keighlee, Keighlei, Keighleigh, Keighley, Keighli, Keighlia, Keighliah, Keighly, Keilea, Keileah, Keilee, Keilei, Keileigh, Keiley, Keili, Keilia, Keiliah, Keilie, Keily, Kelea, Keleah, Kelee, Kelei, Keleigh, Keley, Keli, Kelia, Keliah, Kelie, Kellea, Kelleah, Kellee, Kellei, Kelleigh, Kelley, Kelli, Kellia, Kelliah, Kellie, Kellina, Kellinah, Kelline, Kelton, Kelula,

Kelulah, Kielea, Kieleah, Kielee, Kielei, Kieleigh, Kieley, Kieli, Kielia, Kieliah, Kielie, Kiely, Kyle (Ir), Kylea, Kyleah, Kylee, Kylei, Kyleigh, Kyli, Kylie (Aust/AustKoor), Kyly

Kelsey (Old Norse) from the ship island.
Kelcea, Kelcee, Kelci, Kelcie, Kellcea, Kellcee, Kellcey, Kellci, Kellcia, Kellciah, Kellcie, Kellcy, Kellsea, Kellsee, Kellsey, Kellsi, Kellsia, Kellsiah, Kellsie, Kellsy, Kelsea, Kelsee, Kelsey, Kelsy

Kemba (Old English) saxon lord.
Kembah, Kembara, Kimba, Kimbah, Kymba, Kymbah

Kenda (African) child of the pure water.
Kendah, Kendal, Kendall, Kendel, Kendela, Kendelah, Kendele, Kendell, Kendella, Kendellah, Kendelle

Kendellana (English/Greek/French) she is the chief of the valley of light.
Kendelan, Kendelana, Kendelanah, Kendelane, Kendellan, Kendellanah, Kendellane, Kendelin, Kendelina, Kendelinah, Kendeline, Kendellyn, Kendellyna, Kendellynah, Kendellyne, Kendelyn, Kendelyna, Kendelynah, Kendelyne

Kendelle (Celtic/French) she is the chief of the valley.
Kendal, Kendala, Kendalah, Kendale, Kendall, Kendalla, Kendallah, Kendalle, Kendel, Kendela, Kendelah, Kendele, Kendell, Kendella, Kendellah

Kendra (English/Teutonic) knowledgeable; understanding.
Kendrah, Kendria, Kendriah, Kendrya, Kendryah

K

Kenisha (African American) beautiful.
Kenishah, Kenysha, Kenyshah

Kenna (Old English) knowledgeable, competent woman.
Kena, Kenah, Kenia, Keniah, Kenis, Kenisa, Kenise, Kennah, Kennis, Kennisa, Kennisah, Kennise, Kenniss, Kennissa, Kennissah, Kenisse, Kenya, Kenyah, Kenys, Kenysa, Kenysah, Kenyse, Kenyss, Kenyssa, Kenyssah, Kenysse, Mackenna, Mackennah, Makenna, Makenneah

Kentigerna (Old English) fair-haired woman. (Gae) royal ruler.
Caintigern, Centigerna, Centigernah, Centigerne, Centygern, Centygerna, Centygerne, Kentigern, Kentigernah, Kentigerne, Kentygern, Kentygerna, Kentygernah, Kentygerne

Kenya (African) jewel.
(Geographical) country in Africa.
Enya (Scot/Gae), Enyah, Kania, Kaniah, Kanja, Kanjah, Kanya, Kanyah, Kenbea, Kenbee, Kenbey, Kenbi, Kenbie, Kenby, Kenia, Keniah, Kenja, Kenjah, Kenyah, Kenyatta, Kenyatte, Kenyetta, Kenyette

Keohi (Hawaiian) woman.

Kerani (Hindi) sacred bells.
Keranee, Keraney, Kerani, Kerania, Keraniah, Keranie, Kerany, Keranya, Keranyah

Keren (Hebrew) beam; ray of light; animal horn.
Caran, Caren, Ceren, Kaaran, Kaaren, Kaarin, Kaaron, Karan (Grk), Karen (Austr/Grk), Karin, Karon, Karina, Karine, Karryn,

Keralyn, Keran, Keren, Kerin, Keron, Kerensa, Kerenza, Kerran, Kerre, Kerren, Kerrin, Kerron, Kieran, Kieren, Kierin, Kieron, Kieryn, Kira, Kiran, Kirana, Kiranah, Kirane, Kirra, Kirran, Kirrana, Kirranah, Kirrane, Kyra, Kyrah, Kyran, Kyrana, Kyranah, Kyrane

Kerensa (Cornish) affection; love.
Karensa, Karensah, Karanza, Karanzah, Kerensah, Kerenza, Kerenzah

Kerenza (Hebrew/Cornish) light.
Karensa, Karensah, Karanza, Karanzah, Kerensa, Kerensah, Kerenzah

Kereru (Polynesian) pigeon.
Kerer

Kerrianne (Hebrew/Celtic) dark-haired graceful one.
Kerian, Keriana, Kerianah, Keriane, Kerriann, Kerri-Ann, Kerri-Anna, Kerriannah, Kerri-Annah, Kerrianne, Kerryann, Kerryanna, Kerryannah, Kerryanne, Kerry-Anne, Keryan, Keryana, Keryanah, Keryane, Keryann, Keryanna, Keryannah, Keryanne

Kerrielle (Celtic/French) she who is dark.
Keriel, Keriela, Kerielah, Keriele, Keriella, Keriellah, Kerielle, Kerriel, Kerriela, Kerrielah, Kerriele, Kerriell, Kerriella, Kerryell, Kerryell, Kerryella, Kerryellah, Kerryelle, Keryel, Keryela, Keryele, Keryell, Keryella, Keryellah, Keryelle

Kerry (Celtic) dark-haired.
Ceree, Cerey, Ceri, Cerie, Cerree, Cerrey, Cerri, Cerrie, Cerry, Cery, Keree, Kerey, Keri, Kerie, Kerree, Kerri, Kerrie, Kery

K

Keshet (Hebrew) rainbow.
Kesetta, Kesettah, Kesette, Kesheta, Keshetah, Keshete, Keshett, Keshetta, Keshettah, Keshette

Keshisha (Arabic) elder.
Keshish, Keshishah

Kesi (Swahili) daughter whose father is difficult.
Kesee, Kesey, Kesie, Kesy

Kesia (African) favourite.
Kesiah, Kessia, Kessiah, Kessya, Kessyah, Kezia, Keziah, Kezzia, Kezziah, Kisai, Kisiah, Kizia, Kiziah, Kizzia, Kizziah, Kyzi, Kyzia, Kyziah, Kyzie, Kyzy, Kyzzi, Kyzzia, Kyzziah, Kyzzie, Kyzzy, Kyzzya, Kyzzah

Ketifa (Arabic) to pick a flower.
Ketifah, Kettifa, Kettifah, Kettyfa, Kettyfah, Ketyfa, Ketyfah

Ketina (Hebrew) girl.
Keteena, Keteenah, Ketinah, Ketyna, Ketynah

Ketura (Hebrew) fragrance; perfume.
Keturah

Ketzia (Hebrew) cinnamon spice.
Ketziah, Ketzya, Ketzyah

Keverne (Irish/Gaelic) handsome. The feminine form of Kevin.
Kevern, Keverna, Kervernah, Kevina, Kevinah, Kevine, Kevirn, Kevirna, Kevirnah, Kevirne, Kevyrn, Kevyrna, Kevyrnah, Kevyrne

Kewanee (Native American) prairie hen.

Kezia (Hebrew) cinnamon spice; the cassia tree.
Hazia, Haziah, Keziah, Kezya, Kezyah

Kia (African) beginning of the season.
Kaea, Kai, Kay, Kaya, Kiah, Kya, Kyah

Kiannah (American/Hebrew) God is gracious. A form of Hannah.
Kiana, Kianah, Kianna, Kyana, Kyanah, Kyanna, Kyannah

Kichi (Japanese) fortunate.
Kichee, Kichie, Kichy

Kiki (Egyptian) castor plant. (Tong) squeak.
Kikee, Kikey, Kikie, Kiky

Kiku (Japanese) the chrysanthemum flower, traditionally given on Mother's Day.

Kilia (Hawaiian) heaven.
Kiliah, Kylia, Kyliah, Kylya, Kylyah

Kilkie (Australian Aboriginal) water hen.
Kilkee, Kilkey, Kilki, Kilky

Killara (Australian Aboriginal) one who is always there.
Killarah

Kim (Old English) royal. The short form of Kimberley.
Kem, Khim, Khime, Khimm, Khym, Khyme, Khymm, Kimm, Kym, Kymm

Kimalina (Old English/Latin) chief who is noble and kind.
Kimalinah, Kimalinda, Kimalindah, Kimalinde, Kimaline, Kimalyn, Kimalyna, Kimalynah, Kimalynda, Kimalynde, Kimalyne, Kymalyn, Kymalyna, Kymalynah, Kymalynda, Kymalyndah, Kymalyne

Kimana (Shoshone) butterfly.
Kimanah, Kymana, Kymanah

K

Kimanna (Old English/Hebrew) chief whose God is gracious.
Kiman, Kimana (Nat/Amer), Kimanah, Kimane, Kimann, Kimannah, Kimanne, Kyman, Kymana, Kymanah, Kymane, Kymann, Kymanna, Kymannah, Kymanne

Kimberley (Old English) from the royal meadow.
Kemberlea, Kemberleah, Kemberlee, Kemberlei, Kemberleigh, Kemberley, Kemberli, Kemberlia, Kemberliah, Kemberlie, Kemberlin, Kemberlina, Kemberlinah, Kemberline, Kemberly, Kemberlyn, Kemberlyna, Kemberlynah, Kemberlyne, Khimberlea, Khimberleah, Khimberlee, Khimberlei, Khimberleigh, Khimberli, Khimberlia, Khimberliah, Khimberlie, Khimberlin, Khimberlina, Khimberlinah, Khimberline, Khimberly, Khimberlyn, Khimberlyna, Khimberlynah, Khimberlyne, Khymberlea, Khymberleah, Khymberlee, Khymberlei, Khymberleigh, Khymberley, Khymberli, Khymberlia, Khymberliah, Khymberlie, Khymberly, Kimbalea, Kimbaleah, Kimbalee, Kimbalei, Kimbaleigh, Kimbalina, Kimbalinah, Kimbaline, Kimbalyn, Kimbalyna, Kimbalynah, Kimbalyne, Kimberlea, Kimberleah, Kimberlee, Kimberlei, Kimberleigh, Kimberli, Kimberlia, Kimberliah, Kimberlie, Kimberlin, Kimberlina, Kimberlinah, Kimberline, Kimberly, Kimberlyn, Kymberlyna, Kymberlynah, Kymberlyne, Kymbalea, Kymbaleah, Kymbalee, Kymbalei, Kymbaleigh, Kymbali, Kymbalia, Kymbaliah, Kymbalie, Kymbalin, Kymbalina, Kymbalinah, Kymbaline, Kymballea, Kymballeah, Kymballee, Kymballei, Kymballeigh, Kymberlea, Kymberleah, Kymberlee, Kymberlei, Kymberleigh, Kymberley, Kymberli, Kymberlia, Kymberliah, Kymberlie, Kymberly

Kimi (Japanese) the best.
Kimee, Kimey, Kimie, Kimiko, Kimmee, Kimmey, Kimmi, Kimmie, Kimmy, Kimy, Kymy

Kimiko (Japanese) heavenly; righteous child.
Kimik, Kimyko, Kymiko, Kymyko

Kimimela (Sioux) butterfly.
Kimimela, Kymimela

Kin (Old English) family.
Kina, Kinah, Kinchen, Kinsey, Kyn, Kyna, Kynah

Kina (Hawaiian) China. The Hawaiian form of Tina, little one.
Kinah, Kyna, Kynah

Kindilan (Australian Aboriginal) happy.
Kindilana, Kindilanah, Kindilane, Kindilina, Kindilinah, Kindiline, Kindilyna, Kindilynah, Kindilyne

Kineta (Greek) active; alert.
Kinet, Kinetah, Kinete, Kinett, Kinetta, Kinette, Kynet, Kyneta, Kynetah, Kynete, Kynett, Kynetta, Kynette

Kinta (Choctaw) beaver. (Aust/Abor) laughing.
Kintah, Kynta, Kyntah

Kioko (Japanese) child born in happiness.
Kioka, Kyoka, Kyokah

Kiona/Kiowa (Native American)
brown hills
Kionah, Kiowa, Kiowah, Kyona,
Kyonah, Kyowa, Kyowah

Kip (Old English) dweller at the
pointed hill; sleep.
Kipp, Kyp, Kypp

Kira (New Zealand Maori) tree bark.
(A/Abor) fire place. (Russ) lady.
(Bulg) throne.
Keara, Kearah, Keera, Keerah, Kiera,
Kierra, Kirah, Kiran, Kiri, Kirianna,
Kirianne, Kirra (A/Koo), Kirrah,
Kirralea, Kirralee, Kirraleigh, Kirri,
Kirrie, Kirrilly, Kirrily, Kyra, Kyrah

Kiran (Hindi) beam; ray of light.
Kearan, Kearen, Kearin, Kearon,
Keeran, Keerana, Keeranah,
Keerane, Keeren, Keerin, Keeron,
Keiran, Keiren, Keirin, Keiron,
Keiryn, Kieran, Kierana, Kieranah,
Kierane, Kieren, Kieron, Kirana,
Kiranah, Kirane, Kyran, Kyrana,
Kyranah, Kyrane, Kyren, Kyrin,
Kyron, Kyryn

Kirby (Old English) from the
church by the farm.
Kerbea, Kerbee, Kerbey, Kerbi,
Kerbie, Kerby, Kirbea, Kirbee,
Kirbey, Kirbi, Kirbie, Kyrbea,
Kyrbee, Kyrbey, Kyrbi, Kyrbie,
Kyrby

Kiri (New Zealand Maori) tree bark.
Kirea, Kiree, Kirie, Kiry, Kyrea,
Kyree, Kyrey, Kyri, Kyrie, Kyry

Kirianne (New Zealand Maori/
Hebrew) tree bark; God is
gracious.
Kirian, Kiriana, Kirianah, Kiriane,
Kiriann, Kirianna, Kiriannah,
Kirianne, Kyrian, Kyriana,
Kyrianah, Kyriane, Kyriann,
Kyrianna, Kyriannah, Kyrianne,
Kyryan, Kyryana, Kyryanah,

Kyryane, Kyryann, Kyryanna,
Kyryannah, Kyryanne

Kirilina (New Zealand Maori/
English) tree bark by the pool of
water.
Kirilin, Kirilinah, Kiriline, Kirilyn,
Kirilyna, Kirilynah, Kirilyne,
Kyrilin, Kyrilina, Kyrilinah,
Kyriline, Kyrilyn, Kyrilyna,
Kyrilynah, Kyrilyne, Kyrylin,
Kyrylina, Kyrylinah, Kyryline,
Kyrylyn, Kyrylyna, Kyrylynah,
Kyrylyne

Kirra (Australian Aboriginal)
magpie (black & white bird).
Kira, Kirah, Kirrah, Kyra (Per),
Kyrah, Kyrra, Kyrrah

Kirsten (Scottish) anointed; covered
in oil.
Kerstai, Kerstain, Kerstaina,
Kerstainah, Kerstaine, Kerstan,
Kerstana, Kerstanah, Kerstane,
Kerstea, Kerstean, Kersteana,
Kersteanah, Kersteane, Kerstee,
Kersteen, Kersteena, Kersteenah,
Kersteene, Kersten, Kerstena,
Kerstenah, Kerstene, Kerstin,
Kerstina, Kerstinah, Kerstine,
Kerstyn, Kerstyna, Kerstynah,
Kerstyne, Kirbea, Kirbee, Kirbey,
Kirbi, Kirbie, Kirby, Kireen, Kireena,
Kireenah, Kireene, Kirstai, Kirstain,
Kirstaina, Kirstainah, Kirstaine,
Kirstan, Kirstana, Kirstanah,
Kirstane, Kirste, Kirstea, Kirstee,
Kirsti, Kirstia, Kirstiah, Kirstie,
Kirstin, Kirstina, Kirstinah, Kirstine,
Kirston, Kirstona, Kirstonah,
Kirstone, Kirsty, Kirstya, Kirstye,
Kirstyn, Kirstyna, Kirstynah,
Kirstyne, Kurstea, Kurstean,
Kursteana, Kursteanah, Kursteane,
Kurstee, Kursteen, Kursteena,
Kursteenah, Kursteene, Kurstai,
Kurstain, Kurstaina, Kurstainah,

K

Kurstaine, Kursti, Kurstia, Kurstin, Kurstina, Kurstinah, Kurstine, Kursty, Kurstyn, Kurstyna, Kurstynah, Kurstyne

Kirstie (Scottish) anointed; covered in oil. The short form of Kiersten.
Cerstea, Cerstee, Cerstey, Cersti, Cerstie, Cersty, Cirstea, Cirstee, Cirstey, Cirsti, Cirstie, Cirsty, Kerstea, Kerstee, Kerstey, Kersti, Kerstia, Kerstiah, Kerstie, Kersty, Kirstea, Kirstee, Kirstey, Kirsti, Kirstia, Kirstiah, Kirsty, Kurstea, Kurstee, Kurstey, Kursti, Kurstia, Kurstiah, Kurstie, Kursty, Kyrstea, Kyrstee, Kyrstey, Kyrsti, Kyrstie, Kyrsty

Kisa (Russian) kitten.
Kisah, Kissa, Kissah, Kysa, Kysah, Kyssa, Kyssah

Kishi (Japanese) brings happiness to the Earth.
Kishee, Kishi, Kishie, Kishhy

Kismet (Arabic) destiny; fate.
Kismeta, Kismetah, Kismete, Kismett, Kismetta, Kismettah, Kismette, Kissmet, Kissmeta, Kissmetah, Kissmete, Kissmett, Kissmetta, Kissmettah, Kissmette, Kysmet, Kysmeta, Kysmetah, Kysmete, Kysmett, Kysmetta, Kysmettah, Kysmette, Kyssmet, Kyssmeta, Kyssmetah, Kyssmete, Kyssmett, Kyssmetta, Kyssmettah, Kyssmette

Kiss (Russian) cat. (Eng) affection.
Kis, Kismet, Kissmet, Kys, Kyss

Kissa (Ugandan) born after twins.
Kisa, Kisah, Kissah, Kysa, Kysah, Kyssa, Kyssah

Kitra (Hebrew) crowned.
Kitrah

Kiu (Tongan) sea bird.

Kiupita (Tongan) cupid; love angel.

Kiva (Hebrew) protected.
Kivah

Kiyoka (Japanese) clear.
Kiyoko

Kizzy (African/African American) favourite; cinnamon. (Heb) cassia tree.
Kessee, Kessey, Kessi, Kessie, Kessy, Kezi, Kezia, Keziah, Kezie, Kezy, Kezzee, Kezzey, Kezzi, Kezzie, Kezzy, Kezy, Kizee, Kizey, Kizi, Kizie, Kizzee, Kizzey, Kizzi, Kizzie, Kizy, Kyzee, Kyzey, Kyzi, Kyzie, Kyzzee, Kyzzey, Kyzzi, Kyzzie, Kyzy

Koana (Hawaiian) God is good.
Koanah, Koanna, Koannah

Kodi (Irish/Gaelic) helpful.
Codea, Codee, Codey, Codi, Codie, Cody, Kodea, Kodee, Kodey, Kodi, Kodie, Kody

Koemi (Japanese) smiling a little.
Koemee, Koemey, Koemie, Koemy

Kogarah (Australian Aboriginal) place where rushes grow.
Kogara

Kohia (Polynesian) passion flower.
Kohiah

Koko (Native American) night. (Jap) stork.
Coco

Kokokoho (Native American) night owl.

Koleyn (Australian Aboriginal) winter.
Kolein, Koleina, Koleine, Koleyna, Koleynah, Koleyne

Kolfinnia (Old Norse) cool; white.
Kolfinia, Kolfiniah, Kolfinna, Kolfinnah, Kolfinnia, Kolfinniah

Kolina (Swedish) young girl.
Colina, Colinah, Coline, Colyn,
Colyna, Colynah, Colyne, Kolinah,
Koline, Kolyn, Kolyna, Kolynah,
Kolyne

Koloa (Tongan) treasure.
Koloah

Kololia (Tongan/Hawaiian) glory.
Kololiah

Kolora (Australian Aboriginal) fresh
lagoon; lake.
Kolorah, Kalori, Kalorie, Kalory

Konol (Australian Aboriginal) sky.
Conol, Conola, Konola

Konrada (Polynesian) bold, wise
counsel. The feminine form of
Conrad.
Conrada

Koo (Greek) purity. A short form of
Katherine.
Coo

Kooanna (Greek/Hebrew) pure one
whose God is gracious.
Kooan, Kooana, Kooanah, Kooane,
Kooannah, Kooanne

Koora (Australian Aboriginal)
plenty.
Koorah

Kora (Australian Aboriginal)
companion; friend. (Grk) girl.
Cora, Corah, Coreta, Coretah,
Corete, Corett, Coretta, Corettah,
Corette, Corey, Corina, Corinah,
Corine, Corinna, Corrinah,
Corrine, Korah, Koret, Koreta,
Koretah, Korete, Korett, Koretta,
Korettah, Korette, Korina, Korinah,
Korine, Korinna, Korinnah,
Korinne, Koryna, Korynah, Koryne,
Korynn, Korynna, Korynnah,
Korynne

Korena (Greek) young girl.
Korana, Koranah, Korane, Koranna,
Korannah, Koranne, Korean,
Koreana, Koreanah, Koreane,
Koreen, Koreena, Koreenah,
Koreene, Koreina, Koreinah,
Koreine, Koren, Korenah, Korene,
Korensa, Korenza, Koreyna,
Koreynah, Koreyne, Korin, Korina,
Korinah, Korine, Koryn, Koryna,
Korynah, Koryne

Korenet (Hebrew) shining.
Corenet, Coreneta, Corenetah,
Corenete, Koreneta, Korenetah,
Korenete, Korenett, Korenetta,
Korenettah, Korenette

Korina (English) girl.
Coreena, Coreenah, Corina,
Corinah, Coryna, Corynah,
Koreena, Koreenah, Korinah,
Koryna, Korynah

Kortanya (Greek/Russian) young
fairy queen.
Cortania, Cortaniah, Cortanya,
Cortanyah, Kotania, Kortaniah,
Kotanyah

Kortina (Greek/English) young
Christian; young girl.
Cortina, Cortinah, Cortine, Cortyn,
Cortyna, Cortyne, Kortinah,
Kortine, Kortyn, Kortyna, Kortyne

Kostya (Russian) faith.
Kostia, Kostiah, Kostyah

Koula (Tongan) gold.
Koulah

Krisandra (Greek) prophet. A form
of Cassandra/Kassandra.
Chrisandra, Chrisandrah,
Crisandra, Crisandrah, Crysandra,
Crysandrah, Khrisandra,
Khrisandrah, Khrysandra,
Khrysandrah, Krisanda, Krishna,
Krishnah, Krizandra, Krizandrah,

Krysandra, Krysandrah, Kryzandra,
Kryzandrah

Kristen (Scandinavian) Christian.
**The Scandinavian form of
Christine.**
Christabel, Christabela,
Christabelah, Christabele,
Christabell, Christabella,
Christabellah, Chrisabelle,
Christain, Christaina, Christainah,
Christaine, Christayn, Christayna,
Christaynah, Christayne, Christan,
Christana, Christanah, Christane,
Christean, Christeana, Christeanah,
Christeane, Christeen, Christeena,
Christeenah, Christeene, Christein,
Christeina, Christeinah, Christeine,
Christin, Christina, Christinah,
Christine, Christyn, Christyna,
Christynah, Christyne, Chrystyn,
Chrystyna, Chrystynah, Chrystyne,
Cristabel, Cristabela, Cristabelah,
Cristabele, Crisabell, Cristabella,
Cristabellah, Cristabelle, Cristain,
Cristaina, Cristainah, Cristaine,
Cristan, Cristana, Cristanah,
Cristane, Cristean, Cristeana,
Cristeanah, Cristeane, Cristeen,
Cristeena, Cristeenah, Cristeene,
Cristein, Cristeina, Cristeinah,
Cristeine, Cristen, Cristena,
Cristenah, Cristene, Cristin,
Cristina, Cristinah, Cristinah,
Cristine, Crystyn, Crystyna,
Crystynah, Crystyne, Khristean,
Khristeana, Khristeanah,
Khristeane, Khristeen, Khristeena,
Khristeenah, Khristeene, Khristein,
Khristeina, Khristeinah, Khristeine,
Khristin, Khristina, Khristinah,
Khristine, Khristyn, Khristyna,
Khristynah, Khristyne, Khrystyn,
Khrystyna, Khrystynah, Khrystyne,
Krista, Kristabel, Kristabela,
Kristabelah, Kristabele, Kristabell,
Kristabella, Kristabellah,

Kristabelle, Kristain, Kristaina,
Kristainah, Kristaine, Kristan,
Kristana, Kristanah, Kristane,
Kristayn, Kristayna, Kristaynah,
Kiystayne, Kristeen, Kristeena,
Kristeenah, Kristeene, Kristein,
Kristeina, Kristeinah, Kristeine,
Kristin, Kristina, Kristinah, Kriston,
Kristyn, Kristyna, Kristynah,
Kristyne, Kristynn, Kristynna,
Kristynnah, Kristynne, Krysta,
Krystal, Krystan, Krystana,
Krystanah, Krystane, Krystean,
Krysteana, Krysteanah, Krysteane,
Krysteen, Krysteena, Krysteenah,
Krysteene, Krystein, Krysteina,
Krysteinah, Krysteine, Krysten,
Krystena, Krystenah, Krystene,
Krystenia, Krystenina, Krystin,
Krystina, Krystinah, Krystine,
Kryston, Krystyn, Krystyna,
Krystynah, Krystyne, Krystynn
Krystynna, Krystynnah, Krystynne

Kristianna (Hebrew) Christian,
whose God is gracious.
Christian, Christiana, Christianah,
Christiane, Christiann,
Christianna, Christiannah,
Christianne, Chrystian, Chrystiana,
Chrystiane, Chrystiann,
Chrystianna, Chrystiannah,
Chrystianne, Crestian, Crestiana,
Crestianah, Crestiane, Crestiann,
Crestianna, Crestiannah,
Crestianne, Cristian, Cristiana,
Cristianah, Cristiane, Cristiann,
Cristianna, Cristiannah, Cristianne,
Cristyan, Cristyana, Cristyanah,
Cristyane, Cristyann, Cristyanna,
Cristyannah, Cristyanne, Crystian,
Crystiana, Crystianah, Crystiane,
Crystiann, Crystianna, Crystiannah,
Crystianne, Crystyan, Crystyana,
Crystyanah, Crystyane, Crystyann,
Crystyanna, Crystyannah,
Crystyanne, Khristian, Khristiana,

Kristianna cont.
Khristianah, Khristiane, Khristiann, Khristianna, Khristiannah, Khristianne, Khristyn, Khristyna, Khristynah, Khristyne, Khristynn, Khristynna, Khristynnah, Khristynne, Khrystin, Khrystina, Khrystinah, Khrystine, Khrystyn, Khrystyna, Khrystynah, Khrystyne, Krestian, Krestiana, Krestianah, Krestiane, Krestiann, Krestianna, Krestiannah, Krestianne, Kristian, Kristiana, Kristianah, Kristiane, Kristiann, Kristiannah, Kristianne, Kristyan, Kristyana, Kristyanah, Kristyane, Kristyann, Kristyanna, Kristyannah, Kristyanne, Krystian, Krystiana, Krystianah, Krystiane, Krystiann, Krystianna, Krystianne, Krystyan, Krystyana, Krystyana, Krystyanah, Krystyane, Krystyann, Krystyanna, Krystyannah, Krystyanne

Kristine (Danish/Norwegian) Christian.
Christean, Christean, Christeen, Christeene, Christein, Christeine, Christeyn, Chrysteyne, Christina, Christinah, Christine (Lat), Chrystean, Chrysteane, Chrysteen, Chrysteene, Chrystein, Chrysteine, Chrysteyn, Chrysteyne, Chrystin, Chrystine, Chrystyn, Chrystyne, Cristean, Cristeane, Cristeen, Cristeene, Cristein, Cristeine, Cristeyn, Cristeyne, Cristin, Cristina, Cristine, Cristyn, Cristyne, Crystean, Crysteane, Crysteen, Crysteene, Crystein, Crysteine, Crysteyn, Crysteyne, Crystin, Crystine, Crystyn, Crystyne, Khristean, Khristeane, Khristeen, Khristeene, Khristein, Khristeine, Khristeyn, Khristeyne, Khristiann, Kristianna, Khristianne, Khristin, Khristyn, Khristyne, Khrystean,

Khrysteane, Khrysteen, Khrysteene, Khrystein, Khrysteine, Khrysteyn, Khrysteyne, Khrystin, Khrystyn, Khrystyne, Khrystynna, Khrystynne, Kristana, Kristane, Kristean, Kristeane, Kristeen, Kristeene, Kristel (Ger), Kristell, Kristelle, Kristein, Kristeine, Kristen (Scan), Kristeyn, Kristeyne, Kristijntje (Dut), Kristin, Kristina (Slav/Lith), Kristyn, Kristyna, Kristyne, Kristynn, Kristynna, Kristynne, Krystean, Krysteane, Krysteen, Krysteene, Krystein, Krysteine, Krysteyn, Krysteyne, Krystin, Krystine, Krystyn, Krystyne, Krysynnah, Krystynne

Krita (Sanskrit) perfection.
Crita, Critah, Cryta, Crytah, Kritah, Kryta, Krytah

Krystal (Latin) clear.
Cristal, Cristall, Cristalle, Cristel, Cristele, Cristell, Cristelle, Crystal, Crystel, Crystele, Crystell, Crystelle, Krista, Kristabel, Kristabele, Kristabell, Kristabella, Kristabelle, Kristal, Kristale, Kristall, Kristalle, Kristel, Kristele, Kristell, Kristella, Kristelle, Krystal (USA), Krystalbel, Krystalbele, Krystalbell, Krystalbella, Krystabelle, Krystel, Krystele, Krystell, Krystella, Krystelle, Krystelina, Krysteline, Krystell, Krystella, Krystelle, Krystle (USA), Krystyl, Krystyle, Krystyll, Krystylle

Kubbitha (Australian Aboriginal) black duck.
Kubbith

Kui (Tongan) grandmother.

Kuini (Tongan) queen.

Kula (Tongan) bird.
Kulah

K

Kulya (Native American) pine nuts burning.
Kulia, Kuliah, Kulyah

Kuma (Tongan) mouse.
Kumah

Kumala (Tongan) sweet potato; yam.
Kumalah

Kumari (Sanskrit) woman.
Kumaree, Kumarey, Kumaria, Kumariah, Kumarie, Kumary, Kumarya, Kumaryah

Kumberlin (Australian Aboriginal) sweet.
Cumberlin, Cumberlina, Cumberline, Cumberlyn, Cumberlyne, Kumberlina, Kumberline, Kumberlyn, Kumberlyne

Kumi (Japanese) to braid; plait.
Kumee, Kumie, Kumy

Kunama (Australian Aboriginal) snow.
Kunam, Kunamah

Kunani (Hawaiian) beautiful.
Kunanee, Kunaney, Kunanie, Kunany

Kuri (Japanese) chestnut.
Curee, Curey, Curi, Curie, Cury, Kuree, Kurey, Kurie, Kury

Kyla (Hebrew) crown.
Kila, Kilah, Kylah

Kyle (Irish) attractive one from the strait.
Kiel, Kiela, Kiele, Kiell, Kiella, Kielle, Kile, Kyel, Kyela, Kyele, Kyell, Kyella, Kyelle

Kylie (Australian Aboriginal) boomerang; one who returns. (Irish/English) from the meadow strait.
Kilea, Kileah, Kilee, Kilei, Kileigh, Kiley, Kili, Kilia, Kiliah, Kilie, Killea, Killeah, Killee, Killei, Killeigh, Killi, Killia, Killiah, Killie, Killy, Kily, Kylea, Kyleah, Kylee, Kylei, Kyleigh, Kyley, Kyli, Kylia, Kyliah, Kyllea, Kylleah, Kyllee, Kyllei, Kylleigh, Kylley, Kylli, Kyllia, Kylliah, Kyllie, Kylly, Kyly, Kylya, Kylyah

Kyna (Irish/Gaelic) intelligent; wise.
Kina, Kinah, Kynah

Kyoko (Japanese) mirror.
Kioko, Kioka, Kyoka, Yoka, Yoko

Kyra (Persian) sun.
Kiara, Kira, Kirah, Kirra, Kirrah, Kyara, Kyarah, Kyrah

Kyrene (Greek) lordly.
Kirena, Kirenah, Kirene, Kyrena, Kyrenah

Kyrie (Irish) dark-haired.
Kiree, Kyree, Kyrey, Kyri, Kyry

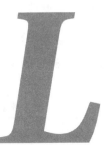

La'a (Tongan) sunny.

Laaka (Tongan) carefree; the lark bird.

Labibi (French/Arabic) lady.
Labiby

Labrenda (Old Norse) sword.
Labreana, Labreanah, Labreann, Labreanna, Labreannah, Labreanne, Labrenna, Labrennah, Labrinda, Labrindah, Labrynda, Labrynah

Lace/Lacey (English) delicate fabric.
Lace, Lacea, Lacee, Laci, Lacia, Laciah, Laciann, Lacianna, Lacianne, Lacie, Lacy, Laicee, Laicey, Laici, Laicia, Laiciah, Laicie, Laicy, Laycee, Laycey, Layci, Layciah, Laycy

Lachandra (American/Sanskrit) the moon.
Lachanda, Lachandah, Lachander, Lachandrah, Lachandrica, Lachandrice, Lachandryce

Lachianina (Scottish) from the land of lakes. The feminine form of Lachlan.
Lachianinah, Lachyanina, Lachyaninah, Lachlanee, Lachlani, Lachlania, Lachlanie, Lachlany, Locklanee, Locklaney, Locklani, Locklanie, Locklany

Lacole (Italian) victory of the people. A form of Nicole.
Lacola, Lacolla, Lacolle, Lecola, Lecole, Lecolla, Lecolle

Lacrecia (Latin) wealthy.
Lacrasha, Lacreash, Lacreasha, Lacreashia, Lacresha, Lacreshah, Lacreshia, Lacreshiah, Lacresia, Lacretia, Lacretiah, Lacretya, Lacretyah, Lacricia, Lacriciah, Lacrisha, Lacrishia, Lacrishiah, Lacrycia, Lacryciah, Lacrychya, Lacrychyah

Lada (Russian) goddess of beauty.
Ladah, Ladia, Ladiah, Ladya, Ladyah

Ladana (Finnish/Celtic) the mother of the gods.
Ladanah, Ladann, Ladanna, Ladannah, Ladanne

Ladancia (French/Slavic) the morning star.
Ladanicah, Ladanicka, Ladanika, Ladanikah, Ladanyca, Ladanycah, Ladanycka, Ladanyka, Ladanykah

Ladasha (American/Russian/Greek) gift of God.
Ladashah

Ladawna (English) the dawning.
Ladawn, Ladawnah, Ladawne, Ladawnee, Ladawni, Ladawnia, Ladawniah, Ladawnie, Ladawny

Ladivina (English) divine.
Ladivinah, Ladivine, Ladivyna, Ladivynah, Ladivyne, Ladyvyna, Ladyvynah, Ladyvyne

Ladonna (Italian/Spanish) lady.
Ladona, Ladonah, Ladonia, Ladoniah, Ladonnah, Ladonnia, Ladonniah, Ladonnya, Ladonnyah, Ladonya, Ladonyah

Laella (French/English) elf.
Lael, Laela, Laele, Laell, Laelle,

Laila, Lailah, Laile, Lailla, Laillah, Laille, Laylla, Laylle

Laetitia (Latin) happy.
Laeticha, Laetichah, Laeticia, Laeticiah, Laetichya, Laetychyah, Laetissma, Laetita, Laetitah, Laetitiah, Laetyta, Laetytah, Laetyte, Laetytia, Laeticha, Laetichah, Laetichia, Laeticiah, Laetycia, Laetyciah, Laetytiah, Laiticia, Laitichiah, Laitichya, Laitichyah, Laitita, Laititah, Laititia, Laititiah, Latita, Latitah, Latite, Latyta, Latytah, Latyte, Latytia, Latytiah, Latytya, Latytyah, Laytita, Laytitah, Laytitia, Laytitiah, Laytyta, Laytytah, Laytytia, Laytytiah, Laytytya, Laytytyah, Leticia, Leticya, Letitia, Lettice, Letizia, Letiziah, Letizya, Letizyah, Letyza, Letyzah, Letyzia, Letyziah, Letyzya, Letyzyah

Laflora (French/Latin) flower.
Laflorah, Leflora, Leflorah

Lafu (Tongan) sea bird that burrows into the hillside.

Lahela (Hawaiian) female deer, doe.
Lahelah

Lahi (Tongan) great.

Laikana (Tongan) lilac.
Laelaka, Laelakah, Lailakah, Laylaka, Laylakah

Laili (Arabic) dark beauty of the night; dark-haired.
Laelea, Laeleah, Laelee, Laelei, Laeleigh, Laeley, Laeli, Laelia, Laeliah, Laelie, Laely, Laelya, Lailea, Laileah, Lailee, Lailei, Laileigh, Lailey, Lailia, Lailiah, Lailie, Laily, Lailya, Laylea, Layleah, Laylee, Laylei, Layleigh, Layli, Laylia, Layliah, Laylie, Layly

Laime (Tongan) lime.
Laem, Laeme, Laim, Laym, Layme

Laine/Lainey (English) light. (Fren) wool. A short form of Elaine.
Laena, Laenah, Laene, Laenee, Laeney, Laeney, Laeni, Laenia, Laeniah, Laenie, Laeny, Laenya, Laenyah, Lain, Laina, Lainah, Laine, Lainee, Laini, Lainia, Lainiah, Lainie, Lainy, Lainya, Lainyah, Layn, Layna, Laynah, Layne, Laynee, Layney, Layni, Laynia, Layniah, Laynie, Layny

Laione (Tongan) lion.
Laeona, Laeonah, Laeone, Laiona, Laionah, Layona, Layonah, Layone

Lais (Greek) happy.
Lays

Lajessica (Hebrew) the wealthy.
Jessica, Jessicah, Jessicka, Jessickah, Jessika, Jessikah, Jessyca, Jessycah, Jessycka, Jessyckah, Jessyka, Jessykah, Lajesica, Lajesicah, Lajesika, Lajesikah, Lajessicah, Lajessika, Lajessikah, Lajessyca, Lajessycah, Lajessycka, Lajessyckah, Lajessyka, Lajessykah

Lajila (Hindi) shy.
Lajilah, Lajilla, Lajillah

Lajoia (Latin) happy.
Lajoiah, Lajoya, Lajoyah

Lajuana (American/Hebrew) God is gracious.
Lajuanah, Lajuanna, Lajuannah, Lajunna, Lawana, Lawanah, Lawanna, Lawanne, Lawanza, Lawanze, Laweania

Lajuliette (Latin) little youthful one.
Lajuliet, Lajulieta, Lajulietah, Lajuliete, Lajuliett, Lajulietta, Lajuliettah, Lajulyet, Lajulyeta, Lajulyete, Lajulyett, Lajulyetta, Lajulyettah, Lajulyette

Laka (Hawaiian) alluring one; Siren.
Lakah

Lakalka (Tongan) ballet dancer.
Laka

Lakeisha/Lakeishia (Swahili/African American) life. (Arab) woman.
Aiesha, Aisha, Ayesha, Keasha, Keashia, Keashiah, Keesha, Keisha, Lakaiesha, Lakaisha, Lakasha, Lakecia, Lakeciah, Lakeesh, Lakeesha, Lakesha, Lakeshia, Lakeshiah, Lakeshya, Lakesia, Lakesiah, Laketia, Laketiah, Lakeysha, Lakeyshia, Lakenzia, Lakenziah, Lakenzya, Lakenzyah, Lakieshia, Lakisha, Lakita, Lakitia, Lakitiah, Lakyta, Lakytah, Lakytia, Lakytiah, Lakytya, Lakytyah

Lakendra/Lakendria (Old English/African American) knowing; understanding.
Kendra, Kendrah, Kendria, Kendriah, Lakanda, Lakandah, Lakendra, Lakendrah, Lakendrya, Lakendryah

Lakenya (African) the jewel.
Kenia, Keniah, Kenja, Kenya, Kanyah, Lakandra, Lakande, Lakeena, Lakeenna, Lakeenya, Lakena, Lakenah, Lakenia, Lakeniah, Lakenja, Lakenyah, Lakin, Lakina, Lakine, Lakinja, Lakinya, Lakinyah, Lakwania, Lakwanya, Lakyna, Lekenia, Lekeniah, Lekenya, Lekenyah

Laketa (Scottish/African American) the woods.
Lakeet, Lakeeta, Lakeetah, Lakeita, Lakeitha, Lakeithia, Laketha, Laketia, Laketiah, Lakett, Laketta, Lakette, Lakietha, Lakita, Lakitra, Lakitri, Lakitrie, Lakitt, Lakitta, Lakitte, Lakyta, Lakytah, Lakyte, Lakytta, Lakyttah, Lakytte

Lakia (Arabic) the treasure.
Lakiah, Lakya, Lakyah

Lakkari (Australian Aboriginal) honeysuckle tree.
Lakaree, Lakarey, Lakari, Lakaria, Lakariah, Lakarie, Lakary, Lakkaree, Lakkarey, Lakkarie, Lakkary, Lakkarya, Lakkaryah

Lakresha (Latin) the rich reward.
Lacresha, Lacreshia, Lacreshiah, Lacresia, Lacresiah, Lacretia, Lacretiah, Lacrisha, Lakresha, Lakreshia, Lakreshiah, Lakrisha, Lakrysha, Lakryshah, Lekresha, Lekresia, Lekreshiah, Lekreshya, Lekresyah

Lakshmi (Sanskrit) mark; success. The Hindi goddess of beauty and good fortune.
Lakme, Lakshmee, Lakshmey, Lakshmie, Lakshmy

Lakya (Hindi) child born on Thursday
Lakia, Lakiah, Lakyah

Lala (Slavic) tulip flower.
Laela, Laelah, Laella, Laellah, Laila, Lailah, Lailla, Laillah, Lalah, Lalla, Lallah, Layla, Laylah, Laylla, Layllah

Lalage (Greek) one who speaks freely.
Lallage

Lalaka (Tongan) walk.
Lalakah

Lalama (Tongan) one who beckons with her eyes.
Lalamah

Lalanga (Tongan) weaver.
Lalangah

Lalasa (Hindi) love.
Lallasa, Lalassa

Lalata (Tongan) tame.
Lalatah

Lali (Spanish/Polynesian) the
highest point of heaven.
(Ton) wooden drum.
Laelea, Laeleah, Laelee, Laelei,
Laeleigh, Laeley, Laeli, Laelia,
Laeliah, Laelie, Laely, Laelya,
Laelyah, Lalea, Laleah, Laelee,
Laelei, Laeleigh, Laeli, Laelia,
Laeliah, Laelie, Laely, Laelya,
Laelyah, Lailea, Laileah, Lailee,
Lailei, Laileigh, Laili, Lailia,
Lailiah, Lailie, Laily, Lailya, Lailyah,
Lalea, Laleah, Lalee, Lalei, Laleigh,
Laley, Lalia, Laliah, Lalie, Lalia,
Laliah, Lalla, Lallah, Lallea,
Lalleah, Lallee, Lallei, Lalleigh,
Lalley, Lalli, Lallia, Lalliah, Lallie,
Lally, Laly, Lalya, Lalyah, Lulanea,
Lulanee, Lulaney, Lulani, Lulanie,
Lulany, Lulanya, Lulanyah

Lalirra (Australian Aboriginal)
talkative.
Lalira, Lalirah, Lalirrah, Lalyra,
Lalyrah, Lalyrra, Lalyrrah, Lirra,
Lirrah, Lyra, Lyrah, Lyrra, Lyrrah

Lalita (Sanskrit) charming; playful;
honest. (Grk) talkative.
Laleata, Laleatah, Laleate, Laleeta,
Laleetah, Laleete, Laleita, Laleitah,
Laleite, Lalitah, Lalite, Lalitt,
Lalitta, Lalitte, Lalyta, Lalytah,
Lalyte, Lalytta, Lalyttah, Lalytte

Lallie (English) talker.
Lalea, Laleah, Lalee, Lalei, Laleigh,
Lalia, Laliah, Lalie, Lallea, Lalleah,
Lallee, Lallei, Lalleigh, Lalley, Lalli,
Lallia, Lalliah, Lally, Lallya,
Lallyah, Laly, Lalya, Lalyah

Lamani (Tongan) lemon.
Lamanee, Lamaney, Lamania,
Lamaniah, Lamanie, Lamany,
Lamanya, Lamanyah

Lamberta (German) bright rich land
or owner of many estates. The
feminine form of Lambert.
Lamberlina, Lamberline,
Lamberlynn, Lamberlynne,
Lambirta, Lambirtah, Lambirte,
Lamburta, Lamburtah, Lamburte,
Lambyrta, Lambyrtah, Lambyrte

Lamesha (Hindi) born under the
sign of Aries.
Lamees, Lameesa, Lameise,
Lameshia, Lameshiah, Lamisha,
Lamysha, Lemesha, Lemisha,
Lemysha

Lami (Tongan) concealer.
Lamee, Lamey, Lamia, Lamie,
Lamy, Lamya

Lamia (German) the bright land.
Lama, Lamah, Lamiah, Lamya,
Lamyah

Lamis (Arabic) softness.
Lamisa, Lamisah, Lamiss, Lamissa,
Lamissah, Lamys, Lamysa, Lamyss,
Lamyssa

Lamora (French/Latin) honour.
Lamorah

Lamorna (Middle English) the
morning. (Fren/Gae) beloved.
Lamornah

Lamya (Arabic) dark-lipped.
Lamia, Lamiah, Lamyah

Lan (Vietnamese) orchid flower.
Lana, Lanah, Lann, Lanna, Lannah

Lana (Latin) woolly. (Haw) light;
airy. The short form of Alannah,
handsome; fair; bright; happy.
The feminine form of Alain/Alan.
Lanae, Lanah, Lanaia, Lanaya,
Lanayah, Lanna, Lannah, Lannaia,
Lannaya, Lanetta, Lanette, Lanne,
Larna, Larnah

Landa (Basque/Hebrew) wished-for; star of the sea; bitter. A form of Mary.
Landah, Landrea

Landra (German/Spanish) counsellor.
Landrada, Landrah, Landrea, Landreah, Landria, Landriah, Landrya, Landryah

Lane (Middle English) narrow lane; little road.
Laen, Laena, Laene, Lain, Laina, Lainah, Laine, Lainee, Lainey, Lanee, Laney, Lannee, Lanni, Lannia, Lanniah, Lannie, Layn, Layna, Laynah, Layne

Laneisha (Swahili/African American) life. (Arab) woman.
Lanecia, Laneciah, Laneesha, Laneise, Lanesha, Laneshe, Laness, Lanessa, Lanesse, Laneysha, Lanisha, Lanysha

Lanelle (Old French) she is from the little road.
Lanel, Lanela, Lanelah, Lanele, Lanell, Lanella, Lanellah

Lanet (Celtic) little graceful one.
Laneta, Lanete, Lanett, Lanetta, Lanette

Langi (Tongan) heaven.
Langia, Langie, Langy

Lani (Hawaiian) sky; heaven.
Lanea, Lanee, Laney, Lania, Laniah, Lanie, Lannee, Lanney, Lanni, Lannia, Lanniah, Lannie, Lanny, Lannya, Lany, Lanya

Lann (Irish) blade.
Lan, Lanita, Lanitah, Lanite, Lanna, Lannah, Lanyt, Lanyta, Lanytah, Lanyte

Lanni (Latin) woolly. (Haw) light; airy. The short form of Alannah, handsome; fair; bright; happy. The feminine form of Alain/Alan.
Lanea, Lanee, Laney, Lani, Lania, Laniah, Lanie, Lannea, Lannee, Lanney, Lannia, Lanniah, Lannie, Lanny, Lannya, Lany, Lanya, Lanyah

Lantha (Greek) purple flower.
Lanthia, Lanthiah, Lanthya, Lanthyah

Lapisi (Tongan) rabbit.

Laqueena/Laquinta (English) the queen.
Laquanda, Laquanta, Laqueen, Laqueene, Laquena, Laquenda, Laquenah, Laquenda, Laquendra, Laquene, Laquenet, Laqueneta, Laquenete, Laquenett, Laquenetta, Laquenette, Laquinta, Laquintah, Laquynta, Laquyntah

Lara (Latin) shining; famous. (A/Abor) hut built on stony ground. (Grk) happy. The short form of Larissa.
Larah, Laria, Lariah, Larra, Larrah, Larrya, Larryah, Larya, Laryah

Laraina/Laraine (Latin) sorrowful. (Ger) famous warrior. (O/Eng) crown of laurel leaves in the rain. (Grk) happy. (Lat) seabird.
Larae, Laraen, Laraena, Laraenah, Laraene, Larain, Larainah, Laraine, Larainee, Larana, Laranah, Larane, Larayna, Laraynah, Larayne, Larein, Lareina, Lareinah, Lareine, Larena, Larenah, Larene, Lareyn, Lareyna, Lareynah, Lareyne, Larrain, Larraina, Larrainah, Larraine, Larrayn, Larrayna, Larraynah, Larrayne, Larrein, Larreina, Larreinah, Larreine, Larreyn,

Larreyna, Larreynah, Larreyne,
Lora, Lorae, Loraen, Loraena,
Loraenah, Loraene, Lorain,
Loraina, Lorainah, Loraine, Lorayn,
Lorayna, Loraynah, Lorayne,
Lorein, Loreina, Loreinah, Loreine,
Loreyn, Loreyna, Loreynah,
Loreyne, Lorraen, Lorraena,
Lorraenah, Lorraene, Lorrain,
Lorraina, Lorrainah, Lorraine,
Lorrayn, Lorrayna, Lorraynah,
Lorrayne, Lorrein, Lorreina,
Lorreinah, Lorreine, Lorreyn,
Lorreyna, Lorreynah, Lorreyne

Larana (Latin) sea bird.
Laranah, Larane, Larann, Laranna,
Larannah, Laranne

Lareina (Spanish) queen.
Larae, Laraen, Laraena, Laraenah,
Laraene, Larain, Laraina, Larainah,
Laraine, Larainee, Larana, Laranah,
Larane, Larayna, Laraynah, Larayne,
Larein, Lareinah, Lareine, Larena,
Larenah, Larene, Lareyn, Lareyna,
Lareynah, Lareyne, Larrain,
Larraina, Larrainah, Larraine,
Larrayn, Larrayna, Larraynah,
Larrayne, Larrein, Larreina,
Larreinah, Larreine, Larreyn,
Larreyna, Larreynah, Larreyne,
Laurain, Lauraina, Laurainah,
Lauraine, Laurayn, Laurayna,
Lauraynah, Laurayne, Lora, Lorae,
Loraen, Loraena, Loraenah,
Loraene, Lorain, Loraina, Lorainah,
Loraine, Lorayn, Lorayna,
Loraynah, Lorayne, Lorein,
Loreina, Loreinah, Loreine, Loreyn,
Loreyna, Loreynah, Loreyne,
Lorraen, Lorraena, Lorraenah,
Lorraene, Lorrain, Lorraina,
Lorrainah, Lorraine, Lorrayn,
Lorrayna, Lorraynah, Lorrayne,
Lorrein, Lorreina, Lorreinah,
Lorreine, Lorreyn, Lorreyna,
Lorreynah, Lorreyne

Lari (Latin) holy. (Lat) crown of
laurel leaves; victory. The short
form of names starting with 'Lari'
e.g. **Lariana.**
Larea, Laree, Larey, Larian,
Larianah, Lariane, Lariann,
Larianna, Lariannah, Larianne,
Larie, Larrian, Larriana, Larrianah,
Larriane, Larriann, Larrianna,
Larriannah, Larrianne, Larrie,
Larryan, Larryana, Larryanah,
Larryane, Larryann, Larryanna,
Larryannah, Larryanne, Lorian,
Loriana, Lorianah, Loriane,
Loriann, Lorianna, Loriannah,
Lorianne, Lorie, Lorrian, Lorriana,
Lorrianah, Lorriane, Lorriann,
Lorrianna, Lorriannah, Lorrianne,
Lorryan, Lorryana, Lorryanah,
Lorryane, Lorryann, Lorryanna,
Lorryannah, Lorryanne, Loryan,
Loryana, Loryanah, Loryane,
Loryann, Loryanna, Loryannah,
Loryanne

Lariana (Latin/Hebrew) graceful;
holy.
Larian, Larianah, Lariane, Lariann,
Larianna, Lariannah, Larianne,
Larrian, Larriana, Larrianah,
Larriane, Larriann, Larrianna,
Larriannah, Larrianne, Larryan,
Larryana, Larryanah, Larryane,
Larryann, Larryanna, Larryannah,
Larryanne, Lorian, Loriana,
Lorianah, Loriane, Loriann,
Lorianna, Loriannah, Lorianne,
Lorrian, Lorriana, Lorrianah,
Lorriane, Lorriann, Lorrianna,
Lorriannah, Lorrianne, Lorryan,
Lorryana, Lorryanah, Lorryane,
Lorryann, Lorryanna, Lorryannah,
Lorryanne, Loryan, Loryana,
Loryanah, Loryane

Laricia (Latin) holy crown of laurel
leaves; victory.
Lariciah, Laricya, Laricyah, Larikia,

Laricia cont.
Larikiah, Larycia, Laryciah, Larycya, Larycyah, Larykia, Laryikiah, Larykya, Larykyah

Lariel (Hebrew) lioness of God.
Lariela, Larielah, Lariele, Lariell, Lariella, Lariellah, Larielle, Laryel, Laryela, Laryelah, Laryele, Laryell, Laryella, Laryellah, Laryelle

Larina/Larine (Latin) sea bird; girl from the sea.
Laren, Larena, Larenah, Larenee, Larinah, Larrine, Larinna, Larinnah, Larrine, Laryn, Laryna, Larynah, Laryne

Larissa (Greek) happy.
Larisa, Larisse, Larysa, Laryssia, Laryssa, Larysse, Latashia, Latahiah, Latoshia, Loriss, Lorissa, Lorisse, Lorysa, Lorysah, Loryssa, Loryssah

Lark (Middle English) carefree; the lark bird. (A/Abor) cloud.
Larke, Larkee, Larkey

Larlene (Celtic) promise.
Larlean, Larleana, Larleanah, Larleane, Larleen, Larleena, Larleenah, Larleene, Larlin, Larlina, Larlinah, Larline, Larlyn, Larlyna, Larlynah, Larlyne

Larmina (German) love. (Per) blue sky. (Hin) born under the sign of Pisces.
Larminah, Larmine, Larmyn, Larmyna, Larmynah, Larmyne, Mina, Minah, Myna, Mynah

Larnelle (Latin) of high degree.
Larnel, Larnela, Larnelah, Larnele, Larnell, Larnella, Larnellah

Laroux (French) red-haired.
Laroux, Laroo

Lasar (Irish) flame; red-haired.
Lasara, Lasarah, Laser, Lazar, Lazer

Lashanda (African American/ Hebrew) God is gracious.
Lashan, Lashana, Lashanay, Lashanee, Lashandra, Lashane, Lashanee, Lashann, Lashanna, Lashanne, Lashannon, Lashanta, Lashante

Lashawna (African American/Irish) God is gracious. The feminine form of Shawn.
Lasean, Laseana, Laseanah, Laseane, Lashaun, Lashauna, Lashaune, Lashaunna, Lashaunnah, Lashaunne, Lashunta, Lashawn, Lashawne, Lashawnda, Lashawndra, Lashawne, Lashawni, Lashawnia, Lashawnie, Lashawny, Lesean, Leseana, Leseanah, Leseane, Leshaughn, Leshaughna, Leshaughnah, Leshaughne, Leshaun, Leshauna, Leshaune, Leshawn, Leshawna, Leshawnah, Leshawne, Seana, Seanah, Seane, Shaun, Shauna, Shaunah, Shaune, Shawn, Shawna, Shawnah, Shawne

Lashonda (African American/Irish) God is gracious. A form of Shona.
Lachonda, Lashaunda, Lashaundra, Lashon, Lashona, Lashond, Lashonda, Lashonde, Lashondia, Lashondra, Lashonna, Lashonta, Lashunda, Lashundra, Lashunta, Lashunte, Leshande, Leshandra, Leshondra, Leshundra, Shonda, Shona, Shonah, Shonia, Shoniah, Shonya, Shonyah

Lasipeli (Tongan) raspberry.

Lass/Lassie (Gaelic) girl.
Lasee, Lasey, Lasi, Lasie, Lasse, Lassee, Lassey, Lassi, Lassy, Lasy

Lata (Hindi) vine.
Latah

L

Latania (French/Russian/African American) queen of the fairies.
Latana, Latanah, Latanda, Latandra, Lataniah, Latanja, Latanna, Latanua, Latanya, Latona, Latonah, Latonee, Latoni, Latonia, Latoniah, Latonie, Latonna, Latonne, Latonshia, Latonya, Latonyah, Tania, Taniah, Tanya, Tanyah, Tonia, Toniah, Tonya, Tonyah

Latara (Irish/African American) rocky hill. A form of Tara.
Latarah, Lataria, Latariah, Latarya, Lotara, Lotarah, Lotaria, Lotarya, Tara, Tarah, Taria, Tariah, Tarya, Taryah

Lataree (Australian Aboriginal) wild fig. (Jap) bending branch.
Latarea, Latarey, Latari, Latarie, Latary, Tarea, Taree

Latasha (Latin) born on Christmas day. A form of Natasha.
Latashah, Latashia, Latisha, Latishah, Latysha, Latyshah

Lateefa (Arabic) to caress.
Lateifa, Lateifah, Lateyfa, Lateyfah

Latia (Latin/African American) latin princess.
Lateena, Lateene, Latiah, Latin, Latina, Latinah, Latja, Latya, Latyah

Latika (Hindi) small creeper plant.
Latik, Latikah, Latyka, Latykah

Latina (French/English) the little one.
Latean, Lateana, Lateanah, Lateane, Lateen, Lateena, Lateenah, Lateene, Latinah, Latine, Latyn, Latyna, Latynah, Latyne

Latisha (Latin) happy.
Laeticia, Laeticiah, Laeticya, Laeticyah, Laetisha, Laetitia, Laetizia, Laetiziah, Laetizya, Laetycia, Laetyciah, Laetyisha, Laetycya, Laetycyah, Laetyshya, Latashia, Lateacha, Lateacia, Lateaciah, Lateacya, Lateacyah, Lateashia, Lateashiah, Lateashya, Lateashyah, Latia, Latiah, Latice, Laticia, Laticiah, Latiesha, Latishia, Latissha, Latitia, Latyca, Latycah, Latycia, Latyciah, Latycya, Latycyah, Latysha, Latyshia, Latyshiah, Latysya, Latysysah

Latona/Latonia (Latin) goddess who gave birth to Diana and Apollo.
Latonah, Latonia, Latoniah, Latonja, Latonya, Latonyah

Latoria (Latin/African American) victory. A form of Victoria.
Latorea, Latoreah, Latoree, Latorey, Latori, Latoriah, Latorie, Latorio, Latorja, Latorray, Latorreia, Latory, Latorya, Latoyra, Latoyria, Latoyrrya

Latoya (Spanish) victory. A form of Latoria.
La Toia, Latoia, La Toiah, La Toya, La Toyah, Latoyia, Latoyiah

Latrice/Latricia (Latin/African American) noble; well born.
Latrecia, Latreciah, Latresh, Latresha, Latreshia, Latreshiah, Latreshya, Latrica, Latricah, Latriciah, Latrisha, Latrishia, Latrishiah, Latrysha, Latryshia, Latryshiah, Latryshya

Lau (Tongan) leaf.

Laukoka (Tongan) yam.
Laumahi

Laulani (Hawaiian) heavenly branch.
Laulanea, Laulanee, Laulaney, Laulania, Laulaniah, Laulanie, Laulany, Laulanya, Laulanyah

Laumanu (Tongan) flock of birds.

Laumarie (Tongan) spirited.
Laumalea, Laumaleah, Laumalee,
Laumalei, Laumaleigh, Laumali,
Laumalia, Laumaliah, Laumaly

Launoa (Tongan) shining moon.
Launoah

Laura (Latin) laurel leaves.
Lara, Larah, Larain, Laraina,
Larainah, Laraine, Lari, Laria,
Lariah, Larie, Larinda, Larindah,
Larinde, Laudra, Launa, Laura,
Laurah, Laurain, Lauraina,
Laurainah, Lauraine, Laural,
Lauralea, Lauraleah, Lauralee,
Lauralei, Lauraleigh, Lauraley,
Laurali, Lauralia, Lauraliah,
Lauralie, Lauralin, Lauralina,
Lauralinah, Lauraline, Lauraly,
Lauralya, Lauralyn, Lauralyna,
Lauran, Laurana, Laurane, Laure
(It), Lauree, Laureen, Laureena,
Laureene, Laurel, Laurelle, Lauren,
Laurena, Laurencia, Laurenia,
Laurene, Laurentia, Laurentiah,
Laurentya, Lawra, Lawrah, Lawrea,
Lawree, Lawrey, Lawri, Lawria,
Lawriah, Lawriah, Lawrie, Lawry,
Lawrya, Lawryah, Lora, Lorah,
Lorayne, Loree, Loreen, Loreena,
Lorel, Lorelea, Lorelee, Loreleigh,
Lorell, Lorelle, Loren, Lorena,
Lorene, Lorenza, Lorettah, Loretta,
Lorette, Lori, Loria, Loriah,
Loriana, Lorianah, Loriane,
Loriann, Lorianna, Loriannah,
Lorianne, Lorie, Loriel, Loriela,
Lorielah, Loriele, Loriell, Loriella,
Loriellah, Lorielle, Lori'elle, Lorin,
Lorind, Lorinda, Lorindah, Lorine,
Lory, Lorya, Loryah, Loryan,
Loryana, Loryanah, Loryane,
Loryann, Loryanna, Loryannah,
Loryanne, Loryel, Loryela,

Loryelah, Loryele, Loryell, Loryella,
Loryelle

Laurel (Latin) laurel leaves.
Laural, Laurala, Lauralah, Laurale,
Lauralea, Lauraleah, Lauralee,
Lauralei, Lauraleigh, Lauralyn,
Lauralyna, Lauralyne, Lauralynn,
Lauralynna, Lauralynne, Laurela,
Laurelah, Laurele, Laurell, Laurella,
Laurellah, Laurelle, Lawrel,
Lawrela, Lawrelah, Lawrele,
Lawrell, Lawrella, Lawrellah,
Lawrelle, Loral, Lorala, Lorel,
Lorela, Lorelah, Lorelea, Loreleah,
Lorelee, Lorelei, Loreleigh, Lorell,
Lorella, Lorellah, Lorelle, Loriel,
Loriela, Lorielah, Loriele, Loriell,
Loriella, Loriellah, Lorielle,
Lori'elle, Loryal, Loryala, Loryalah,
Loryale, Loryale, Loryall, Loryalla,
Loryallah, Loryalle, Loryel, Loryela,
Loryelah, Loryele, Loryell, Loryella,
Loryellah, Loryelle

Lauren (Latin) laurel tree.
Lauran, Laurana, Lauranah,
Laurane, Laurann, Lauranna,
Laurannah, Lauranne, Lauree,
Laureen, Laureena, Laureenah,
Laureene, Laurena, Laurenah,
Laurene, Laurencia, Laurenciah,
Laurenna, Laurennah, Laurenne,
Laurentia, Laurentiah, Lauret,
Lauretah, Laurete, Laurett, Lauretta,
Laurettah, Laurette, Lauryn,
Lauryna, Laurynah, Laurynn,
Laurynna, Laurynnah, Laurynne,
Lawra, Lawrah, Lawran, Lawrana,
Lawranah, Lawrane, Lawre, Lawren,
Lawrena, Lawrenah, Lawrene,
Lawrin, Lawrina, Lawrinah,
Lawrine, Lawryn, Lawryna,
Lawrynah, Lawryne, Loren, Lorena,
Lorenah, Lorene, Lorenza, Loret,
Loreta, Loretah, Lorete, Lorett,
Loretta, Lorettah, Lorett, Lorette,

L

Lorin, Lorina, Lorinah, Lorine,
Lorind, Lorinda, Lorine, Lorren,
Lorrena, Lorrenah, Lorrene, Lorrin,
Lorrina, Lorrinah, Lorrine, Lorryn,
Lorryna, Lorrynah, Lorryne

Laurie (Latin) crown of laurel
leaves; victory.
Lari, Larie, Lary, Laure, Lauree,
Laureen, Laureena, Laurelea,
Laurelee, Laureleigh, Laurene,
Lauri, Laurice, Laurina, Laurinah,
Laurine, Laurissa, Laury, Lauryna,
Lurynah, Lauryne, Lawrea, Lawree,
Lawrey, Lawri, Lawrie, Lawry,
Lorea, Loree, Lorey, Lori, Loria,
Loriah, Lory, Lorya, Loryah

Lautoka (Tongan) plains.
Lautokah

Lavani (Tongan) necklace.
Lavanea, Lavanee, Lavaney,
Lavania, Lavaniah, Lavany, Lavanya

Lave (Tongan) touch.
Lav

Laveda (Latin) purity.
Lavedah, Laveta, Lavetah, Lavete,
Lavett, Lavetta, Lavette

Lavelle (Latin/French) she is purity.
Lavel, Lavela, Lavelah, Lavele,
Lavell, Lavella, Lavellah

Lavender (English) (Botanical) the
lavender shrub; a pale lilac
colour.
Lavenda, Lavendah

Laveni (Tongan) the lavender shrub;
a pale lilac colour.
Lavenee, Laveney, Lavenia,
Laveniah, Lavenie, Laveny, Lavenya,
Lavenyah

Lavenita (Tongan) the lavender
scent.
Lavenit, Lavenitah, Lavenyt,
Lavenyta, Lavenytah, Lavenyte

Laverne (Old French) from the
alder tree grove. (Lat) spring.
Lavern, Laverna, Lavernia,
Laverniah, Lavernya, Laverynah,
Laveryne

Lavina (Latin) purity.
Lavena, Lavenah, Lavania,
Lavaniah, Lavenia, Laveniah,
Lavinah, Lavinia, Laviniah, Lavinie,
Lavyna, Lavynah, Lavyne, Lavyni,
Lavynia, Lavyniah, Lavyny,
Lavynya, Lavynyah, Levenia,
Leveniah, Levinia, Leviniah,
Livinia, Liviniah, Louvinia,
Louviniah, Lovina, Lovinah,
Lovinia, Loviniah, Lovynia,
Lovyniah, Lovynya, Lovynyah,
Lyvina, Lyvinah, Lyvinia, Lyviniah,
Lyvynya, Lyvynyah

Lavinia (Latin) purity.
Lavena, Lavenah, Lavania,
Lavaniah, Lavenia, Laveniah,
Lavinia, Laviniah, Lavinie, Lavyna,
Lavynah, Lavyne, Lavyni, Lavynia,
Lavyniah, Lavyny, Lavynya,
Lavynyah, Levenia, Leveniah,
Levinia, Leviniah, Livinia, Liviniah,
Louvinia, Louviniah, Lovina,
Lovinah, Loviniah, Lovynia,
Lovyniah, Lovynya, Lovynyah,
Lyvina, Lyvinah, Lyvinia, Lyviniah,
Lyvynya, Lyvynyah

Lavonna (French/African American)
young archer.
Lavon, Lavona, Lavonah, Lavonda,
Lavonde, Lavonder, Lavondria,
Lavone, Lavonee, Lavoney, Lavonia,
Lavoniah, Lavonica, Lavonika,
Lavonie, Lavonn, Lavonna,
Lavonnah, Lavonne, Lavonee,
Lavonney, Lavonni, Lavonnie,
Lavonny, Lavonnya, Levon, Levona,
Levonah, Levone, Levonee, Levoni,
Levonia, Levoniah, Levonna,
Levonnah, Levonne, Levony,

Lavonna cont.
Levonya, Levonyah, Lovon, Lovona, Lovonah, Lovoni, Lovonia, Lovoniah, Lovonie, Lovonna, Lovonnah, Lovonne, Lovony, Lovonya, Lovonyah

Lawan (Thai) pretty.
Lawana, Lawane

Lawanda (German/African American) wanderer. A form of Wanda.
Lawandah, Lawinda, Lawindah, Lawynda, Lawyndah

Layaleeta (Australian Aboriginal) ocean; sea.
Laialeeta

Layla/Leila (Swahili) child born during the night. (Per/Arab) dark-haired.
Laela, Laelah, Laeli, Laelia, Laeliah, Laelie, Laely, Lailah, Laili, Lailia, Lailiah, Lailie, Laleh, Layli, Laylia, Layliah, Laylie, Layly, Laylya, Laylyah, Leila, Leilah, Lela, Lelah, Lelia, Leliah, Leyla, Leylah

Layna (Greek) light.
Laena, Laenah, Laina, Lainah, Laynah, Laynie (Grk)

Lazalea (Greek) ruling eagle.
Lazaleah, Lazalee, Lazalei, Lazaleigh, Lazaley, Lazali, Lazalia, Lazaliah, Lazalie, Lazaly, Lazalya

Le (Vietnamese) pearl.
Lea, Leah, Lee, Lei, Leigh, Ley

Lea/Leah/Lee/Leigh (English) meadow. (Heb) tired. (Lat) lioness.
Alea, Aleah, Alee, Alei, Aleia, Aleiah, Aleigha, Aleighah, Aleya, Aleyah, Leah, Leaha, Lee, Lei, Leigh, Li, Lia, Liah, Ly, Lya, Lyah

Leaf (English) the leaf of a tree or plant.
Leaff, Leif, Leiff, Leyf, Leyff

Leakiki (Polynesian) ocean waves.
Leekiki, Leikiki, Leykiki

Leala (Old French) faithful; loyal.
Leal, Lealia, Lealiah, Leanna, Leanne, Leel, Leela, Leelah, Lela, Lelah, Loyale, Loyola

Leandra (Latin) like a lioness; faithful; loyal.
Leandra, Leanka, Leeandra, Leeandrah, Leianda, Leiandah, Leighandra, Leighandrah, Leodora, Leodorah, Leoine, Leolina, Leoline, Leonanie, Leonelle, Leyandra, Leyandrah

Leanna/Leanne (English) from the graceful meadow. (Fren) bounded; legal.
Lea-ann, Lea-anne, Leann, Leanna, Leannah, Leandra, Leandria, Leanka, Leeann, Leeanna, Leeanne, Leeona, Leeonah, Leiana, Leianah, Leiane, Leianna, Leiannah, Leianne, Leighana, Leighanah, Leighane, Leighann, Leighanna, Leighanne, Leyan, Leyana, Leyanah, Leyane, Leyann, Leyanna, Leyannah, Leyanne, Lian, Liana, Lianah, Liane, Liann, Lianna, Liannah, Lianne, Lyan, Lyana, Lyanah, Lyane, Lyann, Lyanna, Lyannah, Lyanne

Leanore (Scottish/Old English) light from the meadow. A form of Eleanor, light.
Leanora, Leanorah, Lanore, Lanoree, Lanorey, Lanori, Lanoriah, Lanorie, Lanory, Lanorya, Lanoryah

Lece (French/Latin) happy.
Lecee, Lecey, Leci, Lecie, Lecy

Lecia (Latin) happy.
Leacia, Leaciah, Leacya, Leacyah, Leasia, Leasiah, Leasie, Leasy, Leasya, Leasyah, Leasye, Leecia, Leeciah, Leecy, Leecya, Leecyah, Leesha, Leesia, Leesiah, Lesha, Leshia, Leshah, Lesia, Lesiah, Lesya, Lesyah

Leda (Greek) lady; happiness.
Leada, Leadah, Leeda, Leedah, Leida, Leidah, Leighda, Leighdah, Leighta, Leightah, Leta, Leyda, Lita, Litah, Lyda, Lydah, Lyta, Lytah

Leeba (Yiddish/Old English) beloved one from the meadow.
Leaba, Leabah, Leebah, Leiba, Leibah, Leighba, Leighbah, Leyba, Leynah, Liba, Libah, Lyba, Lybah

Leena (Australian Aboriginal) water; possum.
Leana, Leanah, Leenah, Leina, Leinah, Leyna, Leynah, Lina, Linah, Lyna, Lynah

Leewan (Australian Aboriginal) wind.
Leawana, Leawanah, Leewana, Leewanah, Leiwana, Leiwanah, Leighwana, Leighwah, Leywana, Leywanah, Liwana, Liwanah, Lywana, Lywanah

Leeza (Hebrew) sacred; holy to God.
Leaza, Leazah, Leezah, Leiza, Leighza, Leighzah, Leyza, Leyzah, Lisa, Lisah, Liza, Lizah, Lyza, Lyzah

Legana (Australian Aboriginal) sea.
Leganah, Leganna, Legannah

Lehua (Hawaiian) sacred.

Lei (Hawaiian) heavenly child; flower. (Tong) ivory; whale's tooth.
Alea, Aleah, Alee, Alei, Aleia, Aleiah, Aleigha, Aleighah, Aleya, Aleyah, Leah, Leaha, Lee, Leigh, Li, Lia, Liah, Ly, Lya, Lyah

Leiko (Japanese) arrogant.
Leako, Leeko, Leyko

Leilani (Hawaiian) child of heavenly flowers.
Lanea, Lanee, Laney, Lani, Lanie, Lany, Lealanea, Lealaneah, Lealanee, Lealaney, Lealani, Lealania, Lealaniah, Lealanie, Lealany, Leelanea, Leelaneah, Leelanee, Leelaney, Leelani, Leelania, Leelanie, Leelany, Leelani, Leelania, Leelaniah, Leelany, Leilanea, Leilanee, Leilaney, Leilani, Leilania, Leilaniah, Leilanie, Leilany, Leighlanea, Leighlanee, Leighlaney, Leighlani, Leighlania, Leighlanie, Leighlany, Lelanea, Lelanee, Lelaney, Lelani, Lelanie, Lelany, Leylanea, Leylanee, Leylaney, Leylani, Leylania, Leylaniah, Leylany

Leire (Basque/Hebrew) wished for; star of the sea; bitter.
Leira, Leyra, Leyrah

Leisi (Polynesian) lace.
Leasi, Leesi, Leysi

Lekasha (Swahili) life. (Arab) woman. A form of Aisha.
Lekeesha, Lekeisha, Lekesha, Lekeshia, Lekeshiah, Lekeshya, Lekesia, Lekesiah, Lekesya, Lekicia, Lekiciah, Lekisha, Lekishah, Lekysha, Lekysia, Lekysya

Lekeleka (Tongan) of the moon.

Lelei (Tongan) wonderful.

Leli (Swiss) from the high tower; from Magdala. The Greek form of Magdalen.
Lelia, Leliah, Lely, Lelya, Lelyah

Lelia (Greek) fair speech.
Lelee, Leli, Lelie, Lelika, Lelita, Lellia, Lelliah, Lellya, Lellyah, Lelya, Lelyah

Lelya (Russian) shining light. The Greek form of Helen.
Leka, Lekah, Lelia, Leliah, Lelyah

Lemana (Australian Aboriginal) she oak tree.
Leaman, Leamanah, Leemana, Leemanah, Leimana, Leimanah, Lemanah, Leymana, Leymanah

Lemula (Hebrew) devoted to God.
Lemulah

Lena (Latin) shining light. A short form of Helen.
Leena, Lenah, Lenee, Lenetta, Lenette, Lina, Linah, Lyna, Lynah

Lenci (Hungarian) shining light. The Greek form of Helen.
Lencea, Lencee, Lencey, Lencia, Lencie, Lency

Lene (German) shining light. A short form of Helen.

Leneisha (Swahili) life. (Arab) woman. A form of Aisha.
Lenece, Lenesha, Lenysha, Lenisa, Lenisah, Lenise, Lenisha, Leniss, Lenissa, Lenissah, Lenisse, Lenysa, Lenysah, Lenyss, Lenyssa, Lenyssah

Leni (Latin) shining light. A short form of Helen.
Lenea, Lenee, Leney, Lenie, Lennee, Lenney, Lenni, Lennie, Lenny, Leny

Lenia (German) like a lioness. The feminine form of Leon.
Lenda, Lendah, Leneen, Leneena, Lenett, Lenetta, Lenette, Lenna, Lennah, Lennett, Lennetta, Lennette, Lenya, Lenyah

Lenice (German) bold; strong like a lioness. The feminine form of Leonard.
Leneace, Lenease, Leneece, Leneese, Lenise, Lenyce, Lenyse

Lenis/Lenita (Latin) smooth; soft.
Lena, Lencia, Lene, Leneta, Lenisa, Lenisah, Lenise, Leniss, Lenissa, Lenissah, Lenisse, Lenita, Lenitah, Lenos, Lenitah, Lenite, Lentia, Lentiah, Lentya, Lentyah, Lenys, Lenysa, Lenysah, Lenyse, Lenyss, Lenyssa, Lenyssah, Lenysse

Lenore (Greek) shining light. A form of Eleanor/Helen.
Leanor, Leanora, Leanorah, Leanore, Lenora, Lenorah, Lenoree, Leonor, Leonora, Leonorah, Leonore

Leoda (German) woman of the people.
Leodah, Leota, Leotah

Leola (Latin) lioness. The feminine form of Leo.
Leolah

Leolina (Old Welsh) lioness. The feminine form of Leo.
Leolinah, Leoline, Leolyn, Leolyna, Leolynah, Leolyne

Leoma (Old English) bright light.
Leomah

Leona (French) lioness.
Leola, Leoma, Leonarda, Leone, Leonel, Leonia, Leonie, Leonina, Leonine, Leonora, Leontina, Leontine, Leontyna, Leontyne

Leonarda (Latin) strong lioness.
Leonardina, Leonardine, Leonardyn, Leonardyna, Leonardyne

Leonie (French) lioness like. The feminine form of Leon.
Leocada, Leocadia, Leokadia, Leokadya, Leona, Leonarda,

L

Leonce, Leoncya, Leondra,
Leondrea, Leondria, Leonee,
Leonela, Leonelah, Leonella,
Leonelle, Leoney, Leonia, Leonice,
Leonni, Leonnie, Leontina,
Leontine, Leontyna, Leontyne

Leonora (Italian) shining light.
A form of Eleanor.
Lenora (Russ), Leonor, Lenore
(Ger), Leonorah, Leonore (Fren),
Leora (Russ), Leorah

Leontina (Latin) like a lioness.
Leontina, Leontine, Leontyn,
Leontyna, Leontyne, Liontin,
Liontina, Liontine, Liontyna,
Liontyne, Lyontina, Lyontine,
Lyontyna, Lyontyne

Leora (Hebrew) shining light.
A form of Eleanor.
Leeora, Leorah, Liora, Liorah,
Lyora, Lyorah

Leota (German) woman of the
people.
Leotah

Leotie (Native American) prairie
flower.
Leotee, Leoti, Leoty

Lepati (Tongan) leopard.
Leapati, Leapatie, Leapaty, Leipati,
Leipatie, Leipaty, Lepatie, Lepaty,
Leypati, Leypatie, Leypaty

Lera (Russian) strong; brave;
healthy. (Eng) from the valley.
The Latin short form of Valerie.
Lerah, Leria, Leriah

Lerato (Botswana) loving.

Lesi (Tongan) the pawpaw fruit.
Lesee, Lesey, Lesie, Lesy

Leslie (Gaelic) from the grey
fortress; low-lying meadow.
Lesil, Leslea, Lesleah, Leslee, Leslei,

Lesleigh, Lesley, Lesli, Lesslie, Lesly,
Leslye, Lesma, Lesney, Lestra,
Lezlea, Lezleah, Lezlee, Lezlei,
Lezleigh, Lezley, Lezli, Lezlie, Lezly

Leta (Latin) happy.
Leata, Leatah, Leeta, Leetah, Leita,
Leitah, Leyta, Leytah, Lyta, Lytah

Letha (Greek) forgetful.
Leda, Lethia, Leitha, Leithia, Leta,
Leythia, Leythiah, Leythya,
Leythyah

Leticia (Latin) happiness.
Latisha, Leisha, Leshia, Leshiah,
Lethia, Lethiah, Letice, Letichia
(Span), Leticya (Pol), Letisha,
Letishah, Letisia, Letisiah, Letita,
Letitah, Letitia (Lat), Letiticia,
Letiza, Letizah, Letizia, Letiziah,
Letycia, Letyciah, Letycya, Letycyah,
Loutitia, Loutitiah, Loutytia,
Loutytiah, Loutytya, Loutytyah

Letifa (Arabic) gentle.
Leitifa, Leitifah, Leitipha,
Leitiphah, Letifah, Letipha,
Letiphah, Letyfa, Letyfah, Letypha,
Letyphah

Letisha (Latin) happiness.
Letish, Letisha, Letishya, Letysha,
Letyshyia, Letysya

Letitia (Latin) happiness.
Latisha, Leisha, Leshia, Leshiah,
Lethia, Lethiah, Letice, Letichia
(Span), Leticya (Pol), Letisha,
Letishah, Letisia, Letisiah, Letita,
Letitah, Letitia (Lat), Letiticia,
Letiza, Letizah, Letizia, Letiziah,
Letycia, Letyciah, Letycya, Letycyah,
Loutitiah, Loutytia, Loutytiah,
Loutytya, Loutytyah

Letricia (Latin) noble.
Letriciah, Letricya, Letrycya

Letty (English) happiness. The English short form of Charlotte, little, strong, courageous woman.
Leta, Letee, Letey, Leti, Letie, Letta, Lettah, Lettee, Lettey, Letti, Lettie, Letty, Lety

Leura (Australian Aboriginal) lava
Lura, Lurah

Levana (Hebrew) white like the moon. (Lat) rising sun.
Levanah, Levanna, Levannah, Levona, Levonah, Levonna, Levonnah, Livana, Livanah, Livanna, Livannah, Lyvana, Lyvanah, Lyvanna, Lyvannah

Levani (Fijian) anointed with oil.
Levanee, Levaney, Levania, Levaniah, Levanie, Levany, Levanya

Levania (Latin) morning sun.
Leavania, Leevania, Leivania, Levannia, Leyvania

Leveni (Tongan) raven.
Levenie, Leveny

Levia (Hebrew) attached; lioness of God.
Leviah, Levya, Levyah

Levina (Middle English) lightning. The feminine form of Levi, united in harmony; promise.
Livinah, Livinna, Lyvina, Lyvinah, Lyvyna, Lyvynah

Levona (Hebrew) spice or incense.
Leavona, Leavonah, Leavonia, Leavoniah, Leavonna, Leavonnah, Leavonnia, Leevona, Leevonah, Leevonia, Leevoniah, Leevonna, Leevonnia, Leevoniah, Leivona, Leivonia, Leivoniah, Leivonna, Leivonna, Leivonnia, Leivonnya, Leighvona, Leighvonah, Leighvonna, Leighvonnah, Leighvonne, Leyvona, Leyvonah,

Leyvone, Leyvonn, Leyvonna, Leyvonnah, Leyvonne, Livona, Livonah, Livone, Livonna, Livonnah, Livonne, Lyvona, Lyvonah, Lyvone, Lyvonna, Lyvonnah, Lyvonne

Lewanna (Hebrew) moon; white.
Leawana, Leawanah, Leawanna, Leawannah, Leewana, Leewanah, Leewanna, Leewannah, Leiwana, Leiwanah, Leiwanna, Leiwannah, Lewana, Lewanah, Lewannah, Leywana, Leywanah, Leywanna, Leywannah

Lexandra (Greek) defender of humankind. A short form of Alexandra. The feminine form of Lex/Alex.
Lexa, Lexah, Lexandrah, Lexandria, Lexandriah, Lexandrya, Lexandryah, Lexi, Lexia, Lexiah, Lexie, Lexy, Lezandra, Lezandrah, Lezandria, Lezandriah, Lisandra, Lisandrah, Lisandria, Lisandriah, Lissandra, Lissandrah, Lissandria, Lissandriah, Lixandra, Lixandrah, Lysandra, Lysandrah, Lyssandra, Lyxandra, Lyxandrah

Leya (Spanish) loyalty; law.
Leia, Leiah, Leyah

Lia (Hebrew/Dutch/Italian) dependent. (Grk) she brings good news. (Eng) meadow.
Alia, Aliah, Liah, Lya, Lyah

Liama (Teutonic) helmet of resolution. (Ir) wilful. The Irish feminine form of Liam/William.
Liamah, Lyama, Lyamah

Liamena (Australian Aboriginal) from the lagoon; lake. (O/Eng/Ger/Dut) from the strong meadow.
Liamenah, Lyamena, Lyamenah

Lian (Chinese) graceful willow.
(Fren) bind.
Lia, Liana, Lianah, Liane, Lianna,
Liannah, Lianne, Lyan, Lyana,
Lyanah, Lyane, Lyann, Lyanna,
Lyannah, Lyanne

Libby (Hebrew) sacred; holy to
God. The short form of Elizabeth.
Libbea, Libbee, Libbi, Libbie,
Libea, Libee, Libey, Libi, Libie,
Liby, Lyb, Lybbea, Lybbee, Lybbey,
Lybbi, Lybbie, Lybby, Lybea, Lybee,
Lybey, Lybi, Lybie, Lyby

Liberty (Latin) freedom.
Libertee, Liberti, Libertie, Libirtee,
Libirtey, Libirti, Libirtie, Libirty,
Librada (Span), Liburtee, Liburtey,
Liburti, Liburtie, Liburty, Libyrtee,
Libyrtey, Libyrti, Libyrtie, Libyrty,
Lybertee, Lybertey, Lyberti,
Lybertia, Lybertyah, Lyberty,
Lybirtee, Lybirtey, Lybirti, Lybirtie,
Lybirty, Lyburtee, Lyburtey, Lyburti,
Lyburty, Lybyrtee, Lybyrtey, Lybyrti,
Lybyrtie, Lybyrty

Libusa (Slavic) darling.
Libusah, Libuse, Lybusa, Lybusah,
Lybuse

Licha (Spanish) noble.
Lycha

Licia (Greek) truthful. (Ger) noble.
Alicia, Aliciah, Alycia, Alyciah,
Alycya, Alycyah, Liciah, Licya,
Licyah, Lycya, Lycyah

Lida (Slavic) she has the people's
love.
Lidah, Lyda, Lydah

Lide (Latin/Basque) life.
Lidee, Lyde, Lydee

Lidia (Greek) beautiful girl.
Lidiah, Lydia, Lydiah, Lydya,
Lydyah

Lien (Chinese) lotus flower.
Liena, Lienn, Lienna, Lienne, Lyen,
Lyena, Lyenn, Lyenna, Lyenne

Liese (German) sacred; holy to God.
A form of Elizabeth.
Liechen, Liechena, Liesa, Liesah,
Liesabet, Liesabeth, Lisbet, Lisbeta,
Lisbete, Lisbeth, Lisbett, Lisbetta,
Lisbette, Lizbet, Lizbeta, Lizbete,
Lizbeth, Lizbett, Lizbetta, Lizbette,
Lyechen, Lyechena, Lyesa, Lyesah,
Lyesabet, Lyesabeth, Lysbet,
Lysbeta, Lysbete, Lysbeth, Lysbett,
Lysbetta, Lysbette, Lyzbet, Lyzbeta,
Lyzbete, Lyzbeth

Liesha (Arabic) woman. (Afr/Swah)
life. A form of Aisha.
Liasha, Liashah, Lieshah, Lyaisha,
Lyaishah, Lyasha, Lyashah,
Lyaysha, Lyayshah, Lyeisha,
Lyeishah, Lyesha, Lyeshah, Lyeysha,
Lyeyshah

Liesl (German/Hebrew) sacred; holy
to God. A form of Elizabeth.
Leasel, Leesel, Leisel, Leysel

Lila (Hindi) unpredictable destiny.
Lilah, Lilla, Lillah, Lyla, Lylah,
Lylla, Lyllah

Lilac (Persian) (Botanical) the lilac
flower; a pale purple colour.
Lila, Lilack, Lilah, Lilak, Lilia,
Liliah, Lylac, Lyack, Lylak

Lile (Tongan) lily.
Lilea, Lilee, Lilei, Liley, Lili, Lilie,
Lillea, Lillee, Lillei, Lelley, Lilli,
Lillie, Lilly, Lily, Lylea, Lyleah,
Lylee, Lyley, Lyli, Lylie, Lylea,
Lyleah, Lylei, Lylee, Lylei, Lyleigh,
Lyley, Lyli, Lylie, Lyllea, Lylleah,
Lyllee, Lyllei, Lylleigh, Lylly

Lilia (Hawaiian) lily.
Liliah, Lilya, Lilyah, Lylia, Lyliah,
Lylya, Lylyah

Lilibeth (English) lily flower; sacred; holy to God. A combination of Lily/Elizabeth.
Lilibet, Lilibeta, Lilibete, Lillibet, Lillibeta, Lillibete, Lillibeth, Lillybet, Lillybeta, Lillybete, Lillybeth, Lillybett, Lillybetta, Lillybette, Lilybet, Lilybeta, Lilybete, Lilybeth, Lilybett, Lilybetta, Lilybette, Lylibet, Lylibeta, Lylibete, Lyllibet, Lillybeta, Lyllibette, Lyllibeth, Lyllybet, Lyllybeta, Lyllybete, Lyllybeth, Lyllybett, Lyllybetta, Lyllybette, Lyllybeth, Lylybet, Lylybeta, Lylybete, Lylybeth, Lylybett, Lylybetta, Lylybette, Lylybeth

Liliko (Tongan) bird.
Lilliko, Lyliko

Lilipili (Australian Aboriginal) the myrtle tree.
Lillipilli

Lilis (Hebrew) spirit of the night.
Lilisa, Lilise, Liliss, Lilissa, Lilisse, Lylis, Lyisa, Lylise, Lyliss, Lylissa, Lylisse, Lylys, Lylysa, Lylyse, Lylyss, Lylyssa, Lylysse

Lilith (Arabic) belonging to the night. (Lat) lily. (Heb) serpent.
Lillis, Lillith, Lyllyth, Lilyth, Lylyth

Lillian (Latin) lily.
Lili, Lilia, Lilianah, Liliana, Lilianah, Liliane, Lilliana, Lillianah, Lilliane, Lillianna, Lilliannah, Lillianne, Lilias, Lilibet, Lilibeth, Lilion, Lilleigh, Lillet, Lillis, Lilyan, Lilybeth, Lyli, Lylia, Lyliah, Lylian, Lyliana, Lylianah, Lyliane, Lyliann, Lylianna, Lyiannah, Lylianne, Lylias, Lylibet, Lylibeta, Lylibeth, Lylion, Lylyon

Lilo (Hawaiian) generous; kind. (Lat) lily.
Lilow

Liluye (Native American) chicken hawk.

Lily (Latin/Arabic) (Botanical) the lily flower.
Lilea, Lileah, Lilee, Lilei, Lileigh, Liley, Lili, Lilia, Liliah, Lilie, Lillea, Lilleah, Lillee, Lillei, Lilleigh, Lelley, Lilli, Lillie, Lilly, Lylea, Lyleah, Lylei, Lyleigh, Lylee, Lylei, Lyleigh, Lyley, Lylie, Lyllea, Lylleah, Lyllee, Lyllei, Lylleigh, Lilli, Lillie, Lylly, Lyly

Lilybelle (Old English) beautiful lily.
Lilibel, Lilibela, Lilibelah, Lilibele, Lilibell, Lilibella, Lilibellah, Lilibelle, Lillibel, Lyllibela, Lylibell, Lyllibellah, Lyllibelle, Lilybel, Lilybela, Lilybelah, Lilybele, Lilybell, Lilybella, Lylibel, Lylibela, Lylibelah, Lylibele, Lylibell, Lylibella, Lylibellah, Lyllibelle, Lyllybel, Lyllybela, Lyllybellah, Lyllybelle, Lylybel, Lylybela, Lylybelah, Lylybele, Lylybell, Lylybella, Lylybelle

Lilybet (English) God's promise. A form of Elizabeth, sacred; holy to God. (Lat) lily.
Lilibet, Lilibeta, Lilibete, Lillibet, Lillibeta, Lillibete, Lillibeth, Lillybet, Lillybeta, Lillybete, Lillybeth, Lillybett, Lillybetta, Lillybette, Lilybet, Lilybeta, Lilybete, Lilybeth, Lilybett, Lilybetta, Lilybette, Lylibeta, Lylibetah, Lylibete, Lyllibet, Lillybeta, Lyllibette, Lyllibeth, Lyllybet, Lyllybeta, Lyllybete, Lyllybeth, Lyllybett, Lyllybetta, Lyllybette, Lyllybeth, Lylybet, Lylybeta, Lylybete, Lylybeth, Lylybett, Lylybetta, Lylybette, Lylybeth

Limber (Tiv) happiness.
Limba, Limbah, Limbera, Lymba,
Lymbah, Lymber, Lymbera

Limu (Tongan) seaweed.

Lin (Chinese) beautiful jade stone.
Lina, Linah, Linn, Linna, Linnah,
Lyn, Lyna, Lynah, Lynn, Lynna,
Lynnah

Lina (Italian/Spanish) light.
Linah, Lyna, Lynah

Linda (Spanish) pretty; beautiful.
Lindah, Lindka, Lynda, Lyndah,
Lynde, Lyndee, Lynden

Lindel (Old English) from the open
valley pool.
Lindal, Lindall, Lindil, Lyndal,
Lyndall, Lyndel, Lyndell, Lyndil

Linden (Old English) flexible
shield.
Lindan, Lindin, Lindon, Lyndan,
Lynden, Lyndin, Lyndon, Lyndyn

Lindie (Spanish) pretty; beautiful.
Lindea, Lindee, Lindey, Lindi,
Lindy, Lyndea, Lyndee, Lyndey,
Lyndi, Lyndie, Lyndy

Lindsay (Old English) from the
linden-tree island; waterside.
Lindsee, Lindsei, Lindsey, Lindsie,
Lindsy, Linzee, Linzey, Linzie,
Lyndsay, Lyndsey, Lyndsie, Lynzy,
Lyndsay, Lyndsey, Lyndzee,
Lyndzey, Lyndzi, Lyndzie, Lyndzy

Lindy (Teutonic) serpent.
(O/Eng) linden tree.
Lindea, Lindee, Lindi, Lindie,
Lyndea, Lyndee, Lyndi, Lyndie,
Lyndy

Linet (English) little, shapely one.
Lineta, Linetah, Linete, Linett,
Linetta, Linettah, Linette, Linnet,
Linneta, Linnetah, Linnete, Linnett,

Linnetta, Linnettah, Linnette,
Lynet, Lyneta, Lynetah, Lynete,
Lynnett, Lynnetta, Lynnettah,
Lynnette

Linette (Celtic) graceful; little.
(O/Fren) linnet bird (finch)
Linet, Lineta, Linetah, Linete,
Linett, Linetta, Linettah, Linnet,
Linneta, Linnetah, Linnete, Linnett,
Linnetta, Linnettah, Linnette, Lynet,
Lyneta, Lynetah, Lynete, Lynnett,
Lynnetta, Lynnettah, Lynnette

Ling (Chinese) delicate.

Linleigh (English) from the pool in
the meadow.
Linlea, Linleah, Linlee, Linlei,
Linley, Linli, Linlia, Linliah, Linlie,
Linly, Lynlea, Lynleah, Lynlee,
Lynlei, Lynleigh, Lynley, Lynli,
Lynlia, Lynliah, Lynlie, Lynly

Linnea (Scandinavian) the linden
tree. (Swed) flower.
Linea, Lineah, Linneah, Lynea,
Lyneah, Lynnea, Lynneah

Liolya (Russian) shining light. A
form of Helen.
Lenuschka, Lenushka, Lenusya,
Liolia, Lioliah, Liolyah, Lyolya,
Lyolyah

Liona (Latin/English) lioness.
Lionah, Lione, Lionee, Lioney,
Lioni, Lionia, Lioniah, Lionie,
Liony, Lyona, Lyonah, Lyone,
Lyonee, Lyoney, Lyoni, Lyonia,
Lyoniah, Lyonie, Lyony, Lyonya,
Lyonyah

Lionetta (Latin/English) little
lioness.
Lionet, Lioneta, Lionetah, Lionete,
Lionett, Lionettah, Lionette,
Lyonet, Lyoneta, Lyonetah,
Lyonete, Lyonett, Lyonetta,
Lyonettah, Lyonette

Liora (Hebrew) light.
Liorah, Lyora, Lyorah

Lira (Australian Aboriginal) river.
Lirah, Lirra, Lirrah, Lyra, Lyrah,
Lyrra, Lyrrah

Lirit (Greek) lyre music.
Lirita, Lirite, Lyrit, Lyrita, Lyrite

Liron (Hebrew) the song is mine.
Lirona, Lironah, Lirone, Lyron,
Lyrona, Lyronah, Lyrone

Lirra (Australian Aboriginal) wren.
Lira

Lis (French) lily.
Lys

Lisa (Greek) honey bee. The short
form of Melissa. A form of
Elizabeth, holy; sacred to God.
Leaca, Leasa, Leasah, Leassa,
Leassah, Leaza, Leazah, Leca,
Lecah, Leeca, Leecah, Leesa,
Leesah, Leeza, Leexah, Leisa,
Leisah, Leisel, Leisl, Lesia, Liesa,
Liesah, Lisah, Lisanna, Lisannah,
Lisanne, Lisay, Lise, Lisett, Lisetta,
Lisette, Lissa, Lissah, Lissay, Lisya,
Liza, Lizah, Lizza, Lizzah, Lysa,
Lysah, Lyssa, Lyssah, Lyza, Lyzah,
Lyzza, Lyzzah

Lisha (Arabic) darkness before
midnight.
Lishah, Lishe, Lysha, Lyshah, Lyshe

Lisle (Old English) from the island.
Leasel, Leasela, Leaselah, Leasele,
Leasle, Leesel, Leesela, Leeselah,
Leesele, Leesle, Leisel, Leisela,
Leiselah, Leisele, Leisle, Lisel,
Lisela, Liselah, Lisele, Lysel, Lysela,
Lyselah, Lysele

Liss (Celtic) from the court.
Lis, Lys, Lyss

Lissa (Greek) honey bee. The short
form of Melissa.
Lissah, Lyssa, Lyssah

Lissilma (Native American) there.

Lita (Spanish/English) strong
woman. The short form of names
ending in 'lita' e.g. Lolita.
Leahta, Leahtah, Leata, Leatah,
Leeta, Leetah, Leita, Leitah, Leighta,
Leightah, Leta, Letah, Leyta,
Leytah, Litah, Lyta, Lytah

Litonya (Moquelumnan) darting
hummingbird.
Litania, Litaniah, Litanya, Litanyah,
Litonia, Litoniah, Lytania,
Lytaniah, Lytanya, Lytanyah,
Lytonia, Lytoniah, Lytonya,
Lytonyah

Liv (Latin) olive. The short form of
Olivia.
Livi, Livie, Livy, Lyv, Lyvi, Lyvie,
Lyvy

Livana (Hebrew) white like the
moon. (Lat) graceful olive.
Livanah, Livane, Livanna,
Livannah, Livanne, Lyvan, Lyvanah,
Lyvane, Lyvanna, Lyvannah,
Lyvanne

Livia (Hebrew) joining. (Lat) olive
tree. The short form of Olivia.
Liviah, Liviya, Liviyah, Lyvia,
Lyviah, Lyvya, Lyvyah, Olivia,
Oliviah, Olivya, Olivyah, Olyvia,
Olyiah, Olyvya, Olyvyah

Liviya (Hebrew) brave lioness;
crown.
Livia, Liviah, Liviyah, Lyvia, Lyviah,
Lyvya, Lyvyah, Olivia, Oliviah,
Olivya, Olivyah, Olyvia, Olyiah,
Olyvya, Olyvyah

Livona (Hebrew) spice.
Livonah, Lyvona, Lyvonah

Liz (English) holy; sacred to God.
A short form of Elizabeth.
Lizz, Lyz, Lyzz

Liza (Hebrew/English) holy; sacred
to God. A short form of
Elizabeth.
Leaca, Leasa, Leasah, Leassa,
Leassah, Leaza, Leazah, Leca,
Lecah, Leeca, Leecah, Leesa,
Leesah, Leeza, Leexah, Leisa,
Leisah, Leisel, Leisl, Lesia, Liesa,
Liesah, Lisa, Lisah, Lisanna,
Lisannah, Lisanne, Lisay, Lise,
Lisett, Lisetta, Lisette, Lissa, Lissah,
Lissay, Lisya, Lizah, Lizza, Lizzah,
Lysa, Lysah, Lyssa, Lyssah, Lyza,
Lyzah, Lyzza, Lyzzah

Lizabeth (English) holy; sacred to
God. A form of Elizabeth.
Lisabet, Lisabeta, Lisabetah,
Lisabete, Lisabeth, Lisabett,
Lisabetta, Lisabettah, Lisabette,
Lisabetth, Lizabet, Lizabeta,
Lizabete, Lizabett, Lizabetta,
Lizabette, Lizbet, Lizbeta, Lizbete,
Lizbeth, Lizbett, Lizbetta, Lizbette,
Lysabet, Lysabeta, Lysabetah,
Lysabete, Lysabeth, Lysabett,
Lysabetta, Lysabettah, Lysabette,
Lyzabet, Lyzabeta, Lyzabetah,
Lyzabete, Lyzabeth, Lyzbett,
Lyzabetta, Lyzabettah, Lyzabette,
Lyzabeth

Lizina (Latvian) holy; sacred to
God. A form of Elizabeth.
Lixena, Lixenah, Lixina, Lixinah,
Lixyna, Lixynah, Lizinah, Lizine,
Lizyna, Lizynah, Lizyne, Lyxina,
Lyxinah, Lyxyna, Lyxynah, Lyzina,
Lyzinah, Lyzine, Lyzyna, Lyzynah,
Lyzyne

Llawella (Welsh) leader; lioness. The
feminine form of Llewelyn, lion-
like friend; lightning.
Lawella

Llian (Welsh) linen.
Lian, Liana, Lianah, Liane, Lliana,
Llianah, Lliane, Lliann, Llianna,
Lliannah, Llianne, Llyan, Llyana,
Llyanah, Llyane, Llylann, Llyanna,
Llyannah, Llyanne

Loa (Tongan) storm clouds.
Loah

Lockett (French) necklace;
keepsake.
Locket, Locketa, Lockete, Locketta,
Lockette

Lodema (Old English) guide.
Lodemah, Lodemai

Lofa (Tongan) storm bird.
Lofah

Loila (Australian Aboriginal) sky.
Loilah, Loyla, Loylah

Lois (Greek) famous warrior. The
feminine form of Louis.
Loiss, Loissa, Loisse, Loys, Loyss,
Loyssa, Loysse

Loiyetu (Native American) flower
blooming.

Lokalia (Hawaiian) rose garland.
Lokaliah, Lokalya, Lokalyah

Loke (Hawaiian) rose.

Lola (Spanish) strong woman.
Lolah

Lole (Tongan) lollies; candy;
attractive.
Lolea, Loleah, Lolee, Lolei, Loleigh,
Loli, Lolie, Loly

Lolita (Spanish) sorrow.
Loleata, Loleatah, Loleate, Loleeta,
Loleetah, Loleete, Loleita, Loleitah,
Loleighta, Loleta, Loletah, Lolit,
Lolitah, Loyta, Lolytah, Lolyte

Lolly (English) sweet one; candy.
Lolea, Loleah, Lolee, Lolei, Loleigh,
Loley, Loli, Lolia, Loliah, Lolie,
Lollea, Lolleah, Lollee, Lollei,
Lolleigh, Lolley, Lolli, Lollie, Loly

Lolotea (Zuni) gift.
Lolotee, Loloti, Lolotia, Lolotie,
Loloty

Lomasi (Native American) pretty
flower.
Lomasee, Lomasey, Lomasie,
Lomasy

Lona/Lone (Middle English/Latin)
solitary.
Alona, Alonah, Alone, Alonna,
Alonnah, Alonne, Ilona, Ilonah,
Ilone, Ilonna, Ilonnah, Ilonne,
Lonee, Loney, Lonlea, Lonleah,
Lonlee, Lonlei, Lonleigh, Lonli,
Lonia, Loniah, Lonlea, Lonleah,
Lonlee, Lonlei, Lonleigh, Lonley,
Lonli, Lonlia, Lonliah, Lonlie, Lonly

Longo (Tongan) quiet.

Loni (English) solitary. (Lat) lioness.
Lonea, Loneah, Lonee, Loney,
Lonia, Loniah, Lonie, Lonnea,
Lonnee, Lonney, Lonni, Lonnia,
Lonniah, Lonnie, Lonny, Lonnya,
Lony, Lonya, Lonyah

Lopeka (Hawaiian) famous;
brightness.

Lopini (Tongan) the robin bird.

Lora (Latin) alluring one; Siren;
wine. (Lat) crown of laurel leaves;
victory.
Laura, Laurah, Lawra, Lawrah,
Lorah, Lorra, Lorrah

Lore/Loree (Latin) alluring one;
Siren; wine. (Lat) crown of laurel
leaves; victory. A form of Lorelei.
Lore, Lorey, Lori, Lorie, Lorre,

Lorree, Lorrey, Lorri, Lorrie, Lorry,
Lory

Lorelei (German) alluring one;
Siren.
Loralea, Loraleah, Loralee, Loralei,
Loraleigh, Loraley, Lorelea,
Loreleah, Lorelee, Loreleigh,
Loralyn, Loralynn, Lorilea,
Lorileah, Lorilee, Lorilei, Lorileigh,
Loriley, Lorili, Lorilia, Loriliah,
Lorilie, Lorily, Lorylea, Loryleah,
Lorylee, Lorylei, Loryleigh, Loryley,
Loryli, Lorylie, Loryly

Loren/Lorena (Latin) crown of
laurel leaves; victory.
Lauran, Lauren, Laurin, Laurina,
Laurinah, Laurine, Lauron, Laurun,
Lauryn, Lauryna, Laurynah,
Lauryne, Lawran, Lawren, Lawrin,
Lawrina, Lawrinah, Lawryn,
Lawryna, Lawryne, Lawron,
Lawrun, Lawryn, Loran, Lorana,
Loranah, Loren, Lorenah, Lorene,
Lorin, Lorina, Lorinah, Lorine,
Loryn, Loryna, Lorynah, Loryne

Lorenza (English) crown of laurel
leaves; victory. The feminine form
of Lorenzo.
Laurensa, Laurensah, Laurenza,
Laurenzah, Lawrensa, Lawrensah,
Lawrenza, Lawrenzah, Lorensa,
Lorensah, Lorenza, Lorenzah,
Lorinsa, Lorinsah, Lorinza,
Lorinzah, Lorynsa, Lorynsah,
Lorynza, Lorynzah

Loret/Loretta (Latin) little crown of
laurel leaves; little victory.
Lauret, Laureta, Lauretah, Laurete,
Laurett, Lauretta, Laurette, Lawret,
Lawreta, Lawretah, Lawrete,
Lawrett, Lawretta, Lawrettah,
Lawette, Loret, Loreta, Loretahj,
Lorete, Loretta, Lorettah, Lorette,
Lorit, Lorita, Loritah, Lorite,

Lorittah, Loritta, Lorittah, Loritte,
Lorreta, Lorettah, Lorrette, Lorrit,
Lorrita, Lorritah, Lorritte, Loryt,
Loryta, Lorytah, Loryte, Lorytt,
Lorytta, Loryttah, Lorytte

Lori (German/Latin/American)
alluring one; Siren. (Lat) crown
of laurel leaves; victory. A form of
Lorelei.
Lawree, Lawrey, Lawri, Lawrie,
Lawry, Lorai (Nat/Amer), Lore,
Loree, Lorey, Lorelea, Loreleah,
Lorelee, Loreleigh, Loria, Loriah,
Lorie, Lorre, Lorree, Lorrey, Lorri,
Lorria, Lorriah, Lorrie, Lorry,
Lorrya, Lorrye, Lory

Loriann (English/Latin/French/
American) graceful, alluring one;
graceful Siren.
Lawreean, Lawreeann,
Lawreenanna, Lawreeanne, Loreean,
Loreeana, Loreeanah, Loreeane,
Loreeann, Loreeanna, Loreeannah,
Loreeanne, Lorian, Loriana,
Lorianah, Loriane, Lorianna,
Loriannah, Lorianne, Loryan,
Loryana, Loryanah, Loryann,
Loryanna, Loryannah, Loryanne

Loric (Latin) armour.
Lorick, Lorik, Loriqu, Loriqua,
Lorique, Loryc, Loryck, Loryk,
Loryqu, Loryqua, Loryque

Lorice (Latin) crown of laurel
leaves; victory.
Loreace, Lorease, Loreece, Loreese,
Lorise, Loryce, Loryse

Loricia (Greek) holy; crown of
laurel leaves; victory.
Lariciah, Laricya, Laricyah, Larikia,
Larikiah, Larycia, Laryciah, Larycya,
Larycyah, Larykia, Laryikiah,
Larykya, Larykyah

Lorielle (Latin) she has a crown of
laurel leaves. (Lat/Fren) she is the
alluring one; Siren.
Loreel, Loreela, Loreelah, Loreele,
Loriel, Loriela, Lorielah, Loriele,
Loriell, Loriella, Loryel, Loryela,
Loryelah, Loryele, Loryell, Loryella,
Loryellah, Loryelle

Lorikeet (Australian Aboriginal)
beautifully coloured bird.
Lorikeat, Lorikeata, Lorikeatah,
Lorikeate, Lorikeeta, Lorikeetah,
Loriket, Loriketa, Loriketah,
Lorikete, Lorikett, Loriketta,
Lorikette, Lorykeet

Lorina (Latin) crown of laurel
leaves; victory.
Lorinah, Lorine, Loryn, Loryna,
Lorynah, Loryne

Lorinda (Spanish) crown of laurel
leaves; victory.
Lorind, Lorindah, Lorinde, Lorynd,
Lorynda, Loryndah, Lorynde

Loris (Greek) pale. (Dut) clown.
Chloris, Chlorys, Loreace, Lorease,
Loreece, Loreese, Lorisa, Lorisah,
Lorise, Loriss, Lorissa, Lorissah,
Lorisse, Loryce, Lorys, Lorysa,
Lorysah, Loryse, Loryss, Loryssa,
Loryssah, Lorysse

Lorissa (Latin) crown of laurel
leaves; victory.
Lorisa, Lorisah, Lorise, Lorissah,
Lorisse, Lorys, Lorysa, Lorysah,
Loryse, Loryss, Loryssa, Loryssah,
Lorysse

Lorna (English) lost love. (Lat)
crown of laurel leaves; victory.
Lornah, Lorne, Lornee, Lorney

Lorraine (Teutonic) famous warrior.
(O/Eng) crown of laurel leaves in
the rain.
Laraen, Laraena, Laraenah,

Lorraine cont.
Laraene, Larain, Laraina, Larainah,
Laraine, Larayn, Larayna, Laraynah,
Larayne, Laurain, Lauraina,
Laurainah, Lauraine, Laurainne,
Lawrain, Lawraina, Lawrainah,
Lawraine, Lawrayn, Lawrayna,
Lawraynah, Lawrayne, Loraen,
Loraena, Loraenah, Loraene,
Lorain, Loraina, Lorainah, Loraine,
Lorayn, Lorayna, Loraynah,
Lorayne, Lorina, Lorinah, Lorine,
Lorrain, Lorraina, Lorrainah,
Lorraine, Lorrayn, Lorrayna,
Lorraynah, Lorrayne, Loryna,
Lorynah, Loryne, Lorynn, Lorynna,
Lorynnah, Lorynne

Lorrelle (Latin/Teutonic) little
crown of laurel leaves; little
victory. (Fren/O/Eng) she is
victory.
Lorel, Lorela, Lorelah, Lorele,
Lorrel, Lorrela, Lorrelah, Lorrele,
Lorrell, Lorella

Losa (Polynesian) rose.
Losah

Losaki (Polynesian) meeting.
Losakee, Losakey, Losakia,
Losakiah, Losaky

Lose (Tongan) rose.
Losa

Loto (Tongan) heart.

Lotta (Swedish) woman.
Lota, Lotah, Lottah

Lotte (French) little, strong,
courageous woman. The short
form of Charlotte.
Lotea, Lote, Lotee, Lotey, Loti,
Lotie, Lottea, Lottee, Lottey, Lotti,
Lottie, Lotty

Lotu (Tongan) admired.

Lotus (Greek) dreamer; the lotus
flower.
Lottus

Lou (Tongan) leaf. (Ger) famous
warrior.
Loulou, Lou-Lou, Lu, Lulu, Lu-Lu

Louam (Ethiopian) sleep well.
Louama

Lough (Irish) lake.
Lou

Louisa/Louise (German) famous
warrior. The feminine form of
Louis.
Aloise, Aloisia, Aloysia, Eloisa,
Eloise, Heloise (Fren), Labhaoise
(Ir), Lasche, Lawis, Lawisa,
Lawisah, Lawise, Lawise, Leot,
Leweese, Leweez, Liudvika, Liusadh
(Scott), Lisette (Fren), Lodoiska,
Loisa, Loisah, Loise, Louisa,
Louisah, Louisetta, Louisette,
Louiz, Louiza, Louizah, Louize,
Louyz, Louyza, Louyzah, Louyze,
Lova, Loyce, Ludoisia, Ludoisya,
Luis, Luisa, Luisah, Luise, Luiz,
Luiza, Luizah, Luize, Luys, Luysa,
Luysah, Luyse, Luyz, Luyza,
Luyzah, Luyze

Lourdes (French/Geographical)
from Lourdes in France.

Lourie (African) bird with bright
feathers.
Louree, Louri, Louria, Louriah,
Loury

Louvaine (French) she-wolf; fierce.
Louvain, Louvaina, Louvayn,
Louvayna, Louvaynah, Louvayne,
Luvain, luvaina, Luvainah, Luvaine,
Luvayn, Luvayna, Luvaynah,
Luvayne

Lovai (Tongan) heavy rain.
(Eng) she is loved.
Lovae, Love, Lovia, Lovie, Lovy,

Lovya, Lovyah, Luv, Luvi, Luvia, Luviah, Luvya, Luvyah

Lovinia (Latin) pure.
Lavina, Lavinia, Laviniah, Laviniya, Laviniyah, Lavynia, Lavyniah, Lavynya, Lavynyah, Levina, Levinah, Levinia, Leviniah, Leviniya, Leviniyah, Levynia, Levyniah, Levynya, Levynyah, Lovena, Lovenah, Lovenia, Loveniah, Lovina, Lovinah, Loviniah, Lovinya, Lovinyah, Lovynia, Lovyinah, Lovynya, Lovynyah

Lovisa (Old English) loved.
Love, Loves, Lovesah, Lovese, Lovessa, Lovessah, Lovesse, Lovisah, Lovissa, Lovissah, Lovisse, Lovys, Lovysa, Lovysah, Lovyse, Lovyss, Lovyssa, Lovyssah, Lovysse

Lovyah (English) she loves you.
Love, Lovee, Lovey, Lovi, Lovia, Loviah, Lovya, Lovyah

Lowana (Australian Aboriginal) girl.
Lowanah, Lowanna, Lowannah

Luana (Teutonic/Hebrew) graceful warrior.
Lewana, Lewanna, Louana, Louanah, Louann, Louanna, Louannah, Louanne, Lovana, Lovanna, Lovanne, Luane, Luann, Luanni, Luannie, Luanny, Luwana, Luwanna

Luca (Italian/Latin) bringer of light. The feminine form of Lucas.
Lucah, Lucka, Luckah, Luka, Lukah

Lucerne (Latin) circle of light.
Lucerina, Lucerinah, Lucerine, Luceryn, Luceryna, Lucerynah, Luceryne

Lucia (Latin) bringer of light. The feminine form of Lucius.
Lleulu, Loucea, Loucee, Loucey,

Louci, Loucia, Louciah, Loucie, Loucy, Luce, Lucea, Lucee, Lucet, Luceta, Lucetah, Lucete, Lucett, Lucetta, Lucettah, Lucette (Fren), Lucey, Luci, Luciah, Luciana, Lucianna, Luciannah, Lucianne, Lucie, Lucienna, Lucienne, Lucile, Lucilla, Lucille (Fren), Lucina, Lucind, Lucinda, Lucindah, Lucine, Lucita (Span), Lucy, Lucya, Lucyah, Lucyee, Lusia, Lusiah, Lusy, Lusya, Lusyah, Luzia, Luziah, Luzina, Luzinah, Luzine, Luzy, Luzya, Luzyah

Lucille (English) bringer of light.
Loucil, Loucila, Loucilah, Loucile, Loucill, Loucilla, Loucillah, Loucille, Lucila, Lucilah, Lucile, Lucill, Lucilla, Lucillah, Lucillah, Lucyl, Lucyla, Lucylah, Lucyle, Lucyll, Lucylla, Lucyllah, Lucylle, Lusil, Lusila, Lusilah, Lusile, Lusill, Lusilla, Lusillah, Lusille, Lusyl, Lusyla, Lusylah, Lusyle, Lusyll, Lusylla, Lusyllah, Lusylle, Luzel, Luzela, Luzelah, Luzele, Luzell, Luzella, Luzellah, Luzelle

Lucinda (Latin) bringer of light.
Loucind, Loucinda, Loucindah, Loucinde, Loucint, Loucinta, Loucintah, Loucinte, Loucynd, Loucynda, Loucyndah, Loucynde, Loucynta, Loucyntah, Loucynte, Lousind, Lousinda, Lousindah, Lousinde, Lousynd, Lousynda, Lousyndah, Lousynde, Lousinta, Lousyntah, Lousynte, Lucind, Lucindah, Lucinde, Lucynd, Lucynda, Lucyndah, Lucynta, Lucyntah, Lucynte, Lusind, Lusinda, Lusindah, Lusinde, Lusinta, Lusintah, Lusinte, Lusynda, Lusyndah, Lusynta, Lusyntah, Lusynte, Luzinda, Luzindah, Luzinde, Luzinta, Luzintah, Luzinte, Luzynda,

Lucinda cont.
Luzyndah, Luzynde, Luzynta, Luzyntah, Luzynte

Lucindee (Latin) bringer of light.
Lucinda, Lucindea, Lucindey, Lucindi, Lucindia, Lucindiah, Lucindie, Lucindy, Lucinta, Lucintah, Lucintea, Lucintee, Lucinti, Lucintia, Lucintiah, Lucintie, Lucinty, Lusintea, Lusintee, Lusintey, Lusinti, Lusintia, Lusintiah, Lusintie, Lusinty, Luzintea, Luzintee, Luzintey, Luzinti, Luzintia, Luzintiah, Luzintie, Luzyntea, Luzyntee, Luzyntey, Luzyti, Luzyntia, Luzyntiah, Luzyntie, Luzinty, Luzynty

Lucine (Arabic) moon.
Lucin, Lucina, Lucinah, Lucyn, Lucyna, Lucynah, Lucyne, Lukena, Lukene, Lusin, Lusina, Lusinah, Lusine, Lusyn, Lusyna, Lusynah, Lusyne, Luzin, Luzina, Luzinah, Luzine, Luzyn, Luzyna, Luzynah, Luzyne

Lucita (Latin) riches; rewards.
Luceata, Luceatah, Luceeta, Luceetah, Lucrece (Fren), Lucrezia (Ital), Lucrecia (Span), Lucyta, Lucytah

Lucky (English) fortunate.
Luckee, Luckey, Lucki, Luckia, Luckiah, Luckie, Luckya, Lukee, Lukey, Luki, Lukia, Lukiah, Lukie, Luky

Lucretia (Latin) one who is rewarded.
Lacrecia, Lacreciah, Lucrece, Lucrecia, Lucreciah, Lucreecia, Lucreeciah, Lucresha, Lucreshia, Lucreshiah, Lucreshya, Lucreshyah, Lucrezia, Lucreziah, Lucrezya,

Lucrezyah, Lucrisha, Lucrishah, Lucrishia, Lucrishiah

Lucy (Latin) bringer of light. The feminine form of Luke.
Liucija, Liusadh (Scott), Lleuleu, Lucasta, Luce (Fren), Lucea, Lucee, Luci, Lucia (Ital/Span), Luciah, Lucian, Luciana, Lucianah, Luciann, Lucianna, Luciannah, Lucianne, Lucie (Fren/Ger), Lucien, Luciena, Lucienah, Luciene, Lucienna, Luciennah, Lucienne (Fren), Lucila, Lucilah, Lucile, Lucilla, Lucille, Lucina, Lucinah, Lucind, Lucinda, Lucindah, Lucine, Lucinta, Lucintah, Lucinte, Lucita, Lucitah, Lucka, Lucya, Lucyah, Lucyan, Lucyana, Lucyanah, Lucyane, Lucyann, Lucyanna, Lucyannah, Lucyanne, Lucye, Lucyee

Ludella (Old English) renowned; cleaver.
Ludela, Ludelah, Ludell, Ludellah

Ludmilla (Slavic) loved by the people.
Ludmila, Ludmilah, Ludmile, Ludmyla, Ludmylah, Ludmylla, Ludmylle, Ludovika

Luella (Old English) famous.
Loella, Loellah, Loelle, Looela, Looelah, Looele, Looella, Looellah, Looelle, Louela, Louelah, Louele, Louella, Louellah, Ludel, Ludela, Ludelah, Ludele, Ludella, Ludellah, Ludelle, Luela, Luelah, Luele, Luell, Luellah, Luelle

Luisa (Spanish/German) famous warrior. A form of Louisa.
Loeasa, Loeasah, Loease, Loeaza, Loeazah, Loeaze, Looesa, Looesah, Looese, Louisa, Louisah, Louise, Luisah, Luiza, Luizah, Luysa,

Luysah, Luyse, Luyza, Luyzah, Luyze

Lulani (New Zealand/Maori) highest point of heaven.
Loulanee, Loulaney, Loulani, Loulanie, Loulany, Lulanee, Lulaney, Lulanie, Lulany

Lulie (Middle English) sleepy.
Lulea, Luleah, Lulee, Lulei, Luleigh, Luley, Luli, Lulia, Luliah, Luly

Lulu (Native American) rabbit. (Tong) owl. (Arab) pearl. (Eng) soothing; fairy.
Looloo, Lolo, Loulou, Lou-Lou, Lulu, Lu-Lu

Lumusi (Ghanian) born with her face down.
Lumusee, Lumusie, Lumusy

Luna (Latin) moon.
Lunah, Lunet, Luneta, Lunetah, Lunete, Lunetta, Lunettah, Lunette, Lunnett, Lunnetta, Lunnettah, Lunnette

Lundy (Welsh) idol.
Lundea, Lundee, Lundey, Lundi, Lundie

Lunetta (Latin) little moon.
Lune, Lunet, Luneta, Lunetah, Lunete, Lunett, Lunettah, Lunette, Lunnett, Lunnetta, Lunnettah, Lunnette

Lupe (Spanish/Mexican) wolf. (Haw) ruby.
Lupee, Lupet, Lupeta, Lupete, Lupett, Lupetta, Lupette

Lupetu (Native American) bear climbing over a person.

Lupi (Tongan) the ruby gem.
Lupee, Lupia, Lupiah, Lupie, Lupy

Lupine (Latin) wolf-like.
Lupina, Lupinah, Lupyna, Lupynah, Lupyne

Lupita (Latin) wolf.
Lupe, Lupeata, Lupeatah, Lupeeta, Lupeetah, Lupeta, Lupete, Lupeeta, Lupette, Lupyta, Lupytah, Lupyte

Luraline (German) alluring one; Siren.
Luralin, Luralina, Luralinah, Luralyn, Luralyna, Luralynah, Luralyne

Lure (Latin) one who attracts.
Lura, Lurah

Lurline (German) alluring one; Siren.
Lura, Luretta, Lurette, Lurlina, Lurlinah, Lurlyn, Lurlyna, Lurlynah, Lurlyne

Lusa (Finnish) holy; sacred to God.
Lusah, Lussa, Lussah

Lusela (Moquelumnan) bear licking its paw.
Luselah, Lusella, Lusellah, Luselle

Lutana (Australian Aboriginal) moon.
Lutanah, Lutane, Lutania, Lutaniah, Lutanna, Lutannah, Lutanne, Lutannia, Lutannya, Lutanya

Lute (Polynesian) friendly.

Luvena (Latin/English) little beloved one.
Louvena, Louvenah, Luvenah, Luvenna, Luvennah

Luyu (Moquelumnan) pecking bird.

Luz (Spanish) light.
Luzee, Luzi, Luzie, Luzija, Luzy

Lycoris (Greek) twilight.
Licoris

M

Lyla (French) from the island. The feminine form of Lyle.
Lila, Lilah, Lylah

Lynda/Linda (Spanish) pretty.
Linda, Lindah, Linnda, Linndah, Lyndah, Lynnda, Lynndah

Lynette (Old French) uncertain. (Wel) idol. (O/Eng) from the little pool.
Linet, Lineta, Linetah, Linete, Linett, Linetta, Linettah, Linette, Linnet, Linneta, Linnetah, Linnete, Linnett, Linnetta, Linnettah, Linnette, Lynet, Lyneta, Lynetah, Lynete, Lynnett, Lynnetta, Lynnettah

Lynfa (Welsh) from the place near the lake.
Linfa, Linfah, Lynfah

Lynn (Old English) pool. The short form of Lynette.
Lin, Linell, Linn, Linne, Linnet, Linnetta, Linnette, Lyn, Lyndel, Lyndell, Lyndelle, Lynna, Lynne, Lynell, Lynelle, Lyneth, Lynett, Lynetta, Lynette, Lynlea, Lynleah, Lynlee, Lynlei, Lynleigh, Lynley, Lynli, Lynlia, Lynliah, Lynlie, Lynly, Lynne, Lynnella, Lynelle, Lynly

Lynx (American) wild cat.
Linx

Lyonella (French) young lioness; cub. The feminine form of Lionel.
Lionela, Lionele, Lionella, Lionelle, Lyonela, Lyonele, Lyonelle

Lyric (English/Latin) song words.
Liric, Lirick, Lirik, Liriqu, Lirique, Lyrick, Lyrik, Lyriqu, Lyrique, Lyryk, Lyryqu, Lyryque

Lyris (Greek) player of the harp; lyrical.
Liris, Lirisa, Lirise, Liriss, Lirissa, Lirisse, Lyra, Lyrah, Lyrisa, Lyrisah, Lyrise, Lyriss, Lyrissa, Lyrisse, Lyrysa, Lyrysah, Lyryssa, Lyryssah

Lysandra (Greek) freedom; defender of humankind.
Lisandra, Lisandrah, Lysanna, Lysannah, Lysanne, Lyshae

Lyzabeth (Hebrew) holy; sacred to God. A form of Elizabeth.
Lisabet, Lisabeta, Lisabetah, Lisabete, Lisabeth, Lisabett, Lisabetta, Lisabettah, Lisabette, Lisabetth, Lizabet, Lizabeta, Lizabete, Lizabett, Lizabetta, Lizabette, Lizbet, Lizbeta, Lizbete, Lizbeth, Lizbett, Lizbetta, Lizbette, Lysabet, Lysabeta, Lysabetah, Lysabete, Lysabeth, Lysabett, Lysabetta, Lysabettah, Lysabette, Lyzabet, Lyzabeta, Lyzabetah, Lyzabete, Lyzbett, Lyzabetta, Lyzabettah, Lyzabette, Lyzabetth

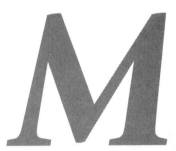

Mab (Celtic) joy; queen of the fairies.
Amabel, Amabela, Amabele, Amabell, Amabella, Amabelle, Mabela, Mabele, Mabell, Mabella, Mabelle, Mabry, Mave, Mavis (Fren), Meave (Ir)

Mabel (Latin) worthy of love. A short form of Amabel, lovable.
Amabel, Amabell, Amabella,

Amabelle, Mab, Mabb, Mabbina(Ir),
Mabele (Lith), Mabell, Mabella
(Eng), Mabelle (Fren), Mabil,
Mabill, Mabilla, Mabille, Mabine,
Mabbit, Mabbo, Maibel (Ir),
Mailbela, Mailbele, Mailbell,
Maibella, Maibelle, Mappin,
Maybel, Maybela, Maybele,
Maybell, Maybella, Maybelle,
Moibeal (Scott)

Macalla (Australian Aboriginal) full
moon.
Macala, Macalah

Macaria (Greek) happy.
Macariah, Macarya, Macaryah

Macawi (Dakota) motherly;
generous.
Macawee, Macawia, Macawie,
Macawy

Macha (Irish) plain.
Machah

Macharios (Greek) blessed.
Macharius, Macharyos

Macia (Polish/Hebrew) bitter.
Macelia, Macee, Macey, Machia,
Maci, Maciah, Macie, Macy, Macya,
Macyah, Masha, Mashia, Mashiah

Maciko (Japanese) beautiful child;
learning truthfully.
Machika, Machikah, Machyka,
Machyko

Mackenna (Gaelic) child of the
handsome one.
Mackena, Mackenah, Makena,
Makenah, Makenna, Makennah,
Mikena, Mikenah, Mikenna,
Mikennah, Mykena, Mykenah,
Mykenna, Mykennah

Mackenzie (Irish/Gaelic) child of
the wise, handsome leader.
Kenzee, Kenzey, Kenzi, Kenzie,
Kenzy, Mackenzee, Mackenzey,

Mackenzi, Mackenz, McKenzee,
McKenzey, McKenzi, McKenzie,
McKenzy

Macra (Greek) long-living.
Macrah, Macrina, Macrine,
Macryna, Macryne

Mada (English) from Magdalen.
(Grk) from the high tower.
Madah, Madda, Maddah, Mahda

Maddie (Greek) from the high
tower. (Eng) from Magdalen.
The short form of names starting
with 'Mad' e.g. Madonna.
Maddea, Maddee, Maddey, Maddi,
Maddie, Maddy, Madea, Madee,
Madey, Madi, Madie, Mady

Maddox (Welsh) lucky.
Madox

Madeleine (Greek) from the high
tower. (Eng) from Magdalen.
Madamain, Madalaina, Madalaine,
Madalayn, Madalayna, Madalayne,
Madelain, Madelaina, Madelaine,
Madelein, Madeleina, Madelena,
Madelene, Madelin, Madelina,
Madelinah, Madeline, Madeleyn,
Madeleyna, Madelyne, Madolonia,
Maighdlin (Ir), Malin (Dan),
Malina, Maline, Marlea, Marleah,
Marlee, Marleen, Marleena,
Marleene, Marlene, Marlene
(Span), Marley, Marli, Marlie,
Marlina, Marline, Marly, Maud,
Maude

Madge (Greek) from the high tower.
(Eng) from Magdalen.
Madgee, Madgey, Madgi, Madgie,
Madgy, Mage, Magee, Magey, Magi,
Magie, Magy

Madira (Sanskrit) the goddess of
wine.
Madirah, Madyra, Madyrah

Madison (English) powerful
warrior.
Maddisan, Maddisen, Maddisin,
Maddison, Maddisun, Maddysyn,
Madisen, Madisin, Madissan,
Madissen, Madissin, Madisson,
Madissyn, Madisun, Madisyn,
Madysan, Madysen, Madysin,
Madyson, Madysun, Madysyn

Madonna (Latin/Italian) my lady.
Maddona, Maddonah, Madonnah

Madra (Latin/Spanish) mother.
Madrah

Maeko (Japanese) truthful child.
Maemi

Maeve (Celtic) intoxicating joy.
(Fren) song bird. (Gae) delicate.
A form of mauve, a pale purple
colour.
Maevi, Maevy, Maive, Mayve

Magda/Magdalen (Slavic/Polish/
Russian/Greek) from the high
tower. (Eng) from Magdalen.
A short form of Madeleine.
Madalana, Madalane, Madalena
(Fren), Madalene, Madalina,
Madaline, Maddelena, Maddelene,
Maddelina, Maddeline, Madelina,
Madeline, Madelon, Madlen,
Magdah, Magdala, Magdalana,
Magdalane, Magdalina, Magdaline,
Magdalena, Magdalene,
Magdaleny, Magdalona,
Magdalonia, Madalyn, Magdalyna,
Magdalyne, Magdelan, Magdelana,
Magdelane, Magdelen, Magdelena,
Magdelene, Magdelin, Magdelina,
Magdeline, Magdelon, Magdelona,
Magdelone, Magdelonia,
Magdolna, Magdelyn, Magdelyna,
Magdelyne, Maud, Maude,
Mazaline

Magena (Native American) the
coming moon.
Magenna

Maggie (Greek) pearl.
Magee, Magey, Maggee, Maggey,
Maggi, Maggia, Maggin, Maggy,
Magy

Magnilda (German) gentle.
Magnildah, Magnylda

Magnolia (Latin) the magnolia tree
blossom.
Magnolea, Magnoleah, Magnoliah,
Magnolya

Mahal (Filipino) love.
Mahala, Mahalah

Mahala (Native American) woman
of power. (Heb) barren.
Mahalah, Mahalar, Mahalla,
Mahela, Mahila, Mahlah, Mahlaha,
Mehala, Mehalah

Mahalia (Hebrew) affectionate;
tender.
Mahala (Nat/Amer), Mahalah,
Mahaliah, Mahalya, Mehalia,
Mehaliah, Mehalya, Mehalyah

Mahesa (Hindi) great lord.
Maheesa, Mahisa, Mahissa,
Mahysa, Mahyssa

Mahila (Sanskrit) woman.
Mahilah, Mahyla, Mahylah

Mahina (Hawaiian/Tongan)
moonlight.
Mahinah, Mahyna, Mahynah

Mahira (Hebrew) energy; speed.
Mahirah, Mahryra, Mahyrah

Mahla (Hebrew) polished; one who
shines.
Mahlah

Mahogany (Spanish) rich in strength; reddish/brown wood.
Mahoganee, Mahoganey, Mahogani, Mahogania, Mahoganie, Mahogny, Mahogonee, Mahogoney, Mahogoney, Mahogoni, Mahogonia, Mahogonie, Mahogonya

Mahola (Hebrew) dancing.
Maholah

Mahwah (Algonquin) beautiful.
Mahwa

Mai (Navajo) coyote. (Jap) bright. (Viet) flower.
Mae, Maie, May, Maye

Maia (Greek) the goddess of spring; bright star; mother. (Eng) woman.
Maea, Maiah, Maie, Maiya, Maya, Mayah, Mya, Myah

Maida (English) woman.
Maeda, Maidah, Mayda

Mailee (Hebrew/English) from the wished-for one's meadow; from the bitter one's meadow; from star of the sea meadow. A combination of Mary/Lee.
Marilea, Marileah, Marilei, Marileigh, Mariley, Marili, Marilia, Marilie, Marily, Marylea, Maryleah, Marylee, Marylei, Maryleigh, Maryley, Maryli, Marylie, Maryly

Maimi (Japanese) smile of truth.
Maemee, Maimee, Maimi, Maymee, Maymi

Maire (Irish/Hebrew) wished for; star of the sea; bitter. A form of Mary.
Mair, Maira, Mairah, Mairi, Mairia, Mairiah, Mairim, Mairin, Mairona, Mairwen, Mairwin, Mairwyn, Mayr, Mayra, Mayrah, Mayre

Mairead (Irish/French) judge.
Maeread, Mayread

Mairi (Hebrew) wished for; star of the sea; bitter. A form of Mary.
Maeree, Maerey, Maeri, Maerie, Maery, Mairee, Mairey, Mairie, Mairy, Maree, Marey, Mari, Marie, Mariel, Mary

Maisie (French) maize, sweet corn. The Scottish form of Margaret, pearl.
Maesee, Maesey, Maesi, Maesie, Maesy, Maisee, Maisey, Maisi, Maisie, Maysee, Maysey, Maysi, Maysie, Maysy

Maita (Aramaic) lady of sorrow. A form of Martha, lady.
Maeta, Maetah, Maite, Maitia, Maitya, Maityah, Mayta, Maytya, Maytyah

Maja (Arabic) delightful; splendid.
Majah, Majal, Majalisa, Majalyn, Majalyna, Majalyne, Majalynn, Majalynne

Majesta (Latin) majestic; great.
Magestic, Magestica, Magesticah, Magestiqua, Magestique, Majestah, Majestic, Majestiqua, Majestique

Majid/Majidah (Arabic) glorious; delightful.
Maja, Majida, Majidah, Majyd, Majyda, Majydah

Makala (Hawaiian) myrtle tree.
Makailea, Makaileah, Makailee, Makailei, Makaileigh, Makailey, Makaili, Makalia, Makaliah, Makalie, Makaily, Makalah, Makalea, Makaleah, Makalee, Makalei, Makaleigh, Makaley, Makali, Makalia, Makaliah, Makalie, Makaly, Makaylea, Makayleah, Makaylee, Makaylei, Makayleigh, Makayley, Makayli,

Makala cont.
Makaylia, Makayliah, Makaylie, Makayly

Makana (Hawaiian) gift.
Makanah, Makanna, Makannah

Makani (Hawaiian) wind.
Makanee, Makania, Makaniah, Makanie, Makany, Makanya, Makanyah

Makara (Hindi) child born under the sign of Capricorn.
Makarah, Makarra, Makarrah

Makayla (Greek/Scottish) child of purity. (Heb) likeness to God. The feminine form of Michael.
Mica, Micah, Micaelah, Micaele, Micala, Micalah, Michaela, Michaelina, Michaeline, Michaella (Ital), Michala, Michalah, Michale, Michelina (Ital), Micheline, Michella, Michellah, Michelle, Miguelina (Span), Mikaela, Mikaelah, Mikelena (Dan), Myca, Mycah, Mycael, Mycaela, Mycaelah, Mycaele, Mycala, Mycalah, Mycale, Mychelina, Mycheline, Mychell, Mychella, Mychelle, Mykaelah, Mykaila, Mykailah, Mykayla, Mykaylah, Mykela, Mykelah, Mykelena

Mal (French) wrong.
Malah, Malana, Malanah, Malia

Malachie (French) angel; messenger of God. The feminine form of Malach.
Malachee, Malachey, Malachi, Malachy

Malala (Tongan) cinders.
Malalah

Malana (Hawaiian) light.
Malanah, Malanna, Malannah

Malania (Greek) dark-haired.
Malanee, Malaney, Malani, Malaniah, Malanie, Malany, Melanee, Melaney, Melani, Melanian, Melanie, Melany, Melana, Melena, Melenee, Meleney, Meleni, Melenie, Meleny, Mellanee, Mellaney, Mellani, Mellanie, Mellany, Mellenee, Melleney, Melleni, Mellenie, Melleny, Melona, Melonee, Meloney, Meloni, Melonia, Melonie, Melony (Corn), Melonya, Melonyah

Malaya (Filipino) freedom.
Malaia, Malaiah, Malaina, Malainah, Malaine, Malayah, Malayna, Malaynah, Malayne

Malfrid (Teutonic) fair worker; fair peace.
Malfreda, Malfredda, Malfrida, Malfryda, Malfrydda

Malha (Hebrew) queen.
Maliah, Malka, Malkah, Malkia, Malkiah, Malkie, Malkiya, Malkiyah, Miliah, Milya, Milyah, Mylia, Myliah, Mylya, Mylyah

Mali (Thai) the jasmine flower.
Malea, Maleah, Malee, Malei, Maleigh, Maley, Maliah, Malie, Maly, Malya, Malyah

Malia/Maliaka (Zuni/Hawaiian) wished for; star of the sea; bitter. A form of Mary.
Malea, Maleah, Maleia, Maleiah, Maleigh, Maleigha, Maliah, Maliaka (Haw), Maliasha, Malie, Maliea, Mallea, Malleah, Mallee, Mallei, Malleia, Malleiah, Malleigh, Malleigha, Malley, Malleya, Malli, Mallia, Malliah, Mallie, Mally, Mallya, Malya

Malie (Tongan) sweet.
Malee, Maley, Mali, Mallee, Malley,
Malli, Mallie, Mally, Maly

Malika (Hungarian) hard-working.
Maleeka, Maleka, Malikah, Malyka,
Malykah

Malina (Hebrew) highly praised.
(Haw) peace.
Malin, Malinah, Maline, Malyn,
Malyna, Malynah, Malyne

Malinda (Greek) gentle.
Malindah, Malynda, Malyndah

Malini (Hindi) gardener; Hindi God
of the Earth.
Malinee, Malinia, Malinie, Maliny,
Malyni, Malynia, Malyniah,
Malynie, Malyny, Malynya

Malka (Arabic) queen.
Malkah, Malkee, Malkeh, Malkey,
Malki (Heb), Malkia, Malkiah,
Malkie, Malkit, Malkya, Malkyah

Mallory (French) armoured;
wild duck. (Lat) hammer.
(O/Ger) army counsel.
Malloree, Mallorey, Mallori,
Mallorie, Mallorree, Mallorrey,
Mallorri, Mallorrie, Mallorry,
Maloree, Malorey, Malori, Malorie,
Malory

Malohi (Tongan) strength.
Malohee

Malu (Hawaiian) peacefulness.
Maloo

Malulani (Hawaiian) under the
skies of peace.
Malulanea, Malulanee, Malulaney,
Malulania, Malulanie, Malulany

Malva (Latin) the mallow flower.
(Grk) tender.
Malvah

Malvina (Latin) sweet friend; sweet
wine; assistant. (Gae) smooth
browed.
Malvinah, Malvinia, Malviniah,
Malvine (Celt), Malvyna,
Malvynah, Malvyne, Malvynia,
Malvyniah, Malvynya, Malvynyah

Mamana (Tongan) sweetheart.
Mamanah

Mamee/Mamie (French) my
sweetheart. A form of
Margaret/Mary, wished for; star of
the sea; bitter.
Maeme, Maemey, Maemi, Maemie,
Maemy, Maimee, Maimey, Maimi,
Maimie, Maimy, Maymee, Maymey,
Maymi, Maymie, Maymy

Mamo (Hawaiian) saffron flower;
yellow bird.

Mana (Tongan) miracle.
(Jap) sensitive.
Manah, Manal, Manali, Manalia,
Manaliah

Manar (Arabic) guiding light.
Manara

Manchu (Chinese) purity.

Manda (Spanish) warrior.
Mandah

Mandara (Hindi) calm.
Mandarah

Manddep (Punjabi) enlightened.
Mandeep

Mandy (American/Latin) worthy of
love. The short form of Amanda.
Amanda, Amandah, Manda,
Mandah, Mandea, Mandee,
Mandey, Mandi, Mandie

Manette (French/Hebrew) little wished for; star of the sea; bitter. A form of Mary.
Manet, Maneta, Manete, Manett, Manetta

Mangaia (Polynesian) peace.
Mangaea, Mangaiah, Mangaya, Mangayah

Mangena (Hebrew) melody.
Mangina, Mangyna

Mani (Chinese) prayer.
Manee, Maney, Manie, Many

Manilla (Australian Aboriginal) winding river.
Manila, Manilah, Manillah, Manille, Manyla, Manylah, Manylla, Manylle

Manisa (Xhosha) sweet.
Mandisah, Mandissa, Mandissah, Mandysa, Mandysah, Mandyssa, Mandyssah

Manka (Polish/Russian/Hebrew) wished for; star of the sea; bitter. A form of Mary.
Mankah

Manon (French/Hebrew) wished for; star of the sea; bitter. A form of Mary.
Manona, Manone, Manyn, Manyne

Manpreet (Punjabi) mind full of love.
Manpret

Mansi (Hopi) plucked flower.
Mancee, Mancey, Manci, Mancie, Mancy, Mansee, Mansie, Mansy

Manuela (Spanish) God is with us. The feminine form of Emmanuel.
Emanuel, Emanuela, Emanuele, Emanuell, Emanuella, Emanuelle, Manuel, Manuela, Manuele, Manuell, Manuella, Manuelle

Manya (Russian/Hebrew) wished for; star of the sea; bitter. A form of Mary.
Mania, Maniah, Manyah

Mapiya (Native American) heaven.
Mapiyah

Mara (Australian Aboriginal) black duck.
Marah, Marra, Marrah

Marabel (English/Hebrew/French) wished for; star of the sea; bitter. A combination of Mary/Mabel.
Marabela, Marabelah, Marabele, Marabell, Marabella, Marabellah, Marabelle, Mareebel, Mareebela, Mareebalah, Mareebele, Mareebell, Mareebella, Mareebellah, Mareebelle, Maribel, Maribela, Maribelah, Maribele, Maribell, Maribella, Maribellah, Maribelle, Marybel, Marybela, Marybelah, Marybele, Marybell, Marybella, Marybellah, Marybelle

Marah (Hebrew) melody.
Mara, Marra, Marrah

Marcaria (Greek) happy.
Marcariah, Marcarya, Marcaryah

Marcella/Marcena (Latin) warrior; warlike one; of Mars. A feminine form of Marc/Mark.
Marceena, Marceenah, Marceene, Marcele (Span), Marcelle (Fren), Marcellina, Marcelline, Marcelia, Marcelinda, Marcena, Marcenah, Marcene, Marcelyn, Marcey, Marcia, Marciana, Marcile, Marcille, Marcilen, Marquita (Span), Marseena, Marseenah, Marseene, Marsha, Marshelle, Marsiella, Marsielle, Markal, Marsha, Marshella, Marshelle

M

Marcia/Marcie (Latin) warrior, warlike one; of Mars. A feminine form of Marc/Mark.
Marcea, Marcee, Marcey, Marchia, Marchiah, Marci, Marcie, Marcial, Marciala, Marsiale, Marcsa, Marcy, Marcya, Marcyah, Marcye, Marsha, Marsia, Martia, Martiah

Mardell (Old English) from the meadow near the marsh.
Mardela, Mardelah, Mardele, Mardella, Mardellah, Mardelle

Marden (Old English) from the valley marsh.
Mardana, Mardanah, Mardane, Mardena, Mardenah, Mardene

Mardi (French) child born on a Tuesday.
March, Mardea, Mardee, Mardey, Mardie, Mardy

Marelda (Teutonic) famous warrior.
Esmarelda, Mareldah, Marilda, Marildah, Marylda, Maryldah

Maren (Latin) sea.
Marena, Marenah, Marin, Marina, Marine, Miren, Mirena, Mirene, Myren, Myrena, Myrenah, Myrene

Maretta (English/Greek) pearl.
Maret, Mareta, Maretah, Marete, Marett, Marette

Marfa (Latin) wished for; star of the sea; bitter. A form of Mary.
Marfah, Marffa, Marffah, Martha

Marg/Margie/Margaret/Margo (Greek) pearl.
Daisy, Gerta, Grethen (Fren), Gretal (Fren), Grete (Fren), Grethel (Fren), Kret, Krot, Madlinka, Madsche (Lett), Maharite (Bret), Mahoul, Maigret, Mairghread (Ir/Scot), Mairgreg, Mairgret, Malgerita (Ital), Malgherita, Malgosia, Malgozata (Pol), Margarete (Ger), Margareth (Dan), Margarethe (Fren/Ger), Margarida (Port), Margarita, Margarite (Lith), Margarta (Hung), Margat, Margaux (Fren), Margen (Ger), Margery (Eng), Margherita (Ital), Marghet (Ger), Margiad, Margit (Hung), Margolis, Margo (Fren), Margot (Fren), Margote, Margrethe (Dan), Margretta (Lett), Margriet (Dut), Margruerita (Fren), Margruerite, Margruta (Lith), Margryta (Lith), Marjarita (Slav), Marjoleine, Marjorie (Scott), Marjory, Marketa, Markete, Marret, Marsali, Maruorie, Meagan, Meagen, Megan, Meghan, Maghann, Metelili, Metje, Vread

Marguerite (French/Greek) pearl. A form of Margaret.
Margaret, Margareta, Margarete, Margaretha, Margarethe, Margarita, Margarite, Margerita, Margerite, Marguareta, Marguarete, Marguaretta, Marguarette, Marguarita, Marguarite, Margueritta, Margueritte, Margueretta, Marguerette, Margurita, Margurite, Marguryt, Marguryta, Marguryte

Mari (Japanese) ball. (Heb) wished for; star of the sea; bitter. The Spanish form of Mary.
Marea, Maree, Maria, Mariah, Mary

Maria/Marie (Hebrew) pearl.
Marea, Maree, Marey, Maria, Marie (Fren) Mariet, Marieta, Mariett, Marietta, Mariette (Ital), Marrea, Marree, Marrey, Marri, Marria, Marrie, Marriet, Marrieta, Marriete, Marrietta, Marriette, Marry, Mary

Mariah (Hebrew) God is my teacher; wished for; star of the sea; bitter. A form of Mary.
Maraia, Maraya, Marayah, Marria, Marriah, Marrya, Marryah, Meria,

Mariah cont.
Meriah, Moria, Moriah, Morya,
Moryah

Marian/Mariana (English/Hebrew)
wished for; star of the sea; bitter.
A form of Mary.
Mariana, Marianah, Mariane,
Mariann, Marianna, Marianne,
Mariena, Mariene, Marion,
Marrian, Marriana, Marriane,
Marriann, Marrianna, Marrianne,
Maryan, Maryana, Maryane,
Maryann, Maryanna, Maryanne

Maribella (English) wished for; star
of the sea; bitter. The Latin form
of Mary.
Mareabel, Mareabela, Mareabele,
Mareabell, Mareabella, Mareabelle,
Mareebel, Mareebela, Mareebele,
Mareebell, Mareebella, Mareebelle,
Maribela, Maribelah, Mariabell,
Mariabelle, Marybel, Marybela,
Marybele, Marybell, Marybella,
Marybelle

Marice (German) marsh flower. A
feminine form of Maurice, dark-
haired; from the moor.
Marica, Maricah, Maryca, Marycah,
Maryce

Mariel (German/Dutch/Hebrew)
wished for; star of the sea; bitter.
A form of Mary.
Marial, Mariala, Marialah, Mariale,
Mariall, Marialla, Marialle,
Marieke, Mariela, Mariele,
Marielin, Marielina, Marieline,
Mariela, Mariele, Mariell, Mariella,
Marielle, Mariellen, Marielsie,
Mariely, Marielys, Marielysa,
Marielyss, Marielyssa, Maryal,
Maryel, Maryil, Maryila, Maryile,
Maryilla, Maryille

Marigold (English) Mary's gold;
flower with yellow/orange petals.
Mareagold, Mareegold, Mariegold,
Marygold

Marika (Dutch/Slavic/Hebrew)
wished for; star of the sea; bitter.
A form of Mary.
Mareeca, Mareecka, Mareeka,
Marica, Maricah, Maricka, Marieka,
Marieke, Marija, Marijke, Marike,
Marikia, Marishka, Mariske,
Marrica, Marricah, Marrika,
Marrike, Maryca, Marycka, Maryka,
Maryk, Maryka, Maryke, Mariqua,
Marique, Merica, Mericah, Merika,
Merikah, Meriqua, Merique

Mariko (Japanese) circle.
Mareako, Makeeco, Mareecko,
Mareeko, Marico, Maricko, Maryco,
Marycko, Maryko

Mariling (Hebrew/Welsh) from the
wished-for one's pool; from the
bitter one's pool; from the star of
the sea pool. The combination of
Mary/Lin.
Marilina, Mariline, Marylina,
Maryline, Maryline, Marylyn,
Marylyna, Marylyne, Marylyng

Marilla (Hebrew/Teutonic) wished
for; star of the sea; bitter. A form
of Mary.
Marila, Marilah, Marillah, Maryla,
Marylah, Marylle

Marilyn (Hebrew/Old English) from
the wished-for one's pool; from
the bitter one's pool; from the
star of the sea pool. The
combination of Mary/Lin.
Maralin, Maralyn, Marilea,
Marileah, Marilena, Marilene,
Marilin, Marilina, Mariline,
Marilynn, Marlana, Marlane,
Marylin, Marylyn, Marylynn,

Merralin, Merralyn, Merrelina,
Merreline, Merrelyn, Merrelynn,
Merrilee, Merrili, Merrill, Merrilli,
Merrillin, Merrillina, Merrilline,
Merrillyn, Merrillynn, Merrylin,
Merrylina, Merryline, Merrylyn,
Merrylyna, Merrylyne

Marina (Latin) of the sea.
Mare, Mareana, Mareanah,
Mareane, Marena, Marenah,
Marianah, Marianna, Mariannah,
Maris, Marisa, Mariss, Marissa,
Marreen, Mareena, Mareenah,
Mareenia, Marrina, Marrinah,
Marrinia, Maryn, Maryna,
Marynah, Maryne, Marynna,
Marynnah, Marynne

Marini (Swahili) healthy; pretty.
Marinee, Mariney, Marinia,
Mariniah, Marinie, Marynee,
Maryney, Maryni, Marynie, Maryny

Marinna (Australian Aboriginal)
song.
Marina, Marinah, Marine,
Marrinah, Marinne, Maryna,
Marynah, Maryne, Marynna,
Marynnah, Marynne

Marion (Hebrew) wished for; star of
the sea; bitter. A form of Mary.
Marian, Mariana (Span), Marianna
(Ital), Marianne (Fren/Ger),
Marien, Maryan, Maryen, Maryin,
Maryon, Maryun

Maris (Latin) from the sea. A
feminine form of Maurice, dark-
haired; from the moor.
(Jap) infinite.
Marisa, Marisah, Marisha (Russ),
Marishah, Mariska (Heb), Marissa,
Marissah, Marris, Marrisa,
Marrisah, Marrisha, Marrishah,
Marrysa, Marrysah, Marryssa,
Marryssah, Meris, Merisa, Merisah,
Merissa, Merissah, Merrisa,

Merrisah, Merrissa, Merrissah,
Merrysa, Merrysah, Merryssa,
Merryssah

Marisol (Spanish) sea which is
sunny.
Marisa, Marise, Marizol, Marysol,
Marysola, Maryzol, Maryzola

Marit/Marita (Aramaic) lady.
(Span) sea.
Marita, Maritah, Marite, Maryt,
Maryta, Maryte

Maritza (Arabic) blessed.
Maritsa, Maritsah, Maritzah,
Marytsa, Marytsah, Marytza,
Marytzah

Marja (Finnish/Hebrew) wished for;
star of the sea; bitter. A form of
Mary.
Marg, Marge, Marjae, Marjah,
Marjatta, Marjatte, Marjie

Marjan (Persian) coral.
(Pol) wished for; star of the sea;
bitter.
Marjana, Marjanah, Marjane

Marjolaine (French) marjoram;
sweet-smelling plant.
Marjolain, Marjolaina, Marjolayn,
Marjolayna, Majolayne

Marjorie (Scottish) pearl. A form of
Margaret.
Margeree, Margerey, Margeri,
Margerie, Magery, Magori, Magorie,
Margory, Marjoree, Marjorey,
Marjori, Marjory

Markeisha (English/Swahili)
warrior; warlike one; of Mars; life.
Markeesha, Markesha, Markeshia,
Markesia, Markesiah, Markeysha,
Markeyshia, Markeysia, Markiesha,
Markieshia, Markiesia, Markisha,
Markishia, Markisia, Markysia,
Markysiah, Markysya, Markysyah

Markie (Latin) warrior; warlike one;
of Mars. A feminine form of
Mark/Marky.
Marke, Markee, Markeeta,
Markeisha, Marketa, Markete,
Marketta, Markette, Markey, Markia,
Markita, Marky, Marquee, Marquey,
Marqui, Marquie, Marquy

Markita (Slavic/Greek) pearl. A
form of Margaret.
Markeata, Markeatah, Markeda,
Markee, Markeeda, Markeeta,
Marketa, Marketta, Markette,
Markia, Markieta, Markitah,
Markitha, Markketta, Markkette,
Markkyt, Markkyta, Markkytah

Marla/Marlee (Hebrew) wished for.
(Aust/Abor) elder tree. (Eng)
from the marsh meadow.
Marlah, Marlana, Marlanah,
Marlania, Marlea, Marleah, Marlee,
Marleigh, Marley, Marli, Malie,
Marlo, Marly

Marlene (Hebrew) praised highly. A
form of Madeline, from the high
tower.
Marlaina, Marlaine, Marlana,
Marlanah, Marlane, Marlayna,
Marlayne, Marlean, Marleana,
Marleanah, Marleane, Marleen,
Marleena, Marleenah, Marleene,
Marleina, Marleine, Marlena,
Marlina, Marlinah, Marline,
Marlyn, Marlyna, Marlynah,
Marlyne

Marlis (English/Hebrew) sacred;
holy to God.
Marlisa, Marlise, Marliss, Marlissa,
Marlisse, Marlys, Marlysa, Marlyse,
Marlyss, Marlyssa, Marlysse

Marlo (English/Hebrew) wished-for
child; star of the sea; bitter. A
form of Mary.
Marlon, Marlona, Marlonah,
Marlone, Marlow, Marlowe

Marmara (Greek) shining.
Marmarah, Marmee

Marmion (Old French) small.
Marmyon

Marney/Marnina (Israeli) happy.
Marna, Marnah, Marnea, Marnee,
Marneena, Marneenah, Marni,
Marnia, Marniah, Marnie, Marnina,
Marninah, Marnique, Marny,
Marnya, Marnyah, Marnyna

Maroula (Greek/Hebrew) wished
for; star of the sea; bitter. A form
of Mary.
Maroulah, Maroullah, Maroullah

Marquise (French) noble.
Markeese, Markese, Marquees,
Marquese, Marquice, Marquies,
Marquiese, Marquisa, Marquisee,
Marquiste, Marquyse

Marquita (French) canopy.
Marqueeda, Marquedia, Marquee,
Marqueita, Marqueite, Marqueta,
Marquete, Marquetta, Marquette,
Marquia, Marquida, Marquietta,
Marquiette, Marquite, Marquitra,
Marquitia, Marquitta, Marquta,
Marquytah, Marquyte, Marquytta,
Marquyttah, Marquytte

Marree (Australian Aboriginal)
place of possums.
Marea, Maree, Marey, Mari, Marie,
Marrea, Marrey, Marri, Marrie,
Marry, Mary

Marsala (Italian) warrior; warlike;
of Mars.
Marsal, Marsali, Marsalla,
Marsallah, Marseilles, Marsela,

Marselah, Marsell, Marsella, Marsellah, Marselle

Marsh (Latin) warrior; warlike; of Mars.
Marcha, Marchah, Marchia, Marchya, Marchyah, Masha, Marshah, Marshia, Marshiah, Marshya, Marshyah

Marta (English/Aramaic) lady of sorrow.
Martah, Marte, Marttaha, Merta, Merte

Martha (Aramaic) lady.
Maita, Marta, Martah, Martaha, Marth, Marthan, Marthe, Marthena, Marthin, Marthina, Marthine, Marthy, Marticka, Martika, Martita, Martushka, Martycka, Martyka

Martina (Latin) warrior; warlike; of Mars. The feminine form of Martin.
Marta, Martah, Martain, Martaina, Martainah, Martaine, Martayn, Martaynah, Martayne, Martana, Martanah, Martane, Martanna, Martannah, Martanne, Marte, Martean, Marteanah, Marteane, Marteen, Marteena, Marteenah, Marteene, Martella, Martin, Martinah, Martine, Martyn, Martyna, Martynah, Martyne

Martiza (Arabic) blessed.
Martisa, Martisah, Martizah, Martysa, Martysah, Martyza, Martyzah

Maru (Polynesian) gentle. (Jap) round.
Maroo

Maruca/Marushka (Spanish/Hebrew) wished for; star of the sea; bitter. A form of Mary.
Maruchka (Pol), Maruja, Maruska (Russ)

Marva (Hebrew) sweet-smelling sage.
Marvah

Marvel (Latin) wonderous.
Marvela, Marvele, Marvell, Marvella, Marvellah, Marvelle, Marvil, Marvila, Marvile, Marvill, Marvilla, Marville, Marvyl, Marvyla, Marvyle, Marvyll, Marvylla, Marvylle

Marvina (French) famous friend. The feminine form of Marvin.
Marvinah, Marvinia, Marviniah, Marvyna, Marvynah, Marvynia, Marvyniah, Marvynya, Marvynyah

Mary (Hebrew) wished for; star of the sea; bitter.
Mae, Maga, Mai, Maida, Maidie, Maija (Finn), Maire (Ir), Maieli (Swed), Maika (Russ), Maillard, Maion (Fren), Mair, Mairee (Celt), Mairi (Scott), Maja (Swed), Malana (Haw), Mame, Mamie, Manetta, Manette (Fren), Manna (Boh), Manon (Fren), Manya, Maon, Mara (Heb), Marda, Mardi (Fren), Mardie, Mare, Marea, Maree, Marella (Fren), Maren, Maresa (Fren), Maret, Maria (Span), Mariah, Mariam (Grk), Mariamna (Russ), Mariamne (Heb), Mariana, Marianna, Marianne (Fren), Marica (Span), Marie (Fren), Maridell (Bav), Marieke (Dut), Mariel (Dut), Marien (Ir), Marika, Marjaka (Boh), Marjatta (Finn),

Mary cont.

Marjetta (Slav), Marij (Dut), Marija (Lith), Marilyn, Marinha (Port), Marintha, Marinyha (Span), Marion, Maris, Marissa, Marita (Span), Mariucca (Ital), Marjanka, Marjeta, Markika (Ger), Marlena, Marlene, Marnia, Maron, Marquilla (Span), Marquite, Marri, Marrije, Marriot, Marsha, Marsia, Mashka (Russ), Maruise, Marushe, Marya (Slav/Arab), Maryke, Marynia, Maryse (Fren), Marysia, Masha, Maura (Ir), Maureen (Ir), Maurene, Maurizia, May, Mearr (Ir), Menia, Mere, Mergen, Meri, Meridel, Merrie, Merry, Mhari, Mie, Miedal, Mieke, Miel, Mietje, Mieze, Mija, Mina, Minetta, Minette, Miriam, Miriamne, Moissey, Molli, Mollie, Molly, Moira (Ir), Moire (Ir/Scott), Moya (Ir), Moyra, Muire (Ir/Scott)

Maryanne (English/Hebrew) graceful; wished for; star of the sea; bitter. A combination of Mary/Ann.
Marian, Mariana, Marianah, Mariane, Mariann, Marianna, Marien, Mariena, Marienah, Mariene, Marienn, Marienna, Mariennah, Marienne, Maryan (Arab), Maryane, Maryannah, Maryanne, Maryen, Maryena, Maryene, Maryenn, Maryenna, Maryenne

Marybeth (Hebrew) wished for; star of the sea; bitter in the house of God. A combination of Mary/Beth.
Mareabeth, Mareebeth, Maribeth, Mariebeth

Maryellen (Hebrew/Greek) shining wished for; star of the sea; bitter. A combination of Mary/Ellen.
Marielen, Mariellen, Maryelen

Maryjo (Hebrew) God's gracious wished for; star of the sea. A combination of Mary/Jo.
Mareajo, Mareejo, Marijo, Marijoe, Marijoh, Maryjoe, Maryjoh

Marylou (Hebrew/German) famous warrior; wished for; star of the sea; bitter in the house of God. A combination of Mary/Lou.
Mareelou, Mareelu, Marilou, Marilu, Marylu

Masada (Hebrew) foundation of strength.
Masadah, Massada, Massadah

Masago (Japanese) the sands of time.
Massago

Masani (Luganda) one with the gap in her tooth.
Masanee, Masaney, Masania, Masaniah, Masanie, Masany, Masanya, Masanyah

Mashika (Swahili) child born during the rainy season.
Marishkah, Maryshka, Maryshkah, Mashyka, Mashykah

Matana (Hebrew) graceful gift.
Matanah, Matania, Mataniah, Matanna, Matannah, Matannia, Matanniah, Matanya, Matanyah, Mathena (Heb), Mathenah

Matilda (Teutonic) strong, powerful warrior.
Machtild (Ger), Mafalda (Span), Maginild, Magtelt (Dut), Matelda, Mathild, Mathilda (Teu), Mathilde, Mathildis, Matilde, Matilly, Mattilda, Mattylda, Mattiwilda, Mattylda, Matyld, Matylda, Matyldah, Matylde, Matusha (Span), Maud (Fren), Mechel (Bav), Mehaut (Fren), Metild, Metilda, Metildah, Metilde, Metyld, Metylda, Metyldah, Metylde

Matrika (Sanskrit) mother.
Matrica, Matricah, Matricka,
Matrickah, Matryca, Matrycah,
Matrycka, Matryckah, Matryka,
Matrykah

Matsuko (Japanese) pine tree child.

Mattea (Hebrew) gift of God. The
feminine form of Matthew.
Matea, Mateah, Mathea, Matheah,
Mathia, Mathiah, Matteah,
Matthea, Matthewe, Matthia,
Matthiah, Mattya, Mattyah

Maud (Teutonic) strong, powerful
warrior. The French form of
Madeline, from the high tower.
Maude, Maudea, Maudee, Maudey,
Maudi, Maudie, Maudy

Mauli (Tongan) Maori, native New
Zealander.
Maulea, Mauleah, Maulee, Maulei,
Mauleigh, Maulia, Mauliah,
Maulie, Mauly

Maura (Latin) dark-haired. The Irish
form of Mary, wished-for child;
star of the sea; bitter.
Maura, Maure (Fren), Mauree,
Mauri, Maurie, Mauritia, Maury,
Mouira, Moirah, Moyra, Moyrah

Maureen (Old French) dark-
skinned.
Maireen, Maireena, Maireene,
Mairin, Mairina, Mairine, Maura,
Maure, Mauree, Maurena,
Maurene, Maurina, Maurine,
Maurisa, Maurise, Maurita,
Mauritah, Mauritia, Maurizia (Ital),
Maurn, Maurya, Morain, Moraina,
Morainah, Moraine, Morayn,
Morayna, Moraynah, Morayne,
Moreen, Moreena, Moreene,
Morena (Span), Moren, Morene,
Morin, Morina, Morinah, Morine,
Moryn, Moryna, Morynah, Moryne

Maurise (French) dark-haired; from
the moor. The feminine form of
Maurice.
Maurisa, Maurisah, Maurisia,
Maurisiah, Maurissa, Maurissah,
Maurisse, Maurita, Mauritah,
Maurite, Maurizia, Maurizaih,
Maurizya, Maurizyah, Mauryzya,
Mauryzyah

Mausi (Native American) plucked
flower.
Mausee, Mausie, Mausy

Mauve (Greek) soft violet colour.
Maeve, Malva, Mauv

Maverick (English) spirited.
Maveric, Maverik, Maveryc,
Maveryck, Maveryk

Mavia (Celtic) happy.
Maviah, Mavie, Mavya, Mavyah

Mavis (French) song bird.
Mavas, Maviss, Mavos, Mavus, Mavys

Maxina/Maxine (Latin) extreme. The
feminine form of Max.
Maxeen, Maxeena, Maxeene,
Maxima, Maxyn, Maxyna, Maxyne,
Mazeen, Mazeena, Mazeene,
Mazin, Mazina, Mazine, Mazyn,
Mazyna, Mazyne

May (Latin) great, pink/white
blossom; child born in the
month of May.
Mae, Mai, Maia, Maiah, Maie,
Maya, Mayah, Maye

Maya (Hindi) the creative power of
God. (Grk) mother; grandmother.
(Lat) great.
Maea, Maia, Maiah, Mayah

Maybell (Latin) great; worthy of
beautiful love. A combination of
May/Bell.
Maebell, Maebella, Maebelle,
Maebelina, Maebeline, Maibell,

Maybell cont.
Maibelle, Maibelle, Maiebell,
Maiebella, Maiebelle, Maibelina,
Maibeline, Maibelyna, Maibelyne,
Maybella, Maybelle, Mayebell,
Mayebella, Mayebelle, Maybelina,
Maybeline, Maybelyna, Maybelyne

Mayda (English) woman.
Maeda, Maida, Maieda, Maydah,
Mayeda

Mayoree (Thai) beautiful.
Mayra, Mayree, Mayaria, Mayariah,
Mayarya, Mayaryah

Mayra (Australian Aboriginal) wind
of spring.
Maera, Maerah, Maira, Mairah,
Mayrah

Maysun (Arabic) beautiful.
Maesun, Maisun, Mason, Mayson

Mazal (Hebrew) lucky star.
Mazal, Mazala, Mazalah, Mazela,
Mazella, Mazelle

Meade (Greek) honey wine.
Mead, Meada, Meadah, Meed,
Meede

Meagan/Megan (Irish/Greek) great.
(Ir) strength. (Fren) daisy. The
Irish/Gaelic form of Margaret.
Maegan, Maegen, Maeghan,
Maeghen, Maeghin, Maeghon,
Maeghyn, Meaegin, Maegon,
Maegyn, Meagen, Meaghan,
Meaghen, Meaghin, Meaghon,
Meaghyn, Meegan, Meegen,
Meeghan, Meeghen, Meeghin,
Meeghon, Meeghyn, Meegin,
Meegon, Meegyn, Megan, Megen,
Meghan, Meghen, Meghon,
Meghyn, Megin, Megon, Megyn,
Meigan, Meigen, Meigin, Meigon,
Meigyn, Meygan, Meygen, Meygin,
Meygon, Meygyn

Meara (Gaelic) from the pool;
laughter.
Mearah, Mearia, Meariah, Mearya,
Mearyah, Meira, Meirah, Meyra,
Meyrah

Meave (Irish) happy.
Meava, Meavah

Meda (Native American) prophet;
priest. (Lat) healer.
Medah, Medea, Media, Mediah,
Medora

Media (Greek) ruling. (Lat) middle
child.
Medea, Medeah, Mediah, Medora,
Medorah, Medya, Medyah

Medina (Arabic) city.
Medeana, Medeanah, Medeena,
Medeenah, Medinah, Medyna,
Medynah

Medora (Greek) ruler.
Medorah

Mee (Chinese) beautiful.
Mee-Mee, Mei, Mei-Mei, Mi-Mi,
My-My

Meee (Australian Aboriginal) stars.
Mee

Meena (Greek) her mother's gift.
Meenah, Mina, Minah, Myna,
Mynah

Meera (Israeli) light.
Meerah, Meira, Meirah, Meyra,
Meyrah

Meg (Greek) little pearl. A short
form of Margaret.
Megg

Megara (Greek) first-born child.
Megarah

Mehadi (Hindi) flower.
Mehadee, Mehadie, Mehady

M

Mehira (Hebrew) energetic; speedy.
Mahira, Mahirah, Mehirah,
Mehyra, Mehyrah

Mehri (Persian) kind; lovable;
happy.
Mehree, Mehrie, Mehry

Mei (Hawaiian) great.
(Chin) beautiful.
Meiko, Meyko

Meiko (Japanese) flower bud.
Meyko

Meinwen (Welsh) slender; fair-
haired.
Meinwin, Meinwyn

Meira (Hebrew) light.
Meirah, Mera, Meerah, Meyra,
Meyrah, Mira, Mirah, Myra, Myrah

Meit (Burmese) affectionate.
Meita, Meyt, Meytah

Meiying (Chinese) beautiful flower.

Mejorana (Spanish) sweet
marjoram.
Mejoranah, Mejoranna,
Mejorannah

Meka (Hebrew) likeness to God.
(Grk/Scott) child of purity. A
form of Makayla.
Mekah

Mel (Portuguese/Spanish) sweet like
honey. The short form of names
starting with 'Mel' e.g. Melissa.
Mell

Mela (Hindi) religious service.
(Pol) dark-haired.
Melah, Mella, Mellah

Melanie (Greek) dark-haired.
Malana, Malanah, Malanee,
Malaney, Malani, Malania,
Malaniah, Malanie, Malany,
Melana (Russ), Melanee, Melaney,
Melani, Melanian, Melanie,
Melantha (Grk), Melanthe, Melany,
Melana, Melena, Melenee,
Meleney, Meleni, Melenie, Meleny,
Mellanee, Mellaney, Mellani,
Mellanie, Mellany, Mellenee,
Melleney, Melleni, Mellenie,
Melleny, Melona, Melonah,
Melonee, Meloney, Meloni,
Melonia, Meloniah, Melonie,
Melony (Corn), Melonya,
Melonyah, Melleny, Melona,
Melonee, Meloney, Meloni,
Melonia, Melonie, Melony (Corn)

Melba (Greek) soft. (Celt) from the
mill stream. (Lat) the mallow
flower.
Malbah, Malva, Malvah, Melba,
Melbah, Melva, Melvah

Meldoy (Greek) choral song.
Meldoi, Melodea, Melodee,
Melodey, Melodi, Melodie, Medosa,
Melody, Melodya, Melodye

Mele (Hawaiian) poem; song.
Melle

Melecent (Greek) honey bee.
(Ger) strength.
Melacent, Melacenta, Melacente,
Melacint, Melacinte, Melecenta,
Melecente, Melecinta, Melecint,
Melicinte, Melycent, Melycente,
Melycint, Melycinta, Melycinte,
Melycynt, Melycynta, Melycynte

Melek (Arabic) angel.
Meleka, Melekah

Meleni (Tongan) melon.
Melenee, Meleney, Melenia,
Meleniah, Meleny, Melenya,
Melenyah

Melesse (Ethiopian) eternal.
Mellesse

Melia (Hawaiian) flower.
Melcia, Melea, Meleah, Meleana,
Meleena, Meleia, Meleisha, Meliah,

Melia cont.
Melida, Melika, Melya, Melyah,
Milica, Milicah, Milika, Milikah,
Miliqua, Milique, Mylia, Myliah,
Mylya, Mylyah

Melina (Greek) song. (Lat) canary
yellow. A form of Melinda, gentle.
(Lat) sweet like honey.
Melaina, Melainah, Melaine,
Melana, Melanah, Melane,
Meleana, Meleanah, Meleane,
Melena, Melenah, Meline,
Melinia, Meliniah, Melinna,
Melinnah, Melinne, Melona,
Melonah, Melyna, Melynah,
Melyne, Melynna, Melynnah,
Melynne

Melinda (Greek) gentle. (Lat) sweet
like honey. A combination of
Mel/Linda, sweet; beautiful.
Malinda, Malindah, Malinde,
Malindea, Malindee, Malindia,
Malynda, Melindah, Melinde,
Melindee, Melindia, Melindiah,
Melynda, Melyndah

Melinga (Australian Aboriginal)
plenty.
Melynga

Melino (Tongan) peace.
Melyno

Meliora (Latin) better.
Mellor, Mellorah, Meliori,
Melioria, Meliorie, Mellear, Melyor,
Melyora, Melyorah

Melisande (German/French)
determined strength.
Lesandra, Lisandra, Melicent,
Melisanda, Melisandra, Melisenda,
Melisent, Melysanda, Melysande,
Millicent, Millicenta, Millicente

Melissa (Greek) honey bee; sweet
like honey.
Malissa, Malessa, Melessa,

Melessah, Melica, Melice, Melicent,
Melisa, Melisah, Melisenda,
Melisent, Melise, Melissah, Melisse,
Melissent, Melissia, Melitta,
Melittah, Mellisa, Mellissa,
Mellissah, Mellosa, Mellosah,
Melosa, Melosah, Melossa,
Melossah, Melysa, Melysah,
Melyssa, Melyssah, Melysse,
Milisa, Milisah, Milissa, Milissah,
Mylisa, Mylisah, Mylissa, Mylissah,
Mylysa, Mylysah, Mylyssa,
Mylyssah

Melita (Greek) balm; aromatic oil;
honey bee. A form of Melissa.
Meleata, Meleatah, Meleatta,
Meleattah, Meleeta, Meleetah,
Meleetta, Meleettah, Melitah,
Melitta, Melittah, Melyta, Melytah,
Melytta, Melyttah

Melody (Greek) beautiful song.
Meloda, Melodah, Melodea,
Melodee, Melodey, Melodi,
Melodia, Melodiah, Melodie,
Melodya, Melodyah

Melora (Greek) golden apple.
Melon, Melona, Melonah, Melone,
Melonee, Meloney, Meloni,
Melonia, Meloniah, Melonie,
Melonora, Melonora, Melonoria,
Melony, Melorah, Melori, Melorie,
Melory, Melorya, Meloryah

Melosa (Spanish) sweet like honey;
beautiful song.
Malosa, Malosah, Malossa,
Melosah, Melossa, Melossah

Melrose (Latin/Greek) sweet rose. A
combination of Mel/Rose.
Melrosa, Melrosah

Melva/Melvina (Irish/Gaelic) Mel's
friend from the mill.
(O/Eng) sword friend.
Malva, Malvah, Malveen,
Malveena, Malveenah, Malvina,

M

Malvinah, Malvinda, Malvindah, Malvine, Melveen, Melveena, Melveenah, Melveene, Melveenia, Melveeniah, Melvinah (Celt), Melvinda, Melvindah, Melvine, Melvinia, Melviniah, Melvyna, Melvynah, Melvyne, Melvynia, Melvyniah, Melvynya, Melvynyah

Mena (German/Dutch) strength.
Meana, Meanah, Meena, Meenah, Meina, Meinah, Menah, Meyna, Meynah

Menora (Hebrew) candle holder.
Menorah, Minora, Minorah, Mynora, Mynorah

Merab (Hebrew) increased greatness.
Meraba, Merabah

Meralda (Latin) emerald. A form of Esmeralda.
Esmaralda, Esmaraldah, Esmeralda, Esmeraldah, Esmerelda, Esmereldah, Meraldah

Mercedees (Spanish) reward; Our Lady of Mercies.
Merceda, Mercede, Mercedeas, Mercedees, Mercedez, Mercee, Mercey, Merci, Mercie, Mercy

Mercer (English/French) merchant.
Mercee, Mercey, Merci, Mercia, Merciah, Mercy, Mercya, Mercyah

Mercia/Mercy (Old English) compassionate. (Lat) reward.
Merce, Mercee, Mercey, Merci, Mercia, Merciah, Mercie, Mercilla, Mercillah, Mercille, Mercina, Mercinah, Mersee, Mersey, Mersi, Mersie, Mersilla, Mersillah, Mersina, Mersinah, Mersille, Mersy

Meredith (Welsh) from the sea.
Meredif, Merediff, Meredyth, Meridith, Meridithe, Meridyth, Merridith, Merridithe, Merridyth, Merridie, Merrydith, Merrydithe, Merrydyth

Mereki (Australian Aboriginal) peace maker.
Merekee, Merekie, Mereky

Meri (Hebrew) rebellious.
Meree, Merey, Merie, Mery

Meriel (Irish) black bird.
Merial, Meriele, Meriella, Merielle, Meryel, Meryela, Meryelah, Meryell, Meryella, Meryellah, Meryelle

Merilyn (English) happy pool. A combination of Meriel/Lyn.
Meralin, Meralina, Meraline, Meralyn, Meralyna, Meralyne, Merelan, Merelen, Merelin, Merelina, Mereline, Merelyn, Merelyna, Merelyne, Merilan, Merilen, Merilin, Merilina, Meriline, Merilyna, Merilyne, Merylan, Merylen, Merylin, Merylina, Meryline, Merylyn, Merylyna, Merylyne

Merinda (Australian Aboriginal) beautiful. (Eng) happy.
Merindah, Merynda, Meryndah

Merit (Latin) deserved.
Merita, Meritah, Merite, Meritt, Meritta, Merittah, Meritte, Meryt, Meryta, Merytah, Merytt, Merytta, Meryttah, Merytte

Merle (Latin/French) black bird.
Mearl, Mearla, Mearle, Merl, Merial, Meriel, Merla, Merlina, Merline, Merril, Merill, Merula (Lat), Meryl, Meryle, Meryll, Morrell, Muriel, Murl, Murle, Myriena, Myriene, Myrl, Myrle

Merpati (Indonesian) dove.
Merpatee, Merpatie, Merpaty

Merrie (Old English) happy.
Marree, Marrey, Marri, Marriann,
Marrianna, Marrianne, Marridee,
Marriella, Marrielle, Marrilee,
Marrie, Marrili, Marry, Marita,
Merree, Merrey, Merri, Merridee,
Merriella, Merrielle, Merrili,
Merilie, Merris, Merrita, Merry,
Mery

Merrina (Australian Aboriginal)
plenty of grass seed; flour.
Merina, Merinah, Meriwa,
Meriwah, Merrin, Merrinah,
Merriwa, Merriwah, Merryn,
Merryna, Merrynah, Merryna,
Merrynah, Merrywa, Merrywah

Merry (Middle English) happy. The
short form of names starting with
'Mer' e.g. Meredith.
Marree, Marri, Marrie, Marrilea,
Marrileah, Marrilee, Marrilei,
Marrileigh, Marylee, Meree, Merey,
Meri, Merie, Merree, Merrey, Merri,
Merrie, Merrile, Merrilee, Merrilei,
Merrileigh, Merriley, Merrili,
Merrill, Merrily, Merrylea,
Merryleah, Merrylee, Merrylei,
Merryleigh, Merryli, Merrylia,
Merrylie, Merryly, Merryn, Merryna,
Merrynah, Merylea, Meryleah,
Merylee, Merylei, Meryleigh,
Meryley, Meryli, Merylie, Meryly,
Meryn, Meryna, Merynah

Merva (Irish/Gaelic) Mel's friend
from the mill. (O/Eng) sword
friend. The feminine form of
Mervin.
Mervah

Meryl (German) famous. (Fren)
black bird. (Ir) shining sea. A
form of Muriel.
Maral, Marel, Marella, Merelle,
Merla, Merlah, Merrel, Merrell,
Merrella, Merelle, Merril, Merrile,
Merryl, Mirel, Mirell, Mirella,

Mirella, Mirl, Mirla, Mirle, Myral,
Myrel, Myrella, Myrelle, Myril,
Myrila, Myrile, Myryl, Myryla,
Myryle

Mesha (Hindi) child born under the
sign of Aries.
Meshah, Meshai

Messina (Latin) middle child;
harvest.
Mesina, Mesinah, Messinah,
Messyna, Messynah, Mesyna,
Mesynah

Meta (Australian Aboriginal) land.
(Lat) ambition.
Metah, Metta, Mettah

Metuka (Hebrew) sweet.
Metukah

Mhairie (Scottish/Hebrew) wished
for; star of the sea; bitter. A form
of Mary.
Mhaire, Mhairee, Mhairey, Mhairi,
Mhairy

Mia (Italian) mine.
Mea, Meah, Miah, Mya, Myah

Miandetta (Australian Aboriginal)
bend in the river.
Miandeta, Myandeta, Myandetta

Micah (Hebrew) likeness to God.
(Grk/Scott) child of purity.
A form of Makayla.
Mica, Mika, Mikah, Myca, Mycah,
Myka, Mykah

Michelle (French) likeness to God.
A feminine form of Michael.
Machell, Machella, Machelle,
Mashell, Mashella, Mashelle,
Mechel, Mechell, Mechella,
Mechelle, Meshell, Meshella.
Meshelle, Mica (Heb), Micaela,
Micah, Mical, Michalina,
Michaline, Michaella, Michaelle,
Michal, Michel, Michele,

Michelina, Micheline, Michell,
Michella, Michellah, Miguela,
Miguelita, Miquela, Miquelah,
Miquella, Miquelle, Mishel,
Mishela, Mishele, Mishell,
Mishella, Mishellah, Mishelle,
Mychel, Mychela, Mychelah,
Mychele, Mychell, Mychella,
Mychelle, Myshel, Myshela,
Myshelah, Myshele, Myshell,
Myshella, Myshellah, Myshelle

Michi (Japanese) the right way.
Miche, Michee, Michey, Michie,
Michiko, Michy

Michiko (Japanese) righteous; child
of beauty.

Micina (Native American) new moon.
Micinah, Mycina, Mycinah

Midgee (Australian Aboriginal)
acacia tree.
Midgey, Midgi, Midgie, Midgy

Midori (Japanese) green.
Madorea, Madoree, Madorey,
Madori, Madorie, Madory,
Midorea, Midoree, Midorey,
Midorie, Midory, Mydorea,
Mydoree, Mydorey, Mydori,
Mydorie, Mydory

Mieko (Japanese) prosperous.
Myeko

Mielikki (Finnish) pleasing.

Miette (French) little sweet one.
Mieta, Mietah, Mietta, Miettah,
Myeta, Myetah, Myett, Myetta,
Myettah

Migdana (Hebrew) gift.
Dana, Danah, Migdanna,
Migdannah, Mygdana, Mygdanah

Migina (Omaha) new moon.
Migeana, Migeanah, Migeena,
Migeenah, Miginah, Mygeana,
Mygeanah, Mygeena, Mygeenah,

Miginah, Migyna, Migynah,
Mygeana, Mygeanah, Mygeena,
Mygeenah, Mygina, Myginah,
Mygyna, Mygynah

Mignon (French) graceful; delicate.
Mignona, Mignone, Mignonetta,
Mignonette, Mygnona, Mygnonah,
Mygnone, Mignonetta, Mygnonette

Mignonette (French) flower.
Mignona, Mignone, Mignonetta,
Mignonettah, Mygnona, Mygnonah,
Mygnone, Mignonetta, Mygnonette

Mika (Japanese) new moon.
Mikah, Myka, Mykah

Miki (Japanese) three trees growing
together. (Haw) quick.
Mika, Mikee, Mikey, Mikia,
Mikiala, Mikie, Mikita, Mikiyo,
Mikka, Mikki, Mikkia, Mikkie,
Mikkiya, Mikko, Miko, Miky

Mila (Slavic) loved by the people.
(Ital) from Milan.
Milah, Milla, Millah, Milo, Myla,
Mylah, Mylla, Myllah

Milada (Slavic) my love. (Eng) my
lady.
Miladah, Miladi, Miladie, Milady,
Mylada, Myladi, Myladie, Mylady

Milagros (Spanish) miracle.
Mila, Milagritos, Milagro,
Milagrosa, Milrari, Milrarie, Milrary

Milcah (Hebrew) queen.
Milca, Mylca, Mylcah

Mildred (Old English) gentle, kind
counsellor; mild power.
Milda, Mildrid, Mylda, Myldred,
Myldreda

Milena (Teutonic) mild.
Milenah, Mylena, Mylenah

M

Mileta (German) merciful. The
feminine form of Milo.
(Lat) miller.
Miletah, Milett, Miletta, Milette,
Milica, Milicah, Milika, Milikah,
Milita, Militah, Milla, Millya,
Myleta, Myletah, Mylita, Mylitah,
Mylyta, Mylytah

Mili (Israeli) she is for me.
Milan, Milana, Milane, Milani,
Milania, Milanie, Milanka, Milanna,
Milanne, Milea, Mileah, Milee,
Milei, Mileigh, Miley, Milia, Miliah,
Milie, Millea, Milleah, Millee, Millei,
Milleigh, Milli, Millia, Milliah,
Millie, Milly, Mylea, Myleah, Mylee,
Mylei, Myleigh, Myli, Mylie, Myllea,
Mylleah, Myllee, Myllei, Mylleigh,
Mylli, Myllie, Mylly, Myly

Milia (German) hard-working.
Mila, Milah, Mili, Milica, Milika,
Milikah, Milla, Millah, Milya,
Milyah, Mylia, Myliah, Myllia,
Mylliah, Myllya, Myllyah

Mililani (Hawaiian) heavenly
caresses.
Mililanee, Mililaney, Mililanie,
Mililany, Mylilanee, Mylilaney,
Mylilani, Myliliania, Mylilianiah,
Mylilanie, Mylilany, Mylylanee,
Mylylaney, Mylylania, Mylylaniah

Milka (Slavic/German) hard-
working. A form of Amelia.
Milkah, Mylka, Mylkah

Millicent (Teutonic) strong worker.
Melicend, Melicent, Melisanda,
Melisande, Melisenda, Melisende,
Melisent, Melita, Mellicent,
Mellisent, Melusina, Melusine,
Milicent, Milicenta, Milissent,
Millisent, Millisenta, Myllicent,
Myllicenta, Myllicente, Myllycent,
Myllycenta, Myllycente, Myllysent,
Myllysenta, Myllysente, Mylycent,

Mylycenta, Mylycente, Mylysent,
Mylysenta, Mylysente

Milly (English/German) hard-
working. A form of Amelia.
Milan, Milana, Milane, Milani,
Milania, Milanie, Milanka,
Milanna, Milanne, Milea, Mileah,
Milee, Milei, Mileigh, Miley, Milia,
Miliah, Milie, Millea, Milleah,
Millee, Millei, Milleigh, Milli,
Millie, Milly, Mylea, Myleah,
Mylee, Mylei, Myleigh, Myli, Mylie,
Myllea, Mylleah, Myllee, Myllei,
Mylleigh, Mylli, Myllie, Mylly, Myly

Mima (Burmese) woman.
Mimah, Mimma, Mimmah, Myma,
Mymah, Mymma, Mymmah

Mimi (Italian) my, my. The French
form of Miriam, strong-willed,
wished for; star of the sea; bitter.
A form Mary.
Mimea, Mimee, Mimey, Mimie,
Mimmea, Mimmee, Mimmey,
Mimmi, Mimmie, Mimmy, Mimy,
Mymea, Mymee, Mymey, Mymi,
Mymie, Mymmea, Mymmee,
Mymmey, Mymmi, Mymmie,
Mymmy, Mymy

Mimiteh (Blackfoot) new moon.

Mina (German) love; loved memory.
(Arab) wish. (Lat) threat.
(Nat/Amer) first-born daughter.
(Eng) little; mine. A short form of
Wilhelmina.
Meena, Meenah, Minah, Minetta,
Minette, Minna, Minnah, Myna,
Mynah, Mynna, Mynnah

Minal (Native American) fruit.
Minala, Minalah, Mynala, Mynalah

Minda (Sanskrit) knowing.
Mindah, Mynda, Myndah

Mindy (Greek) gentle.
Mindea, Mindee, Mindey, Mindi,
Mindie, Mindy, Myn, Mynd,
Myndee, Myndea, Myndey, Myndi,
Myndie, Myndy

Mine (Japanese) wisdom.
Minee, Miney, Mini, Minee, Miney,
Miniver, Myna, Mynah, Myne,
Mynee, Myney, Myni, Mynie, Myny

Minerva (Greek) wisdom.
Minervah, Mynerva, Mynervah

Minette (French) faithful defence.
Minetta, Minnette, Minitta,
Minitte, Mynetta, Mynette,
Mynnetta, Mynnette

Minikin (Dutch) darling.
Minikina, Minikinah, Minikine,
Minikyna, Minikynah, Minikyne,
Mynikin, Mynikina, Mynikinah,
Mynikine

Miniti (Tongan) mint.
Myniti

Minka (Polish/German) little
determined guardian. A form of
Wilhelmina.
Minkah, Mynka, Mynkah

Minkie (Australian Aboriginal) day
light.
Minkee, Minkey, Minki, Minky,
Mynkee, Mynkey, Mynki, Mynkie,
Mynky

Minna (Teutonic) loved memory;
tender; affectionate.
Mina, Mineal, Minetta, Minette,
Minnah, Minta, Mintah, Myna,
Mynah, Mynna, Mynnah

Minnehaha (Native American)
waterfall.
Minehaha, Mynehaha, Mynnehaha

Minnesota (Native American)
cloudy water.
Minesota, Mynnesota, Mynesota

Minnie (Latin) tiny.
Minee, Miney, Mini, Minie,
Minnee, Minney, Minni, Minny,
Miny, Mynee, Myney, Myni, Mynie,
Mynnee, Mynney, Mynni, Mynnie,
Mynny, Myny

Minnta (Australian Aboriginal)
shadow.
Minta, Mintah, Minntah, Mynta,
Myntah, Mynnta, Mynntah

Minore (Australian Aboriginal)
white flower.
Minora, Minoree, Mynora,
Mynorah, Mynoree

Minowa (Native American) singer.
Minowah, Mynowa, Mynowah

Minta (Greek) the mint plant.
Mintah, Mynta, Myntah, Yaminta
(Nat/Amer), Yamintah, Yamynta,
Yamyntah

Minya (Osage) eldest sister.
Minta, Mintah, Minyah,Myna,
Mynah, Yiminta, Yiminya, Mynta,
Mynya

Mio (Japanese) strength three times
over.
Myo

Mira/Mirabel (Latin) spectacular;
beautiful.
Miriam, Mira, Mirabela, Mirabele,
Mirabell, Mirabella, Mirabellah,
Mirabelle, Mirah, Miran, Mireille,
Mirella, Mirelle, Miriell, Miriella,
Mirielle, Mirra, Mirrah, Myra,
Myrabell, Myrabella, Myrabellah,
Myrabelle, Myrah, Myrilla, Myrille

Mirabrook (Australian Aboriginal)
the Southern Cross star
constellation.
Myrabook

Miranda (Latin) worthy of love; mermaid. A form of Amanda.
Maranda, Marandah, Meranda, Merandah, Miran, Mirandah, Myranda, Myrandah

Mireil (Hebrew) God has spoken. (Lat) wonderful.
Mirela, Mirele, Mirella, Mirelle, Mirelys, Mirelyss, Mirelyssa, Mirelysse, Mireya, Mireeyda, Miriella, Mirielle, Mirilla, Mirille, Myrella, Myrelle, Myrilla, Myrelle

Mirena (Hawaiian) loved.
Mirenah, Myrena, Myreanah

Miri (Gypsy/Hebrew) wished for; star of the sea; bitter. A form of Mary.
Miria, Miriah, Myri, Myria, Myriah, Myry, Myrya, Myryah

Miriam (Hebrew) strong-willed, wished for; star of the sea; bitter. A form of Mary.
Mariamne, Meriamne, Miriamne, Myriam, Myriamne, Myryam, Myryamne

Mirica (Latin/English) miracle child.
Miracle, Miricah

Mirna (Irish) polite.
Merna, Mernah, Mirnah, Myrna, Myrnah

Mirrin (Australian Aboriginal) cloud.
Mirrina, Mirrine, Mirryn, Mirryna, Myrrine, Myrryn, Myrryna, Myrryne

Missy (Old English) little miss. A short form of Melissa, honey bee; sweet like honey.
Misee, Misey, Misi, Misie, Missee, Missey, Missi, Missie, Mysea, Mysee, Mysey, Mysi, Mysie, Myssea, Myssee, Myssey, Myssi, Myssie, Myssy, Mysy

Misty (Old English) covered with a mist; concealed.
Mistea, Mistee, Mistey, Misti, Mistie, Mystea, Mystee, Mystey, Mysti, Mystie, Mysty

Mitzi (German) strong-willed. The German form of Maria. A short form of Miriam.
Mitzee, Mitzey, Mitzie, Mitzy, Mytzee, Mytzey, Mytzi, Mytzie, Mytzy

Miwa (Japanese) wise eyes.
Miwah, Miwako, Mywa, Mywah, Mywako

Miya (Japanese) three arrows; temple.
Miyah, Miyana, Miyanna, Mya, Myah

Miyo (Japanese) generation of beauty.
Miyoko, Miyuki, Miyuko, Myo

Miyoko (Japanese) generation's beautiful child.
Myyoko, Yoko

Miyuki (Japanese) deep snow.
Miyukee, Myyukee, Myyuki

Moana (Hawaiian) ocean. (Tong) deep sea.
Moanah, Moane, Moann, Moanna, Moannah, Monanne

Mocha (Arabic) chocolate-flavoured coffee.
Mochah, Moka, Mokah

Modesty (Latin) gentle; modest.
Modesta (Ital), Modestah, Modestee, Modesteen, Modesteena, Modesteene, Modestey, Modestia (Span), Modestina, Modestine (Fren), Modestyn, Modestyna, Modestyne

M

Moesha (Hebrew) saved; taken from the water. (Egypt) child. The feminine form of Moses.
Moeisha, Moeysha

Mohala (Hawaiian) flowering.
Moala, Mohalah

Mohini (Sanskrit) enchantress.
Mohinee, Mohiney, Monhinie, Mohiny, Mohynee, Mohiney, Mohyni, Mohynie, Mohyny

Moina/Mona (Celtic/Irish) gentle; soft. (Grk) solitary. (Arab) wish. (Lat) advice. (O/Eng) month. A form of Mona, sweet, noble angel.
Moness, Monessa, Monessah, Moina, Moinah, Monah, Monic, Monique, Monna, Monnah, Moyna, Moynah, Muna, Munah

Moira (Irish/Gaelic) great. The Irish form of Mary, wished-for child; star of the sea; bitter. (Grk) fate.
Maira, Maura, Moirae, Moirah, Moyra, Moyrah, Myra, Myrah

Molara (Basque/Hebrew) wished-for child; star of the sea; bitter. A form of Mary.
Molarah, Molarra, Molarrah

Moledina (Australian Aboriginal) creek.
Moledin, Moledinah, Moledine, Moledyn, Moledyna, Moledynah, Moledyne

Moli (Tongan) the colour orange.
Molea, Molee, Molei, Moleigh, Moley, Molie, Moly

Molly (Hebrew) wishing.
Molea, Moleah, Molee, Molei, Moleigh, Moley, Moli, Molie, Mollea, Molleah, Mollee, Mollei, Molleigh, Molley, Molli, Mollie

Momi (Hawaiian) pearl. A form of Margaret.
Momee, Momie, Momy

Monet (Greek/French) solitary.
Monae, Monay, Monaye

Monica (Greek) solitary. (Lat) advisor.
Monca, Monia, Moniah, Monic, Monicah, Monice, Monicia, Monicka, Monika, Monikah, Moniqua, Monique, Monisa, Monise, Monnica, Monnicah, Monnicka, Monnika, Monniqua, Monnique, Monnyca, Monnyka

Monifa (Yoruba) lucky.
Monifah, Monyfa, Monyfah

Monique (French) wise counsellor.
Monch (Ir), Moncha, Monchah, Monche, Moneeca, Moneecah, Moneeka, Moneekah, Monica, Monicah, Monicia, Monicka, Monika (Pol), Monikah, Monike (Ger), Moniqua, Monyca, Monycah, Monycka, Monyka, Monykah, Monyqua, Monyque

Monroe (Irish) from the red marsh.
Monrow

Monserrat (Latin) jagged mountain.
Monserat

Montana/Montee/Montina (Latin/Spanish) mountain.
Montanah, Montania, Montaniah, Montanna, Montannah, Montea, Monteen (Fren), Monteena, Monteenah, Montey, Monti, Montia, Montie, Montina. Montinah, Montine (Fren), Monty, Montyn, Montyna, Montynah, Montyne

Moon (English) moon.
Moona, Moonah, Moone, Moonee, Mooney, Mooni, Moonia, Mooniah, Moonie, Moony

Moona (Australian Aboriginal)
plenty. (Eng) moon.
Moonah, Moonia, Mooniah,
Moonya, Moonyah

Mora (Spanish) blueberry.
Morah, Morea, Moreah, Moria,
Moriah, Morita, Morite, Moryta,
Morytah, Moryte

Morag (Gaelic) sun.
Moragg

Morasha (Hebrew) inheritance.
Morash, Morashah

Moree (Australian Aboriginal)
water.
Morey, Mori, Moria, Moriah,
Morie, Mory, Morya, Moryah

Moreen (Irish) great.
Morain, Moraina, Morainah,
Moraine, Morayn, Morayna,
Moraynah, Morayne, Moreena,
Moreenah, Moreene, Morein,
Moreina, Moreinah, Moreine,
Morenah, Morene, Morin, Morina,
Morinah, Morine, Mooreen,
Mooreena, Mooreenah, Mooreene,
Moryn, Moryna, Morynah, Moryne

Morela (Polish) apricot.
Morelah, Morell, Morella,
Morellah, Morelle

Morena (Spanish) brown-haired.
Morain, Moraina, Morainah,
Moraine, Morayn, Morayna,
Moraynah, Morayne, Moreena,
Moreenah, Moreene, Morein,
Moreina, Moreinah, Moreine,
Morenah, Morene, Morin, Morina,
Morinah, Morine, Mooreen,
Mooreena, Mooreenah, Mooreene,
Moryn, Moryna, Morynah, Moryne

Morgan (Celtic) sea bright; of the
sea. (O/Wel) white sea dweller.
Morgain, Morgaina, Morgainah,
Morgana, Morganah, Morgann,

Morganna, Morganne, Morgayn,
Morgayna, Morgaynah, Morgayne,
Morgen, Morgin, Morgon, Morgyn

Morgwen (Welsh) great fair hair.
Morgwena, Morgwenah

Moriah (French) dark-haired.
(Heb) God is my teacher.
Maria, Mariah, Marya, Maryah,
Moria, Morya, Moryah

Morialta (Australian Aboriginal)
ever flowing.
Morialtah

Morie (Japanese) bay.
Morea, Moree, Morey, Mori, Mory

Morina (Irish) mermaid.
Morinah, Morinna, Morinnah,
Moryna, Morynah, Morynna,
Morynnah

Morissa (Latin) dark-haired; from
the moor. The feminine form of
Maurice.
Morica, Morisa, Morisah, Morissah,
Moriset, Morisett, Morisetta,
Morisette, Morysa, Moryssa, Morysse

Morit (Hebrew) teacher.
Moritt, Moritta, Morittah, Morryt,
Morryta, Morrytah, Morryte, Moryt,
Moryta, Moryte, Morytt, Morytta,
Moryttah, Morytte

Morna (Gaelic) affectionate; gentle;
beloved. (Eng) dawn, morning.
Mornah, Mornina, Mornine,
Morning, Mornyng

Morowa (Akan) queen.
Morowah

Morrin (Irish) long-haired.
Morin, Morina, Morinah, Morine,
Moryn, Moryna, Morynah, Moryne

Morrissa (Latin) dark-haired; from the moor. The feminine form of **Morris.**
Morisa, Morisah, Morissah, Morrisa, Morrisah, Morrissa, Morrissah, Morysa, Morysah, Moryssa, Moryssah

Morwenna (Welsh) waves of the sea.
Morwena, Morwenah, Morwennah

Moselle/Mosina (Hebrew/French) saved; taken from the water. (Egypt) child. A feminine form of **Moses.**
Mosel, Mosela, Moselah, Mosele, Mosella, Mosellah, Mosina, Mosinah, Mosine, Mozel, Mozela, Mozelah, Mozele, Mozella, Mozellah, Mozelle, Mozina, Mozinah, Mozine, Mozyna, Mozynah, Mozyne

Mosi (Swahili) first-born child.
Mosea, Mosee, Mosey, Mosie, Mosy

Moswen (Tswana) white.
Moswena, Moswenah, Moswin, Moswina, Moswinah, Moswyn, Moswyna, Moswynah

Motepa (Australian Aboriginal) girl child.
Motepah

Mouche (French) beauty spot.
Mouch, Moush, Moushe

Mouna (Arabic) wish.
Moona, Moonah, Moonia, Mounah, Mounia, Muna, Munah, Munia

Mozelle (Hebrew) little fountain.
Mosel, Mosela, Moselah, Mosele, Mosella, Mosellah, Mozel, Mozela, Mozelah, Mozele, Mozella, Mozellah

Mrena (Slavic) white eyes.
Mren, Mrenah

Mulga (Australian Aboriginal) acacia tree.
Mulgah

Mullion (Australian Aboriginal) eagle.
Mulion

Muluk (Indonesian) praised highly.
Muluka, Mulukah

Muna (Basque) saint.
Munah

Mundai (Australian Aboriginal) pretty.
Mundae, Munday

Mungo (Irish) lovable.

Mura (Japanese) village.
Murah

Muriel (Arabic) myrrh. (Ir/Gae) sea bright. (Grk) fragrant.
Marial, Mariel, Mariella, Marielle, Maryal, Maryel, Maryella, Maryelle, Meriel, Meriella, Merielle, Merl, Merle, Meryl, Mira, Murial, Muriella, Murielle, Muryel, Muryela, Muryele, Muryell, Muryella, Muryelle

Murphy (Celtic) from the sea.
Merffee, Merffey, Merffi, Merffie, Merffy, Murffee, Murffey, Murffi, Murffie, Murffy, Murphee, Murphey, Murphi, Murphie

Musa (Arabic) saved; taken from the water. (Egypt) child. A feminine form of **Moses.**
Musah

Musetta/Musette (Old French/English) little muse; inspiration. (O/Fren) of thought; little bagpipe. In Greek mythology, nine sister goddesses of the arts.
Muse, Muset, Museta, Musetah, Musete, Musettah, Musette

Musidora (Greek) beautiful muse.
Musidorah, Musidore, Musydor,
Musydora, Musydorah, Musydore

Musika (Tongan) music.
Music, Musica, Musicah, Musicka,
Musickah, Musikah, Musyca,
Musycah, Musycka, Musyckah,
Musyka, Musykah

Mya (Burmese) emerald.
Mea, Meaha, Meia, Meiah, Mia,
Miah, Myah

Myer (Hebrew) light.
Myar, Myir, Myyr

Mykaela (American/Hebrew)
likeness to God. A form of
Makayla.
Mica, Micah, Micaelah, Micaele,
Micala, Micalah, Michaela,
Michaelina, Michaeline, Michaella
(Ital), Michala, Michalah, Michale,
Michelina (Ital), Micheline,
Michella, Michellah, Michelle,
Miguelina (Span), Mikaela,
Mikaelah, Mikelena (Dan), Myca,
Mycah, Mycael, Mycaela, Mycaelah,
Mycaele, Mycala, Mycalah, Mycale,
Mychelina, Mycheline, Mychell,
Mychella, Mychelle, Mykaelah,
Mykaila, Mykailah, Mykayla,
Mykaylah, Mykela, Mykelah,
Mykelena

Myla (English) merciful.
Mila, Milah, Milla, Millah, Mylah,
Mylla, Myllah

Myra (Old French) soft song.
(Lat) scented oil; wonderful.
(Grk) plenty.
Mira, Mirah, Myrah, Myrena,
Myria, Myriah, Myrra, Myrrah,
Myrrha

Myrna (Irish/Gaelic) polite; gentle.
(Arab) myrrh.
Merna, Mernah, Mernahm, Mirna,
Mirnah, Moina, Moinah, Morna,
Mornah, Moyna, Moynah, Murna,
Murnah, Myrna, Myrnah

Myrrine (Australian Aboriginal)
wind.
Myrrina, Myrrinah, Myrrine,
Myryna, Myrynah, Myrryna,
Myrrynah

Myrtle (Greek) myrtle tree; victory;
crowned. (Lat) flower.
Mertal, Mertel, Mertell, Mertella,
Mertelle, Mirtal, Mirtel, Mirtil,
Mirtyl, Murtal, Murtel, Murtella,
Murtelle, Myrta, Myrtia, Myrtice,
Myrticia

Myune (Australian Aboriginal) clear
water.
Miunah, Miunah, Myunah

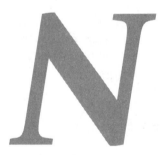

Naarah (Hebrew) girl of my heart.
Naara, Nara, Narah

Nabila (Arabic) born to nobility.
Nabilah, Nabyla, Nabylah

Nachine (Spanish) fiery.
Nachina, Nachinah, Nachyna,
Nachynah, Nachyne

Nada/Nadia/Nadine (Russian) hope
Nada, Nadah, Nadan, Nadana,
Nadanah, Nadean, Nadeana,
Nadeanah, Nadeane, Nadeen,

Nadeena, Nadeenah, Nadeene,
Nadiah (Fren), Nadie, Nadin,
Nadina, Nadine, Nady, Nadya,
Nadyah, Nadyn, Nadyna,
Nadynah, Nadyne,

Nadalia (Australian Aboriginal) fire.
Nandalea, Nandaleah, Nandalee,
Nandalei, Nandaleigh, Nandaley,
Nandali, Nandalia, Nandaliah,
Nandaly, Nandalya, Nandalyah

Nadda (Australian Aboriginal) camp
site. (Arab) generous.
Nada, Nadah, Naddah

Nadira (Arabic) precious.
Nadirah, Nadria, Nadriah, Nadyra,
Nadyrah

Naeva (French/Hebrew) life. A form
of Eve.
Naeve, Nahvon

Nafuna (Luganda) child born feet
first.
Nafunah

Nagida (Hebrew) noble;
prosperous.
Nagda, Nagdah, Nageeda, Nagyda

Nahid (Persian) goddess of love;
Venus.
Nahyd

Naia (Hawaiian) dolphin.
Naiah, Naya, Nayah

Naiad (Greek) water fairy.
Naida, Nayad, Nyad

Nailah (Arabic) successful.
Naila, Nayla, Naylah

Nairi (Armenian) from the land
with the canyons.
Nairia, Nairiah, Nairie, Nairee,
Nairey, Nairy

Nairne (Scottish) from the alder
tree river.
Nairn

Najam (Arabic) star.
Naja, Najma

Najila (Arabic) child with the
brilliant eyes.
Najilah

Nakeisha (Swahili/African
American) life. (Arab) woman. A
form of Keisha.
Nakeasha, Nakeesha, Nakesha,
Nakeshea, Nakeshia, Nakeysha,
Nakiesha, Nakisha, Nakishia,
Nakishiah, Nakishya, Nakishyah,
Nakysha, Nakyshah

Nakeita/Nakia (Russian/Greek)
victory of the people. A form of
Nicole. A feminine form of
Nicholas.
Nakeata, Nakeatah, Nakeea,
Nakeeah, Nakeeta, Nakeitah,
Nakeitha, Nakeithia, Nakeithiah,
Nakeitra, Nakeitress, Nakeitta,
Nakeitte, Nakeittia, Naketta,
Nakette, Nakieta, Nakitha, Nakitia,
Nakitta, Nakitte, Nakyta, Nakytta,
Nakytte, Nikeeta, Nikia, Nikiah,
Nikita, Nikitah, Nikitta, Nikitte,
Nykeita, Nykeitah, Nykeyta,
Nykeytah, Nykia, Nykiah, Nykita,
Nykitah, Nykyta, Nykytah

Nalani (Hawaiian) calm heavens.
Nalanea, Nalaneah, Nalanee,
Nalaney, Nalania, Nalaniah,
Nalanie, Nalany, Nalanya,
Nalanyah

Nami (Japanese) wave.
Namee, Namey, Namie, Namy

Nan (Hebrew) graceful.
Nanet, Naneta, Nanetah, Nanete,
Nanett, Nanetta, Nanettah,
Nanette, Nana, Nanah, Nann,
Nanna, Nannah, Nannet, Nanneta,
Nannetah, Nannete, Nannett,
Nanetta, Nannettah, Nannette

Nana (English/Australian/American) grandmother. (Haw) spring; graceful. (Heb) bitter. (O/Nrs) young woman.
Nanah, Nanna, Nannah

Nanala (Hawaiian) sunflower.
Nanalah

Nancy (English/Hebrew) graceful. A form of Ann.
Nancea, Nancee, Nancey, Nanci, Nancia, Nanciah, Nancie, Nancya, Nancyah, Nancye

Nanda (Australian Aboriginal) lake.
Nandah, Nanda, Nanndah

Nanetta/Nanette (French) little graceful one. A form of Annetta.
Nana, Nanah, Nanet, Naneta, Nanetah, Nanete, Nanett, Nanettah, Nanette Nann, Nanna, Nannah, Nannet, Nanneta, Nannetah, Nannete, Nannett, Nanetta, Nannettah, Nannette

Nani (Hawaiian) beautiful. (Grk) charming.
Nanee, Naney, Nania, Naniah, Nanie, Nannee, Nanney, Nanni, Nannie, Nanny, Nany, Nanya, Nanyah

Nanon (French/Hebrew) graceful bitterness. A form of Ann.
Nanona, Nanonah, Nanone, Nononia, Nononiah, Nanonya, Nanonyah

Naomi (Hebrew) pleasant.
Naoma, Naomah, Naomee, Naomey, Naomia, Naomiah, Naomie, Naomy, Navit, Neoma, Neomah, Neomee, Neomi, Neomie, Neomy, Noma, Nomah, Nomee, Nomey, Nomi, Nomia, Nomiah, Nomie, Nyoma, Nyomee, Nyomey, Nyomi, Nyomia, Nyomiah, Nyomie, Nyomy, Nyomya, Nyomyah

Napea (Latin) from the valley.
Napeah

Nara (Irish) happy. (Jap) oak.
Narah, Narra, Narrah

Narcisse (Greek/French) daffodil; self-love.
Narcissa, Narcissah, Narciska, Narcissus

Narda (Latin) fragrant oil.
Nardah

Nardoo (Australian Aboriginal) clover.
Nardo

Narelle (Australian Aboriginal) light; woman from the sea.
Narel, Narela, Narelah, Narele, Narell, Narella, Narellah

Nari (Japanese) thunder bolt.
Narea, Naree, Narey, Naria, Nariah, Narie, Nary, Narya, Naryah

Narlala (Australian Aboriginal) lookout.
Narla, Narlalah

Narmanda (Hindi) giver of pleasure.
Narmandah

Narooma (Australian Aboriginal) magical stone.
Naroomah

Nashota (Native American) second born of twins.
Nashotah

Nasya (Hebrew) miracle of God.
Nasia, Nasiah, Nasyah

Nata (Native American) creator; speaker. (Sans) dancer. (Hin) rope. (Lat) swimmer.
Natah, Natia, Natiah, Natka, Natya, Natyah

N

Natalie (Latin) born on Christmas Day; nativity.
Natala, Natale (Ital), Natalea, Nataleah, Natalean, Nataleana, Nataleanah, Nataleane, Natalee, Nataleena, Nataleenah, Nataleene, Natalei, Nataleigh, Nataley, Natali, Natalia (Russ/Span), Nataliah, Natalena, Natalenah, Natalene, Natalija (Russ), Natalina, Natalinah, Nataline, Natala, Natalah, Natale, Natall, Natalla, Natallah, Natalle, Nataly, Natalya, Natalyah, Natalyn, Natalyna, Natalynah, Natalyne, Natelea, Nateleah, Natelee, Natelei, Nateleigh, Nateley, Nateli, Natelia, Nateliah, Natelie, Nately, Natelya, Natelyah, Nathalea, Nathaleah, Nathalee, Nathalei, Nathaleigh, Nathaley, Nathali, Nathalia, Nathaliah, Nathalie, Nathaly, Nathalya, Nathalyah, Natilea, Natileah, Natilee, Natilei, Natileigh, Natili, Natilia, Natiliah, Natilie, Natily, Natilya, Natilyah, Natlea, Natleah, Natlee, Natlei, Natleigh, Natley, Natli, Natlia, Natliah, Natlie, Natly, Nattalea, Nattaleah, Nattalee, Nattalei, Nattaleigh, Nattaley, Nattaleya, Nattaleyah, Nattali, Nattalia, Nattaliah, Nattalie, Nattaly, Nattalya, Nattalyah, Nattlea, Nattlee, Nattlei, Nattleigh, Nattley, Nattlia, Nattliah, Nattlie, Nattly, Nattlya, Nattlyah, Natylea, Natyleah, Natylee, Natylei, Natyleigh, Natyley, Natyli, Natylia, Natyliah, Natylie, Natyly, Natylya, Natylyah

Natane (Arapaho) daughter.
Natana, Natanah, Natanna, Natannah, Natanne

Natania (Russian) fairy queen found on Christmas Day. (Heb) gift of God. The feminine form of Nathaniel.
Nataniah, Natanja, Natanjah, Natanya, Natanyah, Natonia, Natoniah, Natonya, Natonyah

Natara (Arabic) sacrifice.
Natarah, Nataria, Natariah, Natarya, Nataryah

Natasha (Russian/Latin) born on Christmas Day.
Nastassia (Rus), Nastassja (Rus), Nastasya, Natashah, Natasia, Natasiah, Natasie, Natashy, Natashya, Natasyah, Nathali, Nathalia, Nathaliah, Nathalie (Fren), Nathaly, Nathalya, Nathalyah

Nathania (Hebrew) gift of God. The feminine form of Nathan.
Natania, Nataniah, Nataniel, Nataniela, Nataniele, Nataniell, Nataniella, Natanielle, Nathaniah, Nathanya, Nathanyah

Natoma (Native American) beautiful girl.
Natomah

Nature (Latin) nature lover.
Natural, Naturala, Naturale, Naturel, Naturela, Naturele, Naturell, Naturella, Naturelle

Naturi (Australian Aboriginal) sandy soil.
Nature, Naturee, Naturey, Naturia, Naturiah, Naturie, Natury, Naturya, Naturyah

Nava/Navit (Hebrew) beautiful.
Navah, Naveh, Navit, Navita, Navitah, Navyt, Navyta, Navytah

Naysa (Hebrew) miracle of God.
Naisa, Naisah, Naysah

Nea (Greek) new.
Neah

Neala (Irish/Gaelic) champion. The feminine form of Neil.
Nealah

Nebraska (Native American) land with flat water.
Nebraskah

Nebula (Latin) mist; cloud.
Nebulah

Nechole (French/Greek) victory of the people. A form of Nicole. A feminine form of Nicholas.
Nechola, Necholah, Necola, Necolah, Necole

Neci (Hungarian) fiery.
Necee, Necey, Necia, Neciah, Necie, Necy

Neda (Slavic) child born on a Sunday. The feminine form of Ned/Edward, wealthy ruling guardian.
Nedah, Nedda, Neddah, Nedeljka (Slav), Nedya, Nedyah

Neema (Swahili) child born in prosperous times.
Neemah

Nefertiti (Egyptian) the beautiful one is coming.
Neferetete

Neheda (Arabic) independent.
Nehedah

Neige (French) snow.
Neig

Nekeisha (Swahili/African American) life. (Hind) woman. A form of Keisha.
Nekeasha, Nekeashia, Nekeashiah, Nekeysha, Nekeayshah, Nekeesha, Nekeeshia, Nekeysha, Nekeyshia, Nekeyshya, Nekeyshyah

Nelda (Old English) from the elder-tree home.
Neldah, Neldda, Nelddah

Nelia/Nell/Nellie (Latin) horn-coloured; horn blower; the cornell tree. The feminine form of Cornelius.
Cornelia, Nel, Nela, Nelah, Nele, Nelee, Nelea, Neleah, Nelei, Neleigh, Neley, Neliah, Nell, Nella, Nellah, Nellea, Nelleah, Nellee, Nellei, Nelleigh, Nelley, Nelli, Nellia, Nelliah, Nellie (O/Eng), Nelly (O/Eng), Nellya, Nellyah, Nelya, Nelyah

Nellwyn (Old English) Nell's friend; friend of the light; friend of the yellow one; friend of the horn blower; friend from the cornell tree.
Nellwin, Nellwina, Nellwinah, Nellwine, Nellwinn, Nellwinna, Nellwinnah, Nellwine, Nellwyna, Nelleynah, Nellwyne, Nellwynn, Nellwynna, Nellwynnah, Nellwynne, Nelwin, Nelwina, Nelwinah, Nelwine, Nelwinn, Nelwinna, Nelwinnah, Nelwyn, Nelwyna, Nelwynah, Nelwyne, Nelwynn, Nelwynna, Nelwynnah, Nelwynne

Nenet (Egyptian) born by the sea.
Neneta, Nenetah, Nenete, Nennet, Nenneta, Nennetah, Nennete, Nennett, Nennetta, Nennettah, Nennette

Neola (Greek) youthful.
Neolah

Neoma (Greek) new moon.
Neomah

Nerida (Australian Aboriginal) blossom; red water lily.
Neridah, Neryda, Nerydah

Nerina (Latin) black.
Nerinah, Nerine, Neryn, Neryna, Nerynah, Neryne, Nerolia, Neroliah, Neryn, Neryna, Nerynah, Neryne

Nerine (Greek) sea fairy.
Nerina, Nerinah, Neryn, Neryna, Nerynah, Neryne, Nerolia, Neroliah, Neryn, Neryna, Nerynah, Neryne

Nerys (Welsh) lady.
Nereace, Nerease, Nereece, Nereese, Nereice, Nereise, Nereyce, Nereyse, Nerice, Nerise, Neryce, Neryl, Neryse

Nessa/Nessy (Norse) headland. A short form of Agnes/Vanessa, purity; butterfly.
Nesee, Nesey, Nesi, Nesie, Nessee, Nessey, Nessi, Nessia, Nessiah, Nessie, Nessy, Nessya, Nessyah, Nesy

Neta (Hebrew) plant.
Netah, Netai, Netia, Netiah, Netta, Nettah, Nettia, Nettiah, Nettya, Nettyah

Netis (Native American) one who is trustworthy.
Netisa, Netisah, Netise, Netissa, Netissah, Nettisse, Nettys, Nettysa, Nettysah, Nettyse, Netys, Netysa, Netysah, Netyse, Netyssa, Netyssah, Netysse

Netta/Nettie (Latin/English) little priceless one. A form of Antoinette.
Net, Neta, Netah, Netee, Netey, Neti, Netiah, Netie, Nett, Nette, Nettee, Nettey, Netti, Nettia, Nettiah, Netti, Nettie, Netty, Nettya, Nettyah, Nety, Netya, Netyah

Neva (Spanish) white.
Nevah

Nevada (Spanish) white like snow.
Nevadah

Neve (Hebrew) life. A form of Eve.
Neiv, Neive, Neva, Nevah, Nevee, Nevein, Nevia, Neviah, Nevin, Neyva, Neyve, Nieve, Nyev, Nyeva, Nyevah, Nyeve

Nevina (Irish) the saint worshipper.
Neveen, Neveena, Neveenah, Neveene, Nevena, Nevenah, Nevinah, Nevine, Nivena, Nivenah, Nivina, Nivinah, Nivine, Nyvina, Nyvinah, Nyvine, Nyvyn, Nyvyna, Nyvynah, Nyvyne

Neylan (Turkish) wish which is fulfilled.
Nealana, Nealanah, Nealanee, Nealaney, Nealani, Nealania, Nealaniah, Nealanya, Nealanyah, Neilana, Neilanah, Neilane, Neilanee, Neilaney, Neilani, Neilania, Neilaniah, Neilany, Neilanya, Neilanyah, Nelana, Nelanah, Nelane, Nelanee, Nelaney, Nelani, Nelania, Nelaniah, Nelanie, Nelany, Nelanya, Nelanyah, Neya, Neyah, Neyla, Neylah, Neylana, Neylanah, Neylane, Neylanee, Neylaney

Neysa/Neza (Greek) purity. A form of Agnes.
Neisa, Neisah, Nesa, Nesah, Nessa, Nessah, Neysah, Neza (Slav/Grk), Nezah, Nezza, Nezzah

Ngaire (Polynesian) family.
Niree, Nyree

Ngoc (Vietnamese) gem.

Nia (Irish) fairy.
Niah, Nya, Nyah

Niabi (Osage) fawn.
Niabia, Niabiah, Niabie, Niaby, Nyabya, Nyabyah

N

Niagara (Native American) thunder water.
Niagra, Niagrah

Niam (Irish) bright.
Niama, Niamah, Nyam, Nyama, Nyamah

Niangala (Australian Aboriginal) eclipse of the moon.
Niangalah

Nichelle (Greek/French) victory of the people; likeness to God. A combination of Michelle/Nicole.
Nechel, Nechela, Nechelah, Nechele, Nechell, Nechella, Nechellah, Nechelle, Nichela, Nichelah, Nichele, Nichell, Nichella, Nichellah, Nishell, Nishella, Nishellah, Nishelle, Nychel, Nychela, Nychelah, Nychele, Nychell, Nychella, Nychellah, Nychelle

Nicki/Nicky (English/Australian/American/Greek) victory of the people. The short form of Nicole. A feminine form of Nick.
Nickee, Nickey, Nickie, Nicky, Nikee, Nikey, Niki, Nikie, Nikk, Nikkee, Nikkey, Nikki, Nikkie, Nikky, Niky, Niquee, Niquey, Niqui, Niquie, Niquy, Nyc, Nyck, Nyckee, Nyckey, Nycki, Nyckie, Nycky, Nyk, Nykee, Nykey, Nyki, Nykie, Nykkee, Nykkey, Nykki, Nykkie, Nykky, Nyky, Nyquee, Nyquey, Nyqui, Nyquie, Nyqy

Nicola/Nicole (Greek) victory of the people. A feminine form of Nick.
Nacol, Nacola, Nacolah, Nacole, Nakita, Nakitah, Necol, Necola, Necolah, Necole, Necoll, Necolla, Necollah, Necolle, Nicia, Niciah, Nickol, Nickola, Nickolah, Nickole, Nicol, Nicola, Nicholah, Nichola, Nicholah, Nichole (Fren), Nicolah, Nicole, Nicolina,

Nicoline, Nikol, Nikola, Nikolah, Nikole, Niquol, Niquola, Niquolah, Niquole, Nocol, Nocola, Nocolah, Nocole, Nycol, Nycola, Nycolah, Nycole

Nicoletta/Nicolette (French/Greek/English) little victory of the people. A form of Nicole. A feminine form of Nicholas.
Necholet, Necholeta, Necholetah, Necholete, Necholett, Necholetta, Necholettah, Necholette, Necolet, Necoleta, Necoletah, Necolete, Necolett, Necoletta, Necolettah, Necolette, Nickolet, Nickoleta, Nickoletah, Nickolete, Nickolett, Nickoletta, Nickolettah, Nickolette, Nicolet, Nicoleta, Nicoletah, Nicolete, Nicolett, Nicoletta, Nicolettah, Nikolet, Nikoleta, Nikoletah, Nikolete, Nikolett, Nikoletta, Nikolettah, Nikolette, Nyckolet, Nyckoleta, Nyckoletah, Nyckolete, Nyckolett, Nyckoletta, Nyckolettah, Nyckolette, Nycolet, Nycoleta, Nycoletah, Nycolete, Nycolett, Nycoletta, Nycolettah, Nycolette, Nykolet, Nykoleta, Nykoletah, Nykolete, Nykolett, Nykoletta, Nykolettah, Nykolette

Nidia (Latin) nest.
Nidiah, Nydia, Nydiah, Nydya, Nydyah

Nidra (Sanskrit) sleeping.
Nidrah, Nydra, Nydrah

Niesha (Scandinavian) friendly fairy. (Afr/Amer) life. A form of Keisha.
Neesha, Neisha, Neysha

Nigella (Latin) black; dark-haired. (Gae) champion.
Nigela, Nigelah, Nigele, Nigell, Nigellah, Nigelle, Nygel, Nygela,

N

Nygelah, Nygele, Nygell, Nygella, Nygelle

Nikah (Russian) belonging to God.
Nicala, Nicalah, Nichala, Nichalah, Nichola, Nicholah, Nickala, Nickalah, Nickola, Nickolah, Nika, Nikah, Nikala, Nikalah, Nikola, Nikolah, Nycala, Nycalah, Nychala, Nychalah, Nychola, Nycholah, Nyckala, Nyckalah, Nyckola, Nyckolah, Nyka, Nykah, Nykala, Nykalah, Nykola, Nykolah

Nike (Greek) victory.
Nikee, Nikey, Niki, Nikie, Niky, Nykee, Nykey, Nyki, Nykie, Nyky

Nikita (Russian/Greek) victory of the people. A form of Nicole. A feminine form of Nicholas.
Nicheata, Nicheatah, Nicheeta, Nicheetah, Nickeata, Nickeatah, Nickeeta, Nickeetah, Nikeata, Nikeatah, Nikeeta, Nikeetah, Nikeita, Nikeitah, Nikitah, Nikkita, Nikkitah, Niquita, Niquitah, Niquite, Nykeata, Nykeatah, Nykeeta, Nykeetah, Nykeita, Nykeitah, Nykeyta, Nykeytah

Nila (Latin) from the Nile in Egypt.
Nilah, Nile, Nilee, Niley, Nili, Nilie, Nilla, Nillah, Nille, Nillee, Nilley, Nilli, Nillie, Nilly, Nily, Nyla, Nylah, Nyle, Nylee, Nyley, Nyli, Nylie, Nylla, Nyllah, Nylle, Nyllee, Nylley, Nylli, Nyllie, Nylly, Nyly

Nili (Hebrew) indigo.
Nilea, Nileah, Nilee, Nilei, Nileigh, Niley, Nilie, Nillea, Nilleah, Nillee, Nillei, Nilleigh, Nilley, Nilli, Nillie, Nilly, Nily, Nylea, Nyleah, Nylee, Nylei, Nyleigh, Nyley, Nyli, Nylie, Nyllea, Nylleah, Nyllee, Nyllei, Nylleigh, Nylley, Nylli, Nyllie, Nylly, Nyly

Nima (Hebrew) thread.
(Arab) blessed.
Neema, Nema, Nemah, Nimah, Nimali, Nimalie, Nimaly, Nyma, Nymah

Nina (Spanish) girl. The Russian form of Ann, graceful.
Neana, Neanah, Neena, Neenah, Ninah, Ninet, Nineta, Ninetah, Ninete, Ninett, Ninetta, Ninette, Ninon (Fren), Nyna, Nynah

Ninetta/Ninette (French) little.
Ninet, Nineta, Ninetah, Ninete, Ninett, Ninetta, Ninettah, Ninon, Ninona, Ninonah, Ninone, Nyet, Nyneta, Nynetah, Nynete, Nynett, Nynetta, Nynettah, Nynette

Ningai (Sumerian) great queen.
Ningae, Ningay

Niree (Australian Aboriginal) family; flax (a plant with blue flowers).
Nyree (Poly)

Nirel (Hebrew) God's light.
Nirela, Nirelah, Nirele, Nirell, Nirella, Nirellah, Nirelle, Nyrel, Nyrela, Nyrelah, Nyrele, Nyrell, Nyrella, Nyrellah, Nyrelle

Nirveli (Hindi) child of the water.
Nirevelea, Nirveleah, Nirvelee, Nirvelei, Nirveleigh, Nirveley, Nirvelie, Nirvely, Nyrevelea, Nyrveleah, Nyrvelee, Nyrvelei, Nyrveleigh, Nyrveley, Nyrvelie, Nyrvely

Nishi (Japanese) west.
Nishee, Nishey, Nishie, Nishy

Nissa (Scandinavian) friendly fairy.
(Heb) sign. (Arab) woman.
Nisa, Nisah, Nissah, Nysa, Nysah, Nyssa, Nyssah

Nita (Choctaw) bear.
Nitah, Nyta, Nytah

Nitara (Hindi) roots run deep.
Nitarah, Nitarra, Nitarrah, Nytara,
Nytarah, Nytarra, Nytarrah

Nitasha (Russian/Latin) child born
on Christmas Day; nativity. A
form of Natasha.
Nitashah, Niteisha, Nitisha,
Nitishah, Nitishia, Nitishiah,
Nytasha, Nytashia, Nytashiah,
Nytashya, Nytashyah

Nitasse (French) resurrection.
Nitase

Nitsa (Greek) shining light. A form
of Helen.
Nitsah, Nytsa, Nytsah

Nituna (Native American) daughter.
Nitunah, Nytuna, Nytunah

Nitza (Hebrew) bud of a flower.
Nitzah, Nitzana, Nitzanit,
Nitzanita, Nytza, Nytzah

Nixie (Teutonic) water fairy.
Nixee, Nixey, Nixi, Nixy, Nyxee,
Nyxey, Nyxi, Nyxie, Nyxy

Noelani (Hawaiian) beautiful one
sent from heaven.
Noelanee, Noelaney, Noelania,
Noelaniah, Noelanie, Noelany,
Noelanya, Noelanyah

Noeline (Latin) born at Christmas
time. A feminine form of Noel.
Noelan, Noelana, Noelanah,
Noelean, Noeleana, Noeleanah,
Noeleane, Noeleen, Noeleena,
Noeleenah, Noeleene, Noeleet,
Noeleeta, Noeleetah, Noeleete,
Noelin, Noelina, Noelinah, Noelit,
Noelita, Noelitah, Noelite, Noell,
Noella, Noellah, Noelle (Fren),
Noellin, Noellina, Noellinah,

Noelline, Noellyn, Noellyna,
Noellynah, Noellyne, Nolein,
Noleina, Noleinah, Noleine,
Noleyn, Noleyna, Noleynah,
Noleyne, Nowel, Nowela,
Nowelah, Nowele, Nowell,
Nowella, Nowelle

Noelle (Latin/French) she was born
at Christmas time. A feminine
form of Noel.
Noel, Noela, Noelah, Noele, Noell,
Noella, Noellah, Noelin, Noelina,
Noelinah, Noeline, Noellyn,
Noellyna, Noellynah, Noellyne,
Nowel, Nowela, Nowelah, Nowele,
Nowell, Nowella, Nowellah,
Nowelle

Noga (Hebrew) light of the
morning.
Nogah

Noicha (Native American) sun.
Nolcha

Nokomis (Native American) moon
daughter; beautiful girl from
heaven. (Chipp) grandmother.
Nokoma, Nokomas, Nokomis

Nola/Nolana (Latin) small bell;
noble. (Gae) white shoulders.
Noelana, Noelanah, Noelanee,
Noelaney, Noelani, Noelania,
Noelaniah, Noelanie, Noelanna,
Noelannah, Noelannee,
Noelanney, Noelanni, Noelannia,
Noelanniah, Noelannie, Noelanny,
Noelannya, Noelannyah, Nolanah,
Nolanee, Nolaney, Nolani,
Nolania, Nolaniah, Nolanie,
Nolany, Nolanya, Nolanyah

Noleta (Latin) unwilling.
Noleata, Noleatah, Noleeta,
Noleetah, Nolita, Nolitah, Nolyta,
Nolytah

Noma/Norma (Hawaiian) rule; pattern. A form of Norma.
Nomah, Normah

Nona (Latin) ninth-born child.
Nonah, Nonia, Noniah, Nonna, Nonnah, Nonya, Nonyah

Noni/Nora (English) honesty. The short form of Noeline/Nona.
Nonee, Noney, Nonia, Noniah, Nonie, Nony, Nonya, Nonyah, Norah, Norra, Norrah

Noora (Australian Aboriginal) camp site.
Noorah

Norberta (Teutonic) brilliant hero.
Norbertah, Norbirta, Norbirtah, Norburta, Norburtah, Norbyrta, Norbyrtah

Nordica/Norell (German) from the north.
Narel, Narell, Narelle (Aust/Abor), Nordic, Nordicah, Nordik, Nordika, Nordikah, Nordiqua, Nordiquah, Nordyca, Nordycah, Nordycka, Nordyckah, Nordyka, Nordykah, Nordyqua, Nordyquah, Norel, Norela, Norele, Norell (Scand), Norella, Norellah, Norrelle

Nori (Japanese) religious teachings; belief; law.
Noree, Norey, Noria, Noriah, Norie, Nory, Norya, Noryah

Norleen (Irish) honest.
Norlan, Norlana, Norlanah, Norlane, Norlean, Norleana, Norleanah, Norleane, Norleena, Norleenah, Norleene, Norlein, Norleina, Norleinah, Norleine, Norleyn, Norleyna, Norleynah, Norleyne, Norlin, Norlina, Norlinah, Norline, Norlyn, Norlyna, Norlynah, Norlyne

Norna (Old Norse) Viking goddess of fate.
Nornah

Nova (Latin) new.
Novah

Novella (Latin) newcomer.
Nova, Novah, Novel, Novela, Novelah, Novele, Novell, Novellah, Novelle

Novia (Latin) youthful. (Lat) new. (Span) sweetheart.
Nova, Novah, Noviah, Novya, Novyah

Nowra (Australian Aboriginal) black cockatoo (black parrot).
Nowrah

Nu (Vietnamese) woman.

Nuala (Irish/Gaelic) fair shoulders.
Nualah

Nui (Maori) great.

Numa (Arabic) beautiful.
Numah

Numilla (Australian Aboriginal) lookout.
Numil, Numila, Numilah, Numile, Numill, Numillah, Numille, Numyl, Numyla, Numylah, Numyle, Numyll, Numylla, Numyllah, Numylle

Nuna (Native American) land.
Nunah

Nunkeri (Australian Aboriginal) excellent.
Nunkerie, Nunkery

Nunziata (Latin/Italian) bearer of news.
Nunziatah

Nura (Aramaic) light.
Noura, Nurah

Nuria (Aramaic) God's light.
Nuriah, Nurya, Nuryah

Nurita (Hebrew) flower with yellow and red blossoms.
Nuritah, Nuryta, Nurytah

Nurla (Australian Aboriginal) plentiful.
Nurlah

Nuru (Swahili) light of day.

Nusi (Hungarian/Hebrew) God is gracious. A form of Hannah.
Nusie, Nusy

Nyah (Australian Aboriginal) river bend.
Nia, Niah, Nya

Nydia (Latin) nest; safe refuge.
Nidia, Nidiah, Nydiah, Nydya, Nydyah

Nyoko (Japanese) gem.
Nioko

Nyora (Australian Aboriginal) cherry tree.
Niora, Niorah, Nyorah

Nyrang (Australian Aboriginal) little.
Nirang

Nyree (Maori) sea.
Niree

Nyssa (Greek) beginning. (Lat) one who has goals.
Nisa, Nisah, Nissa, Nissah, Nysa, Nysah, Nyssah

Nyusha (Russian/Greek) purity. A form of Agnes.
Nyushenka, Nyushka

Nyx (Greek) night. (Lat) one with the snow-white hair.

Oake (Old English) oak tree.
Oak

Oba (Yoruba) goddess of the rivers.
Obah

Obelia (Greek) strength.
Obeliah, Obelya, Obelyah

Ocean (Greek) sea.
Oceana, Oceanah, Oceane

Octavia (Latin) eighth-born child. The feminine form of Octavius.
Aktavija, Octaviah, Octavian, Octavianos, Octavie (Fren), Octavio, Octavious, Octawia (Poly), Ofeliga (Lith), Oktavia, Okatvija, Ottavia (Ital), Ottaviah, Ottavya, Ottavyah

Odda (Old Norse) wealthy.
Oda, Odah, Oddah, Oddia, Oddiah

Ode (Nigerian) born while parents were travelling.
Odee, Odey, Odi, Odia, Odiah, Ody, Odya, Odyah

Odeda (Hebrew) strong; courageous.
Odeada, Odeadah, Odedah

Odele (French) melody; song.
Odel, Odela, Odelah, Odell, Odella, Odellah, Odelle

Odelette (French) little song lyric.
Odelet, Odelatt, Odelatta,
Odelattah, Odelet, Odeleta,
Odeletah, Odelete, Odelett,
Odeletta

Odelia (Hebrew) praise to God.
(Scan) wealthy; little. (O/Eng)
one who lives in the valley. The
feminine form of Odell.
Odele, Odeliah, Odelina,
Odelinah, Odeline, Odell, Odella,
Odellah, Odelle, Odetta, Odette,
Odila, Odilia, Odille, Odyla,
Odylah, Odyle, Odyll, Odylla,
Odyllah, Odylle, Otha, Othelia,
Othilia, Ottilie, Uta

Odessa (Greek) journey; one who is
in search of a quest.
Odesa, Odessah, Odissa, Odissah,
Odysa, Odysah, Odyssa, Odyssah

Odette (German) of the fatherland.
(O/Fren) home lover. The
feminine form of Odin, ruler.
Oddet, Oddeta, Oddete, Oddett,
Oddetta, Odett, Odetta, Odettah,
Odet, Odeta, Odetah, Odete

Odile (French) rich battle.
Odila, Odilah, Odyla, Odylah

Odina (Algonquin) mountain.
Odeana, Odeanah, Odeane, Odeen,
Odeena, Odeenah, Odinah, Odyn,
Odyna, Odynah, Odyne

Odiya (Hebrew) God's song.
Odiyah

Ofa (Polynesian) love.
Ofah

Ofira (Hebrew) golden.
Ofara, Ofarra, Ofarrah, Ophira,
Ophirah, Ophyra, Ophyrah

Ofra (Hebrew/Greek) first born. A
form of Alpha.
Ofrah, Ofrat, Ophra, Ophrah

Ogin (Native American) wild rose.
Ogina, Ogyn, Ogyna, Ogynah

Ohanna (Hebrew) God is gracious.
A form of Hannah.
Hana, Hanah, Hanna, Hannah,
Johana, Johanah, Johanna,
Johannah, Ohana, Ohanah,
Ohannah

Ohara (Japanese) small field.
Oharah

Oheo (Iroquois) beautiful.

Ohnicio (Irish) honourable.
Onicio

Okalani (Hawaiian) sent from
heaven.
Okalana, Okalanah, Okalanea,
Okalanee, Okalaney, Okalania,
Okalaniah, Okalanie, Okalany,
Okalanya, Okalanyah

Oketa (Tongan) orchid.
Oketah

Okiilani (Hawaiian) heaven.
Okiianee, Okiianey, Okiianie,
Okiiany

Ola (Scandinavian) ancestral relic;
family keepsake. (Haw) life; well
being. (Nig) precious.
Olah

Olabisi (Nigerian) increasing.
Olabisie, Olabisie, Olabisy

Olaf (Scandinavian) ancestral
heritage.
Olav, Olava

Olalla (Greek) speaking sweetly.
Olallah

Olanthe (Native American)
beautiful.
Olanth, Olantha, Olanthah,
Olanthye

O

Oldina (Australian Aboriginal) snow.
Oldeena, Oldeenah, Oldenia, Oldeniah, Oldinah, Oldine, Oldyn, Oldyna, Oldynah, Oldyne

Oleander (English/American) evergreen tree with red or white flowers.
Oleanda, Oleandah, Oleeanda, Oleeandah, Oliana, Olianah, Oliane, Oliann, Olianna, Oliannah, Oliannda, Olianndah, Oliannde, Olianne, Olyan, Olyana, Olyanah, Olyane, Olyann, Olyanna, Olyannah, Olyanne

Oleatha (English/Scandinavian) light.
Alethea, Oleanthah, Oleanthe, Oleta, Oletah

Olena (Russian) light.
Alena, Olenah, Olenia, Oleniah, Olina, Olinah, Olyna, Olynah

Olesia (Polish) protector of human kind.
Olesiah, Olesya, Olesyah

Olethea (Latin) truthful.
Aleathea, Aleatheah, Oleathea, Oleatheah, Oleathya, Oleathyah

Olga (Scandinavian) holy.
Elga, Helga, Olenka, Olgah, Olgy, Olia, Olive, Olivia, Oliviah, Olva, olvah

Oliana (Hawaiian) evergreen in flower.
Olianah, Olyana, Olyanah

Olien (Russian) deer.
Olian, Oliene, Olienah, Oliene, Olyan, Olyana, Olyanah, Olyane, Olyen, Olyena, Olyenah, Olyene

Olienka (Russian) holy.
Olienkah, Olyenka, Olyenkah

Olina (Hawaiian) happy.
Olinah, Olyna, Olynah

Olinda (Latin/Hawaiian) sweetly scented.
Olindah, Olinka, Olinkah, Olynda, Olyndah, Olynka, Olynkah

Olisa (Ibo) God.
Olisah, Olysa, Olysah, Olyssa, Olyssah

Olive (Latin) olive tree.
Olave, Oliv, Olliv, Ollive, Ollyv, Ollyve, Olyv, Olyve

Olivia (Latin) olive tree.
Elva, Nola, Nolana, Nolanah, Olga, Olia, Oliah, Olida (Lat), Olive, Olivetta, Olivette, Olva, Olyvia, Olyviah, Olyvya, Olyvyah

Olono (Australian Aboriginal) hill.
Olonno

Olwyn (Welsh) white footprints. (O/Eng) old friend.
Olwen, Olwena, Olwenah, Olwene, Olwenn, Olwenna, Olwennah, Olwenne, Olwin, Olwina, Olwinah, Olwine, Olwinn, Olwinna, Olwinnah, Olwinne, Olwyna, Olwynah, Olwyne, Olwynn, Olwynna, Olwynnah, Olwynne

Olympia (Greek) of Olympus; heavenly.
Olimpe (Fren), Olimpia (Ital), Olimpiah, Olimpias, Olympias, Olympie (Ger), Olympy, Olympya, Olympyah, Olympie, Olympy, Olympiah, Olympya, Olympyah

Oma (Arabic) high commander. The feminine form of Omar, first born; follower of the prophet, speaker.
Omah

O

Omaira (Arabic) red.
Omara, Omarah, Omaria,
Omariah, Omarya, Omaryah

Omega (Greek) large. The last-born
child.
Omegah

Omemee (Native American) pigeon.
Omeme

Ona (Latin/Irish/Gaelic) unity.
(Lith) graceful. (Grk) donkey.
Onah, Oona (Irish), Oonagh
(Irish), Una (lith)

Onatah (Iroquois) daughter of the
spirits of the earth and corn.
Onata

Onawa (Native American) wide-
awake girl.
Onaiwa, Onaiwah, Onaja, Onajah,
Onawah, Onowa, Onowah

Ondine (Latin) wave of water.
Ondina, Ondinah, Undina,
Undinah, Undine, Ondyn,
Ondyna, Ondynah, Undyn,
Undyna, Undynah, Undyne

Ondrea (Slavic) brave woman.
Andrea, Andreah, Andreea,
Andreeah, Andri, Andria, Andriah,
Andrie, Andrya, Andryah, Ondra,
Ondrah, Ondri, Ondrie, Ondry,
Ondrya, Ondryah

Oneida (Native American) one who
is expected.
Oneidah, Oneyda, Oneydah,
Onidah, Onyda, Onydah

Onella (Hungarian/Greek) shining
light. A form of Helen.
Onela, Onelah, Onellah

Onesta (English) honest; reliable.
Esta, Honesta

Ongo (Tongan) spirited.

Oni (Yoruba) born on holy ground.
Onee, Oney, Onie, Ony

Onida (Native American)
Desired.
Onidah, Onyda, Onydah

Onike (Tongan) the onyx gem.
Onika, Onikah, Onikee

Onora (English) honesty.
Ornora, Ornorah, Onoria,
Onoriah, Onorina, Onorine,
Ornoryn, Ornoryna, Onorynah,
Onoryne

Ontario (Native American) beautiful
lake.
Oniatario, Ontaryo

Onyx (Latin) precious black gem.
Onix

Oola (Australian Aboriginal) fire
place.
Ollah

Oona (Irish) lamb.
Oonagh (Ir), Una, Unah

Oonta (Australian Aboriginal) star.
Oontah

Opa (Choctaw) owl.
Opah

Opal (Sanskrit) precious jewel;
justice; hope.
Opala, Opalah, Opalia, Opalina,
Opaline, Opalyn, Opalyna,
Opalynah, Opalyne, Opell, Opella,
Opelle

Opalina (Hindi) jewel.
Opala, Opalah, Opaleana,
Opaleena, Opalin, Opalinah,
Opaline, Opalyn, Opalyna, Opalyne

Opeli (Tongan) opal gem.
Opelea, Opeleah, Opelee, Opelei,
Opeleigh, Opelia, Opeliah, Opelie,
Opely, Opelya, Opelyah

O

Ophelia (Greek) wisdom; immortality.
Ofelia, Ofellia, Ofilia, Opheliah, Ophelie (Fren), Orphellia, Orphellya, Orphillia, Orphylla, Orphyllia, Orphylliah, Orphyllya, Orphyllyah, Phelia, Pheliah, phelya, Phelya, Phelyah

Ophra (Hebrew) deer; place of dust.
Ophrah, Oprah

Oprah (Hebrew) little deer; fawn.
Opra

Ora (Latin) golden prayer. (Eng) coastal shore line. (Heb) golden light.
Aura, Aurah, Ohah, Orabel, Orabell, Orabella, Orabelle, Oralee, Orit, Orlee, Orlice, Orly

Orabel (French) golden beauty.
Orabela, Orabele, Orabell, Orabella, Orabelle, Oribel, Oribela, Oribele, Oribell, Oribella, Oribelle, Orybel, Orybela, Orybele, Orybell, Orybella, Orybelle

Orah (Hebrew) light.
Ora

Oralee (Hebrew) light. (O/Eng) speaker from the meadow.
Oralea, Oraleah, Oralei, Oraleigh, Oraley, Orali, Oralie, Oraly

Oralia (Latin) golden.
Oraliah, Oralie, Oriel, Orielda, Orielle, Orlene, Oriola, Oriole, Orlena, Oralya, Oralyah, Oralye, Oryel, Oryela, Oryelda, Oryell, Oryella, Oryelle

Orana (Australian Aboriginal) welcome.
Oran, Oranah, Orann, Oranna, Orannah

Orazia (Italian) time keeper.
Orazya, Orazyah, Orzaiah, Orzaya, Orzayah

Orchio (Italian) orchid flower child.
Orchiot, Orchyo

Orea (Greek) from the mountain.
Oreah

Orela (Latin) divine announcement.
Orelah

Orell (Old English) from the hill of ore. (Russ) eagle. (Lat) listener.
Orel, Orela, Orelah, Orella, Orellah, Orelle

Orenda (Iroquois) possessor of magic powers.
Orendah

Oretha (Greek) virtuous.
Oreta, Oretah, Oretta, Orettah, Orette

Oriana (Latin) the gold dawn.
Oriane, Orianna, Oriannah, Oryan, Oryana, Oryanah, Oryane, Oryann, Oryanna, Oryannah, Oryanne

Oriel (German/Latin) fire.
Orial, Oriala, Orialah, Oriale, Oriall, Orialla, Oriallah, Orialle, Oriela, Orielah, Oriele, Oriell, Oriella, Oriellah, Orielle, Oryal, Oryala, Oryalah, Oryale, Oryall, Oryalla, Oryallah, Oryalle, Oryel, Oryela, Oryelah, Oryele, Oryell, Oryella, Oryellah, Oryelle

Oriella (Celtic) white-skinned.
Oriel, Oriela, Oriele, Oriell, Orielle, Oryel, Oryela, Oryelah, Oryele, Oryell, Oryella, Oryellah, Oryelle

Orina (Russian/Greek) peaceful.
Orinah, Oryna, Orynah

O

Orinda (Hebrew) pine tree.
(Ir) light-skinned.
Orenda, Orendah, Orynda,
Oryndah

Orino (Japanese) worker in the
field.
Oryno

Oriole (Latin) fair-haired, blond;
black and orange bird.
Oriel, Oriell, Oriellah, Orielle,
Oriol, Oriola, Oriolah, Orioll,
Oriolla, Oriollah, Oriolle, Oryel,
Oryela, Oryelah, Oryele, Oryell,
Oryella, Oryellah, Oryelle, Oryol,
Oryola, Oryolah, Oryoll, Oryolla,
Oryollah, Oryolle

Orla (Irish) golden.
Orlah

Orlena (Latin) golden.
Orlana, Orlanah, Orleana,
Orleanah, Orleen, Orleenah,
Orleene, Orlene, Orlina, Orlinah,
Orline, Orlyn, Orlyna, Orlynah,
Orlyne

Orlenda (Russian) eagle.
Orlanda, Orlandah, Orlendah

Orli (Hebrew) light.
Orlea, Orleah, Orlee, Orlei,
Orleigh, Orley, Orlia, Orliah,
Orlice, Orlie, Orly, Orlya, Orlyah

Ormanda (Latin) noble.
(Ger) sailor.
Ormandah, Ormandia,
Ormandiah, Ormandya,
Ormandyah

Orna (Irish) pale olive colour.
(Lat) decorated.
Ornah

Ornat (Irish) green.
Ornait, Ornaita, Ornaitah, Ornata,
Ornatah, Ornate

Ornice (Hebrew) cedar tree.
(Ir) olive colour.
Orna, Ornah, Ornat, Ornata,
Ornete, Ornetta, Ornette, Ornit,
Ornita, Ornitah, Ornite, Ornyt,
Ornita, Ornitah, Ornite, Ornitt,
Ornitta, Ornittah, Ornitte, Ornyt,
Ornyta, Ornytah, Ornyte, Ornytt,
Ornytta, Ornyttah, Ornytte

Orpah (Hebrew) plucked.
Orpa

Orsa (Greek) little she-bear. A form
of Ursula. A feminine form of
Orson.
Orsa, Orsalin, Orsalina, Orsalinah,
Orsaline, Orsalyn, Orsalyna,
Orsalynah, Orsalyne, Orsel,
Orselina, Orselinah, Orseline,
Orselyna, Orselynah, Orselyne,
Orsola, Orsolah

Orseline (Dutch) little she-bear. A
form of Ursula. A feminine form
of Orson.
Orsa, Orsalin, Orsalina, Orsalinah,
Orsaline, Orsalyn, Orsalyna,
Orsalynah, Orsalyne, Orsel, Orselina,
Orselinah, Orselyna, Orselynah,
Orselyne, Orsola, Orsolah

Ortrude (Old German) golden
woman.
Ortrud, Ortruda, Ortrudah

Orva (French) worth gold. The
feminine form of Orvin, friend
with a spear.
Orvah

Orwin (Hebrew) boar friend.
Orwina, Orwinah, Orwine, Orwyn,
Orwyna, Orwynah, Orwyne

Orya (Russian) peaceful.
Oria, Oriah, Oryah

Osanna (Latin) prayer; merciful.
Osana, Osanah, Osannah

P

Osen (Japanese) one thousand.
Osena, Osenah

Oseye (Benin) happy.
Osey

Osita (Spanish) divine strength.
Ositah, Osith, Ositha, Osithah,
Osithe, Ositah, Osyta, Osytah,
Osyth, Osytha, Osythah, Osyta,
Osytah

Osith (German) divine protector.
The feminine form of Osmond.
Ositha, Osithe, Osyth, Osytha,
Osythe

Osma (English) divine protector.
Osmah, Ozma, Ozmah

Osvalda (English) divinely ruled by
God; God of the forest. The
feminine form of Oswald.
Osvaldah, Oswalda, Oswaldah

Osyka (Choctaw) eagle.
Osika, Osikah, Osykah

Otaybe (Australian Aboriginal) bird.
Otaiba, Otaibah, Otaybah

Otilie (Slavic) lucky.
Otila, Otilah, Otka, Ottili, Otylia,
Otyla, Otylah, Ottyli, Ottyllia,
Ottylliah, Ottylya, Ottylyah

Ottavia (Italian) eighth-born child.
Otavia, Otaviah, Otavya, Otavyah,
Ottaviah, Ottavya, Ottavyah

Otylia (Polish) wealthy.
The feminine form of Otto.
Ottylia, Ottyliah, Ottylya, Ottylyah,
Otyliah, Otylya, Otylyah

Ovia (Latin/Danish) egg.
Ova, Ovah, Oviah, Ovya, Ovyah

Owena (Welsh) young warrior. The
feminine form of Owen, well-
born one.
Owenah, Owina, Owinah, Owyna,
Owynah

Oya (Moquelumnan) to come forth.
Oia, Oiah, Oyah

Oz (Hebrew) strength.
Ozz

Ozara (Hebrew) treasured.
Ozarah, Ozarra, Ozarrah

Ozera (Hebrew) helper.
Ozerah, Ozira, Ozirah, Ozyra,
Ozyrah

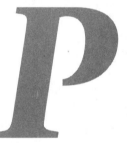

Paame (Tongan) palm tree.
Pam, Pame

Pacifica (Italian) from the Pacific
Ocean.
Pacificah, Pacifyca, Pacifycah,
Pacyfyca, Pacyfycah, Pacykika (Pol)

Padma (Sanskrit) lotus flower.
Padmah, Padmar

Padmani (Sri Lankan) flower.
Padmanee, Padmaney, Padmanie,
Padmania, Padmaniah, Padmanie,
Padmany

Pagan (English/Latin) country
dweller.
Pagen, Pagin, Pagon, Pagun, Pagyn

Paige (Old English) attendant;
young child.
Page, Paget, Payg, Payge

P

Paka (Swahili) kitten.
Pakah

Pala (Native American) water.
Palah, Palla, Pallah

Palila (Polynesian) bird.
Palilah, Palyla, Palylah

Pallas (Greek) goddess of wisdom and knowledge.
Palac, Palaca, Palace, Pallass, Pallassa

Palm/Palma (English) palm tree.
Palma, Palmah, Palmar, Palmara, Palmarah, Palmaria, Palmariah, Palmarya, Palmaryah

Palmela (Greek) like honey; sweet.
Palmelah, Palmelia, Palmeliah, Palmelina, Palmeline, Palmelyn, Palmelyna, Palmelyne

Palmira (Greek/Latin) born on Palm Sunday, the Sunday before Easter.
Palma, Palmir, Palmirah, Palmirar, Palmyra, Palmyrah

Paloma (Spanish/Latin) dove.
Palomah, Palomar, Palomara, Palomarah, Palomaria, Palomariah, Palomarya, Palomaryah

Pam/Pamela (Greek) loving. The short form of Pamela, like honey; sweet.
Pamala, Pamalah, Pamalia, Pamaliah, Pamalya, Pamalyah, Pamela, Pamelia, Pameliah, Pamelya, Pamelyah, Pami, Pamie, Pamm, Pammi, Pammie, Pammy. Pamy

Pana (Native American) partridge bird.
Panah, Panna, Pannah

Panacea (Greek) healer.
Panaceah

Pancha (Spanish) freedom. A form of Frances.
Panchah

Panchali (Sanskrit) princess of Panchala.
Pancha, Panchalea, Panchaleah, Panchalee, Panchalei, Panchaleigh, Panchaley, Panchalie, Panchaly

Pandora (Greek) all gifted.
Pandorah

Pania (Maori) sea woman.
Paniah, Panya, Panyah

Panisi (Tongan) the pansy flower.
Pansy (Grk)

Panola (Choctaw) cotton.
Panolah, Panolla, Panollah

Pansofia (Greek) possessor of wisdom or knowledge.
Pansofee, Pansofey, Pansofee, Pansoffey, Pansoffi, Pansoffia, Pansofi, Pansofiah, Pansofie, Pansophee, Pansophey, Pansophi, Pansophia, Pansophiah, Pansophie, Pansophy, Pansophya, Pansophyah

Pansy (Greek) little flower. (Fren) idea.
Pansea, Panseah, Pansee, Pansey, Pansi, Pansia, Pansiah, Pansie, Pansya, Pansyah

Panthea (Greek) all gods.
Panfia, Panfiah, Pantheah, Panthia, Panthiah, Panthya, Panthyah

Papahi (Tongan) mischievously smart.
Papahee, Papahey, Papahie

Papina (Miwok) oak tree with a vine.
Papinah, Papyna, Papynah

P

Paques (French) born at Easter time.
Pascha

Paramita (Sanskrit) virtuous; good; perfect.
Paramitah, Paramyta, Paramytah

Paris (French) (Geographical) the capital of France.
Parice, Parisa, Parise, Pariss, Parissa, Parisse, Parys, Parysa, Paryse, Paryss, Paryssa, Parysse

Parnel (Old English) stone.
Parnela, Parnelah, Parnele, Parnell, Parnella, Parnellah, Parnelle, Pernel, Pernela, Pernelah, Pernele, Pernell, Pernella, Pernellah, Pernelle

Parthena (Greek) purity.
Parthena, Parthene, Parthenia, Partheniah, Parthenope, Parthenya, Parthenyah

Parvati (Sanskrit) mountain climber.
Parvatee, Parvatey, Parvatia, Parvatiah, Parvatie, Parvaty, Parvatya, Parvatyah

Pascale/Pascha (Latin) born at Easter time.
Pascal, Pascala, Pascalina, Pascaline, Pascalyn, Pascalyna, Pascalyne, Paschah, Paschal, Pasche, Pashel, Pashela, Pashelah, Pashele, Pashell, Pashelle, Pasqua, Pasquah

Pasifiki (Tongan) the Pacific Ocean.
Pacific, Pacifica, Pacificah, Pacificka, Pacifiqua, Pacifiquah, Pacifique, Pacifyqua, Pacifyquah, Pacifycque, Pacyfica, Pacyficah, Pacyficka, Pacyficka, Pacyfiqua, Pacyfiquah, Pacyfique, Pacyfyca, Pacyfycah, Pacyfycka, Pacyfyqua, Pacyfyquah, Pacyfyque

Pat/Patsy/Patty (Latin) little noble one. The short form of Patricia.
Patee, Patey, Pati, Patie, Patsee, Patsey, Patsey, Patsi, Patsie, Patsy, Patt, Pattee, Pattey, Patti, Pattie, Patty, Paty

Patam (Sanskrit) city.
Patem, Patim, Patom, Pattam, Pattem, Pattim, Pattom, Pattym, Patym

Pati (Miwok) twisted willows.
Patee, Patey, Patie, Paty

Patience (Latin) enduring; patient.
Patia, Patiah, Patient, Patya, Patyah

Patrice/Patricia (Latin/English) little noble one.
Patreeza, Patria, Patriah, Patricah, Patricah, Patrice (Fren), Patriciah, Patrisha, Patrishah, Patriza, Patrizah, Patrizia (Ital), Patryce, Patrycya, Patrycyah, Patrycyka (Pol), Patryse

Patya (Australian Aboriginal) flower.
Patia, Patiah, Patyah

Paula/Paulette/Paulina/Pauline (Latin) small. The feminine form of Paul.
Pacyencya (Pol), Pala (Span), Palva (Czech/Illy), Paola (Span/Ital), Paoleta, Paolina (Ital), Paoline, Paule (Lith/Fren), Paulet, Pauleta, Pauletah, Paulete, Paulett, Pauletta, Paulettah, Paulette (Fren), Pauli, Paulia, Pauliah, Paulica, Paulie, Pauliina (Finn), Paulina (Lat/Span), Pauline (Fren), Pauly, Paulya, Paulyah, Paulyn, Paulyna, Paulynah, Paulyne

Payton (Old English) from the toll collector's town.
Paitan, Paiten, Paitin, Paiton, Paityn, Paytan, Payten, Paytin,

Payton, Paytyn, Peitan, Peiten,
Peitin, Peiton, Peityn, Petan,
Peyten, Peytin, Peyton, Peytyn

Paz (Spanish) peaceful.
Pazz

Pazia/Pazice (Hebrew) gold;
golden-haired.
Paza, Pazise, Pazit, Pazya, Pazyah,
Pazyce, Pazyse

Peace (Middle English) tranquil.
Peece

Peach/Peaches (English) peach tree.
Peacha, Peachee, Peachey, Peachia,
Peachy

Pearl (Latin/English) pearl; precious
gem.
Helmi, Pearla, Pearle, Pearlea,
Pearleah, Pearlee, Pearlei,
Pearleigh, Pearley, Pearli, Pearlie,
Pearlina, Pearline, Perl, Perla,
Perlah, Perle, Perli, Perlie, Perly,
Perry, Pery

Peata (Maori) one who brings joy.
Peatah, Peeta, Peetah, Peita, Peitah,
Peyta, Peytah, Pita, Pitah, Pyta,
Pytah

Peg/Peggy (French) daisy. The short
form of Margaret, pearl.
Pegee, Pegey, Pegg, Peggee, Peggey,
Peggi, Peggie, Peggy, Pegi, Pegie,
Pegy

Peilla (Spanish) God has added.
Pepillah, Pepita (Span), Pepyla,
Pepylah, Pepylla, Pepyllah

Peita/Peta (Greek) stone. The
feminine form of Peter.
Peata, Peatah, Peeta, Peetah,
Peitah, Peyta, Peytah, Pita, Pitah,
Pyta, Pytah

Pekabo (Native American) shining
waters.
Peakabo, Peakaboo, Pekaboo

Peke (Hawaiian) bright.

Pelagia (Greek) sea.
Pelagiah, Pelagya, Pelagyah

Penda (Swahili) love.
Pandah, Pendan, Pendana,
Pendant

Peneli/Penelope/Penny (Greek)
weaver; bobbin; penny coin.
Pelcha, Pena, Penah, Penee, Peney,
Penelopa, Peneli (Gyp), Penelia,
Peneliah, Penelie, Penelopa,
Penelopea, Penelopee, Penelopey,
Penelopia, Penelopiah, Penelopie,
Penelopy, Peni, Penie, Penina,
Penine, Pennee, Penney, Penni,
Pennia, penniah, Pennie, Penny,
Penneloppea, Pennelopee,
Pennelopey, Pennelopi,
Pennelopia, Pennelopiah,
Pennelopie, Pennelopy, Peny

Penina (Hebrew) pearl; coral.
Paninah, Panine, Penina, Peninah,
Penine, Penyna, Penynah, Penyne

Pentecosta (Greek) born on the
fiftieth day.
Pentecostah, Pentecoste

Penthea (Greek) fifth-born child.
Pentheah, Penthia, Penthiah,
Penthya, Penthyah

Peony (Greek) god of healing; giver
of praise; flower.
Peonee, Peoney, Peoni, Peonie,
Peony

Pepe (Tongan) butterfly.
Peppe

Pepinga (Australian Aboriginal)
stringy bark tree.
Pepingah, Pepynga, Pepyngah

Pepita (Spanish) bountiful.
Pepee, Pepi, Pepie, Pepitah, Pepite,

Pepita cont.
Pepitta, Pepitte, Pepy, Pepyta,
Pepytah, Pepyte

Perdita (Latin) lost.
Periditah, Perdyta, Perdytah

Perette (English/French) little
stone. The feminine form of
Peter.
Peronne (Fren), Perpetta, Perettah

Perfecta (Spanish) accomplished;
perfection.
Perfect, Perfection

Peri (Greek) prosperous.
Perea, Peree, Perey, Perie, Pery

Peridot (Arabic) precious.
Peridota, Peridotah, Perydota,
Perydotah

Perilla (Latin/Greek) stone.
Perila, Perilah, Perillah, Peryla,
Perylah, Peryll, Perylla, Peryllah

Perizada (Persian) born of the
fairies.
Perizadah, Perizade, Peryzada,
Peryzadah, Peryzade

Perlita (Italian) pearl.
Perleta, Perletta, Perlitta, Perlyta,
Perlytta

Pernella (Greek) stone.
Pernel, Pernela, Pernele, Pernell,
Pernellah, Pernelle

Perpetua (Latin) eternal.
Perpetual, Perpetuala

Perry (French) pear tree.
Perea, Peree, Perey, Peri (Grk),
Peria, Periah, Perie, Perree, Perrey,
Perri, Perrie, Pery, Perya, Peryah

Persis (Greek) woman from Persia.
Persia, Persiah, Persys, Persysa,
Persysah

Petica (Latin) noble.
Peticah, Petrissa (Ger), Petyca,
Petycah

Petra (Greek) stone.
Perrine (Fren), Petrah, Peta, Petrea,
Petrina, Petrissa, Petronia, Petronie,
Petronella, Petronille (Ger), Pier,
Piera, Pierett (Fren), Pierina, Pietra
(Ital), Peytra

Petrina (Greek) steady. The
feminine form of Peter, stone.
Petrin, Petrine, Petriss, Petrissa,
Petrisse, Petroni, Petronie, Petrony,
Petryn, Petryna, Petryne

Petronilla (Latin) stone. The
feminine form of Peter.
Peita, Peretta, Perette, Perilla,
Perinna, Perinnah, Pernel, Pernell,
Pernelle, Peronel, Peronella,
Peronelle, Peronne, Perrine, Petra
(Illy), Petrenela (Pol), Petrija,
Petrina, Petrinah, Petrisse (Ger),
Petronelle (Fren), Petronilha
(Port), Petronilka, Petronylka

Petula (Latin) seeker.
Petulah

Petunia (Native American) sweetly
scented flower.
Petuniah, Petunya, Petunyah

Phaedra (Greek) bright.
Phaedra, Phadra, Phadrah

Phanessa (Greek) butterfly. A form
of Vanessa.
Fanessa, Vanessa

Phedra (Greek) brightly shining.
Faydra, Phaedra, Phaidra, Phedra,
Phedre

Phelia (Greek) immortal wisdom.
Felia, Feliah, Feliah, Felya, Felyah,
Pheliah, Phelya, Phelyah

P

Phemie (Greek/Scottish) of good reputation. The short form of Euphemia.
Phemea, Phemee, Phemey, Phemi, Phemia, Phemiah, Phemy, Phemya, Phemyah

Philana (Greek) lover of humankind.
Filana, Phila, Phileen, Philene, Philida, Philina, Philine, Phillane, Phylana, Phylanah, Phylane, Phyllan, Phyllana, Phyllanah, Phyllane

Philantha (Greek) lover of flowers.
Philanthe, Phylantha, Phylanthe

Philberta (Old English) brilliant intelligence.
Filberta, Filbertah, Filberte, Philberta, Philbertah, Phylbert, Phylberta, Phylbertah, Phylberte, Phyllberta, Phyllbertah, Phyllberte

Philippa (Greek) one who loves horses.
Felipa (Span), Felipe, Felippa, Filippa (Ital), Filipa, Phileen, Phileene, Philene, Philina, Philine, Philipa, Philipine, Philippe, Philippina, Phillipa, Phillipe, Phillippine (Ger), Phylipa, Phylipah, Phyllipa, Phyllipah, Phyllypa, Phyllypah

Philomela (Greek) lover of songs.
Filomela, Filomelah, Philomelah, Phylomela, Phylomelah

Philomena (Greek) she is loved.
Filomena, Filomene, Filomina, Filominah, Filomyna, Filomyne, Fylomina, Fylomine, Fylomyna, Fylomyne, Philomina, Philomine, Phylomina, Phylomine, Phylomyna, Phylomyne

Philothea (Greek) one who loves God.
Filothea, Fylothea, Phylothea

Philyra (Greek) the lime tree.
Philira, Philirah, Phylyrah

Phoebe (Greek) shining; pure; bright.
Feba, Febe, Feebea, Feebee, Fibee, Phebe (Ital), Phebea, Pheebea, Pheebee, Pheibee, Pheibey, Pheybee, Pheybey, Theba, Thebea, Thebee

Phoenix (Greek) purple; immortal.
Feenix, Foenix, Pheenix

Photina (Greek) light. (Egypt) eagle; immortal.
Fotin, Fotina, Fotine, Fotyna, Fotyne, Photine, Photyna, Photyne

Phryne (Greek) lacking colour.
Phrina, Phrine, Phyrne

Phylicia (Latin/Greek) happy one from the green town.
Felicia, Feliciah, Filicia, Filiciah, Philicia, Philiciah, Phyliciah

Phyllida (Greek) loving; leafy.
Philida, Philidah, Phillida, Phillidah, Phillyda, Phillydah, Phylida, Phylidah, Phyllidah, Phylyda, Phylydah, Phyllyda, Phyllydah

Phyllis (Greek) green; leafy branch.
Filide, Fillis, Philis, Phillisla, Phillis, Phillo, Philica, Phylicia, Phyliciah, Phyllicia, Phylliciah, Phyllys

Pia (Italian) devout.
Piah, Pya, Pyah

Piedad (Spanish) devoted.
Piedadah

P

Pierette (French) little steady one.
(Grk) stone. The feminine form
of Pierre/Peter.
Perett, Peretta, Perette, Pieret,
Pierett, Pieretta, Pierin, Pierina,
Pierine, Pieryn, Pieryna, Pieryne

Pilar (Latin/Spanish) pillar;
column.
Peela, Peelah, Peeler, Pilla, Pillar,
Pylar, Pyllar

Pililani (Hawaiian) near to heaven.
Pililanee, Pililaney, Pililanie,
Pililany

Pineki (Hawaiian) peanut.
Pinekee, Pinekey, Pineky

Ping (Chinese) duckweed plant.
(Viet) peaceful.

Pinga (Hindi) bronze.
Pingah

Pinterry (Australian Aboriginal)
star.
Pinterree, Pinterrey, Pinterri,
Pinterrie

Piper (Old English) pipe player.
Pipa, Pipar, Pipper, Pippor, Pypa,
Pypah, Pyper

Pipipa (Australian Aboriginal) sand
piper.
Pipipah, Pypa, Pypah, Pyper,
Pypipa, Pypipah

Pippa (Greek) one who loves
horses. The feminine form of
Philip.
Pipa, Pipah, Pipee, Pipi, Pipie,
Pippah, Pippee, Pippey, Pippi,
Pippie, Pippy, Pipy, Pypa, Pypah,
Pyppa, Pyppah

Pippi (French) rosy-cheeked.
Pipee, Pipey, Pipi, Pipie, Pippee,
Pippie, Pippy, Pipy

Pirrit (Estonian) high.
Pirrita, Pirritah, Pyrrita, Pyrritah

Piscina (Italian) pool of water.
Pischina, Pishinah, Pycina,
Pycinah, Pychina, Pychinah,
Pychyna, Pychynah, Pyshina,
Pyshinah, Pyshyna, Pyshynah

Pita (African) fourth-born child.
Peata, Peatah, Peeta, Peetah, Peita,
Peitah, Peyta, Peytah, Pitah, Pyta,
Pytah

Pixie (English) little fairy.
Pixee, Pixey, Pixi, Pixy, Pyxee,
Pyxey, Pyxi, Pyxie, Pyxy

Placidia (Latin) gentle; serene.
Placida, Placide, Placinda, Placyda,
Placydah, Placynda (Pol)

Platona (Greek) broad; flat-
shouldered. The feminine form
of Plato.
Platonah, Platonia, Platoniah,
Platonya, Platonyah

Pocahontas (Native American)
playful.
Pocohonta

Poeta (Italian) poetry.
Poetah, Poetree, Poetrey, Poetri,
Poetrie, Poett, Poetta, Poette,
Poetry

Pola (Greek) sunlight. The short
form of Apollonia.
Polah, Polar

Polla (Arabic) the poppy flower.
Pollah

Polly (Hebrew) wished for; star of
the sea; bitter. A form of Mary.
Polea, Poleah, Polee, Polei,
Poleigh, Poley, Poli, Polie, Pollea,
Polleah, Pollee, Polleigh, Polley,
Polli, Pollie, Polly, Pollyann,
Pollyanna, Pollyannah, Pollyanne,
Poly

P

Pollyanna (Hebrew) graceful; wished for; star of the sea; bitter. A combination of Polly/Anna.
Polian, Poliana, Polianah, Poliane, Poliann, Polianna, Poliannah, Polianne, Polliann, Pollianna, Polliannah, Pollianne, Polyana, Polyanah, Polyane, Pollyann, Pollyannah, Pollyanne, Polyan, Polyana, Polyanah, Polyane, Polyann, Polyanna, Polyannah, Polyanne

Poloma (Native American) bow.
Polomah, Polome

Polyxena (Greek) one who makes welcome.
Polyxeena, Polyxeenah, Polyxenah, Polyxina, Polyxinah, Polyxyna, Polyxynah, Polyzeena, Polyzeenah, Polyzena, Polyzenah, Polyzina, Polyzinah, Polyzyna, Polyzynah

Pomme/Pomona (French) apple.
Pomma, Pommah, Pomonah (Lat)

Poni (African) second-born child.
Ponee, Poney, Ponie, Pony

Poppy (Latin/English) the poppy flower.
Popea, Popee, Popey, Popi, Popie, Poppea, Poppee, Poppey, Poppi, Poppie

Poria (Hebrew) fruitful.
Pora, Poriah, Porya, Poryah

Porsche (German/Latin) offering.
Porsha, Porshe

Portia (Latin) offering; sweet fortified wine; the left side. (O/Eng) from the town by the water.
Porta, Portah, Portiah, Portya, Portyah

Posala (Miwok) flower.
Posalah

Posy (English) small bunch of flowers.
Posee, Posey, Posi, Posia, Posiah, Posie, Posya, Posyah

Premilla (Sanskrit) girl of love.
Premila, Premilah, Premillah, Premyla, Premylah, Premylla, Premyllah

Preya (Latin/English) prayer.
Praya, Prayah, Preyah

Prima (Latin) first-born child.
Primah, Primara, Primaria, Primariah, Pryma, Prymah, Prymaria, Prymariah, Prymarya, Prymaryah

Primavera (Latin) first born of spring; new life.
Primaverah, Prymavera, Prymaverah

Primrose (English/Scottish) the primrose flower.
Primrosa, Prymrosa, Prymrose

Princess (English) daughter of the queen and king.
Princessa, Pryncess, Pryncessah

Prioska (Hungarian) blushing.
Pryosha

Priscilla (Latin) ancient.
Piroshka, Precilla, Prescilla, Pricila, Pricilia, Prisca, Priscella, Priscila, Priscill, Priscillie, Prisella, Prisila, Prisilla, Prissilla, Prysilla, Prysillah, Prycyla, Prycylah, Prysylla, Prysyllah

Prisma (Greek) to cut; saw.
Prysma

Priya (Hindi) beloved; sweet-natured.
Priyah

Promisee (English) promise.
Promise, Promisea, Promisey, Promisi, Promisie, Promissa, Promisse, Promissee, Promissey,

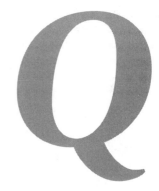

Promisee cont.
Promissi, Promissie, Promissy, Promisy

Prospera (Latin) prosperity.
Prosperitee, Prosperitey, Prosperiti, Prosperitie, Prosperity

Pru/Prudence/Prue (Latin) discreet; cautious. The short form of Prudence, foresight.
Prudance, Prudi, Prudie, Prudy, Prue

Pruity (Middle English) purity.
Pruitee, Pruitey, Pruiti, Pruitie

Prunella (Latin/French) the colour of little plums.
Prunel, Prunela, Prunelah, Prunele, Prunell, Prunellah, Prunelle

Psyche (Greek) mind and soul.
Psyk, Psyke, Syche, Syk, Syke

Pua (Hawaiian) flower.
Puah

Puakai (Hawaiian) sea flower.
Puakay

Puakea (Hawaiian) white flower.
Puakia, Puakiah, Puakeah, Puakya, Puakyah

Pualani (Hawaiian) heavenly flower.
Pualanee, Pualaney, Pualania, Pualaniah, Pualanie, Pualany

Purity (English) purity.
Pura, Purah, Pure, Pureza, Purisima, Puritee, Puritey, Puriti, Puritia, Puritiah, Puritie, Puritya

Pyralis (Greek) fire.
Piralis, Piralissa, Pyralissa

Pyrena (Greek) fiery.
Pirena, Pirenah, Pyrenah

Pythis (Greek) prophet.
Pithea, Pitheah, Pithia, Pithiah, Pythea, Pytheah, Pythiah, Pythya, Pythyah

Qadesh (Egyptian) Egyptian goddess.
Qadesha, Qadeshah, Quedesh, Quedesha

Qadira (Arabic) powerful.
Kadira, Kadirah, Qadirah, Qadyra

Qamra (Arabic) moon.
Kamra, Qamrah

Qitarah (Arabic) fragrant.
Qitara, Qyntara, Qyntarah

Quaashie (Ewe) born on a Sunday.
Quashi, Quashie, Quashy

Quahah (Pueblo) beads of white coral.
Quaha

Quaneisha (Swahili) life. (Arab) woman.
Quanecia, Quanesha, Quanesia, Quanisha, Quanishia, Quansha, Quarnisha, Queisha, Quenisha, Quenishia, Quynecia, Quynesha, Quynesia, Quynisha, Quynishia, Quynsha, Qynecia, Qynisha, Qynysha

Quanika (Russian) dedicated to God. A form of Nikah, belonging to God.
Quanikka, Quanikki, Quanique, Quanyka, Quanykka, Quanykki,

Q

Quanyque, Quantenique,
Quantenyque, Quaqanica,
Quaqanyca, Quawanika, Quawanyka

Quarralia (Australian Aboriginal)
star.
Quaralia, Quaraliah, Quarraliah,
Quaralya, Quaralyah, Quarralya,
Quarralyah

Quartilla (Latin) fourth-born child.
Quartila, Quartilah, Quartile,
Quartillah, Quartille, Quartyla,
Quartylah, Quartyle, Quartylla,
Quartyllah, Quartylle, Quintila,
Quintilah, Quintile, Quantilla,
Quintillah, Quantille, Quintyla,
Quintylah, Quintylla, Quintyllah,
Quyntila, Quyntilah, Quyntile,
Quyntilla, Quyntillah, Quyntille,
Quyntyla, Quyntylah, Quyntyle,
Quyntylla, Quyntyllah, Quyntylle

Qubilah (Arabic) harmony.
Quabila, Quabilah, Quabyla,
Quabylah, Qubila, Quybla,
Quyblah

Queanbeyan (Australian Aboriginal)
clear water.
Queenbeyan

Queen/Queena/Queenie (English)
queen.
Quean, Queana, Queanah,
Queanee, Queaney, Queani,
Queania, Queaniah, Queanie,
Queany, Queanya, Queanyah,
Queen, Queena, Queenah,
Queenation, Queenee, Queenet,
Queeneta, Queenete, Queenett,
Queenetta, Queenette, Queeney,
Queeni, Queenia, Queeniah,
Queenie, Queenika, Queenique,
Queeny, Queenya, Queenyah,
Quenna, Quennah

Queisha (Swahili) life.
(Arab) woman.
Qeyshia, Qeyshiah, Qeysha,
Queishah, Queshia, Queshiah,
Queshya, Queshyah, Queysha

Quelita (American) queen of joy.
Queleata, Queleatah, Queleeta,
Queleetah, Queleta, Queletah,
Quelitah, Quelyta, Quelytah

Quella (Old English) quiet.
Quela, Quele, Quellah, Quelle

Quenby (Swedish) from the
woman's estate.
Queenbea, Queenbee, Queenbey,
Queenbi, Queenbie, Quenbye

Quenna (English) queen.
Quenell, Quenella, Quenelle,
Quenessa, Quenesse, Queneta,
Quenete, Quenetta, Quenette,
Quenna, Quennah

Querida (Swedish) beloved.
(Span) asked for.
Queridah, Queryda, Querydah

Questa (French) searcher; on a
quest.
Quest, Questah, Queste

Queta (Spanish) ruler of the house.
The feminine form of Henry.
Quetah

Quiana (Hebrew) graceful. A form
of Anna.
Quianah, Quiane, Quiann,
Quianna, Quiannah, Quianne,
Quyana, Quyanah, Quyane,
Quyann, Quyanna, Quyannah,
Quyanne

Quieta (English) quiet.
Quietah, Quiete, Quietta,
Quiettah, Quiette, Quyeta,
Quyetah, Quyete, Quyetta,
Quyettah, Quyette

Q

Quilla (Incan) goddess of the moon.
Quila, Quilah, Quill, Quillah, Quille, Quyla, Quylah, Quyle, Quylla, Quyllah, Quylle

Quinby (Scandinavian) dweller by the queen's estate.
Quinbea, Quinbee, Quinbey, Quinbi, Quinbie, Quynbea, Quynbee, Quynbey, Quynbi, Quynbia, Quynbie, Quynby

Quincy (Latin) from the fifth son's estate; fifth-born child.
Quincee, Quincey, Quinci, Quincie, Quinncee, Quinncey, Quinnci, Quinncie, Quinncy, Quyncee, Quyncey, Quynci, Quyncie, Quyncy, Quynncee, Quynncey, Quynnci, Quynncie, Quynncy

Quinella (Latin) fifth-born child. (Eng) from the queen's lawn.
Quinel, Quinela, Quinelah, Quinell, Quinella, Quinelle, Quynel, Quynela, Quynele, Quynell, Quynella, Quynelle

Quinn (Irish/Gaelic) wisdom.
Quin, Quina, Quinah, Quinna, Quinnah, Quiyn, Quyn, Quynn

Quinta (Latin) fifth-born child. The feminine form of Quentin.
Quintah, Quintana, Quintanah, Quintane, Quintann, Quintanna, Quintannah, Quintanne, Quynta, Quyntah, Quyntana, Quyntanah, Quyntann, Quyntanna, Quyntannah, Quyntanne

Quintana (Latin) fifth-born child. (Eng) from the queen's lawn.
Quinntina, Quinntinah, Quinntine, Quinta, Quintah, Quintanah, Quintara, Quintarah, Quintia, Quintiah, Quintila, Quintilla, Quintina, Quintinah, Quintine, Quintona, Quintonah, Quintonica, Quintonice, Quintyna, Quintynah, Quyntana, Quyntanah, Quyntara, Quyntarah, Quyntia, Quyntiah, Quyntila, Quyntilah, Quyntilla, Quyntina, Quyntinah, Quyntine, Quyntonica, Quyntonice, Quyntyna, Quyntynah

Quintessa (Latin) essence.
Quintesa, Quintessah, Quintesse, Quintice, Quyntesa, Quyntesah, Quyntessa, Quyntessah, Quyntesse

Quintina (Latin) fifth-born child.
Quintinah, Quintine, Quintyn, Quintyna, Quintynah, Quintyne, Quyntin, Quyntina, Quyntinah, Quyntine, Quyntyn, Quyntyna, Quyntynah, Quyntyne

Quipolly (Australian Aboriginal) water full of fish.
Quipoly, Quypolly, Quypoly

Quiric (Greek) child born on a Sunday.
Quirick, Quiryc, Quiryck, Quiryk, Quyric, Quyrick, Quyryk

Quirita (Latin) citizen.
Quiritah, Quirite, Quiritta, Quirittah, Quiritte, Quiryta, Quirytah, Quirytta, Quirytte, Quyryta, Quyrytah, Quyrytta, Quyryttah, Quyrytte

Quiterie (Latin/French) tranquil.
Quita, Quitah, Quiteree, Quiteri, Quiteria, Quiteriah, Quitery, Quyta, Quytah, Quyteree, Quyteri, Quyteria, Quyteriah, Quyterie, Quytery

Quoba (Australian Aboriginal) good.
Quobah

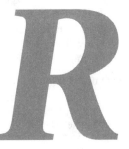

Raama (Hebrew) one who trembles.
Raamah, Rama, Ramah

Raanana (Hebrew) fresh.
Ranana, Rananah

Rabab (Arabic) cloud.
Rababa, Rababah

Rabi (Arabic) breeze; spring harvest.
Rabia, Rabiah, Raby, Rabya, Rabyah

Rachav (Hebrew) big baby.
Rachev

Rachelle/Rachel/Raquel (French/ Hebrew) ewe; lamb.
Rachael, Rachaele, Rachela (Pol), Rachele (Ital), Rachelle (Fren), Racquel, Racquele, Raquell, Racquelle, Rahel (Ger), Raichel, Raichele, Raichell, Raichelle, Raishel, Raishele, Raishell, Raishelle, Rakal, Raoghnailt (Scott), Raquel (Span), Raquele, Raquell, Raquelle, Raychela, Raychele, Raychell, Raychelle, Rayshel, Rayshele, Rayshell, Rayshelle

Radella (Old English) counsellor.
Radela, Radelah, Radelia, Radeliah, Radellah, Radelle, Radiliah, Radillia, Radilliah, Radyla, Radylah, Radyllya, Radyllyah

Radha (Hindi) success.
Radhah

Radhiya (Swahili) to agree.
Radhiyah

Radinka (Slavic) full of life; playful.
Radinkah, Radynka, Radynkah

Radmilla (Slavic) worker for the people.
Radmila, Radmilah, Radmilah, Radmile, Radmill, Radmillah, Radmille, Radmyl, Radmyla, Radmylah, Radmyle, Radmyll, Radmylla, Radmyllah, Radmylle

Radomira (Czech) famous.
Radomirah, Radomyra, Radomyrah

Radwa (Arabic) mountain.
Radwah

Rae (Old English) doe. The short form of names starting with 'Ra' e.g. Rachel.
Ra, Rai, Raii, Ray, Raye

Raelene (Latin/French) royal temptress.
Raelean, Raeleana, Raeleanah, Raeleane, Raeleen, Raeleena, Raeleenah, Railean, Raileana, Raileanah, Raileane, Raileen, Raileena, Raileenah, Raileene, Ralean, Raleana, Raleanah, Raleane, Raleen, Raleena, Raleenah, Raleene, Ralin, Ralina, Ralinah, Raline, Ralyn, Ralyna, Ralynah, Ralyne, Raylean, Rayleana, Rayleanah, Rayleane, Rayleen, Rayleena, Rayleenah, Rayleene

Rafa (Arabic) happy.
Rafah, Raffa, Raffah

Rafaela/Raphaela (Hebrew) God has healed. The feminine form of Raphael.
Rafael, Rafaelah, Rafaele, Rafaelia, Rafaeliah, Rafaell, Rafaella,

R

Rafaela/Raphaela cont.
Rafaellah, Rafaelle, Raffaela,
Raffaelah, Raffaele, Raffaell,
Raffaella, Raffaellah, RaffaelleRafia,
Rafiah, Rafya, Rafyah, Raphaelah,
Raphaele, Raphaell, Raphaella,
Raphaellah, Raphaelle

Ragnild (Norse) warrior of
judgment. (Ger) powerful.
Ragna, Ragnah, Ragnel, Ragnela,
Ragnele, Ragnell, Ragnella,
Ragnelle, Ragnhild, Ragnida,
Ragnidah, Ragnyld, Ragnylda,
Rainel, Rainela, Rainele, Rainell,
Rainella, Rainelle, Renilda, Renilde,
Renyld, Renylda, Renylde

Raidah (Arabic) leader.
Raeda, Raedah, Raida, Raidah,
Rayda, Raydah

Rain (English) precipitation; rain.
Raen, Raena, Raenah, Raene,
Raenee, Raeney, Raeni, Raenie,
Raeny, Raina, Rainah, Raine,
Rainee, Rainey, Raini, Rainie, Rainy,
Rayn, Rayna, Raynah, Rayne

Raina (Teutonic) powerful. A form
of Regina, queen.
Raena, Raenah, Raenia, Raeni,
Raenie, Raeny, Raheen, Raheena,
Raheene, Rain, Rainah, Raine, Rainia,
Rainiah, Rainie, Rainna, Rainnah,
Rainnia, Rainiah, Reann, Reanna,
Reanne, Rein, Reina, Reinah, Reine,
Reyn, Reyna, Reynah, Reyne

Rainbow (Old English) rainbow.
Raenbo, Raenbow, Rainbeau,
Rainbeaux, Rainbo, Rainebow,
Rainebo, Rainebow, Raynbow,
Reinbow, Reynbow

Raine (Latin) queen. (O/Eng) rainy.
Raen, Raena, Raenah, Raene,
Raenee, Raeney, Raeni, Raenie,
Raeny, Rain, Raina, Rainah, Rainee,

Rainey, Raini, Rainie, Rainy, Rana,
Rane, Reina, Reinah, Reine, Reini,
Reinie, Reiny, Reyn, Reyna, Reyne,
Reynee, Reyni, Reynie, Reyny

Rainelle (English/French) she is like
rain.
Rainel, Rainela, Rainele, Rainella,
Rainelle, Raynel, Raynell, Raynella,
Raynelle

Rainfreda (German) advice; peace.
Rainfredah, Rainfrida, Rainfridah,
Raynfreda, Raynfrida, Raynfryda

Raisa/Raizel (Hebrew) rose.
Raizela, Raizelah, Raizele, Rayzil,
Rayzila, Rayzile, Rayzill, Rayzilla,
Rayzille, Rayzyl, Rayzyla, Rayzylah,
Rayzyle, Razil, Razila, Razile, Razill,
Razilla, Razille, Razyl, Razyla,
Razylah, Razyle, Razyll, Razylla,
Razyllah, Razylle

Raissa (Old French) thinker;
believer.
Raisa, Raisah, Raissah, Raysa,
Raysah, Rayssa, Rayssah

Rajani (Hindi) evening.
Rajanee, Rajaney, Rajanie, Rajany

Ramah (Hebrew) highly praised.
Rama

Ramia (African) teller of fortunes.
Ramiah, Ramya, Ramyah

Ramona (Spanish) mighty, wise
protector. The feminine form of
Ramon.
Raema, Raemonda, Raemona,
Raimaona, Raimonah, Raimone,
Raonda, Ramondah, Rayma,
Raymona, Raymonah, Romona,
Romonda

Ramose (Latin) branches.
Ramosa, Ramosah

Ran (Japanese) water lily. (Scand) the sea goddess; destroyer.
Rana, Ranah

Rana (Scandinavian) catcher. (Sans) royal. (Arab) to gaze. (Span) frog.
Rahna, Rahnah, Rahnee, Rahney, Rahni, Rahnie, Rahny, Ranah, Ranee, Raney, Rani, Rania, Raniah, Ranie, Ranna, Rannah, Rannee, Ranney, Ranni, Rannie, Ranny, Rany, Ranya, Ranyah

Ranait (Irish) graceful.
Ranaita, Ranaitah, Ranaite, Ranayt, Ranaytah, Ranayte

Randa (Arabic) tree.
Randah

Randall (English) protected.
Randah, Randal, Randala, Randalah, Randale, Randalea, Randaleah, Randalee, Randelei, Randaleigh, Randaley, Randali, Randalie, Randaly, Randel, Randela, Randelah, Randele, Randella, Randelle

Randi (English) invincible. The short form of Miranda, worthy of love. The feminine form of Randy/Randell/Randolph, shield; wolf.
Rande, Randea, Randean, Randeana, Randeane, Randee, Randeen, Randeena, Randeene, Randena, Randene, Randey, Randie, Randin, Randina, Randine, Randy, Randyn, Randyna, Randyne

Rane (Scandinavian) queen.
Raen, Raena, Raenah, Raene, Rain, Raina, Rainah, Raine, Rayn, Rayna, Raynah, Rayne

Ranger (English) protector of the forest.

Rangi (Maori) sky.
Rangee, Rangia, Rangiah, Rangie, Rangy

Rani/Rania (Sanskrit) queen. (Heb) happy.
Raen, Raena, Raenah, Raene, Raenee, Raeni, Raenia, Raeniah, Raeny, Raenya, Raenyah, Rain, Raina, Rainah, Raine, Rainee, Rainey, Raini, Rainia, Rainiah, Rainie, Rainy, Rainya, Rainyah, Rana, Ranah, Rania, Raniah, Ranie, Ranice, Ranicia, Raniqua, Raniquah, Ranique, Rayna, Raynah, Rayne, Raynee, Raynell, Raynella, Raynelle, Rayney, Rayni, Raynia, Rayniah, Raynie, Rayny, Raynya, Raynyah

Ranielle (Hebrew/African American) God is my judge. A form of Danielle.
Rannielle, Rannyelle, Ranyelle

Ranita (Hebrew) my song of happiness.
Raneata, Raneatah, Raneate, Raneatt, Raneatta, Raneattah, Raneatte, Raneet, Raneeta, Raneetah, Raneete, Ranit, Ranitah, Ranite, Ranitta, Ranittah, Ranitte, Ranyta, Ranytah, Ranyte, Ranytta, Ranyttah, Ranytte

Raniyah (Arabic) gazing.
Raniya

Ranjana (Hindi) loved.
Ranjanah

Rapa (Hawaiian) moonbeam.
Rapah

Rasha (Arabic) young gazelle.
Rahshea, Rahshia, Rahshiah, Rashea, Rashya, Rashyah

Rashawna (Irish/Hebrew) God is gracious. The feminine form of Shawn.
Raseana, Raseanah, Raseane, Rashaun, Rashauna, Rashaunah, Rashaune, Rashawn, Rashawnah, Rashawne, Roseana, Roseanah, Roshauna, Roshaunah, Roshawna, Roshawnah

Rasheda (Swahili) righteous.
Rasheada, Rasheadah, Rashedah, Rasheeda, Rasheedah, Rashida, Rashidah, Rashidee, Rashidi, Rashidie, Rashyda, Rashydah

Rashieka (Arabic) descended from royalty.
Rasheeka, Rasheekah, Rasheika, Rasheka, Rasekah, Rashika, Rashikah, Rasike, Rasiqua, Rasiquah, Rasique, Rasyqua, Rasyquah, Rasyque

Rasia (Greek) rose.
Rasiah, Rasya, Rasyah

Ratana (Thai) crystal.
Ratania, Rataniah, Ratanya, Ratna, Ratnah, Rattan, Rattana, Rattane

Ratna (Sanskrit) jewel.
Ratnah

Ratri (Hindi) night.
Ratree, Ratrey, Ratria, Ratriah, Ratrie, Ratry, Ratrya, Ratryah

Raula (French) famous wolf. The feminine form of Raoul.
Raoula, Raolah, Raole, Raulla, Raullah, Raulle

Raven (Old English) black; raven, the bird; black-haired.
Ravan, Ravana, Ravanah, Ravanna, Ravannah, Raveen, Raveena, Raveenah, Raveene, Ravena, Ravenah, Ravenn, Ravenna, Ravenah, Ravenna, Ravennah,

Ravenne, Ravin, Ravina, Ravinah, Ravine, Ravon, Ravyn, Ravyna, Ravynah, Ravyne

Ravine (English) deep valley.
Ravina, Ravinah, Ravyn, Ravyna, Ravynah

Ravva (Hindi) sun.
Rava, Ravah, Ravvah

Rawiya (Arabic) storyteller.
Rawiyah

Rawnie (Gypsy) lady.
Rawna, Rawnah, Rawnee, Rawney, Rawni, Rawnia, Rawniah, Rawnii, Rawny, Rawnya, Rawnyah,, Rhawna, Rhawnah, Rhawnee, Rhawney, Rhawni, Rhawnie, Rhawny, Rhawnya, Rhawnyah

Raya (Hebrew) friend.
Raea, Raeah, Raia, Raiah, Rayah

Rayann (French/Hebrew) royal grace.
Raean, Raeana, Raeanah, Raeane, Raeann, Raeanna, Raeannah, Raeanne, Raiana, Rainanah, Rainane, Raiann, Raianna, Raiannah, Raianne, Rayana, Rayanah, Rayane, Rayanna, Rayannah, Rayanne

Rayleen (French) from the royal meadow.
Raelean, Raeleana, Raeleane, Raeleen, Raeleena, Raeleenah, Raeleene, Raelin, Raelina, Raelinah, Raeline, Raelyn, Raelyna, Raylinah, Rayline, Raelyn, Raelyna, Raelynah, Raelyne, Railean, Raileana, Raileanah, Raileane, Raileen, Raileena, Raileenah, Raileene, Railin, Railina, Railinah, Railine, Railyn, Railyna, Railynah, Railyne, Raylean, Rayleana, Rayleanah, Rayleane, Rayleena, Rayleenah, Rayleene, Raylin, Raylina, Raylinah,

R

Rayline, Raylyn, Raylyna, Raylynah, Raylyne

Raymonde (German) wise protector. The feminine form of **Raymond**.
Raemond, Raemonda, Raemondah, Raemonde, Raimond, Raimonda, Raimondah, Raimonde, Rayma, Raymae, Ratmay, Raymond, Raymonda, Raymondah

Rayna (Hebrew) purity. (Scan) mighty.
Raen, Raena, Raenah, Raene, Rain, Raina, Rainah, Raine, Raynah, Reina, Reinah, Reyna, Reynah

Raz/Razi/Razilee (Aramaic/Hebrew) my secret. (O/Eng) secret meadow.
Razi, Razia, Raziah, Raziela, Razilea, Razileah, Razilee, Razilei, Razileigh, Raziley, Razili, Razilia, Raziliah, Razilie, Razilla, Razillah, Razille, Razyl, Razyla, Razylah, Razylea, Razyleah, Razylee, Razylei, Razyleigh, Razyley, Razyli, Razylia, Razyliah, Razylie, Razyly

Raziya (Swahili) agreeable.
Raziyah

Rea (Greek) poppy flower.
Reah

Reade (Old English) advisor.
Read, Reid, Reyd

Reanna (German/English) mighty grace.
Rean, Reana, Reanah, Reane, Reann, Reannah, Reanne, Reian, Reiana, Reianah, Reiane, Reiann, Reianna, Reiannah, Reianne, Reyan, Reyana, Reyanah, Reyane, Reyann, Reyanna, Reyannah, Reyanne, Rhean, Rheana, Rheanah, Rheane, Rhian, Rhiana, Rhianah, Rhiane, Rhiann, Rhianna, Rhiannah, Rhianne, Rhyan,

Rhyana, Rhyanah, Rhyane, Rhyann, Rhyanna, Rhyannah, Rhyanne, Rian, Riana, Rianah, Riane, Riann, Rianna, Riannah, Rianne, Ryan, Ryana, Ryanah, Ryan, Ryana, Ryanah, Ryane, Ryann, Ryanna, Ryannah, Ryanne

Reba (Hebrew) bound; faithful. A form of **Rebecca**.
Reaba, Reabah, Rebah, Reeba, Reebah, Reiba, Reibah, Reyba, Reybah, Rheba, Rhebah, Rheiba, Rheibah, Rheyba, Rheybah

Rebecca (Hebrew) bound; faithful.
Rabbecca, Rabbeca, Rabbecah, Rabbecca, Rebbeca, Rebbecah, Rebbecca, Rebeca (Span), Rebecah, Rebeccea, Rebeccka, Rebecckah, Rebecka, Rebeckah, Rebecqua, Rebecquah, Rebeque, Rebeka, Rebekah, Rebekka (Ger), Rebekkah, Rebequa, Rebequah, Rebeque, Revecca (Slav), Reveccah, Revecka (Slav), Reveckah, Reveka (Slav), Revekah, Revequa, Revequah, Reveque

Rechaba (Hebrew) rider of horses.
Rechabah

Reena (Greek) peace.
Rean, Reana, Reanah, Reen, Reenah, Reene, Reenia, Reeniah, Reenie, Reeny Reenya, Reina, Reinah, Reine, Rena, Renah, Rene, Reyna, Reynah, Reyne

Reet (Estonian/Greek) pearl. A form of **Margaret**.
Reat, Reata, Reatah, Reate, Reeta, Reetah, Reete, Reit, Reita, Reitah, Reite, Reyt, Reyta, Reytah, Reyte

Regan (Irish/Gaelic/Latin) queen.
Raga, Reagan, Reagen, Reagin, Reagon, Reagyn, Regana, Reganah, Regane, Regann, Reganna, Reganne, Regen, Regin, Regina, Reginah,

Regan cont.
Regine, Reigan, Reigana, Reiganah,
Reigane, Reygan, Reygana,
Reyganah, Reygane

Regina (Latin) queen.
Regan, Regana, Reganah, Regane,
Regeana, Regeanah, Regeane,
Regeena, Regeenah, Regeene, Regia,
Regiah, Reginah, Regine, Reginta,
Regintah, Regine, Regyna, Regynah,
Regyne, Reina (Span), Reinah,
Reine (Fren), Reinetta, Reniette,
Reygin, Reygina, Reyginah,
Reygine, Reygyn, Reygyna,
Reygynah, Reygyne, Reyna, Reyna

Rei (Japanese) well-behaved; polite.
Rey

Reiko (Japanese) grateful.
Reyko

Reina (Spanish) queen.
Reana, Reanah, Reane, Reena,
Reenah, Reene, Reinah, Reine,
Reinet, Reineta, Reinete, Reinett,
Reinetta, Reinette, Reiny, Reiona,
Renia, Reyna, Reynah, Reyne

Reka (Maori) sweet.
Rekah

Rekha (Hindi) thin line.
Reka, Rekah, Rekia, Rekiah, Rekiya,
Rekiyah

Remy (French) from the
Champagne town of Rheims.
Reims, Remee, Remey, Remi,
Remia, Remiah, Remie, Remmee,
Remmey, Remmi, Remmia,
Remmiah, Remmie, Remmy, Remy

Ren (Japanese) lotus.

Rena (Hebrew) joyful song. A short
form of Irene, peaceful.
Erena, Erenah, Erene, Irena, Irenah,
Irene, Reana, Reanah, Reanna,
Reannah, Reena, Reenah, Reenna,

Reennah, Reina, Reinah, Reinna,
Reinnah, Renata, Renata, Reyna,
Reynah, Reynna, Reynnah

Renata (Hebrew) song of joy.
Rena, Renae, Renah, Renai,
Renarta, Renartah, Renatah, Renate
(Ger), Renay, Renaye, Rene (Fren),
Renea (Bret/Austr), Reneah,
Reneata, Reneatah, Renee (Fren),
Reneeta, Reneetah, Renita, Renitah,
Renyta, Renytah

Rene (Greek) peace. A short form of
Irene. The French form of Renata,
song of joy.
Rean, Reana, Reanah, Reane,
Reanee, Reaney, Reen, Reena,
Reenah, Reene, Reenee, Reeney,
Renea (Bret/Austr), Renee (Fren),
Rina, Rinah, Rinea, Rinee, Riney,
Rini, Rinie, Rinn, Rinna, Rinnah,
Rinne, Rinnee, Rinney, Rinni
Rinnie, Rinny, Riny, Ryn, Ryna,
Rynah, Ryne, Rynea, Rynee, Ryney,
Ryni, Rynie, Ryny

Renee (French) reborn.
Rena, Renae, Renah, Renai, Renaia,
Renaiah, Renay, Renaya, Renaye,
Rene, Renea (Bret/Austr), Reneah,
Renata, Renatah, Renisha, Renitta,
Renittah, Renitte, Renna, Rennah,
Rennae, Rennah, Rennay, Rennaya,
Rennaye, Renne, Rennea, Renneah,
Wrenae, Wrenai, Wrenay, Wrennae,
Wrennai, Wrennay

Renita (Latin) rebel.
Reneata, Reneatah, Reneate,
Reneeta, Reneetah, Reneetae,
Reneita, Reneitah, Renitah, Renitta,
Renittah, Renyta, Renytah, Renyte

Renni (Hebrew) song.
Renea (Bret/Austr), Rene, Renee
(Fren), Reney, Reni, Renie, Rennea,
Rennee, Renney, Rennie, Renny,
Reny

R

Renny (Irish) prosperous one.
A short form of names starting
with 'Ren' e.g. Renee.
Renea (Bret/Austrl), Rene, Renee
(Fren), Reney, Reni, Renie, Rennea,
Rennee, Renney, Renni, Rennie,
Reny

Rere (Polynesian) watchful one.
Reree

Reseda (Latin) healing one.
(Span) the Mignonette flower.
Reseada, Reseadah, Reseeda,
Reseedah, Resedah, Resida,
Residah, Resyda, Resydah, Seda,
Sedah

Reshawna (Irish/Hebrew) God is
gracious. The feminine form of
Shawn.
Reschauna, Reschaunah,
Reschaune, Reschawna,
Reschawnah, Reschawne,
Rescheana, Rescheanah, Rescheane,
Reseana, Reseanah, Reshauna,
Reshaunah, Reshawnah, Roseana,
Roseanah, Roshauna, Roshaunah,
Roshawn, Roshawnah

Resi (German/Greek) harvester. A
form of Teresa.
Resee, Resey, Resie, Ressee, Ressi,
Ressie, Ressy, Resy, Rezee, Rezey,
Rezi, Rezie, Rezy, Rezzee, Rezzey,
Rezzi, Rezzie, Rezzy, Rezy

Reta (African) shaking.
Reata, Reatah, Reeta, Reetah, Reita,
Reitah, Retah, Retta, Rettah, Reyta,
Reytah, Rheta, Rhetah, Rhetta,
Rhettah, Rita, Ritah, Ryta, Rytah

Retha (Greek) the best.
Areatha, Areathah, Areata, Areatta,
Areatte, Aretha, Arethah, Areta,
Aretah, Aretta, Arette, Reata, Reate,
Reatee, Reatey, Reati, Reatie, Reaty,
Ret, Reta, Retah, Retee, Retey,

Rethah, Rethia, Rethiah, Rethya,
Rethyah, Reti, Retie, Rety

Reubena (Hebrew) behold, a
daughter.
Reubina, Reubinah, Reuvena,
Reuvanah, Rubena, Rubenah,
Rubenia, Rubeniah, Rubina,
Rubinah, Rubine, Rubyna,
Rubynah

Reumah (Hebrew) love pearl.
Reuma

Reva (Latin) renewed strength.
(Heb) rain.
Reava, Reavah, Reeva, Reevah,
Revah, Revia, Reviah, Revida,
Revidah, Revya, Revyah, Revyda,
Revydah

Revaya (Hebrew) satisfaction.
Revaia, Revaiah, Revayah

Reverie (English) dream.

Revital (Hebrew) God is my dew;
God will provide; God is my life.
Revita, Revitah, Revyta, Revytah

Rewa (Polynesian) slender; tall.
Rewah

Rewuri (Australian Aboriginal)
spring.
Rewuree, Rewurey, Rewurie,
Rewury

Rexana (Latin/Old English) God's
gracious queen. A feminine form
of Rex.
Rexanah, Rexann, Rexanna,
Rexannah, Rexanne, Roxana,
Roxanah, Roxane, Roxanna,
Roxannah, Roxanne

Reyhan (Turkish) sweet-smelling
flower.
Reihan, Reihana, Reihanah,
Reihane, Reyhana, Reyhanah,
Reyhane

Reynald (German) advisor of the king. The feminine form of Reynold, powerful; mighty.
Reinald, Reinalda, Reinaldah, Reinalde, Reynalda (Scan), Reynaldah, Reynalde

Rez (Latin/Hungarian) red-haired; copper.
Res, Rezz

Reza (Slavic) harvester. The short form of Teresa.
Rezah, Rezi, Rezie, Rezka, Rezza, Rezzah

Rgea (Greek) flowing stream; protector; the mother of all Greek gods.
Rea, Reana, Reanah, Reane, Reann, Reanna, Reanne, Rheah, Rhean, Rheana, Rheanah, Rheane, Rheann, Rheanna, Rheannah, Rheanne, Rheannon, Ria, Riah, Rian, Riana, Rianah, Riane, Riann, Rianna, Riannah, Rianne, Ryan, Ryana, Ryanah, Ryane, Ryann, Ryanna, Ryannah, Ryanne

Rhedyn (Welsh) fern.
Readan, Readen, Readin, Readon, Readyn, Reedan, Reeden, Reedin, Reedon, Reedyn, Rheadan, Rheaden, Rheadin, Rheadon, Rheadyn, Rhedan, Rheden, Rhedin, Rhedon, Rheedan, Rheeden, Rheedin, Rheedon, Rheedyn

Rheta (Greek) well spoken; pearl. (Wel) ardent; enthusiastic. The feminine form of Rhett, mighty; red.
Reata, Reatah, Reeta, Reetah, Reita, Reitah, Reta, Retah, Retta, Rettah, Reyta, Reytah, Rheata, Rheatah, Rheeta, Rheetah, Rhetah, Rhetta, Rhettah, Rita, Ritah, Ryta, Rytah

Rhiamon (Welsh) goddess; wisdom.
Rheamon, Rheemon, Rhyamon

Rhian (Welsh/Old English) God's gracious woman.
Rhean, Rheana, Rheann, Rheanna, Rheannah, Rheanne, Rheean, Rheeana, Rheeanah, Rheeann, Rheeanna, Rheeannah, Rheeanne, Rhiana, Rhianah, Rhiane, Rhianna, Rhiannah, Rhianne, Rhyan, Rhyana, Rhyane, Rhyann, Rhyanna, Rhyannah, Rhyanne

Rhiangar (Welsh) beloved woman.
Rhyangar

Rhiannon (Gaelic/Welsh) sorceress.
Reana, Reanah, Reane, Reann, Reanna, Reannah, Reanne, Rehann, Rehanna, Rehannah, Rehanne, Rheann, Rheanna, Rheannah, Rheanan, Rheanne, Rhian, Rhiana, Rhianah, Rhiane, Rhiann, Rhianna, Rhiannah, Rhianne, Rhiannan, Rhianne, Rhiannen, Rhianon, Rhianyn, Rhyanan, Rhyane, Rhyann, Rhyanna, Rhyanne, Riamma, Riammah, Riamme, Riana, Rianah, Riann, Rianna, Riannah, Rianne, Rioann, Rioanna, Rioannah, Rioanne, Ryan, Ryana, Ryanah, Ryanan, Ryanen, Ryanin, Ryanyn, Rhyann, Rhyanna, Rhyannah, Rhyanne

Rhianvyen (Welsh) fair-haired woman.
Rhianvien

Rhodah (Greek) from where the roses grow; from Rhodes.
Rhodah, Rhode, Rhodia, Rhodiah, Rhodya, Rhodyah

Rhodelia (Greek) rosy-cheeked; rose.
Rhodeliah, Rhodelya, Rhodelyah, Rodelia, Rodeliah, Rodelya, Rodelyah

Rhody (Greek) rose.
Rhodea, Rhode, Rhodee, Rhodey,
Rhodi, Rhodia, Rhodiah, Rhodie,
Rhodya, Rhodyah

Rhonda (Welsh/Teutonic) powerful,
fierce river.
Rhona, Rhondah, Rhondia,
Rhondiah, Rhondya, Rhondyah,
Ronda, Rondah, Ronet, Roneta,
Ronetah, Ronete, Ronett, Ronetta,
Ronettah, Ronette

Rhonwen (Celtic) rose; white
friend. A form of Bronwyn.
Rhonwena, Rhonwenah, Rhonwin,
Rhowina, Rhowinah, Rhowine,
Rhonwinn, Rhowinna,
Rhowinnah, Rhowinne, Rhonwyn,
Rhonwyna, Rhonwynah,
Rhonwyne, Rhonwyyn,
Rhonwynna, Rhonwynnah,
Rhonwynne, Ronwen, Ronwena,
Ronwenah, Ronwene, Ronwin,
Ronwina, Ronwinah, Ronwine,
Ronwyn, Ronwyna, Ronwynah,
Ronwyne, Ronwynn, Ronwynna,
Ronwynnah, Ronwynne

Rhu (Hindi) purity.

Ria (Spanish) small river.
Riah, Rhia, Rhiah, Rhya, Rhyah,
Rya, Ryah

Riana (Irish) virtuous strength.
Rhiana, Rhianah, Rhiane, Rhiann,
Rhianna, Rhiannah, Rhianne,
Rhyana, Rhyanah, Rhyane,
Rhyanna, Rhyannah, Rhyanne,
Rianah, Riane, Riann, Rianna,
Riannah, Rianne, Ryan, Ryana,
Ryanah, Ryane, Ryann, Ryanna,
Ryannah, Ryanne

Riane (Irish/Gaelic) little queen.
The feminine form of Ryan.
Rhiana, Rhianah, Rhiane, Rhiann,
Rhianna, Rhiannah, Rhianne,

Rhyana, Rhyanah, Rhyane,
Rhyanna, Rhyannah, Rhyanne,
Riana, Rianah, Riann, Rianna,
Riannah, Rianne, Ryan, Ryana,
Ryanah, Ryane, Ryann, Ryanna,
Ryannah, Ryanne

Ricarda (Teutonic) powerful, hard
ruler. A feminine form of
Richard.
Rica, Ricah, Ricca, Riccah, Riccarda,
Riccardah, Richa, Richarda,
Richardah, Richardena,
Richardenda, Richardina, Richella,
Richelle, Richen, Richena,
Richendra, Richenza, Richenzah,
Richmal, Rickarda, Rickardah,
Rikarda, Rikardah, Ritcarda,
Ritcharda, Ritchardia, Rycarda,
Rycardah, Rycharda, Rychardah,
Ryckarda, Ryckardah, Rykarda,
Rykardah

Ricca (Spanish) ruler. A form of
Erica/Frederica/Ricarda.
Rhica, Rhicah, Rhicca, Rhiccah,
Rhika, Rhikah, Rhikka, Rhikkah,
Rica, Ricah, Riccah, Ricka, Rickah,
Rika, Rikah, Rikka, Rikkah, Riqua,
Riquah, Rique, Ryca, Rhycah,
Rycca, Ryccah, Rycka, Ryckah,
Ryka, Rykah, Rykka, Rykkah,
Ryqua, Ryquah, Ryque

Riccadonna (Italian) rich lady.
Ricadona, Ricadonah, Ricadonna,
Ricadonnah, Riccadona,
Riccadonah, Riccadonnah,
Rickadona, Rickadonah,
Rickadonna, Rickadonnah,
Rikadona, Rikadonah, Rikadonna,
Rikadonnah, Rycadona,
Rycadonah, Rycadonna,
Rycadonnah, Ryccadona,
Ryccadonah, Ryccadonna,
Ryccadonnah, Ryckadona,
Ryckadonah, Ryckadonna,
Ryckadonnah, Rykadona,

R

Riccadonna cont.
Rykadonah, Rykadonna,
Rykadonnah

Richael (Irish) saint.
Ricael, Rickael, Rikael, Rycael,
Ryckael, Rykael

Richelle (German/French) she is
rich and powerful. A feminine
form of Richard. A form of
Rachelle.
Richel, Richelah, Richele, Richell,
Richella, Richellah, Rishel, Rishela,
Rishelah, Rishele, Rishell, Rishella,
Rishellah, Rishelle, Rychel,
Rychela, Rychelah, Rychele,
Rychell, Rychella, Rychelle, Ryshel,
Ryshela, Ryshelah, Ryshele, Ryshell,
Ryshella, Ryshellah, Ryshelle

Ricki (English) rich, powerful ruler.
The feminine form of Ricky.
Rica, Ricah, Ricka, Rickah, Rickee,
Rickey, Rickie, Ricky, Rikee, Rikey,
Riki, Rikie, Rikkee, Rikkey, Rikki,
Rikkie, Rikky, Riky, Ryckee, Ryckey,
Rycki, Ryckie, Rykee, Rykey, Ryki,
Rykie, Ryky

Rickma (Hebrew) woven; given to a
child who looks like both her
parents.
Rickmah, Ricma, Ricmah, Ryckma,
Ryckmah, Rycma, Rycmah, Rykma,
Rykmah

Rida (Arabic) God has favoured her.
Ridah, Ryda, Rydah

Riddhi (Sanskrit) prosperous.
Ridhi

Rihana (Arabic) sweet basil herb.
Rhiana, Rhianah, Rhiane, Rhiann,
Rhianna, Rhiannah, Rhianne,
Rhyan, Rhyana, Rhyanah, Rhyane,
Rhyann, Rhyanna, Rhyannah,
Rhyanne, Riana, Rianah, Rianna,
Riannah, Rianne, Ryan, Ryana,
Ryanah, Ryane, Ryann, Ryanna,
Ryannah, Ryanne

Rika (Swedish) ruler.
Rhica, Rhicah, Rhicca, Rhiccah,
Rhika, Rhikah, Rhikka, Rhikkah,
Rica, Ricah, Ricca, Riccah, Ricka,
Rickah, Rikah, Rikka, Rikkah,
Riqua, Riquah, Rique, Ryca,
Rhycah, Rycca, Ryccah, Rycka,
Ryckah, Ryka, Rykah, Rykka,
Rykkah, Ryqua, Ryquah, Ryque

Riley (Irish) valiant; courageous.
Rilea, Rileah, Rilee, Rilei, Rileigh,
Rili, Rilie, Rily, Rylea, Ryleah,
Rylee, Rylei, Ryleigh, Ryley, Ryli,
Rylie, Ryly

Rilla (Teutonic) stream.
Rila, Rilah, Rillah, Rhila, Rhilah,
Rhilla, Rhillah, Rhyla, Rhylah,
Rhylla, Rhyllah, Ryla, Rylah, Rylla,
Ryllah

Rima (Spanish) poetry; rhyme.
Reama, Reamah, Reema, Reemah,
Rema, Remah, Rheama, Rheamah,
Rheema, Rheemah, Rheyma,
Rheymah, Rhima, Rhimah, Rhima,
Rhimah, Rhime, Rhyma, Rhymah,
Rimah, Ryma, Rymah

Rimona (Arabic) pomegranate, a
shrub with red fruit.
Reamona, Reamonah, Reamone,
Reemona, Reemonah, Reemone,
Remona, Remonah, Remone,
Rheimona, Rheimonah, Rheimone,
Rheymona, Rheymonah,
Rheymone, Rhimona, Rhimonah,
Rhimone, Rhymona, Rhymonah,
Rimonah, Rimone, Rymona,
Rymonah, Rymone

Rimu (Polynesian) red pine tree.
Rymu

Rin (Japanese) park.
Rini, Ryn, Ryny

Rina (Hebrew) happy; song.
Reana, Reanah, Reena, Reenah,
Reina, Reinah, Reyna, Reynah,
Rheana, Rheanah, Rheena,
Rheenah, Rheina, Rheinah, Rheyna,
Rheynah, Rinah, Ryna, Rynah

Riona (Irish) queen; saintly.
Reaona, Reaonah, Reeona,
Reeonah, Reona, Reonah, Rheaona,
Rheaonah, Rheeona, Rheeonah,
Rheiona, Rheionah, Rheona,
Rheonah, Rheyona, Rheyonah,
Rhionah, Rhyona, Rhyonah,
Rionah, Ryona, Ryonah

Risa (Latin) laughing.
Reasa, Reasah, Reesa, Reesah, Reisa,
Reisah, Resa, Resah, Rysa, Rysah

Risha (Hindi) born in the month of
Taurus.
Rishah, Rysha, Ryshah

Rishona (Hebrew) first-born child.
Rishonah, Ryshona, Ryshonah

Rissa (Greek) sea fairy.
Risa, Risah, Rissah, Rysa, Rysah,
Ryssa, Ryssah

Rita (French) daisy. (Grk) pear.
(Hin) brave strength.
Reata, Reatah, Reatta, Reattah,
Reeta, Reetah, Reetta, Reettah,
Reita, Reitah, Reitta, Reittah, Reta,
Retah, Retta, Rettah, Reyta, Reytah,
Reytta, Reyttah, Ritah, Ritta, Rittah,
Ryta, Rytah, Rytta, Ryttah

Ritsa (Greek) defender of
humankind. A form of Alexandra.
Ritsah, Rytsa, Rytsah

Riva/River (French) from the river
bank.
Riva (Fren), Rivah, Rivana,
Rivanah, Rivane, Rivanna,
Rivannah, Rivanne, Ryva, Ryvah,
Ryvana, Ryvanah, Ryvane, Ryvanna,
Ryvannah, Ryvanne, Ryver

Riverlea (Latin/Old English) from
the river meadow.
Riverleah, Rivalee, Rivalei,
Rivaleigh, Rivaley, Rivali, Rivalia,
Rivaliah, Rivaly, Rivalya, Rivalyah,
Ryva, Ryvah, Ryvalea, Ryvaleah,
Ryvalee, Ryvalei, Ryvaleigh, Ryvali,
Ryvalia, Ryvaliah, Ryvalie, Ryvaly,
Ryvalya, Ryvalyah

Rivkah (French) shore.
Riva, Rivah, River, Rivka, Ryva,
Ryvah, Ryvka, Ryvkah

Riza (Greek) harvester. A short form
of Teresa.
Riesa, Riesah, Rieser, Reiser, Rizus,
Rizah, Rizza, Rizzah, Ryza, Ryzah,
Ryzza, Ryzzah

Rizpah (Hebrew) hot stone.
Rizpa, Ryzpa, Ryzpah

Roannah (Hebrew) graceful rose.
Roan, Roana, Roanae, Roanah,
Roane, Roann, Roanna, Roannae,
Roannah, Rhoann, Rhoanna,
Rhoannah, Rhoanne

Roberta (Teutonic) brilliant;
famous. (O/Eng) bright flame.
The feminine form of Robert.
Bobina, Bobine, Bobinetta.
Bobinette, Robena, Robenah,
Robenia, Robeniah, Robertah,
Robertha, Robett, Robetta, Robette,
Robettia, Robettiah, Roben, Robin,
Robinatta, Robinette, Robinia,
Robiniah, Roburta, Roburtah,
Robyn, Robyna, Robynah, Robyne,
Ruberta, Ruperta

Robin (Old English) the robin bird.
Rebin, Rebina, Rebinah, Rebine,
Rebyna, Rebynah, Rebyne, Robban,
Robbana, Robbanah, Robbane,
Robben, Robbena, Robbenah,
Robbene, Robbin, Robbina,
Robbinah, Robbine, Robbon,
Robbyn, Robbyna, Robbynah,

Robin cont.
Robbyne, Robina, Robinah,
Robine, Robine, Robena, Robenah,
Robenia, Robinett, Robinetta,
Robinette, Robon, Robbon, Robyn,
Robynett, Robynetta, Robynette

Rochelle (Old French) she is little
like a rock.
Rachell, Rachella, Rachelle,
Rachetta, Rachette, Rashell,
Rashella, Rashelle, Rashetta,
Rashette, Rochel, Rochele, Rochell,
Rohcel, Rohcell, Rohcelle, Roshel,
Roshele, Roshell, Roshelle

Rocio (Latin) dew.
Rocyo

Roda (Polish) rose.
Rodah

Roderica (Teutonic) famous ruler.
The feminine form of Roderick.
Roderocah, Roderick, Rodericka,
Roderik, Roderika, Roderyc,
Roderyca, Roderycah, Roderyck,
Roderycka, Roderykya

Rodnae (English) from the island
clearing.
Rodna, Rodnah, Rodnai, Rodnay,
Rodneisha, Rodnesha, Rodneta,
Rodnete, Rodnett, Rodnetta,
Rodnette

Roesia (Old French) rose.
Rodica, Rodice, Rodicia, Roeesha,
Roedicia, Rohesia

Rohana (Hindi) sandalwood.
Rochana, Rochanah, Rohanah,
Rohanna, Rohannah, Rohena,
Rohenah

Rohini (Hindi) woman.
Rohinee, Rohiney, Rohinie, Rohiny,
Rohynee, Rohyney, Rohyni,
Rohynie, Rohyny

Roisin (Latin/Irish) rose.
Roisina, Roisinah, Roisine, Roisyn,
Roisyna, Roisynah, Roisyne,
Roysin, Roysina, Roysinah, Roysine,
Roysyn, Roysyna, Roysynah,
Roysyne

Rokeya (Persian) dawn.
Rokey, Rokeyah

Rokuko (Japanese) sixth-born child.

Rolanda (Teutonic) from the
famous land. The feminine form
of Roland.
Rolandah, Rolandia, Rolandiah,
Rolande (Fren), Rolandya,
Rolandyah, Orlanda (Ital),
Orlandah, Orlande

**Roma/Romaine/Romana/Romilda/
Romina** (Italian) from Rome.
Romah, Romain, Romaina,
Romainah, Romana, Romanah,
Romanda, Romanel, Romanela,
Romanele, Romanella, Romanelle,
Romanique, Romayna, Romaynah,
Romayne, Romel, Romela,
Romelah, Romele, Romelle,
Romilda, Romildah, Romilde,
Romina, Rominah, Romine,
Romyn, Romyna, Romynah,
Romyne

Romelda (German) roman warrior.
Romeld, Romeldah, Romelde,
Romilda, Romildah, Romilde,
Romildia, Romildiah, Romylda,
Romyldah, Romylde

Romia (Hebrew) highly praised.
Roma, Romiah, Romit, Romya,
Romyah

Romola (Latin) lady from Rome.
Romela, Romelah, Romele, Romell,
Romella, Romellah, Romelle,
Romellia, Romelliah, Romila,
Romilah, Romile, Romilla,
Romillah, Romille, Romillia,

R

Romolah, Romole, Romolla, Romollah, Romolle, Romyla, Romylah, Romyle, Romylla, Romyllah, Romylle

Romy (French) from Rome. The short form of Romaine.
Romee, Romey, Romi, Romia, Romiah, Romie, Romy, Romya, Romyah

Rona (Irish/Gaelic) seal. (Heb) song of joy. (Scand) powerful. The feminine form of Ronald.
Ronah, Ronna, Ronnah

Ronaele (Greek) shining light. Eleanor spelt backwards.

Ronalda (Old Norse) powerful. The feminine form of Ronald.
Rhonala, Rhonaldah, Rhonaldia, Rhonaldiah, Ronaldah, Ronaldia, Ronaldiah, Ronaldya, Ronaldyah

Roneisha (Welsh/Swahili) grand life.
Ronecia, Ronee, Roneeka, Roneice, Roneshia, Ronessa, Ronesse, Roneysha, Ronichia, Ronicia, Roniesha, Ronisha, Ronnesa, Ronnesha, Ronnisa, Ronnisha, Ronnishia, Ronnysha, Ronysha

Ronelle (Welsh/French) she is grand.
Ronel, Ronela, Ronelah, Ronele, Ronell, Ronella, Ronelle, Ronnel, Ronnela, Ronnelah, Ronnele, Ronnell, Ronella

Ronena (Hebrew) my song is happiness.
Ronenah, Ronenna, Ronennah

Roni (Hebrew) happy.
Rani, Rania, Raniah, Ranit, Ranita, Ranitah, Rany, Ranya, Ranyah, Renana, Renanit, Ronea, Ronee, Roney, Ronia, Roniah, Ronie, Ronit, Ronli, Ronilie, Ronnit. Rony, Ronya, Ronyah, Ronye

Roniya (Hebrew) God's happiness.
Ronia, Roniah, Roniyah, Ronya, Ronyah

Ronli (Hebrew) happy. (O/Eng) from the happy meadow.
Ronlea, Ronleah, Ronlei, Ronleigh, Ronley, Ronlia, Ronliah, Ronlie, Ronly, Ronoia, Roniah, Ronice, Ronit, Ronita, Ronite, Ronlea, Ronleah, Ronnlee, Ronnlei, Ronnleigh, Ronnley, Ronnli, Ronnliah, Ronnlie, Ronnly

Ronnette (Welsh) little grand one.
Ronet, Roneta, Ronetah, Ronete, Ronett, Ronetta, Ronettah

Roo (Australian/Australian Aboriginal) kangaroo. (O/Eng) compassionate. A form of Ruth, kind-hearted vision of beauty.
Ru, Rue

Roondeau (French) poem.

Rori/Rory (Latin) aurora; dawn. (Ir) famous ruler.
Roarea, Roaree, Roaorey, Roari, Roarie, Roary, Rorea, Roree, Roria, Roriah, Rorie, Rory, Rorya, Roryah

Rosa (Latin) rose.
Rois (Ir), Roosje (Dut), Rosah, Rosabel, Rosabela, Rosabelah, Rosabele, Rosabele, Rosabell, Rosabella, Rosabellah, Rosabelle, Rosan, Rosana, Rosanah, Rosane, Rosann, Rosanna, Rosannah, Rosanne, Rosea, Rosean, Roseana, Roseanah, Roseane, Roseann, Roseanna, Roseannah, Roseanne, Rosebel, Rosebela, Rosebelah, Rosebele, Rosebell, Rosebella, Rosebelle, Rosebud, Rosey, Rosia, Rosiah, Rosie, Rosy, Rosya, Rosyah

Rosabelle (Latin) beautiful rose.
Rosabel, Rosabela, Rosabelah, Rosabele, Rosabell, Rosabella,

Rosabelle cont.
Rosabellah, Rosabellia,
Rosabelliah, Rosebel, Rosebela,
Rosebelah, Rosebele, Rosebell,
Rosebella, Rosebellah, Rosebelle,
Rosebellia, Rosebelliah, Rozabel,
Rozabela, Rozabelah, Rzabele,
Rozabell, Rozabella, Rozabellah,
Rozabelle, Rozebel, Rozebela,
Rozebelah, Rozebele, Rozebell,
Rozebella, Rozebellah, Rozebelle

Rosalba (Latin) white rose.
Rosalbah

Rosalee (Latin/Old English) from
the rose meadow.
Rosalea, Rosaleah, Rosalei,
Rosaleigh, Rosali, Rosalia,
Rosaliah, Rosalie, Roselea,
Roseleah, Roselee, Roselei,
Roseleigh, Roseli, Roselia, Roseliah,
Roselie, Rosely, Rozalea, Rozaleah,
Rozalee, Rozalei, Rozaleigh,
Rozaley, Rozali, Rozalia, Rozaliah,
Rozalie, Rozaly, Rozlea, Rozleah,
Rozlee, Rozlei, Rozleigh, Rozley,
Rozli, Rozlia, Rozliah, Rozlie, Rozly

Rosalind (Irish) little rose. (Span)
lovely rose. (O/Ger) horse.
Rosalean, Rosaleana, Rosaleanah,
Rosaleane, Rosaleen, Rosaleena,
Rosaleenah, Rosaleene, Rosalinda,
Rosalindah, Rosaline, Rosalyn,
Rosalyna, Rosalynah, Rosalynda,
Rosalyndah, Rosalynde, Rosalyne,
Rosalynda, Rosalyndah, Roselean,
Roseleane, Roseleen, Roseleena,
Roselin, Roselina, Roselinah,
Roseline, Roslan, Roslana,
Roslanah, Roslane, Roslain,
Roslane, Roslin, Roslina, Roslinah,
Rosline, Roslinia, Rosliniah,
Rosliniah, Roslyn, Roslynda,
Roslyndah, Roslyne, Rozalan,
Rozalana, Rozalanah, Rozalane,

Rozalain, Rozalaina, Rozalainah,
Rozalaine, Rozalin, Rozalina,
Rozalinah, Rozalind, Rozalinda,
Rozalindah, Rozalinde, Rozelan,
Rozelana, Rozelanah, Rozelane,
Rozelain, Rozelaina, Rozelainah,
Rozelaine, Rozelan, Rozelanah,
Rozelane, Rozelin, Rozelina,
Rozelinah, Rozelinda, Rozelindah,
Rozeline, Rozelyn, Rozelyna,
Rozelynah, Rozelynd, Rozelynda,
Rozelyndah, Rozelynde, Rozelyne,
Rozlain, Rozlaina, Rozlainah,
Rozlaine, Rozlayn, Rozlaynah,
Rozlin, Rozlina, Rozlinah, Rozline,
Rozlyn, Rozlynah, Rozlyne,
Rozlynn, Rozlynna, Rozlynnah,
Rozlynne

Rosamond (Teutonic) famous
prophet. (Lat/Fren) rose of the
world; rose of purity.
Rosamonda, Rosamondah,
Rosamonde, Rosamund (Span),
Rosamunda, Rosamundah,
Rosemonda, Rosemondah,
Rosemonde (Fren), Rosemund,
Rosemunda, Rosemundah,
Rosiemond, Rosiemund,
Rosiemunda, Rozamond,
Rozamonda, Rozmond (Dut),
Rozmonda, Rozmondah,
Rozmonde, Rozmund, Rozmunda,
Rozmundah, Rozmundah,
Rozmunde

Rosanna (English) graceful rose. A
combination of Rose/Ann.
Rosana, Rosanah, Rosane, Rosann,
Rosannah, Rosanne, Roseann,
Roseanna, Roseannah, Roseanne

Rosaria/Rosario (Italian) rosary.
Rosariah, Rosarya, Rosaryah,
Rozaria, Rozariah, Rozarya,
Rozaryah, Rozaryo (Span)

Roschan (Hindi) sunrise.

Roscrana (Celtic) rosebush.
Roscranah

Rose/Rosie (Latin/Irish/English) the
rose flower.
Rosa, Rosae, Rosah, Rosan, Rosana,
Rosanae, Rosanah, Rosane, Rosani,
Rosania, Rosaniah, Rosanie,
Rosalea, Rosaleah, Rosalean,
Rosaleana, Rosaleanah, Rosaleane,
Rosalee, Rosaleen, Rosaleena,
Rosaleenah, Rosaleene, Rosalei,
Rosaleigh, Rosalein, Rosaleina,
Rosaleinah, Rosaleine, Rosaley,
Rosali, Rosalia, Rosaliah, Rosalie,
Rosalin, Rosalina, Rosalinah,
Rosaline, Rosall, Rosalla, Rosallah,
Rosalle, Rosaly, Rosalyna,
Rosalynah, Rosalyne, Rosann,
Rosanna, Rosannae, Rosannah,
Rosanne, Rosea, Roseah, Rosean,
Roseana, Roseanah, Roseane,
Roseann, Roseanna, Roseannah,
Roseanne, Rosee, Roselea,
Roseleah, Roselean, Roseleana,
Roseleanah, Roseleane, Roselee,
Roseleen, Roseleena, Roseleenah,
Roseleene, Roselei, Roseleigh,
Roseley, Roseli, Rosleia, Roseliah,
Roselie, Roselin, Roselina,
Roselinah, Roseline, Rosely,
Roselyn, Roselyna, Roselynah,
Roselyne, Rosey, Rosi, Rosia,
Rosiah, Rosian, Rosiana, Rosianah,
Rosiane, Rosiann, Rosianna,
Rosiannah, Rosianne, Rosie, Rosy,
Rosya, Rosyah, Rosyan, Rosyana,
Rosyanah, Rosyane, Rosyann,
Rosyanna, Rosyannah, Rosyanne,
Rosye, Roza, Rozah, Rozalea,
Rozaleah, Rozalee, Rozalei,
Rozaleigh, Rozaley, Rozali, Rozalia
(Pol), Rozaliah, Rozalie, Rozan,
Rozana, Rozanah, Rozane, Rozann,
Rozanna, Rozannah, Rozannia,
Rozanniah, Rozannie, Rozanny,
Rozannya, Roze, Rozea, Rozeah,
Rozean, Rozeana, Rozeanah,
Rozeann, Rozeanna, Rozeannah,
Rozel, Rozela, Rozelah, Rozele,
Rozell, Rozella, Rozellah, Rozelle,
Rozellia, Rozelliah, Rozet, Rozeta,
Rozetah, Rozete, Rozett, Rozetta,
Rozettah, Rozette, Rozanne, Rozin,
Rozina (Slav), Rozsi (Hung),
Rozzann, Rozzanna, Rozzannah,
Rozzanne, Rozzannia, Rozzanniah,
Rozzanya, Rozzanyah

Roseanne (Latin) pretty rose.
Rosan, Rosana, Rosanah, Rosania,
Rosaniah, Rosann, Rosanna,
Rosannah, Rosannia, Rosanniah,
Rosean, Roseana, Roseanah,
Roseania, Roseaniah, Roseann,
Roseanna, Roseannah, Roseannia,
Roseanniah, Rozan, Rozana,
Rozanah, Rozane, Rozann,
Rozanna, Rozannah, Rozanne,
Rozannia, Rozanniah, Rozanny,
Rozannya, Rozean, Rozeana,
Rozeanah, Rozeane, Rozeann,
Rozeanna, Rozeannah, Rozeanne

Rosedale (Latin/Old English) from
the valley of the roses.
Rosedalia, Rosedaliah, Rosedail,
Rosedailia, Rosedayl, Rosedayla,
Rosedayle

Roselani (English/Filipino)
heavenly rose.
Roselana, Roselanah, Roselanea,
Roselanee, Roselaney, Roselani,
Roselania, Roselaniah, Roselanie,
Roselany, Roselanya, Roslan,
Roslana, Roslanah, Roslanea,
Roslanee, Roslaney, Roslania,
Roslaniah, Roslanie, Roslain,
Roslane, Roslany, Roslanya, Roslin,
Roslina, Roslinah, Rosline, Roslyn,
Roslyna, Roslynah, Roslyne

Rosemary (Latin) the rosemary herb.
Rosemarea, Rosemaree, Rose-Maree, Rosemarey, Rose-Marey, Rosemari, Rose-Mari, Rosemaria, Rose-Maria, Rosemariah, Rose-Mariah, Rosemarie, Rose-Marie, Rosemarya, Rose-Marya, Rosemaryah, Rose-Maryah, Rozmaree, Rozmarey, Rozmari, Rozmaria, Rozmariah, Rozmarie, Rozmary, Rozmarya, Rozmaryah

Rosetta (Latin) little rose.
Roset, Roseta, Rosetah, Rosete, Rosett, Rosettah, Rosette, Rozet, Rozeta, Rozetah, Rozete, Rozett, Rozettah, Rozette

Roshan (Sanskrit) shining light.
Roshaina, Roshainah, Roshaine, Roshana, Roshanah, Roshane, Roshani, Roshania, Roshaniah, Roshanie, Roshany, Roshanya, Roshanya, Roshanyah

Rosina (English) rose.
Roseana, Roseanah, Roseane, Roseena, Roseenah, Roseene, Rosena, Rosenah, Rosene, Rosheen, Rosheena, Rosheene, Rosinah, Rosine, Rosyna, Rosynah, Rosyne, Roxina, Roxinah, Roxine, Roxyna, Roxynah, Roxyne, Rozeana, Rozeanah, Rozeane, Rozeena, Rozeenah, Rozeene, Rozena, Rozenah, Rozene, Rozina, Rozinah, Rozine, Rozyna, Rozynah, Rozyne

Rosita (Spanish) rose.
Roseat, Roseata, Roseatah, Roseate, Roseet, Roseeta, Roseetah, Roseete, Roset, Roseta, Rosetah, Rosete, Rosetta, Rosettah, Rosette, Rosit, Rositah, Rosite, Rositt, Rositta, Rosittah, Rositte, Rosyt, Rosyta, Rosytah, Rosyte, Rozeta, Rozetah, Rozete, Rozetta, Rozettah, Rozette, Rozit, Rozita, Rozitah, Rozite,

Rozyt, Rozyta, Rozytah, Rozyte, Rozytt, Rozytta, Rozyttah, Rozytte

Rossalyn (Scottish) from the cape; headland meadow. (O/Eng) from the rose pool.
Rosalin, Rosaline, Rosalyn, Rosalyne, Rossalin, Rossaline, Rossalyn, Rossalyne

Roto (Maori) lake.

Rouge (French) blush.

Roula (Greek) rebel.
Roulah

Rowan (Old Norse) mountain ash tree. (Celt) little red-haired one.
Rhoan, Rhoana, Rhoanah, Rhoane, Rhoann, Rhoanna, Rhosnnah, Rhoanne, Rhoen, Rhoin, Rhoina, Rhoinah, Rhoine, Rhoinn, Rhoinna, Rhoinnah, Rhoinne, Rohan, Rohana, Rohanah, Rohane, Rohann, Rohanna, Rohannah, Rohanne, Rowana, Rowanah, Rowane, Rowen, Rowena, Rowenah, Rowene, Rowin, Rowina, Rowinah, Rowine, Rowon, Rowona, Rowonah, Rowone, Rowyn, Rowyna, Rowynah, Rowyne, Rowynn, Rowynna, Rowynnah, Rowynne

Rowena (Old English) famous friend. (Celt) slender; light-haired; white.
Rana, Ranah, Ranna, Rannah, Rena, Renah, Renna, Rennah, Rhoina, Rhoinah, Rohena, Rohenah, Rohenia, Roweana, Roweanah, Roweena, Roweenah, Rowein, Roweina, Rowen, Rowena, Rowina, Rowinah, Rowyna, Rowynah, Rowyne, Rowynna, Rowynnah

Roxanne (Persian) sunrise.
Rexan, Rexana, Rexanah, Rexane, Rexann, Rexanna, Rexannah,

R

Rexanne, Roxan, Roxana, Roxanah,
Roxane, Roxann, Roxanna,
Roxannah, Roxanne, Roxannia,
Roxanniah, Roxannie, Roxanny

Royale (Old French) royal. A
feminine form of Roy.
Roial, Roiala, Roiale, Roiell,
Roielle, Royal, Royala, Royel, Royel,
Royela, Royele, Royell, Royella,
Royelle

Royanna (English) gracious queen.
A feminine form of Roy.
Roiana, Roianah, Roiane, Roianna,
Roiannah, Roianne, Royana,
Royanah, Royane, Royannah,
Royanne

Roz (English/Spanish) fair rose. The
short form of Rosalind, little
rose.
Ros, Ross, Rozz

Roza (Slavic) rose.
Rosa, Rosah, Rozah, Rozalia,
Rozaliah, Rozel, Rozela,Rozele,
Rozell, Rozella, Rozellah, Rozelle,
Rozita, Rozite, Rozyta, Rozyte,
Ruzuna, Ruzunah, Ruzune,
Ruzena, Ruzenah, Ruzene,
Ruzenka, Ruzha, Ruzsa, Ruzsah

Rozelle (Greek/French) she is a
rose.
Rosel, Rosela, Roselah, Rosele,
Rosell, Rosella, Rosellah, Roselle,
Rozel, Rozela, Rozekah, Rozele,
Rozell, Rozella, Rozellah, Rozin,
Rozina, Rozinah, Rozine, Rozyn,
Rozyna, Rozynah, Rozyne

Rozena (Native American) rose
blossom.
Rozeana, Rozeanah, Rozeane,
Rozeena, Rozeenah, Rozeene,
Rozenaa, Rozenah, Rozina,
Rozinah, Rozine, Rozyn, Rozyna,
Rozynah, Rozyne

Ruana (Hindi) musical instrument.
Ruanah, Ruane, Ruann, Ruanna,
Ruannah, Ruanne, Ruon

Rubena (Hebrew) behold, a
daughter.
Reubena, Rubenah, Rubenia,
Rubeniah, Rubina, Rubinah,
Rubibia, Rubibiah, Rubyna,
Rubynah

Rubina/Ruby (French) the ruby
gem. (Lat) red.
Rube, Rubea, Rubee, Rubet, Rubett,
Rubetta, Rubette, Rubey, Rubi,
Rubia, Rubiah, Rubie, Rubina,
Rubine, Rubinia, Rubiniah, Rubis,
Rubyn, Rubyna, Rubynah, Rubyne,
Rubis, Rubys

Ruchi (Hindi) wanting to please.
Ruchee, Ruchey, Ruchie, Ruchy

Ruchika (Hindi) pretty.
Ruchikah

Rudee (German) famous wolf. A
feminine short form of Rudolph.
Rudea, Rudey, Rudi, Rudia, Rudiah,
Rudie, Rudy, Rudya, Rudyah

Rudelle (Teutonic/French) she is
famous.
Rudel, Rudela, Rudele, Rudell,
Rudella, Rudellah

Rudi/Rudy (German) famous wolf;
flame. The feminine form of
Rudy.
Rudea, Rudee, Rudey, Rudia,
Rudiah, Rudie, Rudya, Rudyah

Rudolfa (Polish) famous wolf. A
feminine form of Rudolph.
Rudolfea, Rudolfee, Rudolfia,
Rudolfiah, Rudophee, Rudolphey,
Rudolphia, Rudolphiah

Rudra (Hindi) seeds.
Rud, Rudee, Rudey, Rudi, Rudia,

Rudra cont.
Rudiah, Rudie, Rudrah, Rudy,
Rudya, Rudyah

Rue (English) strong herbs; regret.
(Ger) famous. (Fren) street.
Roo (Aust), Ru, Ruey

Ruel (Old English) path.
Rual, Ruela, Ruelah, Ruele, Ruell,
Ruella, Ruellah, Ruelle

Rufina (Italian) red-haired. The
feminine form of Rufus.
Rufeana, Rufeanah, Rufeane,
Rufeena, Rufeenah, Rufeene,
Rufinah, Rufinia, Rufiniah,
Rufynia, Rufyniah, Rufynya,
Rufynyah, Ruphina, Ruphinah,
Ruphinia, Ruphiniah, Ruphynia,
Ruphyniah, Ruphynya, Ruphynyah

Rui (Japanese) affectionate; tears.
Ru

Rukan (Arabic) steady; confident.
Rukana, Rukanah, Rukane, Rukann,
Rukanna, Rukannah, Rukanne

Rukiya (Swahili) rising.
Rukiyah

Rukmini (Hindi) gold.
Rukminie, Rukminy

Rula (Latin) ruler.
Ruela, Ruelah, Rulah, Rular, Rule,
Ruler, Rulla, Rullah, Rulor

Rumer (Gypsy) gypsy.
Rouma, Roumah, Roumar, Ruma,
Rumah, Rumar, Rumor

Runa (Old Norse) flowing secret.
Runah, Rune, Runes, Runna,
Runnag, Runne

Rupal (Hindi) beauty.

Ruri (Japanese) emerald.
Ruriko

Rusalka (Russian) mermaid.
(Slavic) a fairy from the forest.
Rusalkah

Russhell (French) red-haired; fox.
The feminine form of Russell.
Rushel, Rushela, Rushelah,
Rushele, Rushell, Rushella,
Rushellah, Rushelle, Russhel,
Russhela, Russhelah, Russhele,
Russhella, Russhellah, Russhelle

Rusty (English) tawny;
reddish/brown-coloured hair.
Ruste, Rustee, Rustey, Rusti, Rustie

Ruta (Hawaiian) friendly.
Rutah

Ruth (Hebrew) kind-hearted;
vision of beauty.
(O/Eng) compassionate.
Rooth, Routh, Rueth, Rute (Lith),
Rutha, Ruthe, Rutherina. Ruthery,
Ruthina

Ruza (Slavic) rose.
Ruz, Ruze, Ruzena, Ruzenah,
Ruzenka (Russ), Ruzenkah, Ruzha,
Ruzsa

Ryann (Irish) little queen. The
feminine form of Ryan.
Rian, Riana, Rianah, Riane, Riann,
Rianna, Riannah, Rianne, Ryana,
Ryanah, Ryane, Ryanna, Ryannah,
Ryanne

Ryba (Slavic) fish.
Riba, Ribah, Rybah

Rylee (Irish) valiant; courageous.
Rilea, Rileah, Rilee, Rilei, Rileigh,
Riley, Rili, Rilie, Rylea, Ryleah,
Rylei, Ryleigh, Ryley, Ryli, Rylie,
Ryly

Ryo (Japanese) dragon.

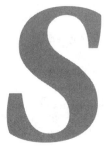

Saada (Hebrew) one who gives support.
Saadah, Sada, Sadah

Saarah (Arabic) princess. A form of Sara.
Saara, Saarra, Saarrah, Sara, Sarah, Sarra, Sarrah

Saba (Hebrew) old. (Grk) woman from Sheba. (Arab) morning.
Sabah, Sabba, Sabbah

Sabara (Hebrew) thorny cactus.
Sabarah, Sabarra, Sabra, Sabrah

Sabbatha (Latin) child born on a Sunday.
Sabbathe

Sabina (Latin) the Sabines (ancient people who once lived in Italy).
Sabiennea, Sabienne, Sabinah, Sabine, Sabinka, Sabinna, Sabiny, Saby, Sabyna, Sabyne, Savina, Savinah, Savine, Savyna, Savynah, Savyne, Sebina, Sebinah, Sebine, Sebyn, Sebyna, Sebynah, Sebyne

Sabiya (Arabic) morning east wind.
Saba, Sabah, Sabaya, Sabayah, Sabya, Sabyah

Sable (English) soft fur.
Sabel, Sabela, Sabelah, Sabele, Sabella, Sabelle

Sabra (Hebrew) thorny.
(Arab) restful.
Sabea, Sabena, Sabenah, Sabene, Sabia, Sabiah, Sabie, Sabin, Sabine, Sabinella, Sabrah, Sabyn, Sabyne, Savina, Savinah, Savine, Savyn, Savyna, Savynah, Savyne

Sabrina (Latin) boundary. (Heb) seventh daughter; promise. A form of Bathsheba/Sheba.
Sabre, Sabreana, Sabreanah, Sabreane, Sabreen, Sabreena, Sabreenah, Sabreene, Sabrin, Sabrinah, Sabrine, Sabrinia, Sabriniah, Sabryna, Sabrynah, Sabryne, Sebrina, Sebrinah, Xabrina, Xabrinah, Xabryna, Xabrynah, Zabrina, Zabrinah, Zabrine, Zabryna, Zabrynah, Zabryne

Sabriyya (Arabic) patient.
Sabriya

Sacha (Greek) defender of humankind. A form of Alexandra.
Sachah, Sahsha, Sasa, Sascha, Saschae, Sasha, Sashah, Sashana, Sashel, Sashenka, Sashia, Sashiah, Sashira, Sashsha, Sashya, Shashyah, Sasjara, Sasshalai, Shashia, Shura, Shurah, Shurka

Sachi (Japanese) bringer of bliss.
Sachiko

Sada (Old English) seed.
Sadah, Sadda, Saddah, Sadel, Sadela, Sadelah, Sadele, Sadell, Sadella, Sadellah, Sadelle

Sade/Sadie (Hebrew) princess. A form of Sara.
Sadea, Sadey, Sadi, Sadie, Sady, Saedea, Saedee, Saedi, Saedie, Saedy, Saidea, Saidee, Saidi, Saidie, Saidy, Saydea, Saydee, Saydi, Saydie, Saydy, Shadae, Shadai, Shaday, Shardae, Shardai, Sharday

Sadhana (Hindi) devoted.
Sadhanah, Sadhanna, Sadhannah

S

Sadira (Persian) lily. (Arab) star.
Sadirah, Sadire, Sadra, Sadrah,
Sadyra, Sadyrah, Sadyre

Sadiya (Arabic) lucky.
Sadia, Sadiah, Sadya, Sadyah

Sadzi (Carrier) sunny; happy.
Sadzee, Sadzey, Sadzia, Sadziah,
Sadzie, Sadzy, Sadzya, Sadyzah

Safa (Arabic) purity.
Safah, Saffa, Saffah

Safaia (Tongan) the sapphire stone;
blue.
Safaiah, Safaya, Safayah

Saffi (Dansih) wisdom.
Safee, Safey, Saffee, Saffey, Saffie,
Safee, Safey, Safi, Safie, Saffy, Safy

Saffron (Arabic) yellow/orange
colour.
Safron, Safrona, Safronah, Safrone,
Saffronna, Saffronnah

Safiya (Arabic) purity; best friend.
Safeia, Safeya, Saffa, Saffah, Safia,
Safiah, Safiya, Safiyah

Sagara (Hindi) sea.
Sagarah

Sage (Latin) healthy wisdom.
Saeg, Saege, Saig, Saige, Sayg, Sayge

Sahar (Arabic) dawn.
Sahara, Saharah

Sahara (Arabic) from the desert.
Sahar, Saharah, Saharra, Saharrah

Sai (Tongan) good. (Jap) talented.
Saiko (Jap), Saisai, Say

Saidah (Arabic) lucky; happy.
Saeda, Saedah, Saida, Sayda, Saydah

Sakae (Japanese) wealthy.
Sakai, Sakaie, Sakay

Sakara (Native American) sweet.
Sakarah, Sakaree, Sakari, Sakaria,

Sakariah, Sakarie, Sakary, Sakarya,
Sakaryah, Sakkara, Sakkarah

Saki (Arabic) giver. (Jap) cloak and
a rice wine.
Sakee, Sakia, Sakiah, Sakie, Saky,
Sakya, Sakyah

Sakti (Hindi) energy.
Saktee, Saktey, Saktia, Saktiah,
Sakty, Sakta, Saktyah

Sakuna (Native American) bird.
Sakunah

Sakura (Japanese) cherry blossom;
wealthy.
Sakurah

Sala (Hindi) the sala tree; sacred
tree.
Salah, Salla, Sallah

Salali (Cherokee) squirrel.
Salalea, Salaleah, Salalee, Salalei,
Salaleigh, Salalia, Salaliah, Salalie,
Salaly, Salalya, Salalyah

Salama (Arabic) peaceful.
Salamah, Zalama, Zalamah,
Zulima, Zulimah, Zulyma,
Zulymah

Salato (Tongan) tree.

Sale (Hawaiian) princess. A form of
Sara.
Saarai, Sera

Salena (Latin) from the salty place.
(Eng) princess. A form of Sally.
Salana, Salanah, Salane, Salean,
Saleana, Saleanah, Saleane, Saleen,
Saleena, Saleenah, Saleene, Salen,
Salenah, Salene, Salina, Salinah,
Saline, Salinee, Salleen, Salleena,
Salleenah, Salleene, Sallin, Sallina,
Sallinah, Salline, Sallyn, Sallyna,
Sallynah, Sallyne, Sallynee, Salyn,
Salyna, Salynah, Salyne, Xalean,
Xaleana, Xaleanah, Xaleane,
Xaleen, Xaleena, Xaleenah,

S

Xaleene, Xalena, Xalenah, Xalina, Xalinah, Xaline, Xalyna, Xalynah, Xalyne, Zalean, Zaleana, Zaleanah, Zaleane, Zaleena, Zaleenah, Zaleene, Zalena, Zalenah, Zalene, Zalina, Zalinah, Zaline, Zalyna, Zalynah, Zalyne

Salette (English) little Sally; little princess.
Salet, Saleta, Saletah, Salete, Salett, Saletta, Salettah, Sallet, Salleta, Salletta, Sallettah, Sallette

Salida (Hebrew) happy.
Salidah, Salyda, Salydah

Salihah (Arabic) purity.

Salima (Arabic) safe.
Salimah, Salyma, Salymah

Salina (French) solemn.
Salana, Salanah, Salane, Salean, Saleana, Saleanah, Saleane, Saleen, Saleena, Saleenah, Saleene, Salen, Salena, Salenah, Salene, Salinah, Saline, Salinee, Salleen, Salleena, Salleenah, Salleene, Sallin, Sallina, Sallinah, Salline, Sallyn, Sallyna, Sallynah, Sallyne, Sallynee, Salyn, Salyna, Salynah, Salyne, Xalean, Xaleana, Xaleanah, Xaleane, Xaleen, Xaleena, Xaleenah, Xaleene, Xalena, Xalenah, Xalina, Xalinah, Xaline, Xalyna, Xalynah, Xalyne, Zalean, Zaleana, Zaleanah, Zaleane, Zaleena, Zaleenah, Zaleene, Zalena, Zalenah, Zalene, Zalina, Zalinah, Zaline, Zalyna, Zalynah, Zalyne

Salliann (English) graceful princess.
Saleann, Saleanna, Saleannah, Saleanne, Saleean, Saleeanah, Saleeane, Saleeann, Saleeanna, Saleeannah, Saleeanne, Saliana, Salianah, Saliane, Saliann, Salianna, Saliannah, Salianne, Salleeann, Salleeanna, Salleeanne,

Sallianna, Salliannah, Sallianne, Sallyann, Sallyanna, Sallyannah, Sallyanne

Sally (Hebrew) princess.
Salea, Saleah, Salee, Salei, Saleigh, Saley, Sali, Salia, Saliah, Salie, Sallea, Salleah, Sallee, Sallei, Salleigh, Salley, Salli, Sallia, Salliah, Sallie, Sallya, Sallyah, Sallye, Saly, Salya, Salyah, Salye

Salma (Swahili) one who is safe.
Salmah

Salome (Hebrew) peaceful.
Salaome (Lith), Saloma, Salomah, Salome, Salomea (Pol), Salomee (Fren), Salomeli (Swed), Salomi, Salomia, Salomiah, Salomya, Salomyah

Salote (Polynesian) lady.

Salvadora (Spanish) saved. The feminine form of Salvadore.
Salvadorah

Salvia (Latin) strong; healthy; wisdom.
Sallvia, Sallviah, Salviah, Salviana, Salvianah, Salviane, Salvianna, Salvianne, Salvina, Salvinah, Salvine, Salvyn, Salvyna, Salvynah, Salvyne

Salwa (Arabic) bringer of comfort.
Salwah

Sam (Hebrew) her name is God; asked for; listening. The short form of names starting with 'Sam' e.g. Samantha.
Sama, Samah, Sami, Samia, Samiah, Samm, Samma, Sammah, Sammi, Sammia, Sammiah, Sammy, Sammya, Sammyah, Samy, Samya, Samyah, Xam, Xama, Xamah, Xami, Xamia, Xamiah, Xamm, Xamma, Xammah, Xammi, Xammia, Xammiah, Xammy,

Sam cont.
Xammya, Xammyah, Xamy, Xamya,
Xamya, Xamyah, Zam, Xama,
Zamah, Zami, Zamia, Zamiah,
Zamm, Zamma, Zammah, Zammi,
Zammia, Zammiah, Zammy,
Zammya, Zammyah, Zamy, Zamya,
Zamya, Zamyah

Samala (Hebrew) her name is God;
asked for.
Samalah, Samale, Sammala,
Sammalah

Samantha (Aramaic) listening.
Samana, Samanath, Samanatha,
Samanfa, Samanffa, Samanitha,
Samanta, Samanthah, Samanth,
Samanthe, Samanthi, Samanthia,
Samanthiah, Sammanfa,
Sammanffa, Sammanth,
Sammantha, Sammanthia,
Sammanthiah, Sammanthya,
Sammanthyah, Semenfa,
Semenfah, Semenffa, Semenffah,
Semantha, Xamanfa, Xamanfah,
Xamanffa, Xamanffah, Xamantha,
Xamanthah, Zamantha, Zamathia,
Zamanthiah, Zammantha,
Zammanthia, Zammanthiah,
Zammanthya, Zammanthyah

Samar/Samara/Samariah (Arabic)
one who talks at night. (Arab)
guarded; ruled by God; watcher.
Samara, Samarah

Sameh (Hebrew) listening.
(Arab) forgiving.
Samaiya, Samaya

Samena (Tongan) secret.
Samenah

Sami (Arabic) praised. (Heb) asked
for. The short form of names
starting with 'Sam' e.g. Samantha.
Samea, Samee, Samey, Sami,
Samie, Samm, Sammea, Sammee,
Sammey, Sammi, Sammie, Sammy,

Samo, Samy, Xamea, Xamee,
Xamey, Xami, Xamie, Xamm,
Xammea, Xammee, Xammey,
Xammi, Xammie, Xammy, Xamo,
Xamy, Zamea, Zamee, Zamey,
Zami, Zamie, Zamm, Zammea,
Zammee, Zammey, Zammi,
Zammie, Zammy, Zamo, Zamy

Samia (Arabic) one who
understands.
Samiah, Samya, Samyah

Samina (Hindi) happiness.
(Eng/Heb) little Sam; little asked-
for one.
Saminah, Samyna, Samynah

Samira (Arabic) entertainer.
Samir, Samirah, Samire, Samyra,
Samyrah, Samyre

Samuela (Hebrew) her name is
God; asked for. The feminine
form of Samuel.
Samala, Samalah, Samelia,
Samella, Samiella, Samielle,
Samilla, Samille, Sammila,
Sammile, Samuella, Samuelle,
Xamuela, Xamuelah, Xamuele,
Xamuell, Xamuella, Xamuellah,
Xamuelle, Zamuel, Zamuela,
Zamuelah, Zamuele, Zamuell,
Zamuella, Zamuellah, Zamuelle

Samya (Hebrew) rising.
Samia, Samiah, Samyh

Sana (Hebrew) lily. (Arab)
mountain top.
Sanaa, Sanah

Sananda (Hindi) happiness.
Sanansah

Sanchia/Sanchia (Latin) sacred
purity.
Sancheska, Sancha, Sanchia,
Sanchiah, Sanchie, Sanchya,
Sanchyah, Sancia, Sanciah, Sancha,
Sanche, Sancta, Saint, Sanctia,

Sanctussa (Ital), Santuzza, Sancya
(Pol), Sancyah, Santussa, Santuzza,
Sanzia, Sanziah, Sanzya, Sanzyah,
Sayntes, Sens, Senses, Synthia,
Synthya, Synthyah

Sandeep (Punjabi) enlightened.

Sandra/Sandre/Sandrica/Sandy
(Greek) defender of humankind.
The short form of Alexandra/
Cassandra.
Sandea, Sandee, Sandey, Sandi,
Sandia, Sandiah, Sandrea,
Sandreah, Sandreana, Sandreanah,
Sandreane, Sandreen, Sandreena,
Sandreenah, Sandreene, Sandreia,
Sandreiah, Sandrella, Sandrellah,
Sandrelle, Sandrenna, Sandrennah,
Sandrenne, Sandria, Sandriah,
Sandrica, Sandricah, Sandricka,
Sandrickah, Sandrika, Sandrikah,
Sandrina, Sandrinah, Sandrine,
Sandryca, Sandrycah, Sandrycka,
Sandryckah, Sandryka, Sandrykah,
Sandryna, Sandrynah, Sandryne,
Sandy, Xandea, Xandee, Xandi,
Xandia, Xandiah, Xandie, Xandrea,
Xandreah, Xandrean, Xandreanah,
Xandreane, Xandreen, Xandreena,
Xandreenah, Xandreene, Xandreia,
Xandreiah, Xandrina, Xandrinah,
Xandrine, Xandryna, Xandrynah,
Xandy, Zandea, Zandee, Zandey,
Zandi, Zandia, Zandiah, Zandrea,
Zandreah, Zandreen, Zandreena,
Zandreenah, Zandreene,
Zandreina, Zandreinah, Zandreine,
Zandrina, Zandrinah, Zandrine,
Zandryna, Zandrynah, Zandryne,
Zandy

Sandyha (Hindi) twilight.
Sandiha

Sangata (Tongan) saint.
Sangatah

Sanjana (Sanskrit) knowing right
from wrong.
Sanjanah, Sanyana, Sanyanah

Sanne (Hebrew/Dutch) lily flower.
Sanneen, Sanneena

Sansana (Hebrew) palm-tree leaf.
Sansanah

Santa (Latin) saint.
Sainta, Saintah, Santah, Saynta,
Sayntah

Santana (Spanish) saint.
Santa, Santah, Santania, Santaniah,
Santaniata, Santanna, Santanne,
Santena, Santenah, Santenna,
Santina, Santinah, Santine,
Santyna, Santynah, Santyne,
Shantana, Shantanna

Santavana (Hindi) hope.
Santavanah

Santillana (Spanish) soft-haired.
Santillanah

Santina (Spanish) little saint.
Santin, Santinah, Santine, Santinia,
Santyn, Santyna, Santynah,
Santyne, Xantina, Xantinah,
Xantine, Xantyna, Xantynah,
Xantyne, Zantina, Zantinah,
Zantine, Zantyna, Zantynah,
Zantyne

Sanura (Swahili) kitten.
Sanurah

Sanuye (Moquelumnan) red clouds
in the sunset.

Sanya (Sanskrit) born on a
Saturday.
Sanyah

Sanyu (Lugandan) happy.

Sapata (Native American) dancing
bear.
Sapatah

Sapphira/Sapphire (Greek)
sapphire jewel; precious gem;
blue.
Saffir, Saffira, Saffirah, Saffire, Safir,
Safira, Safirah, Safire, Safyr, Safyra,
Safyrah, Saphir, Saphira, Saphirah,
Saphire, Sapir, Sapira, Sapphir,
Sapphirah, Sapphire, Sapphyr,
Sapphyra, Sapphyre, Sapphyrah,
Sapyr, Sapyra, Sapyrah

Sappi (Lithuanian) wisdom.
Sapee, Sapey, Sapi, Sapia, Sapiah,
Sapie, Sappee, Sappey, Sappie,
Sappy, Sappya, Sappya, Sapya,
Sapyah

Sapta (Sanskrit) seventh-born child.
Saptah

Sara (Hebrew) princess.
Morag, Saara, Saarah, Sada, Sadah,
Sadel, Sadela, Sadelah, Sadele,
Sadell, Sadella, Sadellah, Sadelle,
Sadea, Sadee, Sadey, Sadi, Sadia,
Sadiah, Sadie, Sahra, Sahrah,
Sahria, Sahriah, Sahrya, Sahryah,
Said, Saida, Saidah, Saide, Saidea,
Saidee, Saidey, Saidi, Saidia, Saidie,
Saidy, Sailea, Sailee, Saileigh,
Sailey, Saili, Sailia, Sailie, Saily,
Sallea, Sallee, Salley, Salli, Sallia,
Sallie, Sally, Salaidth, Saydea,
Saydee, Saydi, Saydia, Saydiah,
Saydie, Saydy, Sadye, Salaidth,
Salilea, Salieah, Saliee, Salilei,
Salileigh, Saliley, Salili, Salilia,
Saliliah, Salilie, Salily, Sallea,
Salleah, Sallee, Sallei, Salleigh,
Salli, Sallia, Salliah, Sallie, Sally,
Saly, Sarah (Eng/Amer), Sarae,
Sarai, Saria, Sariah, Saraid, Saran,
Sarana, Saranah, Sarane, Sarann,
Saranna, Sarannah, Saranne, Sarea,
Sareah, Sareana, Sareanah, Sareane,
Saree, Sareen, Sareena, Sareenah,
Sareene, Sarena, Sarenah, Sarene,
Saret, Sareta, Saretah, Sarete, Sarett,
Saretta, Sarettah, Sarette, Sari,
Saria, Sariah, Sarie, Sarina, Sarinah,
Sarine, Sarita, Saritah, Sarite,
Saritta, Sarittah, Saritte, Sarolta
(Hung/Heb/Arab), Sarot, Sarota,
Sarotah, Sarote, Sarott, Sarotta,
Sarottah, Sarotte (Fren/Heb/Hung/
Arab), Sary, Sarya, Saryah, Sarye,
Sarya, Saryah, Saryna, Sarynah,
Saryne, Sarynna, Sarynna,
Sarynnah, Sarynne, Sasa (Hung),
Sasah, Sayra, Sayrah, Sayria,
Sayriah, Sayrya, Sayryah, Xahra,
Xahrah, Xara, Xarah, Xarra, Xarrah,
Zahra, Zahrah, Zahria, Zahriah,
Zara, Zarah, Zarra, Zarrah

Sarab (Arabic) dream.

Sarala (Hindi) straight.
Saralah

Saranu (Sanskrit) fast runner.
Saran, Sarana, Saranah

Saree/Sari/Sarice/Sarika (Hebrew)
princess. A form of Sara.
Sarea, Sareaka, Sareakah, Sareeka,
Sareekah, Sareka, Sarekah, Sari,
Saria, Sariah, Sarie, Sarika, Sarikah,
Sarise, Sarka, Sarkah, Sarri, Sarria,
Sarriah, Sarrie, Sarry, Sary, Sarya,
Saryah, Saryce, Saryse, Xarea,
Xareaka, Xareakah, Xareeka,
Xareekah, Xareka, Xarekah, Xari,
Xaria, Xariah, Xarie, Xarika,
Xarikah, Xarka, Xarkah, Xarri,
Xarria, Xarriah, Xarrie, Xarry, Xary,
Xarya, Xaryah, Zarea, Zareaka,
Zareakah, Zareeka, Zareekah,
Zareka, Zarekah, Zari, Zaria,
Zariah, Zarie, Zarika, Zarikah,
Zarka, Zarkah, Zarri, Zarria,
Zarriah, Zarrie, Zarry, Zary, Zarya,
Zaryah

Saril (Turkish) flowing water.
Sarill, Sarille, Saryl, Saryll, Sarylle

Sarila (Turkish) waterfall.
Sarilah, Sarilla, Sarillah, Saryla, Sarylah, Saryle, Sarylla, Saryllah, Sarylle

Sarina (Hebrew/Arabic) princess. A form of Sara.
Sareana, Sareanah, Sareane, Sareena, Sareenah, Sareene, Sarena, Sarenah, Sarene, Sarinah, Sarine, Sarinna, Sarinnah, Sarinne, Saryna, Sarynah, Saryne, Sarynna, Sarynnah, Xareana, Xareanah, Xareane, Xareena, Xareenah, Xareene, Xarena, Xarenah, Xarene, Xarinah, Xarine, Xarinna, Xarinnah, Xarinne, Xaryna, Xarynah, Xaryne, Xarynna, Xarynnah, Zareana, Zareanah, Zareane, Zareena, Zareenah, Zareene, Zarena, Zarenah, Zarene, Zarinah, Zarine, Zarinna, Zarinnah, Zarinne, Zaryna, Zarynah, Zaryne, Zarynna, Zarynnah

Sarinha (Amazonian) princess of the jungle.
Sarita

Sarita (Hebrew/Arabic) princess. A form of Sara.
Saeata, Sareatah, Sareate, Sareatta, Sareattah, Sareatte, Sareeta, Sareetah, Sareete, Sareta, Saretah, Saretta, Sarettah, Sarette, Saritah, Saritia, Saritah, Sarolta, Sarotta, Sarotte, Saryta, Sarytah, Saryte, Sarytta, Saryttah, Sarytte

Saroja (Hindi) born near a lake.

Sarolta (Hungarian/Hebrew/Arabic) princess. A form of Sara.
Saroltah

Saronna (African American/ Hebrew) princess; from the plains. A form of Sharon.
Sarona, Saronah, Saronnah

Sarotte (French/Hebrew/ English/Arabic) little princess. A form of Sara.
Sarot, Sarota, Sarotah, Sarote, Sarott, Sarotta, Sarottah

Sarwin (Kurdish) flower.

Sasa (Hungarian/Hebrew/Arabic) princess. A form of Sara.
Sasah

Sasha (Greek/Russian) defender of humankind. A form of Alexandra/Sandra.
Sacha, Sahsha, Sasa, Sasah, Sascha, Saschae, Sashah, Sashana, Sashel, Sashenka, Sashia, Sashiah, Sashira, Sashsha, Sashya, Sasjara, Sasshalai, Shashia, Shura, Shurah, Shurka

Sasona (Hebrew) happy.
Sasonah

Sass (Irish) Saxon; bright; cheeky. (Heb) life. The short form of Sasson.
Sas, Sasi, Sasie, Sassi, Sassie, Sassy, Sasy

Satara (Hebrew/Arabic/Irish) princess from the rocky hill.
Satarah, Sataria, Satariah, Satarra, Satarrah, Satarya, Sataryah, Sateria, Sateriah, Saterra, Saterria, Saterriah, Saterya, Sateryah

Satin (French) smooth; shiny.
Satean, Sateana, Sateane, Sateen, Sateena, Sateene, Satina, Satinah, Satinda, Satinder, Satine, Satyn, Satyna, Satynah, Satyne

Satini (Tongan) satin.
Satinia, Satiniah, Satine, Satiny, Satyna, Satynah

Satinka (Native American) sacred dancer.
Satinkah

Sato (Japanese) sugar; sweet.
Satu

Satoria (African American/Japanese) bird. A form of Tori, victory.
Satori, Satoriah, Satory, Satorya, Satoryah

Satuna (Tongan) Saturn, the planet.
Satunah

Saturnia (Latin) planting.
Saturn, Saturna, Saturne, Saturniah, Saturnya, Saturnyah

Sauda (Swahili) dark-skinned.
Saudah

Saula (Hebrew) asked for. The feminine form of Saul, borrowed; soul.
Saulah

Saundra (English/Greek) defender of humankind. A form of Sandra.
Saundea, Saudee, Saundey, Saundi, Saundia, Saundiah, Saundie, Saundy, Saundya, Saundyah

Saura (Hindi) worshipper of the sun.
Saurah

Savanna (Latin) open grassland.
Sahvana, Sahvanah, Sahvanna, Sahvannah, Savan, Savana, Savanah, Savanha, Savania, Savann, Savannah, Savannia, Savanniah, Savannha, Sevana, Sevanah, Sevanna, Sevannah, Zavana, Zavanah, Zavanna, Zavannah, Zevana, Zevanah, Zevanna, Zevannah

Savina (Latin) from Sabines (an ancient Italian tribe).
Savean, Saveana, Saveanah, Saveane, Saveen, Saveena, Saveenah, Saveene, Savinah, Savine, Savyn, Savyna, Savynah, Savyne

Savitri (Sanskrit) inciter; one who provokes.
Savitree

Sawa (Moquelumnan) stone. (Jap) swamp.
Sawah

Sawni (Seminole) echo.
Sawnee, Sawney, Sawnie, Sawny

Sawson (Arabic) lily.
Sawsen, Sawsin, Sawson, Sawsyn

Saxon (German/Latin) large stone. (O/Eng) saxon.
Sasanch, Sassunn, Saxona, Saxonah

Sayo (Japanese) born during the night.
Saio, Sao (Aust)

Scarlett (Middle English) brilliant red colour.
Scarlet, Scarleta, Scarlete, Scarletta, Scarlette, Scarlit, Scarlitt, Scarlyt, Scarlyta, Scarlyte

Schuyler (Dutch) scholar.
Schiler, Schyler, Schyler, Skiler, Sky, Skye, Skyla, Skylah, Skyler

Scientia (Latin) knowledgeable; scientist.
Scientiah, Scientya, Scientyah, Scyentia, Scyentiah, Scyentya, Scyentyah

Scotia (English/Hebrew) princess from Scotland. A combination of Scott/Tia. The feminine form of Scott.
Scotea, Scoteah, Scotea, Scotee, Scotey, Scoti, Scotiah, Scotie, Scottea, Scotteah, Scottee, Scottey, Scotti, Scottia, Scottiah, Scottie, Scotty, Scoty, Scotya, Scotyah

Seana (Irish/Hebrew) God is gracious. The feminine form of Sean.
Seanah, Seandra, Seane, Seanetta,

Seanette, Seann, Seanna, Seannah,
Seannalisa, Seante, Seantell,
Seantella, Seantelle, Shauna,
Shaunah, Shawna, Shawnah

Season (Latin) the season.
Seazon

Sebastiana/Sebastiane (Greek)
honoured above all others. The
feminine form of Sebastian.
Sebastianah, Sebastiann,
Sebastianna, Sebastianna,
Sebatianne, Sebastienne,
Sebastyana (Pol), Sebastyann,
Sebastyanna, Sebatyanne, Sebesta
(Boh), Seevastyana (Russ)

Seble (Ethiopian) born in
autumn/fall.

Secilia/Seelia (Latin) unseeing. A
form of Cecilia. The feminine
form of Cecil.
Saselia, Saseliah, Sasilla, Seciliah,
Secylia, Secyliah, Secylya, Secylyah,
Sesilia, Sesiliah, Sesylia, S;esyliah,
Sesylya, Sesylyah, Sileas, Syleas

Secunda (Latin) second-born child.
Seconda, Secondah, Secondea,
Secondee, Secondia, Secondiah,
Secondya, Secondyah

Seda (Armenian) one who hears the
voices of the forest.
Sedah

Sedna (Eskimo) well fed; the
goddess of sea animals.
Sednah

Seema (Greek) symbol; sign.
Cyma, Seama, Seamah, Seemah,
Seena, Seenah, Senaldy, Sima,
Simah, Syma, Symah

Sefa (Swiss) God will increase; God
has added a child. A feminine
form of Joseph.
Sefah, Seffa, Seffah

Seiko (Japanese) accomplished.

Seini (Polynesian) God is gracious.
Seinie

Seiran/Seirol (Welsh) sparkling;
bright.
Seiriola, Seiriole, Seiryan

Sekhmet (Egyptian) mighty.
Sekhmeta

Seki (Japanese) wonderful.
Seka, Sekah, Sekee, Sekey, Sekia,
Sekiah, Sekie, Seky, Sekya, Sekyah

Sela (Hebrew) stone.
Selah, Sella, Sellah

Selam (Ethiopian) peace.
Selama, Selamah

Selda (Old English) rare.
Seldah, Zelda, Zeldah

Selena/Selene/Selina (Greek)
moon; heavenly.
Celeana, Celeanah, Celeane,
Celeen, Celeena, Celeenah,
Celeene, Celena, Celenah, Celene,
Celina, Celine, Celinda, Celindah,
Celinde, Celine, Celyn, Celyna,
Celynah, Celyne, Cilina, Cilinah,
Ciline, Cillina, Cillinah, Cilline,
Coelina, Coelinah, Coeline,
Coelyn, Coelyna, Coelynah,
Coelyne, Sela, Selah, Selean,
Seleana, Seleanah, Seleane, Seleen,
Seleena, Seleenah, Seleene, Selena,
Selenah, Selene, Selia, Seliah, Selie,
Selin, Selinah, Seline, Selyn,
Selyna, Selynah, Selyne, Sena,
Senah, Silina, Silinah, Siline,
Sillina, Sillinah, Silline, Sillyn,
Sillyna, Sillynah, Sillyne, Sylin,
Sylina, Sylinah, Syline, Sylyn,
Sylyna, Sylynah, Sylyne, Zelean,
Zeleana, Zeleanah, Zeleane, Zeleen,
Zeleena, Zeleenah, Zeleene, Zelen,
Zelena, Zelenah, Zelene, Zelina,

Selena/Selene/Selina cont.
Zelina, Zelinah, Zeline, Zelyn,
Zelyna, Zelynah, Zelyne

Selima (Hebrew) peace. A feminine
form of Solomon.
Selimah, Selyma, Selymah

Selma (Scandinavian) divinely
protected; guarded. (Arab) secure.
(Celt) fair-haired. A feminine
form of Solomon, peace.
Annselma, Anselm, Anselma,
Anselme, Selmah, Zelma, Zelmah

Selo/Sema (Tongan/Latin) heaven.
Sello, Semah, Semaj

Semira (Hebrew) tall as the
heavens.
Semirah, Semyra, Semyrah

Sen (Japanese) magical forest fairy.

Sena (Greek) hospitable; guest. A
form of Xenia.
Senah, Senia, Seniah, Senya,
Senyah, Xenia, Xeniah, Xenya,
Xenyah, Zena, Zenia, Zeniah,
Zenya, Zenyah

Senalda (Spanish) symbol; sign.
Sena, Senda, Senna, Sennah

Senga (Scottish) purity. Agnes spelt
backwards.
Sengah

Seona/Seonaid (Scottish/Hebrew)
God is gracious. The Scottish
form of Jane.
Seonah, Seonia, Seoniah, Seonya,
Seonyah, Shinaed, Shinaid, Sinead
(Ir), Shynaed, Shynaid

Septima (Latin) seventh-born child.
Septime, Septyn, Septyna, Septyne,
Sevann, Sevanna, Sevanne,
Sevantha, Sevanthe, Sevena,
Sevenah, Seventeen, Seventeena,
Seventeene, Seventina, Seventine,
Seventyn, Seventyna, Seventyne

Sequoia (Cherokee) redwood tree.
Sequora, Sequoya, Sikoya

Serah (Hebrew) to pour.
Sera, Serra, Serrah

Seraphina (Hebrew) Seraph, the
highest order of the angels. The
feminine form of Serafino.
Seafia, Seafin, Seafina, Seafine,
Seaphia, Seaphin, Seaphina,
Seaphine, Serafeen, Serafeena,
Serafeene, Serafin, Serafina,
Serafine, Serapheen, Serapheena,
Serapheene, Serapheene, Seraphin,
Seraphina, Seraphynah, Seraphine
(Fren), Seraphita (Span), Serephyn,
Serephyna, Serephynah

Serena/Serene/Serenity (Latin)
peace.
Careana, Careanah, Careena,
Careenah, Cereana, Cereanah,
Cereena, Cereenah, Sareana,
Sareanah, Sareena, Sareenah,
Savina, Savinah, Serean, Sereana,
Sereanah, Sereane, Serene (Fren),
Serenitee, Serenitie, Serenity,
Serepta, Serin, Serina, Serinah,
Serine, Seryn, Seryna, Serynah,
Seryne, Siren, Sirena, Sirenah,
Sirene, Syreana, Syreanah, Syreane,
Syreen, Syreena, Syreenah, Syreene,
Syrin, Syrina, Syrinah, Syrine,
Syryn, Syryna, Syrynah, Syryne

Serica (Greek) silky.
Sarica, Saricah, Saricka, Sarickah,
Sarika, Sarikah, Saryca, Sarycah,
Sarycka, Saryckah, Saryka, Sarykah,
Sericah, Sericka, Serickah, Serika,
Serikah, Seryca, Serycah, Serycka,
Seryckah, Seryka, Serykah

Serilda (Teutonic) armoured for
battle; woman warrior.
Sarilda, Sarildah, Serildah, Serylda,
Seryldah

Serita (Italian/Hebrew) little
princess. A form of Sara.
Sareata, Sareatah, Sareeta, Sareetah,
Sarita, Saritah, Sarite, Saritt, Saritta,
Sarittah, Saritte, Saryt, Saryta,
Sarytah, Saryte, Sarytt, Sarytta,
Saryttah, Sarytte, Seri, Seritah,
Serite, Seritt, Seritta, Serittah,
Seritte, Seryt, Seryta, Serytah,
Seryte, Serytt, Serytta, Seryttah,
Serytte

Sesheta (Egyptian) goddess of stars.
Seshetah

Setsu (Japanese) faith.

Sevilla (Spanish) prophet; wise
woman. The Spanish form of
Sibyl.
Sevil, Sevila, Sevilah, Sevile, Sevill,
Sevillah, Seville, Sevyl, Sevyla,
Sevyle, Sevyll, Sevylla, Sevylle

Shaanana (Hebrew) peace.
Shanana

Shaba (Spanish) rose.
Shabah, Shabana, Shabanah,
Shabina, Shabinah, Shabine,
Shabyna, Shabynah, Shabyne

Shada (Native American) pelican.
Shadae, Shadea, Shadeana, Shadee,
Shadi, Shadie, Shadiya, Shaida,
Shaida, Shaidah, Shaiday, Shaide,
Shayda, Shaydah

Shade/Shadoe (Old English)
shadow cover; dweller from the
shady doe enclosure.
Shada, Shadah, Shadoe, Shadow,
Shaid, Shaida, Shaidah, Shaide,
Shayd, Shayda, Shaydah, Shayde

Shadrika (Swedish/English) ruler of
the shadows.
Shadreeka, Shadreka, Shadrica,
Shadricah, Shadricka, Shadrikah,
Shadrica, Shadricah, Shadricka,
Shadrickah, Shadrikah, Shadriqua,

Shadriquah, Shadrique, Shadryca,
Shadrycah, Shadrycka, Shadryckah,
Shardrica, Shardricah, Shardricka,
Shardrickah, Shardryka,
Shardrykah, Shardryqua,
Shardriquah, Shardryque

Shadya (Arabic) one who sings.
Shadia, Shadiah, Shadyah

Shae/Shay/Shea (Irish) from the
fairy palace. A form of Shea/Shay.
QShaeen, Shaeena, Shaeina,
Shaeine, Shaela, Shaelea, Shaeleah,
Shaelee, Shaeleigh, Shaelie, Shaely,
Shaelyn, Shaena, Shaenah,
Shaenel, Shaeya, Shai, Shaiah,
Shailea, Shaileah, Shailee, Shailei,
Shaileigh, Shailey, Shaili, Shailia,
Shailiah, Shailie, Shaily, Shaya,
Shayah, Shayla, Shaylah, Shaylea,
Shayleah, Shaylee, Shaylei,
Shayleigh, Shayli, Shaylia,
Shayliah, Shaylie, Shayly

Shaelea (Irish/Australian/English)
from the fairy palace in the
meadow. A combination of
Shae/Lea.
Shaeleah, Shaelee, Shaelei,
Shaeleigh, Shaeley, Shaeli, Shaelia,
Shaeliah, Shailie, Shaely, Shailea,
Shaileah, Shailee, Shailei,
Shaileigh, Shailey, Shaili, Shailia,
Shailiah, Shailie, Shaily, Shalea,
Shaleah, Shalee, Shalei, Shaleigh,
Shaley, Shali, Shalie, Shaly,
Shaylea, Shayleah, Shaylee, Shaylei,
Shayleigh, Shayley, Shayli, Shaylia,
Shayliah, Shaylie, Shayly

Shaelyn (Irish) from the fairy palace
pool. A combination of Shae/Lyn.
Shaelean, Shaeleana, Shaeleanah,
Shaeleane, Shaeleen, Shaleena,
Shaeleenah, Shaeleene, Shaelena,
Shaelenah, Shaelene, Shaelin,
Shaelina, Shaelinah, Shaeline,
Shaelyn, Shaelyna, Shaelynah,

Shaelyn cont.
Shaelyne, Shailean, Shaileana,
Shaileanah, Shaileane, Shaileen,
Shaileena, Shaileenah, Shaileene,
Shailin, Shailina, Shailinah,
Shailine, Shailyn, Shailyna,
Shailynah, Shailyne, Shaylean,
Shayleana, Shayleanah, Shayleane,
Shayleen, Shayleena, Shayleenah,
Shayleene, Shaylin, Shaylina,
Shaylinah, Shayline, Shaylyn,
Shaylyna, Shaylynah, Shaylyne

Shafira (Swahili) distinguished.
Shafirah, Shafyra, Shafyrah

Shahar (Arabic) born on a moonlit
night.
Sharharah, Sharharia, Sharhariah,
Sharharya, Sharharyah

Shahina (Arabic) the falcon bird.
Shahean, Shaheana, Shaheanah,
Shaheane, Shaheen, Shaheena,
Shaheenah, Shaheene, Shahi,
Shahia, Shahiah, Shahin, Shahina,
Shahinah, Shahyna, Shahynah,
Shahyne

Shahira (Arabic) famous.
Shahirah, Shahyra, Shahyrah

Shahla (Afghani) beautiful eyes.
Shahlah, Sharla, Sharlah

Shaila (Hindi) mountain that is
small.
Shailah, Shayla, Shaylah

Shaina/Shaine (Hebrew/Irish)
beautiful. The feminine form of
Shane, God is gracious.
Shaena, Shaenah, Shainah, Shaine,
Shainna, Shanja, Shania, Shaniah,
Shanie, Shayna, Shaynah,
Shayndel, Shaynee, Sheina,
Sheindel

Shajuana (Spanish/African
American) God is gracious. A
form of Juanita. A feminine form
of Juan.
Shajana, Shajanah, Shajuan,
Shajuanda, Shajuanita, Shajuanitte,
Shajuanna, Shajuanne, Shajuanza

Shaka (Hindi) divine woman.
Shakah, Shakha, Shakia, Shakiah,
Shakya, Shakyah, Shikah, Shikha

Shakara (Danish/American) she is
purity. A form of Katherine.
Shacara, Shacarah, Shacari,
Shacaria, Shacariah, Shaccara,
Shaccarah, Shaka, Shakah,
Shakarah, Shakari, Shakaria,
Shakariah, Shakarya, Shakaryah,
Shakkara, Shikara, Shykara,
Shykarah

Shakeena (Irish/American) she is
brave; quick. A form of Keena.
Shaka, Shakah, Shakean, Shakeana,
Shakeanah, Shakeane, Shakeen,
Shakeena, Shakeenah, Shakeene,
Shakein, Shakeina, Shakeinah,
Shakeine, Shakeyn, Shakeyna,
Shakeynah, Shakeyne, Shakin,
Shakina, Shakinah, Shakine,
Shakyn, Shakyna, Shakynah,
Shakyne

Shakeia/Shakia (African/Blackfoot)
unknown; beginning of the
season. (Sans) energy circle. A
form of Chakra. A form of Kia.
Chakiah, Chakira, Chakria,
Chakriya, Chakya, Chakyah,
Chakyra, Chakyrah, Shakeeia,
Shakeeiah, Shakeeya, Shakeeyah,
Shakeia, Shakeiah, Shakeya,
Shakiya, Shakiyah, Shakya,
Shakyah, Shekela, Shekia, Shekiah,
Shekya, Shekyah

Shakeita (Scottish/African
  American) she is from the woods.
  Shakeata, Shakeatah, Shakeatia,
  Shakeatiah, Shakeeta,Shakeetah,
  Shakeetia, Shakeetia, Shekeita,
  Shakeitah, Shakeitha, Shakeithia,
  Shaketa, Shaketah, Shaketha,
  Shakethia, Shaketia, Shaketiah,
  Shakeyta, Shakeytah, Shakita,
  Shakitah, Shakitra, Shakyta,
  Shakytah, Shakytia, Shakytiah,
  Sheketa, Sheketah, Sheketia,
  Shekita, Shekitah, Shikita, Shikitha,
  Shikyta, Shikytah, Shykita,
  Shykitah, Shykitia, Shykitiah,
  Shykyta, Shykytah, Shykytia,
  Shykytiah, Shykytya, Shykytyah

Shakela (African American/Irish)
  warrior; dweller from the farm
  near the woods. A form of Kelly.
  Shakleah, Shakella, Shakellah

Shakila (Arabic) she is the pretty
  one.
  Shakeala, Shakealah, Shakeela,
  Shakeelah, Shakeena, Shakeenah,
  Shakela, Shakila, Shakilah,
  Shakyla, Shakylah, Shikila

Shakira (Arabic) she is thankful.
  Shaakira, Shakera, Shakerah,
  Shakeria, Shakeriah, Shakeriay,
  Shakeyra, Shakir, Shakirah,
  Shakirat, Shakirra, Shakyra,
  Shakyrah, Shekiera, Shekira,
  Shikira, Shikirah, Shikyra,
  Shikyrah, Shykira, Shykirah,
  Shykyra, Shykyrah

Shakti (Hindi) she is divine.
  Saktea, Saktee, Saktey, Sakti, Saktia,
  Saktiah, Saktie, Sakty, Shaka,
  Shakah, Shaktea, Shaktee, Shaktey,
  Shakti, Shaktia, Shaktiah, Shaktie,
  Shakty

Shalana (Irish) attractive. (Haw)
  light; airy; awakening; handsome;
  harmony; happy; peaceful. A
  short form of Alannah. The
  feminine form of Alan,
  handsome; fair; bright; cheery.
  Shalain, Shalaina, Shalainah,
  Shalaine, Shalana, Shaland,
  Shalanda, Shalandah, Shalane,
  Shalanna, Shalannah, Shalanne,
  Shalaun, Shalauna, Shalaunah,
  Shallan, Shallana, Shallanah,
  Shalyn, Shalyna, Shalynah,
  Shalyne, Shelan, Shelana,
  Shelanah, Shelanda, Shelane,
  Shelayna, Shelaynah, Shelayne,
  Sholaina, Sholainah, Sholaine,
  Sholana, Sholanah, Sholane,
  Sholayna, Sholaynah, Sholayne

Shaleisha (Swahili) life. (Arab)
  woman. A form of Aisha.
  Shalesha, Shaleshah, Shalesia,
  Shalesiah, Shalicia, Shaliciah,
  Shalisha, Shalishah, Shalysha,
  Shalyshah

Shalena (Norwegian) famous;
  distinguished. (Heb) dwelling.
  Shalain, Shalaina, Shalainah,
  Shalan, Shalana, Shalanah,
  Shalane, Shalaine, Shalayn,
  Shalayna, Shalaynah, Shalayne,
  Shalean, Shaleana, Shaleanah,
  Shaleane, Shaleen, Shaleena,
  Shaleenah, Shaleene, Shalen,
  Shalenah, Shalene, Shalenna,
  Shalennah, Shalenne, Shelayna,
  Shelaynah, Shelayne, Shelena,
  Shelenah

Shalgia (Hebrew) snow white.
  Shalgiah

Shalisa (Hebrew) honey bee. A form
  of Melissa/Elizabeth, holy; sacred
  to God.
  Shalesa, Shalesah, Shalese, Shalice,
  Shalisah, Shalise, Shalisia,

Shalisa cont.
Shalisiah, Shalissa, Shalissah,
Shallisse, Shalys, Shalysa, Shalysah,
Shalyse, Shalyss, Shalyssa, Shalysse

Shalita (Latin) happy.
(Afri/Swa) one who brings.
Shaleata, Shaleatah, Shaleeta,
Shaleetah, Shaleta, Shaletah,
Shaletta, Shalettah, Shalida,
Shalidah, Shalitta, Shalittah,
Shalyta, Shalytah, Shalytta,
Shalyttah

Shalona (Latin) lioness. A form of
Lona, solitary.
Shalonah, Shalonna, Shalonnah,
Shalonne

Shalonda (Latin) water fairy.
Shalondah, Shalonde, Shalondina,
Shalondine, Shalondyna,
Shalondyne

Shalva (Hebrew) peace.
Shalvah

Shalyn (Welsh) from the shade
pool. (Eng) from the fairy pool.
Shalin, Shalina, Shalinda, Shaline,
Shalyna, Shalynda, Shalyne,
Shalynn, Shalynna, Shalynne

Shamara (Arabic) battle-ready
warrior.
Shamar, Shamarah, Shamari,
Shamaria, Shamariah, Shamarra,
Shamarri, Shamarria, Shamarya,
Shamaryah, Shammara, Shamora,
Shamorah, Shamorra, Shamorah,
Shamoria, Shamoriah, Shamorya,
Shamoryah

Shameena (Hindi) beautiful.

Shameka (Hebrew) likeness to God.
A feminine form of Michael.
Shameca, Shamecca, Shamecha,
Shameeka, Shameika, Shameke,
Shamekia, Shamekiah, Shamekya,
Shamekyah, Shamica, Shamicah,

Shamicka, Shamickah, Shamika,
Shamikah, Shamyca, Shamycah,
Shamycka, Shamyckah, Shamyka,
Shamykah

Shamika (Native American) wise
raccoon.
Shameca, Shamecca, Shamecha,
Shameeka, Shameika, Shameka,
Shamekah, Shameke, Shamekia,
Shamekiah, Shamekya,
Shamekyah, Shamica, Shamicah,
Shamicka, Shamickah, Shamikah,
Shamyca, Shamycah, Shamycka,
Shamyckah, Shamyka, Shamykah

Shamira (Latin) wonderful.
(Span) to gaze.
Shamir, Shamirah, Shamiran,
Shamiria, Shamyra, Shamyrah,
Shamyria, Shamyriah, Shamyrya,
Shamyryah

Shammara (Arabic) battle-prepared
warrior.
Shamara, Shamarah, Shammarah

Shana/Shanae (Hebrew) God is
gracious. The feminine form of
Shane.
Shaana, Shaanah, Shanah, Shanay,
Shanda, Shandah, Shandi,
Shandie, Shane, Shanee, Shanna,
Shannah, Shauna, Shawna

Shanasa (Hindi) wish.
Shanasah

Shanda (Sanskrit) great goddess.
Chanda, Shana, Shanah, Shandah,
Shandra

Shandra (African American/Greek)
defender of humankind. A form
of Sandra.
Shandrah

Shandy (Old English) noisy.
Shandea, Shandee, Shandei,
Shandeigh, Shandey, Shandie,
Shanta, Shantee, Shantey, Shanti,

Shantia, Shantiah, Shantie, Shanty,
Shantya, Shantyah

Shane (Irish) God is gracious.
Chaen, Chaena, Chaenah, Chaene,
Chain, Chaina, Chainah, Chaine,
Chayn, Chayna, Chaynah, Chayne,
Cheyn, Cheyna, Cheynah, Cheyne,
Schain, Schaina, Schainah,
Schaine, Schayn, Schayna,
Schaynah, Schayne, Shaen, Shaena,
Shaena, Shaenah, Shaene, Shain,
Shaina, Shainah, Shaine, Shayn,
Shayna, Shaynah

Shanea/Shani (African/African
American) wonderful.
Shanea, Shanee, Shaney, Shani,
Shania (Nat/Can/Ojib), Shaniah,
Shanie, Shany, Shanya, Shanyah

Shaneisha (Swahili/African
American/Hebrew) God's
gracious life. (Arab) woman. A
combination of Shane/Aisha.
Shanesha, Shaneshia, Shanessa,
Shanesse, Shaneysa, Shaneysah,
Shanisha, Shanishia, Shanishiah,
Shanissa, Shanysha, Shanyssa,
Shanysse

Shaneka (Russian) belonging to
God.
Shaneaca, Shaneacah, Shaneacka,
Shaneackah, Shaneaka, Shaneakah,
Shaneaqua, Shaneaquah,
Shaneaque, Shaneca, Shenecka,
Shaneeca, Shaneecah, Shaneecka,
Shaneeckah, Shaneequa,
Shaneequah, Shaneeque, Shaneika,
Shaneikah, Shaneiqua,
Shaneiquah, Shaneique, Shaneka,
Shanekah, Shanekia, Shanekiah,
Shanequa, Shanequah, Shaneque,
Shaneyka, Shanica, Shanicah,
Shanicka, Shanickah, Shanika,
Shanikah, Shaniqua, Shaniquah,
Shanique, Shanyca, Shanycah,
Shanycka, Shanyckah, Shanyka,

Shanykah, Shanyqua, Shanyquah,
Shanyque

Shanelle (English/French) she is
from the channel.
Schanel, Schanela, Schanelah,
Schanele, Shanel, Shanela,
Shanelah, Shanele, Shanell,
Shanella, Shannel, Shannela,
Shannelah, Shannele, Shannell,
Shannella, Shannellah, Shannelle,
Shenel, Shenela, Shenelah,
Shenele, Shenell, Shenella,
Shenelle, Shonel, Shonela,
Shonelah, Shonele, Shonell,
Shonella, Shonelle

Shaneta (Hebrew) plant. A form of
Neta.
Shaneata, Shaneatah, Shaneate,
Shaneeta, Shaneetah, Shanetha,
Shanethia, Shanithis, Shanetta,
Shanette, Shanita, Shanitah,
Shanitt, Shanitta, Shanittah,
Shanitte, Shanyt, Shanyta,
Shanytah, Shanyte, Shanytt,
Shanytta, Shanyttah, Shanytte

Shania (Ojibway) I'm on my way.
Shaniah, Shanya, Shanyah

Shanice (Hebrew) God is gracious.
A form of Janice.
Shaneace, Shanease, Shaneece,
Shaneese, Shanece, Shaneice,
Shaneise, Shaniece, Shaniss,
Shanissa, Shanisse, Shanneice,
Shannice, Shannyce, Shanyce,
Shanyse, Sheneice, Shenyce

Shanida (English) prosperous.
(Ger) hard-working.
Shaneeda, Shaneedah, Shannida,
Shannidah, Shanyda, Shanydah

Shanie (Hebrew) beautiful.
Chaenea, Chaenee, Chaeney,
Chaeni, Chaenie, Chaeny, Chainea,
Chainee, Chainey, Chaini, Chainie,
Chainy, Chaynea, Chaynee,

Shanie cont.
Chayney, Chayni, Chaynie,
Chayny, Shaenea, Shaenee,
Shaeney, Shaeni, Shaenia,
Shaeniah, Shaenie, Shaeny,
Shaenya, Shaenyah, Shaenye,
Shaina, Shainah, Shainea, Shainee,
Shainey, Shaini, Shainia, Shainiah,
Shainie, Shainy, Shainya, Shainyah,
Shanee, Shaney, Shani, Shania
(Nat/Amer), Shaniah, Shany,
Shanya, Shanyah

Shanika (Russian) belonging to
God.
Shaneaca, Shaneacah, Shaneacka,
Shaneackah, Shaneaka, Shaneakah,
Shaneaqua, Shaneaquah,
Shaneaque, Shaneca, Shenecka,
Shaneeca, Shaneecah, Shaneecka,
Shaneeckah, Shaneequa,
Shaneequah, Shaneeque, Shaneika,
Shaneikah, Shaneiqua,
Shaneiquah, Shaneique, Shaneka,
Shanekah, Shanekia, Shanekiah,
Shanequa, Shanequah, Shaneque,
Shaneyka, Shanica, Shanicah,
Shanicka, Shanickah, Shanika,
Shanikah, Shaniqua, Shaniquah,
Shanique, Shanyca, Shanycah,
Shanycka, Shanyckah, Shanyka,
Shanykah, Shanyqua, Shanyquah,
Shanyque

Shaningo (Algonquin) beautiful.

Shanisa (Hebrew) God is gracious.
(Scand) God's gracious, friendly
fairy. (Heb) sign. A combination
of Shane/Nissa.
Shanisah, Shanissa, Shanissah,
Shaysa, Shanysah, Shanyssa,
Shanyssah

Shanita (Choctaw) bear.
(Heb) planter.
Shaneata, Shaneatah, Shaneate,
Shaneeta, Shaneetah, Shaneta,

Shanetah, Shanetha, Shanethia,
Shanethis, Shanetta, Shanette,
Shanitah, Shanitt, Shanitta,
Shanittah, Shanitte, Shanyt,
Shanyta, Shanytah, Shanyte,
Shanytt, Shanytta, Shanyttah,
Shanytte

Shanley (Irish/Gaelic) child of the
hero from the meadow.
Shanlea, Shanleah, Shanlee,
Shanlei, Shanleigh, Shanli, Shalie,
Shanly

Shanna (Celtic) slow water.
(Ir/Heb) God is gracious. The
feminine form of Shane.
Shana, Shanah, Shannah

Shannon (Irish/Gaelic) small
wisdom; slow-moving stream.
Channa, Channon, Shana, Shandy,
Shane, Shanna, Shannah,
Shannahn, Shannen, Shannin,
Shannyn, Shanon, Shanyn

Shanta (French) song. A form of
Chantal.
Shantae, Shantah, Shantai,
Shantay, Shantaya, Shantaye,
Shantea, Shantee

Shantaina (Spanish/African
American) saintly. A form of
Shantana.
Shantana, Shantanah, Shantainah,
Shantayna, Shantaynah

Shantana (Spanish) saint.
Shanta, Shantah, Shantania,
Shantaniah, Shantaniata,
Shantanna, Shantanne, Shantanya,
Shantanyah, Shantena, Shantenah,
Shantenna, Shantina, Shantinah,
Shantine, Shantyna, Shantyne,
Shentana, Shentanna

Shantara (Irish/American) she is from the rocky hill. (Heb/Ir) from God's gracious rocky hill. A form of Tara.
Shantarah, Shantaria, Shantariah, Shantarra, Shantera, Shanteria, Shanterra, Shantieria, Shantira, Shantirea, Shantrya, Shantyah

Shanteca (Hungarian/Greek) harvester. A form of Teresa.
Shantecca, Shantecka, Shanteka, Shantika, Shantikia, Shantikiah, Shantyca, Shantycah, Shantycka, Shantyckah, Shantyka, Shantykah

Shantelle/Shantille (French) song.
Chantal, Chantala, Chantalah, Chantale, Chantel, Chantela, Chantelah, Chantele, Chontel, Chontela, Chontelah, Chontele, Chontell, Chontella, Chontellah, Chontelle, Shantal, Shantel, Shantela, Shantelah, Shantele, Shantell, Shantella, Shantellah, Shontel, Shontela, Shontelah, Shontele, Shontell, Shontella, Shontellah, Shontelle

Shantesa (Greek) harvester. A form of Teresa.
Shantesah, Shantessa, Shantessah, Shantesse

Shantia (Greek) God's gracious princess. A combination of Shane/Tia.
Shanteia, Shanteya, Shanti, Shantiah, Shantida, Shantie, Shantya, Shantyah, Shaunteya, Shauntia, Shauntah, Shauntya, Shauntyah

Shantina (English) little song. (Lat) little Christian.
Shanteana, Shanteanah, Shanteena, Shanteenah, Shanteina,

Shanteinah, Shanteyna, Shanteynah, Shantinah, Shantyna, Shantynah

Shantora (Latin/American) victorious. A combination of Shane/Tori, God's gracious victory; God's gracious bird.
Shantola, Shantoree, Shantorey, Shantori, Shantoria, Shantoriah, Shantorie, Shantory, Shantorya, Shantoryah, Shantoya, Shanttoria

Shantrice (French) song. A form of Chantrice.
Shantreace, Shantrease, Shantreece, Shantreese, Shantriece, Shantriese, Shantrisa, Shantrisah, Shantrissa, Shantrisse, Shanrtyce, Shantryse

Shappa (Native American) red thunder.
Shapa, Shapah, Shappah

Shaquanda (German/African American) wanderer. A form of Wanda.
Shaquan, Shaquana, Shaquanah, Shaquand, Shaquandah, Shaquandra, Shaquandrah, Shaquanera, Shaquani, Shaquania, Shaquaniah, Shaquanna, Shaquannah, Shaquanne, Shaquantia, Shaquanitah, Shaquonda, Shaquondah, Shaquondra, Shaquondrah

Shaqueita (Scottish/African American) from the woods. (Arab) handsome. The feminine form of Shaquille.
Shaqueta, Shaquetah, Shaquetta, Shaquettah, Shaquette, Shaquita, Shaquitah, Shequida, Shequidah, Shequita, Shequitah, Shequittia, Shequittiah, Shequitya, Shequityah, Shequytya, Shequytah

S

Shara (Hebrew) princess. A form of
Sharon, from the plains.
Sharae, Sharah, Sharai, Sharay,
Sharra, Sharrah, Sharrai, Sharray

Sharae (Hebrew) princess.
Sharae, Sharai, Sharay

Sharda (English) one who runs
away.
Shardah

Shardae (Punjabi) charitable.
(Yor) honoured by royalty.
(Arab) runaway.
Sade, Shadae, Sharda, Shardah,
Shardai, Sharday, Shardea, Shardee,
Shardey, Shardi, Shardie, Shardy

Sharenne (Hebrew/English) from
the graceful plains. A
combination of Sharron/Anne.
Sharen, Sharena, Sharenah,
Sharene, Sharenn, Sharenna,
Sharennah

Shari (French) beloved. The
Hungarian form of Sara, princess.
Sharea, Shareah, Sharee, Sharian,
Shariana, Sharianah, Shariann,
Sharianna, Shariannah, Sharianne,
Sharie, Sharra, Sharrah, Sharri,
Sharria, Sharriah, Sharrie, Sharry,
Sharrya, Sharryah, Shary, Sharya,
Sharyah

Sharice (French/American) song of
happiness. A form of Caroline,
little woman.
Shareace, Sharease, Shareece,
Shareese, Sharese, Sharica,
Sharicen, Sharicena, Sharicka,
Sharicke, Shariece, Sharis, Sharise,
Sharisha, Shariss, Sharissa,
Sharisse, Sharyce, Sharyse

Sharik (African) child of God.
Sharika, Sharike, Shariqua,
Shariquah, Sharique, Sharyka,

Sharykah, Sharyqua, Sharyquah,
Sharyque

Sharleen (French/American) song
of happiness. A form of Caroline,
little woman.
Charla, Charlah, Charlean,
Charleana, Charleanah, Charleane,
Charleen, Charleena, Charleenah,
Charleene, Charlin, Chalina,
Charlinah, Charline, Charlyn,
Charlyna, Charlynah, Charlyne,
Sharla, Sharlah, Sharlean,
Sharleana, Sharleanah, Sharleane,
Sharleena, Sharleenah, Sharleene,
Sharlina, Sharlinah, Sharline,
Sharlyn, Sharlyna, Sharlynah,
Sharlyne

Sharlotte (French) little, strong,
courageous woman. A form of
Charlotte.
Charlot, Charlota, Charlotah,
Charlote, Charlott, Charlotta,
Charlottah, Charlotte, Sharlet,
Sharleta, Sharletah, Sharlete,
Sharlett, Sharletta, Sharlettah,
Sharlette, Sharlot, Sharlota,
Sharlotah, Sharlote, Sharlotta,
Sharlottah

Sharmaine (Latin/French) song.
Charma, Charmae, Charmah,
Charmain, Charmaina,
Charmainah, Charmaine,
Charmayn, Charmayna,
Charmaynah, Charmayne, Sharma,
Sharmae, Sharmah, Sharmain,
Sharmaina, Sharman, Sharmane,
Sharmanta, Sharmayn, Sharmayna,
Sharmayne, Sharmeen, Sharmeena,
Sharmena, Sharmene, Sharmese,
Sharmin, Sharmina, Sharmine,
Sharmon, Sharmona Sharmone,
Sharmyn, Sharmyna, Sharmyne

Sharman (Old English) divided.
Charman, Charmana, Charmane,
Charmain, Charmaina, Charmayn,

Charmayna, Sharmana, Sharmane, Sharmain, Sharmaina, Sharmayn, Sharmayna, Sharmayne

Sharna (Hebrew) from the plains.
Sharnae, Sharnah, Sharnai, Sharnay, Sharnah, Sharne, Sharnea, Sharnease, Sharnee, Sharneesa, Sharneese, Sharnesa, Sharnese, Sharneta, Sharnete, Sharnetta, Sharnette, Sharnice, Sharnisa, Sharnise, Sharnissa, Sharnisse, Sharnyc, Sharnyca, Sharnycah, Sharnyce, Sharnys, Sharnysa, Sharnysah, Sharnyse

Sharolyn (Celtic/Hebrew) princess from the pool.
Sharolean, Sharoleana, Sharoleanah, Sharoleane, Sharoleen, Sharoleena, Sharoleenah, Sharoleene, Sharolin, Sharolina, Sharolinah, Sharoline, Sharolyna, Sharolynah, Sharolyne, Sharolynn, Sharolynna, Sharolynnah, Sharolynne

Sharon (Hebrew) from the plains.
Charan, Charen, Charin, Charyn, Cheran, Cheren, Cherin, Cheron, Cheryn, Shara, Sharai, Sharea, Sharean, Shareana, Shareane, Sharee, Shareen, Shareena, Shareene, Shari, Sharie, Sharin, Sharina, Sharine, Sharla, Sharlah, Sharne, Sharnee, Sharney, Sharnie, Sharolyn, Sharolyna, Sharolyne, Sharolynn, Sharolynna, Sharolynne, Sharona, Sharonah, Sharonda, Sharonah, Sharone, Sharran, Sharrana, Sharrane, Sharren, Sharenna, Sharrene, Sharrin, Sharrina, Sharrinae, Sharryn, Sharryna, Sharryne

Shatara (Irish) from the rocky hill.
Shatarah, Shataria, Shatariah, Shatarra, Shatarrah, Shataura, Shateira, Shaterah, Shateria,

Shateriah, Shatherian, Shatierra, Shatiria, Shatyra, Shatyrah

Shatoria (Latin/African American) God's gracious victory. A combination of Shane/Tori.
Shatora, Shatorah, Shatoriah, Shatorria, Shatorya, Shatoryah, Shatoya, Shatoyah

Shauna (Irish/Hebrew) God is gracious. The Irish form of Jane.
Schean, Scheana, Scheanah, Schaun, Schauna, Schaunah, Seana, Seanah, Seanee, Shaunah, Shaunee, Shawna, Shawnah, Shawnee (Nat/Amer)

Shaunta (Irish/Hebrew) God is gracious. A feminine form of Shaun.
Schaunta, Schuntae, Shauntah, Schauntay, Shaunte, Shauntea, Shauntee, Shaunteena, Shauntel, Shauntela, Shauntele, Shauntell, Shauntella, Shauntelle, Shauntia, Shauntier, Shauntrel, Shauntrella, Shauntrelle, Shawnta, Shawntah, Shawntel, Shawntela, Shawntelah, Shawntele, Shawntell, Shawntella, Shawntellah, Shawntelle

Shavonda (Irish/Hebrew/African American) admired. The Irish form of Joanna/Siobhain, God is gracious.
Shavona, Shavonah, Shavondah

Shawanna (German/African American) wanderer. A form of Wanda.
Shawana, Shawanah, Shawanda, Shawannah, Shawanta, Shawante

Shawn/Shawna (Hebrew) God is gracious. The feminine form of Sean/Shaun.
Schaun, Schaunah, Schaune, Schaunee, Schawn, Schawna, Schawnah, Schawne, Schawnee,

Shawn/Shawna cont.
Sean, Seana, Seanah, Shaun,
Shauna, Shaunah, Shaune,
Shaunee, Shawna, Shawnah,
Shawndel, Shawndel, Shawndell,
Shawdelle, Shawnee (Nat/Amer),
Shawney, Shawni, Shawnie, Siana,
Sianah, Sianna, Siannah, Sion,
Syon

Shawndelle (Irish/Canadian) God is
gracious to her. A feminine form
of Shawn.
Schaundel, Schaundela,
Schaundele, Schaundell,
Schaundelle, Schawndel,
Schawndele, Schawdell,
Schawndelle, Seandel, Seandela,
Seandele, Seandell, Seandella,
Seandelle, Shaundel, Shaundela,
Shaundele, Shaundell, Shaundella,
Shaundelle, Shawndel, Shawndela,
Shawndele, Shawndella

Shayla (Irish) from the fairy palace.
Shaela, Shaelah, Shaila, Shailah,
Shaylah

Shayna (Hebrew) beautiful one
from the fairy palace. The
feminine Irish form of Shane,
God is gracious.
Shaena, Shaenah, Shaina, Shainah,
Shaynae, Shaynah, Shayne,
Shaynee, Shayney, Shayni, Shaynia,
Shaynie, Shayny

Sheba (Hebrew) queen; seventh
daughter; promise. The short
form of Bathsheba.
Saba, Sabah, Sheaba, Sheabah,
Shabeah, Sheeba, Sheebah, Sheiba,
Sheibah, Sheyba, Sheybah

Sheena (Irish) God has favoured.
The feminine form of Sean. The
Irish form of Jane, God is
gracious.
Sheana, Sheanah, Sheenah, Sheina,

Sheinah, Shena, Shenah, Sheyna,
Sheynah

Sheha (Irish/Latin) from the
boundary. (Heb) seventh
daughter; promise. A form of
Sabrina.
Shehah

Sheila (Australian/English)
feminine. The Irish form of
Cecilia, unseeing.
Sela, Selia, Sheelag, Sheelagh,
Sheelah, Sheilah, Shelag (Ir),
Shelagh (Ir), Shelia, Sheliah,
Sheilah, Sheilla, Sheilia, Sheillah,
Sheilliah, Shela, Shelagh, Shelah,
Shelia, Sheliah, Shielah, Shyla,
Shylah

Sheina (Hebrew) gift from God.
Sheana, Sheanah, Sheena,
Sheenah, Sheina, Sheinah, Shena,
Shenah, Sheyna, Sheynah

Shekeda (Hebrew) almond tree.
Shekedah

Shelby (Old English) dweller at the
estate by the shell meadow.
Shelbea, Shelbee, Shelbi, Shelbie,
Shellbea, Shellbee, Shellbey,
Shellbi, Shellbie, Shellby

Shelley (Old English) belonging to
the meadow of shells. The short
form of Michelle/Roshelle.
Chellea, Chelleah, Chellee, Chellei,
Chelleigh, Chelley, Chelli, Chellie,
Chelly, Sheilla, Sheillah, Shelea,
Sheleah, Shelee, Shelei, Sheleigh,
Sheley, Sheli, Shelie, Shell, Shellea,
Shelleah, Shellee, Shellei, Shelleigh,
Shelli, Shellie, Shelly, Shely

Shenandoa (Algonquin) beautiful
star girl.
Shenandoah

Sheona (Irish/Latin/French) she is
unity.
Sheonah, Sheowna, Sheownah

Sher (Old English) shrine.
Cher, Cherr, Sherr

Shera (Aramaic) light.
Sheara, Shearah, Sheera, Sheerah,
Sherae, Sherah, Sheralea, Sheralee,
Sheraley, Sheralla, Sheralle, Sheralin,
Sheralina, Sheraline, Sheralyn,
Sheralyna, Sheralyne, Sheray,
Sheraya, Shira, Shirah, Shyra, Shyrah

Sherelle (French) she is the
beloved.
Sherel, Sherela, Sherelah, Sherele,
Sherell, Sherella

Sheri (French) beloved.
Scherea, Scheree, Scherey, Scheri,
Scherie, Schery, Sheree, Sherey,
Sheria, Sheriah, Sherie, Sherree,
Sherrea, Sherree, Sherrey, Sherri,
Sherria, Sherriah, Sherrie, Sherry,
Shery

Sheridan (Irish/Gaelic) wild
butterfly. (Celt) from the wild
one's lair. The combination of
Sherry/Danielle, God is the judge
of the cherished one.
Cheridan, Cheriden, Sheriden,
Sheridin, Sheridon, Sherisyn,
Sherridan, Sherridana, Sherridane,
Sherridanne, Sherrydan,
Sherrydana, Sherrydane, Sherrydin,
Sherrydon, Sherrydyn, Sherydan,
Sherydana, Sherydane

Sherika (Arabic) one who listens.
(M/East/Pun) relation; family.
Shereka, Sherekah, Sherica,
Shericah, Shericka, Sherikah,
Sheriqua, Sheriquah, Sherique,
Sharyca, Sherycah, Sherycka,
Sheryckah, Sheryqua, Sheryquah,
Sheryque

Sherilyn (Celtic/Hebrew) from the
beloved pool.
Cherilyn, Cherilynn, Cherilynne,
Sherilin, Sherilina, Sherilinah,
Sheriline, Sherilyna, Sherilynah,
Sherilyne, Sherilynn, Sherilynna,
Sherilynnah, Sherilynne, Sherylin,
Sherylina, Sherylinah, Sheryline,
Sherylyn, Sherylyna, Sherylynah

Sherissa (French) beloved.
Shereesa, Shereese, Shereeza,
Shereeze, Sherisa, Sherisah, Sherise,
Sheriss, Sherissah, Sherisse,
Sheriza, Sherizah, Sherize,
Sherizza, Sherizzah, Sherizze,
Sherys, Sherysa, Sherysah, Sherys;e,
Sheryss, Sheryssa, Sheryssah,
Sherysse

Sherita (French) beloved.
Chereata, Chereatah, Chereeta,
Cherettah, Cherita, Cheritah,
Cheryta, Cherytah, Shereata,
Shereatah, Shereeta, Shereetah,
Shereta, Sheritah, Sheryta, Sherytah

Sherry (French) cherished. A short
form of Charlotte/Sheridan, wild
satyr butterfly.
Cher, Cherea, Cheree, Cherey,
Cheri, Cherie, Cherianne, Cherilyn,
Cherilynn, Cherilynne, Cherr,
Cherrea, Cherree, Cherrey, Cherri,
Cherriann, Cherrianna,
Cherrianne, Cherrie, Cherry,
Sharea, Sharee, Sharey, Shari,
Sharie, Sheerea, Sheeree, Sheerey,
Sheeri, Sheerie, Sheery, Sher,
Sherea, Sheree, Sherey, Sheri,
Sherie, Sheriann, Sherianne,
Sheridan, Shery, Sherye

Sheryl (Welsh) beloved.
Cheril, Cherile, Cherill, Cherille,
Cheryl, Cheryle, Cheryll, Cherylle,
Sheril, Sherile, Sherill, Sherille,
Sheryle, Sheryll, Sherylle

Sheyenne (Cheyenne) a tribal name. (O/Fren/Hebrew) graceful oak tree.
Cheyanne, Cheyenne, Sheyan, Shiana, Shiane, Shiann, Shianna, Shianne, Shienn, Shienna, Shienne, Shyan, Shyana, Shyanah, Shyann, Shyanna, Shyanne

Shifra (Hebrew) beautiful.
Schifra, Shifrah, Shyfra, Shyfrah

Shika (Japanese) gentle deer.
Shikah

Shilo (Hebrew) gift of God.
Shiloh, Shylo, Shyloh

Shimra (Hebrew) to keep safe from harm.
Shimrah, Shimria, Shimriah, Shymra, Shymrah, Shymria, Shymriah

Shina (Japanese) victorious.
Shinah, Shine, Shineeca, Shineese, Shinella, Shinelle, Shinequa, Shineta, Shiniqua, Shinique, Shinita, Shinitah, Shiona, Shionah, Shymra, Shymrah, Shyna, Shynah

Shinae (Irish/Gaelic/Latin) God is gracious; reborn. A combination of Renee/Shane.
Shenae, Shenai, Shenaia, Shenaiah, Shenaie, Shenay, Shinae, Shinay, Shinaya, Shinayah, Shinaye, Shynae, Shynai, Shynaia, Shynaiah, Shynaie, Shynay

Shino (Japanese) stalk of bamboo.
Shyno

Shiona (Hebrew) God is gracious.
Shionah, Shyona, Shyonah

Shiquita (Spanish) little girl. A form of Chiquita.
Shiquata, Shiquatah, Shiquitta, Shyquita, Shyquitah, Shyquyta, Shyquytah

Shiri (Hebrew) my song.
Shira, Shirah, Shiree, Shirey, Shirie, Shiry, Shyree, Shyrey, Shyri, Shyrie, Shyry

Shirley (Old English) from the bright meadow and the sunny clearing.
Sher, Sheril, Sherila, Sherilah, Sherill, Sherlea, Sherleah, Sherlee, Sherlei, Sherleigh, Sherley, Sherli, Sherlie, Sherly, Shirlea, Shirleah, Shirlee, Shirlei, Shirleigh, Shirillea, Shirilleah, Shirillee, Shirilei, Shirilleigh, Shirilley, Shirleen, Shirleena, Shirleene, Shirlei, Shirlein, Shirleina, Shirleinah, Shirleine, Shirleyn, Shirleyna, Shirleynah, Shirleyne, Shirli, Shirlin, Shirlina, Shirlinah, Shirline, Shirly, Shirlyn, Sherlyna, Sherlynah, Sherlyne, Shyrlea, Shyrleah, Shyrlee, Shyrlei, Shyrleigh, Shyrley, Shyrli, Shyrlie, Shyrly

Shirna (Japanese) good virtue.
Shirnah, Shyrna, Shyrnah

Shizu (Japanese) quiet.
Shizue, Shizuka, Shizuko, Shizuyo, Shyzu

Shona (Irish) God has favoured. The feminine form of Sean/Shane, God is gracious.
Sinead (Ir), Shain, Shaina, Shainah, Shaine, Shana, Shanah, Shane, Shanee, Shaney, Shani, Shanie, Shannon, Shany, Sharona, Sharonah, Shayn, Shayna, Shayne, Shonah, Shonee, Shoney, Shoni, Shonia, Shoniah, Shonie, Shonna, Shonnah, Shonya, Shonyah, Showna, Shownah

Shonak (Native American) stream.

Shonda/Shonta (Irish) God is
gracious. A form of Shona.
Shondah, Shondel, Shondela,
Shondele, Shondell, Shondella,
Shondelle, Shondreka, Shonta,
Shontae, Shontah, Shontia,
Shontiah, Shontya, Shontyah

Shoshana (Hebrew) graceful,
flowering lily. A form of Susanna.
Shosha, Shoshan, Shoshanah,
Shoshane, Shoshann, Shoshanna,
Shoshanne, Shoshaun,
Shoshaunah, Shoshi, Shoshia,
Shoshiah, Shoshy, Shoshya,
Shoshyah

Shoshi (Hebrew) flowering lily.
Shoshee, Shoshey, Shoshia,
Shoshoah, Shoshie, Shoshy,
Shoshya, Shoshyah

Shoshona (Hebrew) graceful,
flowering lily. A form of Susanna.
Shoshonah, Shoshonna,
Shoshonnah, Shoshowna,
Shoshownah

Shu (Chinese) kind; gentle.

Shua (Hebrew) enough.
Shuah

Shula (Arabic) bright flame.
Shulah

Shumana (Native American) rattle-
snake girl.
Chumana, Chumani, Shumani

Shunta (Irish) God is gracious. A
form of Shona.
Shuntah

Shura (Russian/Greek) defender of
humankind. A form of Alexandra.
Shurah

Shyama (Hindi) dark; beautiful.
Shiama

Shyla (English) shy.
Shila, Shilah, Shylah

Siaina (Tongan) from China.
Siainah, Syaina, Syainah

Siale (Tongan) flowering bush.
Sial, Syal, Syale

Sialea-lea (Navajo) little blue bird;
good dreamer.
Sialee, Sialey, Sialei, Sialeigh, Sialey,
Sialia, Sialiah, Sialie, Sialea-Leah,
Sialea-Lee, Sialea-Lei, Sialea-Leigh,
Sialea-Ley, Sialea-Li, Sialea-Ly

Siany (Irish) health.
Syany

Sibena (Greek) alluring; Siren.
Sibean, Sibeana, Sibeanah,
Sibeane, Sibeen, Sibeena,
Sibeenah, Sibeene, Sibenah,
Sibene, Sybean, Sybeana,
Sybeanah, Sybeane, Sybeena,
Sybeenah, Sybeene, Sybena,
Sybenah, Sybene

Sibeta (Moquelumnan) found a fish
under a rock.
Sibetta, Sibettah, Sybeta, Sybetah,
Sybetta, Sybettah

Sibley (Middle English) sister from
the meadow.
Ciblea, Cibleah, Ciblee, Ciblei,
Cibleigh, Cibley, Cibli, Ciblia,
Cibliah, Ciblie, Cibly, Siblea,
Sibleah, Siblee, Siblei, Sibleigh,
Sybley, Sybli, Syblia, Sybliah,
Syblie, Sybly

Sibyl (Greek) prophet; wise woman.
Cebel, Cebele (Fren), Cebell,
Cebelle, Cibal, Cibel, Cibell,
Cibelle, Cibil, Cibyl, Cybal, Cylbel,
Cybele, Cybell, Cybelle, Cybil,
Cybill, Cybyl, Sevilla, Sevillia,
Sibeale (Ir), Sibel, Sibelle, Sibelle,
Sibette, Sibila, Sibilla (Ital), Sibille

Sibyl cont.
(Fren), Sibillie, Sibillina, Sibla, Sibley, Sibylle (Fren/Ger), Sibyllina, Ssevilla, Sybelle, Sybelle

Sidba (Latin) shining like a star.
Sidbah, Sydba, Sydbah

Sidonia (Greek) cloth of fine linen. (Phoe) enchantress.
Sidnea, Sidneah, Sidnee, Sidney, Sidona, Sidonah, Sidonee, Sidoney, Sidoni, Sidoniah, Sidonie (Ger), Sidony, Sydona, Sydonah, Sydonia, Sydoniah, Sydnee, Sydney, Sydny, Sydonee, Sydoney, Sydoni, Sydonie, Sydony, Zedena, Zidonia, Zidoniah, Zidonya, Zidonyah, Zydona, Zydonah, Zydonia, Zydoniah, Zydonya, Zydonyah

Sidra (Latin) star.
Sidrah, Sydra, Sydrah

Sierra (Spanish/Arabic) mountain. (Ir) black. (Span) saw-like toothed.
Seara, Searah, Searria, Searriah, Seera, Seerah, Seirra, Siara, Siarah, Siarra, Siarrah, Sieara, Siearra, Siera, Sieria, Sierrah, Sierria, Sierriah, Syera, Syerah, Syerra, Syerrah

Siete (Tongan) the jet stone; dark; black.
Siet

Sigfreda (German) victorious peace. The feminine form of Sigfried.
Sigfreida, Sigfrida, Sigfrieda, Sigfryda, Sygfreda, Sygfredah, Sygfrida, Sygfridah, Sygfryda, Sygfrydah

Sigmunda (German) victorious protector. The feminine form of Sigmund.
Sigmona, Sigmonah, Sigmuna, Sigmunah, Sigmundah, Sygmon, Sygmonda, Sygmondah, Sygmuna, Sygmunah, Sygmundah

Signa/Signe (Norse) conquering guardian. (Lat) sign; symbol.
Signee, Signey, Sygne, Sygnee, Sygney

Signy (Scandinavian) victory.
Signee, Signey, Signi, Signie, Sygnee, Sygney, Sygni, Sygnie, Sygny

Sigourney (English) conqueror who is victorious. A form of Susan, lily.
Sigornee, Sigorni, Sigornie, Sigorny, Sygournee, Sygourney, Sygourni, Sygournie, Sygourny

Sigrid (Old Norse/Teutonic) beautiful victory.
Sigrida, Sigryd, Sigryda, Sygrid, Sigrida, Sygryd, Sygryda

Sigrun (Scandinavian) victory; secret.
Sygrun

Siham (Arabic) arrow.
Syham

Sihu (Native American) flower.
Syhu

Sikopio (Tongan) scorpion.
Sykopio

Sikota (Tongan) the kingfisher bird.
Sikotah, Sykoya, Sykotah

Sikueli (Tongan) squirrel.

Silafi (Tongan) giraffe.

Silika (Tongan) silk.
Silikah

Siliva (Tongan) silver.
Silivah

Silvana (Italian/Latin) silver; girl
from the woods. The Italian form
of Sylvia.
Silvanah, Silvania, Silvaniah,
Silvanna, Silvannah, Silvanne,
Silvannia, Silvanniah, Silvannya,
Silvannyah, Sylvana, Sylvanah,
Sylvania, Sylvaniah, Sylvanie,
Sylvany, Sylvanya, Sylvanyah

Silver (Old English) silversmith,
silver worker.
Silvia, Silviah, Sylver, Sylvia,
Sylviah, Sylvya, Sylvyah

Silvia (Latin) silver; girl from the
woods.
Silviah, Sylvia, Sylviah, Sylvyah

Sima (Aramaic) treasure.
Simah, Syma, Symah

Simcha (Hebrew) happiness.
Symcha

Simone (Hebrew) listening. The
feminine form of Simon.
Samon, Samone, Semoan,
Semmoan, Semmon, Semmone,
Semon, Semona, Semonah,
Semone, Simoan, Simoane,
Simmona, Simmone, Simona
(Fren), Simonna, Simonne,
Simonetta (Ital), Simonette (Fren),
Symon, Symone, Ximenia,
Ximoan, Ximon, Ximone, Xymon,
Xymone, Zimon, Zimone, Zymon,
Zymone

Simoriah (Hebrew) watcher.
Samaria, Samariah, Samarya,
Samaryah, Simaria, Simariah,
Simoria, Simorya, Simoryah,
Symoria, Symoriah, Symorya,
Symoryah

Sina (Irish) God is gracious.
Seana, Seanah, Sinah, Syna, Synah

Sinamoni (Tongan) the cinnamon
spice.
Cinamoni, Cynamoni, Synamoni

Sindy (Greek) little ashes. A short
form of Cinderella.
Cindea, Cindee, Cindey, Cindi,
Cindia, Cindiah, Cindie, Cindy,
Sinda, Sindah, Sindea, Sindee,
Sindey, Sindi, Sindia, Sindiah,
Sindie, Syndea, Syndee, Syndey,
Syndi, Syndia, Syndiah, Syndie,
Syndy

Sinead (Irish/Hebrew) God has
favoured. The Irish form of Jane,
God is gracious.
Shinad, Shinade, Shinaid, Shynade,
Shynaid

Sinitalela (Tongan) little one from
the ashes. A form of Cinderella.
Cinitalela

Sinopa (Blackfoot) fox.
Sinopah

Sinou (Tongan) snow.
Synou

Siobhain (Irish/Hebrew) admired.
The Irish form of Joanna, God is
gracious.
Chavaughn, Chavon, Chavona,
Chavonah, Chavonn, Chavonna,
Chavonne, Shavaugn, Shavaughn,
Shavon, Shavona, Shavonah,
Shavone, Shavondra, Shavonn,
Shavonna, Shavonnah, Shavonne,
Shiobain, Shivaun, Shivawn, Shyvon,
Shyvona, Shyvonah, Shyvone,
Shyvonn, Shyvonna, Shyvonnah,
Shyvonne, Sibhan, Sibraon, Siobhan,
Sobraon, Sybhan, Syvon, Syvona,
Syvonah, Syvone, Syvonn, Syvonna,
Syvonnah, Syvonne

Siola'a (Tongan) sunflower.

Sipalo (Tongan) sparrow.
Sypalo

Sipeta (Native American) fish.
Sipetah

Sirena (Greek) alluring; Siren.
Cereana, Cereanah, Cereane,
Cereena, Cereene, Cerena,
Cerenah, Cerene, Cireena,
Cireenah, Cireene, Cyreana,
Cyreanah, Cyreane, Sereana,
Sereanah, Sereane, Sereen, Sereena,
Sereene, Serena, Serene, Serin,
Serina, Serinah, Serine, Sireana,
Sireanah, Sireane, Sireen, Sireena,
Sireenah, Sireene, Sirenah, Sirene,
Sirin, Sirina, Sirenah, Sirine,
Syreana, Syreanah, Syreane,
Syreena, Syreenah, Syreene, Syrena,
Syrenah, Syrene

Siri (Scandinavian) tranquil. The
Scandinavian form of Serena.
Siree, Sirey, Sirie, Siry, Syri, Syrie,
Syry

Sirios (Greek) burning; glowing
star.
Cirios, Ciryos, Cyrios, Cyryos,
Siryos, Syrios, Syryos

Sirri (Finnish/Hebrew) princess.
The Finnish form of Sara.
Sirree, Sirrey, Sirrie, Sirry, Syrry,
Syry

Sisika (Native American) songbird.
Siskah, Syska, Syskah

Sissy (English/American) sister. The
short form of Cecilia, unseeing.
Sisee, Sisey, Sisi, Sissee, Sissey, Sissi,
Sissie, Sysee, Sysey, Sysi, Sysie, Syssee,
Syssey, Syssi, Syssie, Syssy, Sysy

Sita (Tongan) the cedar tree.
(Sans) trench.
Seata, Seatah, Seeta, Seetha, Sitah,
Syta, Sytah

Siti (Swahili) woman of respect.
Sitee, Sitey, Siti, Sitie, Sity, Sytee,
Sytey, Syti, Sytie, Syty

Sitoake (Tongan) stork.
Sytoake

Sivanah (Israeli) born during the
ninth month of the Jewish year.
Savanna, Savannah, Sivana,
Sivanna, Sivannah, Syvana,
Syvanah, Syvanna, Syvannah

Sivia (Hebrew) deer.
Siviah, Sivya, Sivyah, Syvia, Syviah,
Syvya, Syvyah

Sky/Skyler (English) blue sky;
heavenly.
Schyler (Dut), Ski, Skila, Skilar,
Skiler, Skye (Dut), Skyla, Skylar,
Skyler

Slany (Irish) healthy.
Slanee, Slaney, Slani, Slanie

Sloane (Scottish/Gaelic) warrior.
Sloan, Sloana, Sloanah, Sloane

Smiljana (Slavic) everlasting flower.
Jana, Janah, Smiljanah, Smyljana,
Smyljanah

Socorro (Spanish) one who helps.
Socoro

Sofia (Greek) wisdom. A form of
Sophia.
Sofeea, Sofeeia, Sofeeiah, Soffia,
Soffiah, Soffie, Soffy, Sofia, Sofiah,
Sofie, Sofya, Sofyah, Sophea,
Sopheea, Sopheia, Sopheiah,
Sopheya, Sopheyah, Zofea, Zofee,
Zofey, Zoffea, Zoffee, Zoffey, Zoffi,
Zoffia, Zoffiah, Zoffie, Zoffy, Zofi,
Zofia, Zofiah, Zofie, Zofy, Zofya,
Zofyah, Zophea, Zophee, Zophey,
Zophi, Zophia, Zophiah, Zophie,
Zophy

Sofronia (Greek) wisdom.
Sofroniah, Sofronya, Sofronyah

Sol (Spanish/Norse) sun.
Sola, Solah, Solar, Solara, Solla,
Sollah, Sollar, Sollara

S

Solace (Latin) bringing of comfort in a time of misery.
Sollace

Solada (Thai) listening.
Soladah

Solana (Spanish) sunshine. (Lat) easterly wind.
Solanah, Solania, Solaniah, Solanna, Solannah, Solanne, Solanya, Solanyah

Solange (French) sun angel. (Lat) alone. (Fren) solemn.
Solang, Solemnia, Solemniah

Soledad (Spanish) alone.
Sole, Soleda

Soleil (French) sunflower.
Soleila, Soleilah, Soleyl, Soleyla, Soleylah

Solenne (French) solemn; dignified.
Solaina, Solainah, Solaine, Solayna, Solaynah, Solayne, Soleana, Soleanah, Soleane, Soleena, Soleenah, Soleene, Solena, Solenah, Solene, Solenna, Solennah, Solina, Solinah, Soline, Solonez, Solyna, Solynah, Solyne, Soulina, Souline, Soulle

Solina (Greek) moon.
Soleana, Soleanah, Soleane, Soleena, Soleenah, Soleene, Solena, Solenah, Solene, Solenna, Solennah, Solina, Solinah, Soline, Solonez, Solyna, Solynah, Solyne, Soulina, Souline

Solita (Latin) accustomed; use to.
Soleata, Soleatah, Soleeta, Soleita, Soleitah, Soleighta, Soleightah, Soleetah, Soleete, Solitah, Solite, Solitta, Solittah, Solitte, Solyta, Solytah, Solytta, Solyttah, Solytte

Solva (Norse) healer.
Solvah, Solvara

Solveig (Norse) healing. (Teut) victorious warrior woman.
Solvig

Soma (Greek) body. (Hin) luna.
Somah, Somar, Somara, Somarah

Sommer (English) summer. (Arab) black.
Somma, Sommar, Sommara, Sommarah, Suma, Sumah, Sumer, Summa, Summah, Summer

Sona (Latin) noisy.
Sonah

Sondra (Greek) defender of humankind. The short form of Alexandra.
Sandra, Sandrah, Sandria, Sandriah, Sondrah, Sondria, Sondriah, Sondrya, Sondryah, Zondra, Zondrah, Zondria, Zondriah, Zondrya, Zondryah

Sonel (Hebrew) lily.
Sonela, Sonele, Sonell, Sonella, Sonelle

Sonia (Greek) wisdom. The Scandinavian/Slavic form of Sophie.
Soniah, Sonja (Dut/Nrs), Sonya (Slav), Sonyah, Zonia, Zoniah, Zonya, Zonyah

Sook (Korean) purity.
Sooki

Sopheary (Cambodian) beautiful.
Sopheaee, Sopheari, Sophearie

Sophia/Sophie (French/German/ Danish/Greek/Dutch) wisdom.
Asofe, Beathag (Scott), Sadhbba (Ir), Sadhbh (Ir), Sapienta, Sappe, Sappi, Sofee, Soffea, Soffee, Soffey, Soffi, Soffia, Soffiah, Soffie, Soffy, Soffya, Soffyah, Sofi, Sofia, Sofiah, Sofie, Sofy, Sonia, Soniah, Sonja (Slav/Nrs), Sonya (Scand/Slav),

Sophia/Sophie cont.
Sophee, Sophey, Sophi, Sophia,
Sophiah, Sophronia, Sophroniah,
Sophy, Sophya, Sophyah, Ssofija
(Russ), Zoffia, Zoffiah, Zoffya,
Zoffyah, Zofia, Zofiah, Zonya,
Zonyah, Zophia (Pol), Zophiah,
Zophie, Zophy, Zophya, Zophyah

Sora (Native American) songbird
chirping.
Sorah

Soraya (Persian) princess.
Soraia, Soraiah, Sorayah, Suraya

Sorcha (Irish/Gaelic) bright. The
Irish form of Sara, princess.
Sorchah

Sorrell (English/French) reddish-
brown colour.
Sorel, Sorela, Sorelah, Sorele,
Sorella, Sorellah, Sorelle (Fren)

Soso (Native American) chubby-
cheeked baby; squirrel eating
pine nuts.

Sospita (Latin) the saving goddess.
Sospitah

Sotiaka (Tongan) zodiac.
Sotiakah

Souzan (Persian) fire.
Souzana, Souzanah, Souzane,
Souzann, Souzanna, Souzannah,
Souzanne, Suzan, Suzana,
Suzanah, Suzane, Suzann,
Suzanna, Suzannah, Suzanne

Spangle (Dutch) sparkling
ornament.
Spangal, Spangela, Spangelah,
Spangele, Spangell, Spangella,
Spangellah, Spangelle

Sparkle (Old English) shining; witty.
Sparkal, Sparke, Sparkela,
Spakelah, Sparkele, Sparkell,
Sparkella, Sparkelle

Speranza (Italian) hope.
Speranah

Spira (Illyrian/Greek) round basket.
Spirah, Spyra, Spyrah

Spirit (Latin) lively; spiritual.
Spiryt, Spyrit, Spyryt

Spring (Old English) springtime.
Spryng

Stacey/Stacia (Greek) resurrection;
springtime. A short form of
Anastasia.
Stace, Stacee, Stacey, Staci, Staciah,
Stacie, Stacy, Stacya, Stacyah,
Stacye, Stacyee, Staicea, Staicee,
Staici, Staicia, Staiciah, Staicie,
Staicy, Staisia, Staisiah, Staisya,
Staisyah, Stasia, Stasiah, Stasha,
Staycea, Staycee, Staycey, Stayci,
Staycia, Stayciah, Staycie, Staycy,
Stasia, Staysiah, Staysya, Staysyah

Star (Old English) celestial body;
star.
Staree, Starey, Stari, Starie, Starla,
Starlea, Starleah, Starlee, Starleen,
Starleene, Starlei, Starleigh, Starley,
Starli, Starlia, Starliah, Starlie,
Starlina, Starline, Starlet, Starleta,
Starlete, Starr, Starrett, Starretta,
Starrette, Starrla, Starrlea, Starrleah,
Starrlee, Starrley, Starrlei,
Starrleigh, Starrly, Staly

Starla (English) star.
Star, Starlah, Starlana, Starlanah,
Starleana, Starleanah, Starleane,
Starleena, Starleenah, Starleene,
Starlena, Starlenah, Starlene,
Starlet, Starleta, Starletah, Starlete,
Starlett, Starletta, Starlettah,
Starlette, Starlin, Starlina, Starlinah,
Starline, Starlyn, Starlyna,
S;tarlynah, Starlyne, Starlynn,
Starlynna, Starlynnah, Starlynne

Starlee (Old English) from the star meadow.
Starlea, Starleah, Starlean, Starleana, Starleanah, Starleane, Starleen, Starleena, Starleenah, Starleene, Starlei, Starleigh, Starley, Starlin, Starlina, Starlinah, Starline, Starly, Starlya, Starlyah, Starlyn, Starlyna, Starlynah, Starlyne, Starrlea, Starrleah, Starrlee, Starrlei, Starrleigh, Starrley, Starrly, Starly

Starling (English) the starling bird.
Starlin, Starlina, Starlinah, Starline, Starlyna, Starlynah, Starlyne, Starlyng

Stefanidia (Russian) crowned.
A feminine form of Steven.
Stefanidiah, Stephanidia

Stefannia (Greek) crowned.
A feminine form of Steven.
Stefania, Stefaniah, Stefanniah, Stefannie, Stefanny, Stefannya, Stefannyah, Stefannye, Stephana, Stephanah, Stephania, Stephaniah, Stephanie, Stephany, Stephanya, Stephanyah, Stephanye, Stephenee, Stepheney, Stephenia, Stepheniah, Stephenniah, Stevania, Stevaniah, Stevanie, Stevannia, Stevanniah, Stevannie, Stevany, Stevanya, Stevanyah, Stevanye

Steffi (Greek) crowned. The short form of Stephanie. A feminine form of Steven.
Stefa, Stefah, Stefea, Stefee, Steffea, Steffee, Steffey, Steffie, Steffy, Stefy, Stephea, Stephee, Stephey, Stephi, Stephie, Stephy

Stella (Latin) star. The short form of Estella.
Estel, Estela, Estelah, Estele, Estell, Estella, Estellah, Estelle, Stela, Stelah, Stele, Stellah, Stelle

Stephanie (Greek) crowned.
A feminine form of Steven.
Estaphania, Etienette, Stefa, Stefah, Stefanea, Stefanee, Stefaney, Stefani, Stefania, Stefaniah, Stefanidia (Rus), Stefanie (USA), Steffane, Steffanea, Steffanee, Steffaney, Steffania, Steffaniah, Steffanie, Steffany, Steffanya, Steffanyah, Staffanye, Steinarna (Nrs), Stepandia (Rus), Stepania (Illy), Stephana, Stephanah, Stephane (Fren), Stephanea, Stephanee, Stephaney, Stephani, Stephania, Stephaniah, Stephanina, Stephanine (Ger), Stephany

Stevana (Greek) crowned.
A feminine form of Steven.
Stefana, Stefanah, Stefane, Stefanna, Stefannah, Steffana, Steffanah, Stephana, Stephanah, Stephanna, Stephannah, Stevanah, Stevann, Stevanna, Stevannah, Stevanne

Stevie (Greek/American) crowned.
The short form of Stephanie.
A feminine form of Steven.
Steavea, Steavee, Steavey, Steavi, Steavia, Steaviah, Steavie, Steavy, Steevea, Steevee, Steevey, Steevi, Steevia, Steeviah, Steevie, Steevy, Steevya, Steevyah, Stevea, Stevee, Stevey, Stevi, Stevia, Steviah, Stevy, Stevya, Stevyah

Stina (German/Greek) Christian.
The short form of names ending in 'stina' e.g. Christina.
Steana, Steanah, Steena, Steenah, Stinah, Styna, Stynah

Stockard (Old English) tree stump.
Stokard

Stonie (Latin/English) little stone.
Stonee, Stony, Stonia, Stoniah, Stony

Storm/Stormy (English) tempest;
storm.
Storm, Storme, Stormea, Stormee,
Stormey, Stormi, Stormia,
Sormiah, Stormie

Suchin (Thai) thoughts of beauty.
Suchina

Sudy (Old English) southerly wind.
Sudan, Sudana, Sudane, Sudea,
Sudee, Sudi, Sudie

Sue (Hebrew) lily. The short form of
Susan.
Soo, Sou, Su

Sue-Ellen (Scottish/Hebrew) lily of
the shining light.
Sooellen, Soo-Ellen, Souellen, Sou-
Ellen, Suellen, Su-Ellen

Suela (Spanish) consolation.
Suelah, Suelita, Suelyta,

Sugar (English) sweet; sugar.
Shug, Shuga, Shugah, Shugar, Suga,
Sugah

Sugi (Japanese) cedar tree.
Sugee, Sugie, Sugy

Suhaila (Arabic) gentle.
Suhailah

Sujata (Hindi) noble.
Sujatah

Suka (Tongan) sugar.
Sukah

Suke/Sukey (Hawaiian) lily. A form
of Susan.
Sukea, Sukee, Sukei, Sukey, Suki,
Sukie, Suky

Suki (Moquelumnan) eagle eye.
(Jap) beloved.
Sukea, Sukee, Sukei, Sukey, Sukie,
Suky

Sukoji (African) first-born daughter
after a son.

Sula (Icelandic) large sea bird.
Sulah

Suletu (Moquelumnan) soaring
bird.

Sulgwyn (Welsh) born on Whitsun,
the seventh Sunday after Easter.
Sulgwin

Sulia (Latin) youthful. A form of
Julia.
Suliah, Sulya, Sulyah

Sulwen (Welsh) bright like the sun.
Sulwena, Sulwenah, Sulwene,
Sulwin, Sulwina, Sulwinah,
Sulwine, Sulayn, Sulwyna,
Sulwynah, Sulwyne

Suma (Tanzanian) asked for.
Sumah

Sumalee (Thai) beautiful flower.
(Eng) from the summer meadow.
Sumalea, Sumaleah, Sumalei,
Sumaleigh, Sumaley, Sumali,
Sumalia, Sumaliah, Sumalie,
Sumaly

Sumati (Hindi) unity.
Sumatee, Sumatie, Sumaty

Sumi (Japanese) elegant.
Sumiko

Sumiko (Japanese) child of
goodness; beautiful child.
Sumi

Summer (Old English) born during
summer time.
Soma, Somah, Somma, Sommah,
Sommer, Sumer, Sunnee, Sunney,
Sunni, Sunnie, Sunny, Suvi (Finn)

Sun (Korean) obedient.
(Eng) bright.
Suncance, Sundai, Sunday, Sundea,
Sundee, Sundeep, Sundi, Sundia,
Sundiah, Sundie, Sunta, Suntah,
Sunya

Sunee (Thai) good. (Eng) sunny; happy.
Suney, Suni, Sunia, Suniah, Sunie, Sunnee, Sunney, Sunni, Sunnia, Sunniah, Sunnie, sunny, Suny

Sun-Hi (Korean) happy; good.

Sunita (Hindi) behaved.
Sunitah

Sunki (Hopi) swift, successful hunter.
Sunkia, Sunkiah, Sunkya, Sunkyah

Sunniva (Scandinavian) sun gift.
Suniva, Sunivah, Sunnivah, Sunnyva

Sunny (Old English) bright; happy.
Sonee, Soney, Soni, Sonia, Soniah, Sonie, Sonnee, Sonney, Sonni, Sonnie, Sonnny, Sunee, Suney, Suni, Sunia, Suniah, Sunie, Sunnee, Sunney, Sunni, Sunnia, Sunniah, Sunnie, Suny

Sunshine (English) shining.
Sunshyn, Sunshyne

Surata (Pakistani) blessed happiness.
Suratah

Suri (Todas) pointy nosed.
Suree, Surey, Surie, Sury

Surya (Pakistani) sun god.
Surra

Susammi (French/Latin/Hebrew) beloved lily.
Susami, Susamy, Suzami, Suzammi, Suzammy

Susan/Susannah (Hebrew) graceful lily. The short form of Susannah.
Santje, Shoshan, Shoshana (Span), Shoshanah, Shushan, Siusan (Scott), Soosan, Soosana, Soosanah, Soosane, Sosan, Sosana, Sosanah, Sosane, Sosann, Sosanna (Ital), Sosannah, Sousan, Sousana, Sousanah, Sousane, Sousann, Sousanna, Sousannah, Sousanne, Suann, Suanna, Suannah, Suanne, Suella, Suelle, Suesan, Suesana, Suesanah, Suesane, Suesann, Suesanna, Suesannah, Suesanne, Susana (Span), Susanah, Susane, Susanka, Susanna (Ital), Susannah, Susanne, Suzan, Suzana, Suzanah, Suzane, Suzann, Suzanna, Suzannah, Suzanne, Suzzan, Suzzana, Suzzanah, Suzzane, Suzzann, Suzzanna, Suzzannah, Suzzanne, Zoosan, Zoosana, Zoosanah, Zoosann, Zoosanna, Zoosannah, Zoosanne, Zoozan, Zoozana, Zoozanah, Zoozane, Zousan, Zousana, Zousanah, Zousane, Zousann, Zousanna, Zousannah, Zousanne, Zouzan, Zouzana, Zouzanah, Zouzane, Zouzann, Zouzanna, Zouzannah, Zouzanne, Zusan, Zusana, Zusanah, Zusane, Zusann, Zusanna, Zusannah, Zusanne, Zuzan, Zuzana, Zuzanah, Zuzane, Zuzann, Zuzanna, Zuzannah, Zuzanne

Susie (Hebrew) little lily. The short form of Susan.
Soosee, Soosey, Soosi, Soosie, Soosy, Sousee, Sousey, Sousi, Sousie, Sousy, Susee, Susey, Susi, Susy, Suzee, Suzey, Suzi, Suzie, Suzy, Zoosee, Zoosey, Zoosi, Zoosie, Zoosy, Zousee, Zousey, Zousi, Zousie, Zousy, Zus, Zusee, Zusey, Zusi, Zusie, Zusy, Zuz, Zuzee, Zuzey, Zuzi, Zuzie, Zuzy

Sutki (Native American) broken pot.

Suzette (French/Hebrew) little lily.
Suzet, Suzeta, Suzetah, Suzete, Suzett, Suzetta, Suzettah

Suzu (Japanese) long-lived. The
crane bird.
Suzue, Suzuko, Zuzu

Suzuki (Japanese) bell tree.
Suzukee

Suzuko (Japanese) born during the
spring or autumn/fall.
Suzu

Svannt (Scandinavian) slim.

Svea (Swedish) southerly wind.
Sveah

Svetlana (Russian/Slavic) star light.
Lana, Sveta, Svetah, Svetlanna,
Svetlannah, Svetochka

Swan/Swana (English) the swan
bird; graceful.
Swana, Swanah, Swania, Swaniah,
Swann, Swanna, Swannah, Swanya,
Swanyah

Sya (Chinese) summer.
Sia, Siah, Syah

Sybil (Greek) prophet.
Cebel, Cebele (Fren), Cebell,
Cebelle, Cibal, Cibel, Cibell,
Cibelle, Cibil, Cibyl, Cybal, Cylbel,
Cybele, Cybell, Cybelle, Cybil,
Cybill, Cybyl, Sevilla, Sevillia,
Sibeale (Ir), Sibel, Sibelle, Sibelle,
Sibette, Sibila, Sibilla (Ital), Sibille
(Fren), Sibillie, Sibillina, Sibla,
Sibley, Sibylle (Fren/Ger),
Sibyllina, Ssevilla, Sybelle, Sybelle

Sydelle (Hebrew) princess.
Cindel, Cindela, Cindele, Cindell,
Cindella, Cindelle, Sindel, Sindela,
Sindele, Sindell, Sindella, Sindelle,
Syndel, Syndela, Syndele, Syndell,
Syndella, Syndelle

Sydney (Old French) from the city
of St Denis.
Sidel, Sidell, Sidelle, Sidnee,
Sidney, Sidni, Sidnie, Sidny,

Sydnee, Sydel, Sydell, Sydelle,
Sydni, Sydnie, Sydny

Sying (Chinese) star.

Syke (Greek) mulberry tree.
Sike

Sylwen (Latin) from the forest.
Silwen, Silwena, Silwenah, Silwene,
Silwin, Silwina, Silwinah, Silwine,
Silwyn, Silwyna, Silwynah,
Silwyne, Sylwena, Sylwenah,
Sylwene, Sylwin, Sylwina,
Sylwinah, Sylwine, Sylwyn,
Sylwyna, Sylwynah, Sylwyne

Syona (Hindi) happiness.
Siona, Sionah, Syonah

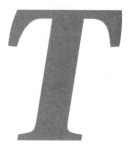

Ta'ahine (Tongan) young woman.
Tahine

Tabia (Swahili) talented.
Tabiah, Tabya, Tabyah

Tabina (Arabic) follower of
Mohammad.
Tabinah, Tabyna, Tabynah

Tabitha (Aramaic) graceful gazelle.
Tabatha, Tabbatha, Tabbetha,
Tabbitha, Tabbytha, Tabetha, Tabytha

Tacey (English) peaceful silence.
Tacea, Tacee, Taci, Tacie, Taicea,
Taicee, Taicey, Taici, Taicie, Taicy,

Taycea, Taycee, Taycey, Tayci, Taycie, Taycy

Taci (Zuni) washing tub.
Tacee, Tacey, Tacia, Taciah, Tacy, Tacya, Tacyah

Tacita (Latin) silence.
Tace, Tacea, Tacee, Taceeta, Taceetah, Tacia, Tacie, Tasie, Tasita, Tasitah, Tayce, Taycita, Taycitah, Taycyta, Taycytah

Taddea/Tadia (Hebrew) praising God. (Grk) courageous. The feminine form of Thaddeus.
Taddeah, Tadea, Tadeah, Tadia (Illy), Tadiah, Tadya, Tadyah

Tadewi (Omaha) wind.
Tadiwi

Tadita (Omaha) running.
Tadeta, Tadetah, Taditah, Tadra, Tadrah, Tadyta, Tadytah

Taesha (Latin/American) happy.
Taheisha, Tahisha, Taiesha, Taisha, Taishae, Tayesha, Teisha, Tesha, Tyeisha, Tyeishia, Tyeshia, Tyeyshia, Tyieshia, Tyishia, Tyishya, Tyshia, Tyshya

Taffy (Welsh) beloved.
Taafe, Taffea, Taffee, Taffey, Taffi, Taffie, Tafy, Tavita, Tevita

Tafline (Welsh) beloved.
A feminine form of David.
Taafe, Taflina, Taflinah, Tafline, Taflyn, Taflyna, Taflynah, Taflyne, Tavita, Tavitah, Tavyta, Tavytah, Tevita, Tevitah, Tevyta, Tevytah

Tafne (Egyptian) goddess of light.
Taffnee, Taffney, Taffni, Taffnie, Taffny, Tafna, Tafnah, Tafnee

Tafotila (Tongan) the daffodil flower.
Dafotila

Tahi (Tongan) sea water.

Tahira (Arabic) purity.
Taheera, Tahirah, Tahyra, Tahyrah

Tahiti (Polynesian) east; rising sun.
Tahitea, Tahitee, Tahitey, Tahitia, Tahitie, Tahity

Tahmoor (Australian Aboriginal) bronze-wing pigeon.
Tahmoora, Tahmoorah, Tammor, Tammora, Tammore, Tamor, Tamora, Tamorah, Tamore

Tahnee (Russian/Slavic) fairy queen. (Eng) little.
Tahne, Tahney, Tahni, Tahnia, Tahniah, Tahny, Tahnya, Tahnyah

Taika (Tongan) tiger.
Tayka

Taima (Native American) loud thunder.
Taimah, Taimy, Taimmy, Tayma, Taymah, Taymi, Taymie, Taymmi, Taymmie, Taymmy, Taymy

Taimani (Tongan) diamonds.
Taimanee, Taimaney, Taimania, Taimaniah, Taimanie, Taimany, Taimanya, Taimanyah

Tain (Omaha) new moon.
Taina, Tainah, Taine, Tayn, Tayna, Taynah, Tayne

Taipa (Moquelumnan) quail flapping its wings during flight.
Taipah, Taypa, Taypah

Tais (Greek) bound together; bond.
Taisa, Taisah, Tays, Taysa, Taysah, Thais, Thays

Taite (English) happy.
Tait, Taita, Taitah, Tate, Tayt, Tayta, Taytah, Tayte

Taiwo (Nigerian) first born of twins.
Taywo

Taja (Hindi) crown. The feminine form of Taj.
Tajah

Taka (Japanese) one who is honoured.
Takah

Takanga (Tongan) friend.
Takangah

Takaniko (Tongan) halo; Angelic.

Takara (Japanese) precious treasure.
Takarah, Takaria, Takariah, Takarya, Takaryah

Takeko (Japanese) bamboo.

Takenya (Moquelumnan) the falcon bird.
Takenia, Takeniah, Takenja, Takenjah, Takenyah

Taki (Japanese) waterfall.
Takee, Takey, Takie, Taky

Takia (Arabic) one who worships.
Takeiah, Takeiya, Takeiyah, Takeya, Takeyah, Takiah, Takija, Takijah, Takiya, Takiyah, Takkia, Takkiah, Takkya, Takkyah, Takya, Takyah, Taqiya, Taqiyah, Taqiyya, Taquaia, Taquaiah, Taquaya, Taquayah, Taquiia, Taquiiah, Tekeyia, Tekiya, Tekiyah, Tekia, Tekiah, Tykeia, Tykeiah, Tykia, Tykiah, Tykya, Tykyah

Takina (Tongan) to be carried away.
Takinah, Takyna, Takynah

Takira (Persian) sun. (Lat) light. A form of Kyra.
Takara, Takarah, Takarra, Takarrah, Takeara, Takearah, Takirah, Takiria, Takiriah, Takyra, Takyrah, Taquera, Taquerah, Taquira, Taquirah, Tekeria, Tekeriah, Tekyria, Tekyriah, Tekyrya, Tikara, Tikarah, Tikira, Tikirah, Tikiria, Tikiriah, Tikirya, Tykira, Tykirah, Tykyra, Tykyrah

Takota (Native American) friendly to all. A form of Dakota/Takoda.
Dakota (Nat/Amer/Dak), Dakotah, Takotah

Tala (Native American) stalking wolf. (Tong) seagull.
Talah

Talal (Hebrew) dew drop.
Talala, Talalah

Talanoa (Tongan) storyteller.
Talanoah

Talasi (Hopi) corn tassel.
Talasea, Talasee, Talasia, Talasiah, Talasy, Talasya, Talasyah

Tale (Botswana) the colour green.

Taleah (English/American) from the meadow with the tall trees.
Talea, Talee, Talei, Taleigh, Taley, Tali, Talia, Taliah, Taly, Talya, Talyah

Taleebin (Australian Aboriginal) new; young.
Taleabin, Taleabina, Taleabine, Taleabyn, Taleabyna, Taleabyne, Taleebina, Taleebyn, Taleebyna, Taleebyne

Taleisha (Swahili) life. A form of Aisha.
Taleasha, Taleashia, Taleashiah, Taleashya, Taleesha, Taleeshia, Taleeshiah, Taleeshya, Taleysha, Taleyshia, Taleyshiah, Taleyshya, Taleyshyah

Talena (Latin) temptress. (Nor) hard-working. (Heb) home.
Taleana, Taleanah, Taleane, Taleena, Taleenah, Taleene, Talena, Talenah, Talene, Talina, Talinah, Taline, Talyna, Talynah, Talyne

Tali (Tongan) waiting. (Heb) dew drops.
Talia, Talie, Tallia, Talliah, Tallie, Tally, Taly

Talia (Greek) flowering. (Heb)
gentle dew drops from heaven.
Tablia, Talea, Taleah, Taliah, Talli,
Tallia, Tallie, Tally, Talya, Talyah,
Thalia, Thaliah, Thalya, Thalyah

Taliba (Arabic) knowledge seeker.
Talibah, Talyba, Talybah

Taliesin (Welsh) glowing brow.
Taliesina, Taliesinah, Taliesine,
Taliesyn, Taliesyna, Taliesynah,
Taliesyne

Talikula (Tongan) fire to keep one
warm.
Talikulah

Talise (Creek) beautiful water.
Taleace, Talease, Taleece, Taleese,
Taleice, Taleise, Taleyce, Taleyse,
Talice, Taliece, Taliese, Talyce,
Talyse

Talissa (African American/English)
honey bee; holy; sacred to God. A
combination of Tally/Lisa.
Talisa, Talisah, Talissah, Talysa,
Talysah, Talyssa, Talyssah

Talite (Tongan) treaty.
Talita, Talitah, Talyt, Talyta, Talyte

Talitha (Hebrew) child.
(Aram) woman.
Talisha, Talith, Talithah (Aram),
Talithe, Talysha, Talyth, Talytha,
Talythe

Tallara (Australian Aboriginal) rain.
Talara, Talarah, Talaria, Talariah,
Talarya, Tallarah, Tallaria, Tallariah,
Tallarya, Tallaryah

Tallis (English/French) from the
woods.
Talisa, Talisah, Taliss, Talissa,
Talissah, Talisse, Talisia, Talisiah,
Talys, Talysa, Talysah, Talyse,
Talysia, Talysiah, Tallisa, Tallisah,
Talliss, Tallissa, Tallissah, Tallisse,

Tallys, Tallysa, Tallysah, Tallyse,
Talys, Talysa, Talysah, Talyss,
Talyssa, Talyssah

Tallulah (Choctaw) leaping,
running water.
Tallis, Tallou, Tallula, Tallula

Tally (Hebrew) child.
Talea, Taleah, Talee, Talei, Taleigh,
Taley, Tali, Talie, Tallea, Tallee,
Tallei, Talleigh, Talley, Talli, Tallie,
Taly

Talma (Native American) crash of
thunder. (Heb) small hill.
Talmah (Heb), Talmar, Talmara,
Talmarah, Talmare, Talmaria,
Talmariah, Talmarya, Talmaryah

Talmor (Arabic) mound of myrrh;
perfume.
Talmoor, Talmoora, Talmoorah,
Talmoore, Talmora, Talmorah,
Talmore

Talor (Hebrew) morning dew drops.
Talora, Talorah, Talore, Talorey,
Talori, Taloria, Taloriah, Talorie,
Talory, Talorya, Taloryah, Talorye

Talutah (Sioux) red.
Taluta

Talya (Hebrew) little lamb.
Talia, Taliah, Talyah

Tam (Vietnamese) heart. The short
form of names starting with 'Tam'
e.g. Tammy.
Tama, Tamah, Tami, Tamia,
Tamiah, Tamie, Tamy, Tamya,
Tamyah

Tama (Hebrew) palm tree; pigeon.
(Jap) well-polished jewel.
Tamah, Tamara, Tamarah

Tamah (Hebrew) wonder.
Tama

Tamaka/Tamaki (Japanese) bracelet.
Tamakah, Tamakia, Tamakiah,
Tamaky, Tamakya, Tamakyah

Tamanna (Hindi) desire.
Tamana, Tamanah, Tamannah

Tamar/Tamara (Hebrew) palm tree;
date fruit. The feminine form of
Tamar.
Ramora, Tama, Tamar, Tamarah,
Tamaree, Tamari, Tamaria,
Tamariah, Tamarie, Tamarind
(Arab), Tamarra, Tamarrah,
Tamarya, Tamaryah, Tamera,
Tamerlain, Tamerlaina, Tamerlaine,
Tamika, Tamma, Tamra, Tamy

Tamas (Hindi) night. (Heb) twin.
A feminine form of Thomas.
Tamass

Tamasina/Tamassa (Aramaic) twin.
A feminine form of Thomas.
Tamas, Tamasa (Heb), Tamasah,
Tamsin, Tamsinah, Tamsine,
Tamsyn, Tamsyna, Tamasynah,
Tamsyne, Tamzin, Tamzina,
Tamzinah, Tamzine, Tamzyn,
Tamzyna, Tamzynah, Tamzyne

Tamath (Arabic) slow pace.
Tamatha, Tamathah, Tamathe,
Tamathia, Tamathiah, Tamathya,
Tamathyah

Tameka (Hebrew) twin. A feminine
form of Thomas.
Tameca, Tamecah, Tamecka,
Tameckah, Tameeca, Tameecah,
Tameeka, Tameekah, Tamekah,
Tamica, Tamicah, Tamicka,
Tamickah, Tamika, Tamikah,
Tamyca, Tamycah, Tamycka,
Tamyckah, Tamyka, Tamykah

Tamesha (Hindi) born under the
sign of Aries.
Tameesha, Tameeshia, Tameeshiah,
Tameeshya, Tameshah, Tameshia,

Tamisha, Tamishah, Tamishiah,
Tamysha, Tamyshah, Tamyshia,
Tamyshiah, Tamyshya, Tamyshyah

Tami (Japanese) people. (Heb)
perfection; palm tree; date fruit.
A form of Tammy.
Tamee, Tamey, Tamie, Tamika,
Tamm, Tammee, Tammey, Tammi,
Tammie, Tammy, Tamo, Tamy

Tamiko (Japanese) the people's
child.
Tameeko, Tameko, Tamyko

Tamila (Russian) dearest.
Tamilah, Tamilla, Tamillah,
Tamyla, Tamylah, Tamylla,
Tamyllah

Tammy/Tamra (Hebrew) perfection;
palm tree; date fruit.
Tamalane, Tamalina, Tamalinah,
Tamaline, Tamara, Tamee,
Tameeka, Tameika, Tamera,
Tamerah, Tamey, Tamia, Tamiah,
Tamika, Tamike, Tamiko, Tamilla,
Tamille, Tamira, Tamisa, Tamisha,
Tamitta, Tamitte, Tamlyn, Tammee,
Tammey, Tammi, Tammia,
Tammiah, Tammie, Tammra,
Tammrah, Tamra, Tamrah, Tamy,
Tamya, Tamyah, Tema, Temah,
Temara, Temarah, Temaria,
Temariah, Temarya, Temaryah,
Tomika, Tomyka

Tamrika (African American/Hebrew)
wealthy perfection. (Heb) wealthy
palm tree; date fruit. A
combination of Tammy/Rick.
Tamrick, Tamrickah, Tamrikah,
Tamriqua, Tamriquah, Tamrique,
Tamryca, Tamrycah, Tamrycka,
Tamryckah, Tamryka, Tamrykah,
Tamryqua, Tamryquah, Tamryque

Tana (Australian Aboriginal)
ceremony.
Tanah

Tanah/Tanasha (Slavic/Russian) fairy queen found on Christmas Day. The combination of Tanya/Natasha.
Taina, Tainah, Tanae, Tanah, Tanasha, Tanashah, Tania, Taniah, Tanya, Tanyah

Tanay/Tanaya (African American/Hindi) daughter.
Tanaya, Tanayah, Tania, Taniah, Tanya, Tanyah

Tandie (Greek) immortal.
Tandea, Tandee, Tandey, Tandi, Tandia, Tandiah, Tandt, Tandy, Tandya, Tandyah, Tandye

Tandy (English) part of a team.
Tandea, Tandee, Tandey, Tandia, Tandiah, Tandya, Tandyah

Taneya (Russian/Slavic) fairy queen.
Taneeia, Taneeiah, Taneeya, Taneeyah, Taneia, Taniah, Tanya, Tanyah

Tangelia (Greek) angel; messenger of God.
Tangel, Tangelah, Tangele, Tangell, Tangellah, Tangelle, Tanjel, Tanjela, Tanjele, Tanjell, Tanjella, Tanjelle

Tangerine (English) girl from the city of Tangier in Morocco; an orange/red colour.
Tangeryne

Tangia (Greek) angel.
Tangiah, Tangya, Tangyah, Tanja, Tanji, Tanjia, Tanjie, Tanjy

Tani (Japanese) valley. (Span) to make famous.
Tanee, Tania, Taniah, Tanie, Tanita, Tannis, Tany, Tanya, Tanyah, Tanys, Tanysa, Tanysah, Tanyta, Tanytah, Tanyte

Tania/Tanya (Russian/English/Australian/American) fairy queen. The short form of Tatiana.
Tana, Tanah, Tanelle, Tahna, Tahni, Tahnia, Tahnee, Taina (Scan), Tanja, Tana, Tanae, Tanaya, Tanea, Tanee, Taneek, Taneisha, Tanhya, Taniah, Tanika, Tanique, Taniya, Taniyah, Tanja, Tanjah, Tanje, Tanneale, Tannia, Tanniah, Tannika, Tannya, Tannyah, Tanthe, Tanya, Tanyah, Tatiana, Tatianah, Tatiania, Tatianiah, Tatiann, Tatianna, Tatiannah, Tawnea, Tawnee, Tawney, Tawni, Tawnia, Tawniah, Tawnie, Tawny, Tawnya, Tawnyah, Tenaya, Teneal, Tenia, Teniah, Tenie, Tenya, Tenyah, Tonia, Toniah, Tonie, Tonya, Tonyah

Taniel (Hebrew) God is my judge. The feminine short form of Nathaniel.
Taniela, Tanielah, Taniele, Taniell, Taniella, Taniellah, Tanielle, Tanyel, Tanyela, Tanyelah, Tanyell, Tanyella, Tanyellah, Tanyelle

Tanisha (Russian/Slavic) fairy queen.
Taneesha, Taneeshah, Tanishah, Tanysha, Tanyshah

Tanita (Hebrew) one who plants.
Taneeta, Taneetah, Tanitah, Tanyta, Tanytah

Tanith (Phoenican) goddess of love.
Tanitha, Tanithah, Tanithe, Tanyth, Tanytha, Tanythah, Tanythe

Tannis (Slavic) fairy queen.
Tanis, Tanisa, Tanisah, Tanissa, Tanissah, Tanisse, Tannisa, Tanniah, Tannisah, Tannissa, Tannisse, Tannys, Tannysa, Tannysah, Tannyssa, Tannyssah

Tansy (English) the tansy herb.
(Lat) persistent. (Grk) immortal.
Tansea, Tansee, Tansey, Tansi,
Tansia, Tanisah, Tansie, Tansya,
Tansyah, Tansye

Tao (Chinese/Vietnamese) peach
flower child.

Tara (Irish/Gaelic) rocky hill.
(Aram) carry. (Arab) measure.
Taria, Tariah, Tarah, Taralyn,
Taralynn, Taralynne, Taran, Tarnia,
Tarniah, Tarra, Tarrah, Tarya,
Taryah, Taryn, Taryna, Tarynah,
Taryne

Taral (Hindi) ripple.
Tarala, Tarala, Tarale, Tarral,
Tarrala, Tarralah, Tarrel

Taralga (Australian Aboriginal)
native friend.
Taralgah

Taraneh (Persian) melody.
Taran, Tarana, Taranah, Tarane

Tarati (Maori) gift of God.
Taratea, Taratee, Taratey, Taratia,
Taratiah, Taratie, Taraty, Taratya,
Taratyah

Taree (Australian Aboriginal) wild
fig. (Jap) branch with an arch.
Tarea, Tarey, Taria, Tariah, Tarie,
Tary, Tarya, Taryah

Tari (Irish) from the rocky hill. A
form of Tara.
Tarea, Taree (Aust/Abor), Tarey,
Taria, Tariah, Tarie, Tary, Tarya,
Taryah

Tarika (Hindi) star.
Tarikah, Taryka, Tarykah

Tarne (English/Scandinavian)
mountain lake.
Tarn, Tarnee, Tarney, Tarni, Tarnia,
Tarniah, Tarnie, Tarny, Tarnya,
Tarnyah, Tarnye

Tarni (Australian Aboriginal) salt
water.
Tarne, Tarnea, Tarnee, Tarney,
Tarnia, Tarniah, Tarnie, Tarny,
Tarnya, Tarnyah, Tarnye

Tarra (Australian Aboriginal) small
stream.
Tara, Tarah, Tarrah

Taryn (Irish/Gaelic) from the
peaceful, rocky hill. A
combination of Tara/Erin.
Taran, Taren, Tarin, Tarina, Tarinah,
Tarine, Tarrin, Tarrina, Tarrinah,
Tarrine, Taron, Tarron, Tarryn,
Tarryna, Tarrynah, Tarryne, Taryna,
Tarynah, Taryne, Tarynn, Tarynna,
Tarynnah, Tarynne

Tasaria (Gypsy) child born at
sunrise.
Tasara, Tasarah, Tasariah, Tasarya,
Tasaryah

Tasarla (Gypsy) child born during
the morning.
Tasarlea, Tasarleah, Tasarlee,
Tasarleigh, Tasarley, Tasarli,
Tasarlia, Tasarliah, Tasarlie, Tasarly,
Tasarlya, Tasarlyah, Tasarlye

Tasha (Latin/English) born on
Christmas Day. A short form of
Natasha, nativity.
Tashi, Tashia, Tashiah, Tashy,
Tashya, Tashyah, Tassam, Tawsha

Tashana (Hebrew) God's gracious
child born on Christmas Day;
nativity. A combination of
Shane/Natasha. A feminine form
of Shane.
Tashanah, Tashani, Tashania,
Tashaniah, Tashanya, Tashanyah

Tashanee (African American/
Swahili) marvellous, wonderful
one born on Christmas Day. A
combination of Shani/Natasha,
nativity.
Tashaney, Tashani, Tashania,
Tashaniah, Tashanie, Tashany,
Tashanya, Tashanyah

Tashawna (Hebrew) God's gracious
child born on Christmas Day;
nativity. A combination of
Shawna/Natasha. A feminine
form of Shawn.
Taseana, Taseanah, Taseania,
Taseaniah, Taseanya, Taseanyah,
Tashaughna, Tashaughnah,
Tashauna, Tashaunah, Tashaunia,
Tashauniah, Tashaunya,
Tashaunyah, Tashawnah,
Tashawnia, Tashawniah,
Tashawnya, Tashawnyah

Tashelle (Hebrew) born on
Christmas Day; nativity; likeness
to God. A combination of
Michelle/Natasha.
Tashel, Tashela, Tashelah, Tashele,
Tashelei, Tashelia, Tasheliah,
Tashelie, Tashell, Tashella,
Tashellah, Tashellea, Tashelleah,
Tashellee, Tashelleigh, Tashelley,
Tashelli, Tashellia, Tashelliah,
Tashelly, Tashellya, Tashellyah

Tashi (Hausa) bird flying.
Tashe, Tashee, Tashey, Tashia,
Tashiah, Tashie, Tashy, Tashya,
Tashyah

Tasia (Slavic/Greek) born on
Christmas day.
Tasiah, Tasija, Tasiya, Tasya, Tasyah

Tasida (Native American) horse
rider.
Tasidah, Tasyda, Tasydah

Tasma (Hebrew) twin. (Slav) born
on Christmas Day. The short
form of Tasmin. A feminine form
of Thomas.
Tasmah, Tasmar, Tasmara,
Tasmarah, Tasmaria, Tasmariah,
Tasmarya, Tasmaryah

Tasmin (Hebrew) twin. A feminine
form of Thomas.
Tamasin, Tamasine, Tammi,
Tammie, Tamsin, Tammy, Tamzin,
Tamzina, Tasma, Tasmyn, Tasmyna,
Tasmynah, Tasmyne, Tasmynn,
Tasmynna, Tasmynnah, Tasmynne,
Tazmin, Tazmina, Tazminah,
Tazmine, Tazmyn, Tazmynah,
Tazmyne, Thomasa, Thomasah,
Thomasin, Thomasina,
Thomasinah, Thomasine,
Thomasyn, Thomasyna,
Thomasynah, Thomasyne,
Tomasin, Tomasina, Tomasinah,
Tomasine, Tomasyn, Tomasyna,
Tomasynah, Tomasyne

Tassie (Australian) from Tasmania,
a state in Australia. (Heb) twin.
A short form of Tasmin.
Tasee, Tasey, Tasi, Tasia, Tasiah,
Tasie, Tassee, Tassey, Tassi, Tassia,
Tassiah, Tassy, Tasy, Tazee, Tazey,
Tazi, Tazia, Taziah, Tazie, Tazy,
Tazzee, Tazzey, Tazzi, Tazzia,
Tazziah, Tazzie, Tazzy

Tassos (Greek) harvester.
Tasos

Tata (Russian) fairy queen.
Tatah, Tatia, Tatiah, Tatja, Tatjah,
Tatya, Tatyah

Tate (Old English) happy.
Tait, Taitam, Taitem, Tiatim,
Taitom, Taitum, Taite, Tatam,
Tatem, Tatim, Tatom, Tatum, Tayt,
Tayta, Tayte

Tatiana (Russian) fairy queen.
Tahna, Tanea, Tanee, Tania, Taniah, Tanja, Tanjah, Tanya, Tatania, Tataniah, Tatgana, Tatianna, Tatiannah, Tatiara (Aust/Abor), Tatiarah, Tatjana, Tatyana, Tatyanah, Tatyane, Tatyann, Tatyanna, Tatyannah, Tatyanne

Tatsu (Japanese) dragon.

Tatum (Old English) happy; from Tate's town; from the spirited, cheerful one's town. (Nat/Amer) long-winded talker.
Tait, Taitam, Taitem, Taitim, Taitom, Taitum, Taitym, Tata, Tatam, Tate, Tatem, Tatim, Tatom, Taytam, Taytem, Taytim, Taytom, Taytum, Taytym

Tauba (German) dove.
Taubah

Taufa (Tongan) storm.

Taula (Tongan) priestess.
Taulah

Taulaki (Polynesian) waiting.
Taulakee, Taulakie, Taulaky

Taura (Latin) child born under the sign of Taurus; bull.
Taurah, Tauri, Tauria, Tauriah, Taurie, Taury, Tauryah

Tautiti (Polynesian) graceful dancer.
Tautitee, Tautitie, Tautity

Tavake (Tongan) white sea bird with black spots, two long feathers in the tail. (Poly) honoured.
Tavakee, Tavakey, Tavaki, Tavakiah, Tavakie, Tavaky, Tavakya, Tavakyah

Tavia (Latin) eighth-born child. A form of Octavia.
Taviah, Tavja, Tavjah, Tavya, Tavyah

Tavie (Scottish) twin. (Aram) good. The feminine short form of Tavi/Tavish.
Tavee, Tavey, Tavia, Taviah, Tavja, Tavya, Tavyah

Tawanna (German/American) wandering. A form of Wanda.
Tawanda, Tawandah, Tawannda, Tawanndah, Tawannah

Tawia (African) child born after twins.
Tawiah, Tawya, Tawyah

Tawny (English) light brown/red complexioned. (Gyp) little.
Tawnea, Tawnee, Tawney, Tawni, Tawnia, Tawniah, Tawnie, Tawnya, Tawnyah, Tawnye

Taya (Japanese) home in the valley field.
Taia, Taiah, Tayah

Tayanita (Cherokee) beaver.
Taianita, Taianitah, Tayanitah, Tayanyta, Tayanytah

Taylea (Old English) from the tall tree meadow.
Tailea, Taileah, Tailee, Tailei, Taileigh, Tailey, Taili, Taailia, Taliah, Tailie, Taly, Talya, Talyah, Tayleah, Taylee, Taylei, Tayleigh, Tayley, Tayli, Taylia, Tayliah, Taylie, Tayly

Taylor (Old English) tailor of clothes.
Tai, Taie, Taila, Tailah, Tailar, Tailara, Tailer, Tailor, Tailora, Tailore, Taurina, Taurine, Tay, Taya, Tayah, Taye, Tayla, Taylah, Taylar, Taylara, Tayler, Taylora, Taylore

Tazu (Japanese) stork; long-lived.
Tazoo

Tea (Welsh) beautiful. The short form of Teagan.
Teah, Tee, Teeh, Teia, Teiah, Teya, Teyah

Teagan/Tegan (English/Irish/Welsh) beautiful. (Celt) doe.
Taegan, Taegen, Taegin, Taegon, Taegun, Taegyn, Teagen, Teahgan, Teahgen, Teahgin, Teahgon, Teahgyn, Teagin, Teagon, Teagun, Teagyn, Teegan, Teegen, Teegin, Teegon, Teegun, Teegyn, Tegan, Tegana, Teganah, Tegane, Teigan, Teigen, Teigin, Teigon, Teigun, Teigyn, Teygan, Teygen, Teygin, Teygon, Teygun, Teygyn, Tigan, Tigen, Tigin, Tigon, Tigun, Tigyn, Tygan, Tygen, Tygin, Tygon, Tygun, Tygyn

Teal (English) sea green/blue.
Teala, Tealah, Teale, Teel, Teela, Teele, Teil, Teila, Teilah, Teyla, Teylah

Teangi (Australian Aboriginal) earthy.
Teeangi

Teanna (English/German/Swedish) graceful.
Teana, Teanah, Teane, Teannah, Teanne, Teiana, Teianah, Teiane, Teiann, Teianna, Teiannah, Teianne, Teyan, Teyana, Teyanah, Teyane, Teyann, Teyanna, Teyannah, Teyanne, Tian, Tiana, Tianah, Tiane, Tiann, Tianna, Tiannah, Tianne, Tyan, Tyana, Tyanah, Tyane, Tyann, Tyanna, Tyannah, Tyanne, Tyanne

Teca (Hungarian) harvester. A form of Theresa.
Tecah, Techa, Techah, Tecka, Teckah, Teka, Tekah, Tica, Ticah, Tika, Tikah, Tyca, Tycah, Tyka, Tykah

Tecia (Greek) God's famous one.
Teciah, Tecya, Tecyah, Tekia, Tekiah, Tekya, Tekyah

Tecla (Greek) divine; famous.
Tecla, Tekla (Swed), Telca, Telka, Thecla, Thecle, Theoclia, Tjokle

Teddi/Teddi-Jo (Old English/American/Greek) wealthy ruling guardian; gift of God; bear; God is gracious. A feminine form of Edward/Theodore.
Teddea, Teddee, Teddey, Teddi, Teddia, Teddiah, Teddie, Teddi-jo, Teddy, Teddy-jo, Tedi, Tedia, Tediah, Tedie, Tedy-jo, Tedy

Tedra (Greek) gift of God. (Eng) divine flame.
Teddra, Teddrah, Tedrah

Tegan-Evvron (Celtic) beautiful doe.
Taegan, Taegen, Taegin, Taegon, Taegun, Taegyn, Teagen, Teahgan, Teahgen, Teahgin, Teahgon, Teahgyn, Teagin, Teagon, Teagun, Teagyn, Teegan, Teegen, Teegin, Teegon, Teegun, Teegyn, Tegan, Tegana, Teganah, Tegane, Teigan, Teigen, Teigin, Teigon, Teigun, Teigyn, Teygan, Teygen, Teygin, Teygon, Teygun, Teygyn, Tigan, Tigen, Tigin, Tigon, Tigun, Tigyn, Tygan, Tygen, Tygin, Tygon, Tygun, Tygyn

Telae (Tongan) fish.

Tellus (Latin) earth.
Tellas, Tellass, Tellassa, Telasse, Tellous

Temima (Hebrew/Arabic) honest.
Tamar, Tamimah, Tamyma, Tamymah

Tempany (Latin/Australian) storm.
A form of Tempest.
Tempanee, Tempaney, Tempani,
Tempania, Tempaniah, Tempanie,
Tempanya, Tempanyah

Temperance (Latin) moderation.
Tempe, Tempee

Tempest (Latin) storm.
Tempesta, Tempestah, Tempeste
(Fren), Tempestt, Tempestta,
Tempestte

Templa (Latin) temple.
Temp, Templa, Templah, Tempe,
Temple

Tennille (Irish/English) champion.
The feminine form of Neil.
Teneal, Teneall, Tenealla, Teanelle,
Tenil, Tenila, Tenilah, Tenile, Tenill,
Tenilla, Tenillah, Tennille, Tennil,
Tennila, Tennile, Tennill, Tennilla,
Tennyl, Tennyla, Tennylah,
Tennylle, Tenyl, Tenyla, Tenylah,
Tenyle, Tenyll, Tenylla, Tenyllah,
Tenylle

Tequila (Spanish) alcoholic drink.
Takila, Takilah, Taquela, Taquella,
Taquila, Taquilla

Tera (Latin) earth.
Terah, Teria, Teriah, Terra, Terrah,
Terria, Terriah, Terrya, Terryah

Teralyn (Latin/English) from the
land by the pool.
Teralin, Teralina, Teralinah,
Teraline, Teralyna, Teralynah,
Teralyne, Terralin, Terralina,
Terralinah, Terraline, Terralyn,
Terralyna, Terralynah, Terralyne

Terelle (Greek/French) she is the
harvester.
Terel, Terela, Terele, Terell, Terella,
Terelle, Terrel, Terrella

Terentia (Greek) smooth; tender;
gracious. The feminine form of
Terrence.
Terentilla, Terentillah, Terentille,
Terentya, Terentyah, Terentyla,
Terentylah, Terentyle, Terentylla,
Terentyllah, Terentylle

Teresa/Teri/Terry/Theresa/Therese
(Greek) harvester.
Terea, Tereasa, Tereasah, Terease,
Teree, Terees, Tereesa, Tereesah,
Tereese, Tereey, Teresah, Terese,
Teresina (Ital), Teresita (Span),
Teressa, Tereza (Illy), Terezia
(Hung), Treza, Terezie (Boh),
Terezija (Slav), Terezon (Fren),
Terezyga (Poly), Teri, Teria, Teriah,
Terie, Terisa, Terisah, Terise, Terrea,
Terreas, Terreasa, Terreasah,
Terrease, Terree, Terreey, Terris,
Terrisa, Terrisah, Terrise, Terry,
Terrys, Terrysa, Terrysah, Terryse,
Tery, Terza (Illy), Thereas, Thereasa,
Thereasah, Therease, Theresa,
Theresah, Therese (Fren/Ger),
Theresia (Ger), Theresie (Ger),
Theris, Therisa, Therisah, Therise,
Therris, Therrisa, Therrisah,
Therrise, Therrys, Therrysa,
Therrysah, Therryse, Therys,
Therysa, Therysah, Theryse, Tracey,
Tracie, Tracy, Tresca, Tresa, Tressa

Terra (Japanese) swiftly moving
arrow. (Lat) land.
Tera, Terah, Teria, Teriah, Terrah,
Terria, Terriah, Terrya, Terryah

Terrand (Latin/Greek) humankind's
Earth.
Teranda, Terandah, Terrandah

Terrene (Latin) smooth; tender;
gracious. The feminine form of
Terrence.
Terean, Tereana, Tereane, Tereen,
Tereena, Tereene, Terin, Terina,
Terine, Terrean, Terreana, Terreane,

T

Terreen, Terreena, Terreene, Terrin,
Terrina, Terrine, Terryn, Terryne,
Terryne

Tertia (Latin) third-born child.
Tertiah, Tertya, Tertyah

Teruma (Hebrew) gift.
Terumah, Teshura, Teshurah

Tess (Greek) harvester; fourth-born
child. A short form of Theresa.
Tes, Tesa, Tesah, Tessa, Tessah,
Tessara

Tessa (Polish) loved by God.
Tesa, Tesah, Tessah

Tetsu (Japanese) iron.
Tetsoo

Tetta (Teutonic) ruler of the house.
A short form of Henrietta.
Teta, Tetah, Tettah

Tevy (Cambodian) angel.
Tevee, Tevey, Tevi, Tevie

Thaddea (Greek) praising God.
(Grk) courageous. The feminine
form of Thaddeus.
Thadia, Thadiah, Thadie, Thadina,
Thadinah, Thadine, Thadya,
Thadyah, Thadyn, Thadyna,
Thadynah, Thadyne

Thai (Greek) bonding.
Thaisa, Thaise, Thays, Thaysa,
Thaysah, Thayse

Thalassa (Greek) from the sea.
Thalassah

Thalia (Greek) flowering.
Thaliah, Thalya, Thalyah

Thamah (Hebrew) honest.
Thama

Thamar (Hebrew) palm tree; the
date fruit. A form of Tamara.
Thamara, Thamarah, Thamare,
Thamaria, Thamariah, Thamarya,
Thamaryah

Thana (Arabic) happy time.
Thaina, Thainah, Thayna, Thaynah

Thandie (Zulu) beloved.
Tandee, Tandey, Tandi, Tandie,
Tandy, Thandee, Thandey, Thandi,
Thandy

Thanh (Chinese/Vietnamese) blue.

Thao (Vietnamese) one who
respects her parents.

Thea (Greek) divine. The short form
of Dorothea, gift.
Fea, Feah, Theah, Theia, Theiah,
Theya, Theyah

Theano (Greek) divine name.
Feano

Thecla (Greek) divine flame.
Tecla (Fren), Tekla, Thecle (Fren),
Thekla, Theoclia, Tjokle (Russ)

Thekla (Greek) famous of God.
Tecla, Teclah, Theklah

Thelma (Greek) wilful.
Telma, Thelmae, Thelmah,
Thelmai, Velma, Velmah

Thema (African) queen.
Themah

Themba (Zulu) trusted.
Thembah

Theodora (Greek) gift of God. The
feminine form of Theodore.
Bohdana, Fedore (Slav), Feodora
(Slav), Feodoria, Feodoriah,
Fjodora, Tedra, Teodora (Ital/Span),
Teodosia, Tewdews (Wel), Thaddea,
Thadine, Theadora, Thedra,
Thedosia, Thedosiah, Thedosya,
Thedosyah, Theklatheo

Theodosia (Greek) God-given.
Feodosia (Slav), Teodosia (Ital),
Teodosiah, Teodosya, Teodosyah,
Theodosiah, Theodosya,
Theodosyah

Theola (Greek) God's name is divine.
Theolah, Theone

Theone (Greek) gift of God.
Theona, Theonah, Theonee

Theophania (Greek) God has appeared; given to girls born at Epiphany (Jan 6th), a Christian festival.
Epiphant, Theophaniah, Theophanie (Fren), Theophano, Theophanya, Theophanyah

Theophila (Greek) beloved of God. The feminine form of Theodore, gift of God.
Teofilia, Tesia, Theofilia, Theofilie, Theophila, Theophyla, Theophylah, Theophylla, Theophyllah

Theora (Greek) watchful.
Theorah

Thera (Greek) wild.
Thereah

Thetis (Greek) determined.
Thetisa, Thetisah, Thetise, Thetiss, Thetissa, Thetisse, Thetys, Thetysa, Thetyse, Thetyss, Thetyssa, Thetyssah, Thetysse

Thi (Vietnamese) poem.
Thia, Thiah, Thy, Thya, Thyah

Thirza (Hebrew) pleasant; acceptable.
Thirzah, Thyrza, Thyrzah

Thomasina/Thomasine (Latin/Greek) twin. A feminine form of Thomas.
Tamasin, Tamasina, Tamasine, Tamsin, Tamzin, Tamzina, Tamzine, Tamzon, Tasasin, Tasin, Thamasa, Thamasin, Thamasina, Thamasine, Thomasa, Thomasin (Ger), Thomasina, Thomasine,
Thomasing, Thomason, Thomassine, Thomassyn, Thomassyna, Thomassynah, Thomassyne, Thomasyn, Thomasyna, Thomasynah, Thomasyne, Tomasin, Tomasinah, Tomasine, Tomasyn, Tomasyna, Tomasynah, Tomasyne, Tommianne, Tommyana, Tommyanah, Tommyane, Tommyann, Tommyanna, Tommyannah, Tommyanne

Thoomie (Australian Aboriginal) silence.
Thoomee, Thoomey, Thoomi, Thoomia, Thoomiah, Thoomy, Thoomya, Thoomyah

Thora (Scandinavian) thunder. The feminine form of Thor.
Thorah, Thordia, Thordiah, Thordis, Thordya, Thordyah, Tira, Tirah, Tyra, Tyrah

Thorberta (Old Norse) the brilliance of Thor; thunder brilliance. The feminine form of Thor.
Thorbertah, Thorbirta, Thorbirtah, Thorburta, Thorburtah, Thorbyrta, Thorbyrtah

Thordis (Old Norse) Thor's spirit; thunder spirit.
Thordia, Thordisa, Thordisah, Thordise, Thordiss, Thordissa, Thordissah, Thordisse, Thordys, Thordysa, Thordyse, Thordyss, Thordyssa, Thordyssah, Thordysse

Thrine (Greek) purity.
Thrina, Thrinah, Thryn, Thryna, Thrynah, Thryne

Thur (Australian Aboriginal) truthful.
Thura, Thurah

Thuy (Vietnamese) gentle.

Thyra (Old Norse) dedicated to the god of war. (Grk) shield bearer.
Thira, Thirah, Thyrah, Tyra, Tyrah

Thyrza (Greek) wand.
Thirza, Thirzah, Thyrzah

Tia (Tongan) deer. (Egypt) princess.
Tea, Teah, Teea, Teeah, Teia, Teiah, Teya, Teyah, Tiah, Tianah, Tiane, Tianee, Tianna, Tiannah, Tianne, Tya, Tyah, Tyana, Tyanah, Tyane, Tyann, Tyanna, Tyannah, Tyanne

Tiana (Russian) fairy queen. (Eng/Heb/Egypt) graceful princess. The short form of Tatiana.
Tianah, Tiane, Tianee, Tianna, Tiannah, Tianne, Tiannee, Tyana, Tyanah, Tyane, Tyann, Tyanna, Tyannah, Tyanne, Tyannee

Tiara (Latin) jewelled crown.
Tiarah, Tyara, Tyarah

Tiba (Navajo) grey.
Tibah

Tibelda (Teutonic) boldest one of all.
Tibeldah, Tybelda, Tybeldah

Tiberia (Latin) from the river Tiber.
Tiberiah, Tyberia, Tyberiah, Tyberya, Tyberyah

Tida (Thai) daughter.
Taj, Tidah, Tyda, Tydah

Tiernan (English) of the Lord.
Tyernan

Tierney (Irish/Gaelic) grandchild of the chief.
Tiernee, Tierni, Tiernie, Tierny, Tyernee, Tyerney, Tyerni, Tyernie, Tyerny

Tifara (Hebrew) happy.
Tifarah, Tifarra, Tifarrah, Tyfara, Tyfarah, Tyfarra, Tyfarrah

Tiffany (Greek) God appears to her.
Teffan, Teffani, Thefania, Theophania, Thiphania, Tifane, Tifainee, Tifanie, Tiffan, Tiffanie, Tiffinie, Tiphane, Tiphanee, Tiphaney, Tiphani, Tiphania, Tiphaniah, Tiphanie, Tiphany, Tyffanee, Tyffaney, Tyffani, Tyffanie, Tyffany

Tigris (Irish) tiger.
Tiger, Tigriss, Tyger, Tygris, Tygriss, Tygrys, Tygryss

Tijuana (Spanish) Mexican town.
Tajuyana, Tajuanah, Tajuanna, Thejuana, Thejuanah, Tiajuana, Tiajuanah, Tiawanna, Tyawanna

Tiki (Maori) green stone ornament; carving. (Poly) a dead person's soul is taken by the gods.
Tikee, Tikey, Tikie, Tiky

Tikvah (Hebrew) hope.
Tikva

Tilda (German) powerful warrior.
Tildah, Tylda, Tyldah

Tilly (Teutonic) strength through the battle. (Grk) fortunate warrior.
Tilda, Tildah, Tildea, Tildeah, Tildee, Tildey, Tildi, Tildie, Tildy, Tillea, Tilleah, Tillee, Tillei, Tilleigh, Tilley, Tilli, Tillie, Tily, Tylda, Tyldah, Tyldee, Tyldey, Tyldi, Tyldie, Tyldy, Tylee, Tylei, Tyleigh, Tyley, Tyli, Tylie, Tyllea, Tyleah, Tylee, Tylei, Tyleigh, Tyley, Tyli, Tylie, Tyllea, Tylleah, Tyllee, Tyllei, Tylleigh, Tylley, Tylli, Tyllie, Tylly, Tyly

Timi (English) she honours God.
Timea, Timee, Timey, Timie, Timmea, Timmee, Timmey, Timmi, Timmie, Timmy, Timy, Tymea, Tymee, Tymey, Tymi, Tymie,

Timi cont.
Tymmea, Tymmee, Tymmi,
Tymmie, Tymmy, Tymy

Timmy (Hebrew) honouring God.
The short feminine form of
Timothy.
Timea, Timee, Timey, Timie,
Timmea, Timmee, Timmey, Timmi,
Timmie, Timy, Tymea, Tymee,
Tymey, Tymi, Tymie, Tymmea,
Tymmee, Tymmi, Tymmie, Tymmy,
Tymy

Timna (Hebrew) one who is
restrained; bound.
Timnah, Tymna, Tymnah

Timone (Hebrew) listening. A form
of Simone. A feminine form of
Simon.
Temon, Temone, Tymon, Tymona

Timothea (Greek) one who honours
God. A feminine form of
Timothy.
Timathea, Timithea, Timythea,
Tymathea, Tymithea, Tymithea,
Tymythea

Tina (English) little. (Lat) Christian.
The short form of names
containing or ending in 'tina' e.g.
Christina.
Teana, Teanah, Teania, Teaniah,
Teanya, Teanyah, Teena, Teenah,
Teenia, Teeniah, Teenya, Teenyah,
Tena, Tenah, Tenia, Teniah, Tenna,
Tennah, Tennia, Tenniah, Tennya,
Tennyah, Tenya, Tenyah, Tiena,
Tienah, Tienna, Tiennah, Tinah,
Tyna, Tynah

Tinble (English) bell.
Tinbla, Tynbal, Tynble

Ting (Chinese) graceful.

Tinka (Australian Aboriginal) day.
Tinkah, Tynka, Tynkah

Tinkerbelle (Middle English) one
who rings the bell.
Tinkabel, Tinkabela, Tinkabelah,
Tinkabele, Tinkabell, Tinkabella,
Tinkabellah, Tinkerbell,
Tinkerbella, Tinkerbellah,
Tinkerbelle, Tinkle, Tynkabel,
Tynkabela, Tynkabelah, Tynkabele,
Tynkabell, Tynkabellah, Tynkabelle

Tiponya (Native American) great
horn owl eating an egg.
Tiponia, Tiponiah, Tiponyah,
Typonia, Typoniah, Typonya,
Typonyah

Tira (Hebrew) enclosure.
(Hind) arrow.
Tirah, Tyra, Tyrah

Tirranna (Australian Aboriginal)
running water; stream.
Tirran, Tirrann, Tirrannah,
Tirranne, Tyran, Tyrana, Tyranah,
Tyrane, Tyrann, Tyranna, Tyrannah,
Tyranne, Tyrran, Tyrrana, Tyrranah,
Tyrrane, Tyrrann, Tyrranna,
Tyrrannah, Tyrranne

Tirza (Hebrew) cypress tree;
pleasant.
Tierza, Thirza, Thirzah, Thyrza,
Tyrza, Tyrzah

Tish/Tisha (English) happy. The
short form of names ending in
'Tisha' e.g. Latisha.
Teasha, Teashia, Teashiah, Teashya,
Teashyah, Teesha, Teeshia,
Teeshiah, Teisha, Tiesha, Tieshia,
Tieshiah, Tishah, Tishia, Tishiah,
Tysha, Tyshah, Tyshia, Tyshiah

Titania (Greek) graceful great one.
The feminine form of Titan.
Titaniah, Titanya, Titanyah, Titia,
Titiah, Tytania, Tytaniah, Tytanya,
Tytanyah

T

Titia (Greek) of great size and power; of the giants. The feminine form of Titus.
Titiah, Titya, Tityah, Tytia, Tytiah, Tytya, Tytyah

Titilayo (Nigerian) forever happy.
Titilaio

Tiulipe (Tongan) the tulip flower.
Tulip

Tivona (Hebrew) fondness for nature.
Tibona, Tiboni, Tivonah, Tivone, Tivoni, Tivonie, Tivony, Tyvona, Tyvonah, Tyvone

Tiwa (Zuni) onion.
Tiwah, Tywa, Tywah

Tobi/Tobia (Hebrew) God is good. The feminine form of Tobias/ Toby.
Toba, Tobe, Tobea, Tobee, Tobelle, Tobey, Tobi, Tobia, Tobiah, Tobias, Tobie, Toby, Tobye, Tobya, Tobyah, Tobyas, Tov, Tova, Tove, Tybi, Tybie, Tyby

Tocarra (Irish/Latin) dearest friend.
Tocara, Tocarah, Tocarrah

Toeris (Egyptian) she is great.
Toerisa, Toerys, Toeryse

Tofe (Tongan) oyster.
Tofee, Tofey

Tofu (Tongan) calm.
Tofoo

Tohuia (Polynesian) flower.
Tohuiah, Tohuya, Tohuyah

Toinette (Greek/Latin) priceless. The short form of Antoinette. A feminine form of Anthony.
Toinet, Toineta, Toinete, Toinett, Toinetta, Toynet, Toyneta, Toynete, Toynett, Toynetta, Toynette

Toki (Japanese) hopeful.
Tokee, Tokey, Toko, Tokoya, Tokyo

Tokoni (Tongan) helper.
Tokonee, Tokoney, Tokonia, Tokoniah, Tokony, Tokonya, Tokonyah

Toku (Japanese) virtue; purity.

Tola (Polish/Greek) flowering.
Tolah, Tolsia, Tolsiah, Tolsya, Tolsyah

Tolla (Polish/Latin/Roman) priceless.
Tola, Tolah, Tollah

Toloa (Tongan) the Southern Cross, group of stars in the southern hemisphere.
Toloah

Tomi (Japanese) wealthy.
Tomea, Tomee, Tomey, Tomie, Tommea, Tommee, Tommey, Tommi, Tommie, Tommy, Tomy

Tomiko (Japanese) child born of wealth and happiness.
Tomika, Tomikah, Tomyko

Tomo (Japanese) intelligent.
Tomoko

Toni/Tonia (Greek) priceless. The short form of Antonia. The feminine form of Tony/Anthony.
Antonia, Antoniah, Tona, Tonah, Tonea, Tonee, Toneea, Tonia, Toniah, Tonie, Tonneli (Swiss), Tonnia, Tonniah, Tonnya, Tonnyah, Tonya, Tonyah

Tonneli (Swiss) priceless. The feminine form of Tony.
Tonelea, Toneleah, Tonelee, Tonelei, Toneleigh, Toneley, Toneli, Tonelia, Toneliah, Tonelie, Tonely, Tonnelea, Tonneleah, Tonnelee, Tonnelei, Tonneleigh, Tonneley, Tonnelie, Tonnely

Toora (Australian Aboriginal) bird.
Toorah

Topaz/Topaza (Latin) the topaz
gem. (Sans) fire.
Topaza, Topazah, Topazia,
Topaziah, Topazz, Topazza,
Topazzah, Topazzia, Topazziah

Topsy (English) the best.
Topsea, Topsee, Topsey, Topsi,
Topsia, Topsie

Tora (Japanese) tiger.
Torah, Torra, Torrah

Tordis (Scandinavian) goddess of
Thor's; goddess of thunder.
Tordiss

Tori (Japanese) bird of victory. A
short form of Victoria, victory.
Torea, Toree, Torey, Toria, Toriah,
Torie, Torree, Torrey, Torri, Torrie,
Torry, Tory, Torya, Toryah

Toriana (English/Latin) graceful
victory.
Torian, Torianah, Toriane, Toriann,
Torianna, Toriannah, Torianne,
Torya, Toryah, Toryan, Toryana,
Toryanah, Toryane, Toryann,
Toryanna, Toryannah, Toryanne

Toshala (Hindi) satisfaction.
Shala, Shalah, Toshalah

Toshi (Japanese) mirror reflection;
she resembles her mother; year.
Toshee, Toshey, Toshi, Toshie, Toshy

Toski (Hopi) squashed beetle.
Toskee, Toskey, Toskie, Toskt

Totara (Irish/Maori) to the rocky
hill. A form of Tara.
Totarah, Totarra, Totarrah

Totsi (Hopi) moccasins.
Totsee, Totsey, Totsia, Totsie, Totsy,
Totsya, Totsyah

Totti (English) little one; baby.
Totee, Totey, Toti, Totie, Tottee,
Tottey, Tottie, Totty, Toty

Tourmaline (Sri Lankan) the
tourmaline gem.
Tourmalina, Tourmalyn,
Tourmalyna, Tourmalyne

Tovah (Hebrew) good.
Tova

Toya/Toyah (Japanese) door that
leads into a valley. (Eng) play
thing.
Latoya, Latoyah, Toia, Toiah, Toyah

Tracey/Tracie/Tracy (Irish/Gaelic)
warrior. (Lat) courageous.
Tracea, Tracee, Tracia, Traciah,
Tracie, Tracinda, Tracinta, Tracy,
Traicee, Traicey, Traici, Traicia,
Traiciah, Traicie, Traicy, Traisea,
Traisee, Traisey, Traisi, Traisia,
Traisiah, Traisie, Traisy, Trasea,
Trasee, Trasey, Trasi, Trasia, Trasiah,
Trasie, Trasy, Trasya, Trasyah,
Traycea, Traycee, Traycey, Traci,
Traycia, Trayciah, Traycya,
Traycyah, Traysea, Traysee, Traysey,
Trasi, Trasia, Trasiah, Trasie, Trasy

Tracta (English) attractive.
Attracta, Attractah, Tractah

Traudl (Bavarian/Teutonic) spear
strength. A short form of
Gertrude.
Trudea, Trudee, Trudey, Trudi,
Trudia, Trudiah, Trudie, Trudy,
Trudya, Trudyah

Trava (Slavic) the first grass of
spring.
Travah

Traviata (Italian) one who strays.
Traviatah, Travyata, Travyatah

Treasure (English) precious.
Treasur, Treasura, Treasurah

Treinel (Bavarian/Greek) purity. A form of Katherine.
Treinala, Treinele, Treinell, Treinella, Treinelle, Trynel, Trynela, Trynelah, Trynele, Trynell, Trynella, Trynellah, Trynelle

Treveen (Welsh) cautious one; large village home. The feminine form of Trevor.
Treveana, Treveanah, Treveane, Treveena, Treveenah, Treveene, Trevin, Trevina, Trevinah, Trevine, Trevora, Trevore, Trevyn, Trevyna, Trevynah, Trevyne

Trevina (Welsh) from the homestead.
Treveana, Treveanah, Treveane, Treveen, Treveena, Treveenah, Treveene, Trevin, Trevinah, Trevine, Trevora, Trevore, Trevyn, Trevyna, Trevynah, Trevyne

Triana (Latin/English) graceful third-born child.
Trianah, Triane, Triann, Trianna, Triannah, Trianne, Tryan, Tryana, Tryanah, Tryane, Tryann, Tryanna, Tryannah, Tryanne

Trifene (Greek) delicate.
Trifena, Trifenah, Trifenna, Trifennah, Tryfena, Tryfenah, Tryfenna, Tryfennah, Tryphena, Tryphenah

Trilby (English) music; soft hat.
Trilbea, Trilbee, Trilbey, Trilbi, Trilbie, Trylbea, Trylbee, Trylbey, Trylbi, Trylbie, Trylby

Trina (Scandinavian) purity. The short form of names ending in 'trina' e.g. Katrina. (Eng) third-born child.
Treana, Treanah, Treanee, Treaney, Treani, Treanie, Treany, Treena, Treenah, Treenee, Treeney, Treeni, Treenia, Treeniah, Treenie, Trinah,

Trini, Trinia, Triniah, Trinie, Triny, Tryna, Trynah, Trynia, Tryniah, Trynya, Trynyah

Trinity (Latin/Hebrew) three; the Father, the Son and the Holy Spirit.
Trinidad, Trinitee, Trinitey, Triniti, Trinitie, Trynitee, Tryniti, Trynitie, Trynity

Trisha (Latin) noble; well born. The short form for names ending in 'trisha' e.g. Patricia.
Tricia, Trish, Trista, Trysha, Tryshah, Trysta, Trystah

Trista (Latin) melancholy; sad; thoughtful. A feminine form of Tristan, bold.
Tristah, Tristar, Trysta, Trystah

Tristanne (Latin/Hebrew) graceful; sad; thoughtful.
Tristan, Tristana, Tristanah, Tristane, Tristann, Tristanna, Tristannah, Trystan, Trystana, Trystanah, Trystane, Trystann, Trystanna, Trystannah, Trystanne

Tristbelle (Latin/French) beautiful; sad; thoughtful.
Tristabel, Tristabela, Tristabelah, Tristabele, Tristabell, Tristabella, Tristabellah, Tystrabel, Trystabela, Trystabelah, Trystabele, Trystabell, Trystabella, Trystabellah, Trystabelle

Tristen (Latin) loud. (Fren) sorrowful. (Wel) bold knight. A feminine form of Tristan.
Trista, Tristah, Tristan, Tristana, Tristanah, Tristane, Tristar, Tristian, Tristiana, Tristianah, Tristiane, Tristiann, Tristianna, Tristiannah, Tristianne, Trystian, Trystiana, Trystianah, Trystiane, Trystiann, Trystianna, Trystiannah, Trystianne, Trystyan, Trystyana, Trystyanah,

Tristen cont.
Trystyane, Trystyann, Trystyanna, Trystyannah, Trystyanne

Tristianna (Celtic) graceful; sad; thoughtful.
Tristiana, Tristianah, Tristiane, Tristiann, Tristiannah, Tristianne, Tristyan, Tristyana, Tristyanah, Tristyane, Tristyann, Tristyanna, Tristyannah, Tristyanne, Trystian, Trystiana, Trystianah, Trystianna, Trystiannah, Trystianne, Trystyan, Trystyana, Trystyanah, Trystyane, Trystyann, Trystyanna, Trystyannah, Trystyanne

Trixi/Trixie (English/Latin) she brings happiness. A form of Beatrice. (Eng) trickster.
Trixe, Trixee, Trixey, Trixie, Trixy, Tryxee, Tryxey, Tryxi, Tryxie, Tryxy

Troya (Irish) warrior.
Troi, Troia, Troiah, Troiana, Troianah, Troiane, Troiann, Troianna, Troiannah, Troianne, Troyan, Troyana, Troyanah, Troyane, Troyann, Troyanna, Troyannah, Troyanne

Truda (Teutonic) loved. (Pol) spear warrior.
Trudah, Trudee, Trudey, Trudi, Trudia, Trudiah, Trudie, Trudy, Trudya, Trudyah

Trudel (Dutch/German) beloved warrior.
Trudela, Trudelah, Trudele, Trudell, Trudella, Trudellah, Trudelle

Trudy (Teutonic) spear strength. A short form of Gertrude.
Truda, Trudah, Trudee, Trudey, Trudi, Trudia, Trudiah, Trudie, Trudya, Trudyah

True/Truley/Truth (Old English/Puritan) truthful.
Trula, Trulea, Truleah, Trulee, Trulei, Truleigh, Trulia, Truliah, Truly, Trulya, Trulyah

Trutta (Australian Aboriginal) star.
Truta, Trutah, Truttah

Tryphena (Greek) delicate.
Trifena, Trifenna, Truffeni, Truffeniah, Tryphosa

Tsomah (Kiowa) fair-haired.
Tsoma

Tsula (Cherokee) fox.
Tsulah

Tu (Chinese) jade stone.

Tuesday (English) born on a Tuesday.
Tuesdae, Tuesdai

Tuhina (Hindi) snow.
Tuhinah, Tuhyna, Tuhynah

Tuki (Japanese) moon.
Tukee, Tukie, Tuky

Tula (Hindi) peace.
Tulah, Tulla, Tullah

Tulip (English) (Botanical) the tulip flower.
Tulip, Tullip, Tullop, Tullyp,Tulop, Tulyp

Tullia (Irish/Gaelic) peaceful.
Tulliah, Tulla, Tullah, Tullya, Tullyah, Tulya, Tulyah

Tully (Irish) mighty people.
Tulea, Tuleah, Tulee, Tulei, Tuleigh, Tuley, Tuli, Tulie, Tullea, Tulleah, Tullee, Tullei, Tulleigh, Tulley, Tulli, Tullie, Tuly

Tulsi (Hindi) the basil herb.
Tulsia, Tulsiah, Tulsy, Tulsya, Tulsyah

U

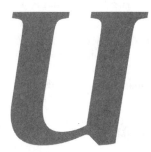

Turquoise (Old French) the Turkish stone; blue/green colour.
Turquois

Tusa (Zuni) prairie dog.
Tusah

Tuwa (Hopi) earth.
Tuwah

Tuyen (Vietnamese) snow.

Tuyet (Chinese) snow white.
Tuyeta, Tuyetah

Twyla (Old English) woven; double thread.
Twila

Tyanna (Latin/English) graceful.
Tian, Tiana, Tianah, Tiane, Tiann, Tianna, Tiannah, Tianne, Tyan, Tyana, Tyanah, Tyane, Tyannah, Tyanne

Tybal (Old English) holy place where sacrifices occur.
Tibal, Tibala, Tibalah, Tybala, Tybalah

Tyler (English) tile layer.
Tiler, Tiller, Tyller, Tylor

Tyne (Old English) river.
Tine

Tyra (Scandinavian) warrior.
Tira, Tirah, Tyrah

U (Korean) gentle.

Ualani (Hawaiian) heavenly rain.
Ualana, Ualanah, Ualanea, Ualanee, Ualaney, Ualania, Ualanie, Ualany, Ualanya, Ualanyah

Ualusi (Tongan) walrus.

Uchenna (Nigerian) God's will.
Uchena

Uda/Udele (Teutonic/Old English) prosperous.
Udah, Udel

Udiya (Hebrew) God's fire.
Udiyah

Ugolina (Teutonic) intelligent. (O/Ger) heart; mind. The feminine form of Hugo/Ugo.
Hugolin, Hugolina, Hugolinah, Hugoline, Hugolyna, Hugolynah, Hugolyne, Ugolin, Ugolinah, Ugoline, Ugolyna, Ugolynah, Ugolyne

Uha (Tongan) rain.

Uha-Tea (Tongan) sun shower.

Uhila (Tongan) lightning.
Uhilah, Uhilla, Uhillah, Uhyla, Uhylah, Uhylla, Uhyllah

Uinise (Polynesian) victory.

Ujana (Breton) noble excellence.
Jana, Janah, Ujanah, Uyana, Uyanah

U

Ujila (Hindi) light that is bright.
Ujilah

Ula (Celtic) jewel of the sea.
(O/Ger) inheritor. (Span)
wealthy.
Eula, Oola, Uli, Ulah, Ulia, Ulla,
Ullah

Ulalia (Greek) speaks sweetly.
Ulaliah, Ulalya, Ulalyah

Ulani (Hawaiian) light-hearted.
Ulana, Ulanah, Ulane, Ulanee,
Ulaney, Ulania, Ulanie, Ulany,
Ulanya, Ulanyah

Ulema (Arabic) wisdom.
Uleama, Uleamah, Uleema,
Uleemah, Ulemah, Ulima, Ulimah,
Ulyma, Ulymah

Ulla (Old French) to fill.
(Ger/O/Nrs) wilful. (Arab)
wisdom.
Ula, Ulah, Ullah

Ulrica (Teutonic) ruling wolf.
(O/Nrs) wolf. The French
feminine form of Ulrich.
Ulricah, Ulricka, Ulrickah, Ulrika
(Russ), Ulrikah, Ulriqua, Ulrique,
Ulriques (Fren), Ulryca, Ulrycah,
Ulrycka, Ulryckah, Ulryka (Pol),
Ulrykah, Ulryqua, Ulryque, Ulva,
Ulvah

Ultima (Latin) great.
Ultimah, Ultyma, Ultymah

Ulu (Nigerian) second-born child.

Uluaki (Polynesian) first-born
child.

Ululani (Hawaiian) heavenly
inspiration.
Ululanee, Ululaney, Ululani,
Ululania, Ululaniah, Ululanie,
Ululany, Ululanya

Ulva (Norse) wolf; courage; fierce
ruler.
Ulvah

Uma (Sanskrit) peace. (Heb) nation.
(Hind) mother.
Umah

Umali (Hindi) generous.

Umay (Turkish) hopeful.
Umai

Umayma (Arabic) little mother.
Umaymah

Ume (Japanese) plum blossom
flower.

Umeko (Japanese) plum blossom
child; patience.

Umiko (Japanese) sea child.

Umina (Australian Aboriginal)
sleeping child.
Uminah, Umyna, Umynah

Umm (Arabic) mother.

Umniya (Arabic) desired.
Umnyah

Umpima (Australian Aboriginal)
water lily.
Umpimah, Umpyma, Umpymah

Una (Hopi) good memory.
(Ir) lamb. (Lat) one.
Juno, Ona, Oona, Oonagh, Unagh,
Unah, Unitee, Unitey, Unity, Wony

Undina (Latin) wave of water.
Ondin, Ondina, Ondinah, Ondine,
Ondyn, Ondyna, Ondynah,
Ondyne, Undinah, Undine,
Undyn, Undyna, Undynah,
Undyne

Undurra (Australian Aboriginal)
silver wattle tree (tree with little
yellow flowers).
Undura, Undurah, Undurrah

Unique (Latin) the only one.
Unica, Uniqua, Uniqua, Unique

Unity (Middle English) together.
Unita, Unite, Unitea, Unitee,
Unitey, Unyt, Unyta, Unytea,
Unytee, Unytey, Unyti, Unytie,
Unyty

Unn (Norwegian) she is loved.
Un, Una, Unah, Unna, Unnah

Unna (Icelandic/German) woman.
Una, Unah, Unnah

Unnea (Old Norse) linden tree.
Unea, Uneah, Unneah

Upala (Hindi) beach.
Upalah

Urana (Australian Aboriginal) quail
flapping its wings in flight.
Uranah, Uranna, Urannah

Urania (Greek) heavenly.
Uraina, Urainah, Urainia,
Urainiah, Uranie, Uraniya, Uranya,
Uranyah

Urbana (Latin) belonging to the
town.
Urbanah, Urbanna, Urbannah

Urbi (Nigerian) princess.
Urbia, Urbiah, Urby, Urbya,
Urbyah

Uri (Hebrew) God's light.
Uree, Urie, Ury

Uriana (Greek) heaven.
Riana, Rianna, Riann, Rianne,
Urianna, Uriannah, Urianne,
Uryan, Uryana, Uryanah, Uryane,
Uryann, Uryanna, Uryanne

Urika (Omaha) useful.
Urica, Uricah, Uricka, Urickah,
Urikah, Uriqua, Uryca, Urycah,
Uryka, Urykah, Uryqua

Urit (Hebrew) light.
Urice, Urita, Uritah, Urith, Uryt,
Urita, Urytah

Urith (Teutonic) deserving.
Uritha, Urithah, Uryth, Urythah

Ursa (Greek) little bear.
Ursah, Ursea, Ursey, Ursi, Ursie,
Ursy

Ursula (Latin) little she-bear.
Orsa, Orscha, Orsche, Orselina,
Orseline, Orsola (Irish), Orsolija,
Sula, Ursa, Ursala, Ursel, Ursina,
Ursine, Ursola (Span), Ursule
(Fren), Ursulina, Ursuline, Ursylyn,
Ursulyna, Ursulyne, Urzsula,
Urzsulah, Urzula (Pol), Urzulah,
Worsola

Urte (Latin) thorny bush.
Urta, Urtah

Usha (Sanskrit) sunrise.
Ushah, Ushas

Ushi (Chinese) ox.
Ushee, Ushie, Ushy

Ushmil (Hindi) warm.

Ut (Vietnamese) from the east.

Uta (German) rich heroine.
(Jap) poem; song.
Utah, Utako

Utah (Spanish) mountain dweller.
Uta, Utar

Utano (Japanese) song field.
Utan, Utana, Utanah

Utatci (Native American) scratching
bear.

Utina (Native American) woman of
my country.
Uteana, Uteanah, Uteena, Uteenah,
Utinah, Utyna, Utynah

Uzza (Arabic) mighty.
Uza, Uzah, Uzzah

Uzzia (Hebrew) God is strong.
Uzia, Uziah, Uzya, Uzyah,
Uzziahm Uzzya, Uzzyah

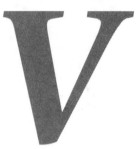

Vach (Sanskrit) speech.
Vac

Vachya (Hindi) speaking.
Vachia, Vachiah, Vachyah

Vaha (Tongan) open sea.
Vah

Vail (English) from the valley.
Vail, Vailee, Vailey, Vaili, Vailie,
Vaily, Vale, Valee, Valey, Valie, Valy,
Vayl, Vayle

Vailea (Polynesian) talking water.
Vaileah, Vailee, Vailei, Vaileigh,
Vailey, Vaili, Vailie, Vaily, Vaylea,
Vayleah, Vaylee, Vaylei, Vayleigh,
Vayley, Vayli, Vaylie, Vayly

Vaino (Latin) self-obsessed; vain.
Vaina, Vainah, Vaine, Vanitee,
Vanitey, Vaniti, Vanitie, Vanity

Vaitafe (Tongan) stream.
Vaytafe

Val (Latin) strength. The short form
of Valerie, strong; brave; healthy.
Vale, Vall, Valle

Vala (Gothic/German) chosen.
Valah, Valla, Vallah

Valancia (Latin) strength.
Valanca, Valence, Valenciah,
Valencya, Valencyah

Valasquita (Teutonic) powerful
protector.
Valasquitah, Valasquitta,
Valasquittah

Valborga (Teutonic) protecting
ruler; guardian.
Valborg, Valborgah

Valda (Old Norse) hero ruler of the
battle.
Valdah, Valma, Valmah

Valencia (Spanish) strong; brave;
healthy.
Valenciah, Valencya, Valencyah

Valene (Latin) strength.
Valaina,Valainah, Valaine, Valean,
Valeana, Valeanah, Valeane, Valeda,
Valeen, Valeena, Valeenah, Valeene,
Valena, Valeney, Valien, Valina,
Valine, Vallan, Vallana, Vallanah,
Vallane, Vallen, Vallena, Valenah,
Vallene, Vallina, Vallinah, Valline,
Vallyna, Vallynah, Vallyne

Valentia (Latin/Italian) strong
princess.
Valena, Valentiah, Valentya,
Valentyah

Valentina/Valentine (Latin) strong;
healthy; brave; powerful.
Valeda, Valencia, Valenteana,
Valenteane, Valenteen, Valenteena,
Valenteene, Valentia, Valentin,
Valentina, Valentine, Valentyn,
Valentyna, Valentyne, Valida,
Validah, Valyda, Valydah

Valerie (Latin) strong; brave; healthy.
Valaree, Valaria, Valariah, Vale,
Valeri, Valeria (Ital), Valeriah,
Valery, Valerye, Valeska, Valry,
Valori, Valorie, Valory, Valorya,
Valoryah

V

Valeska (Polish/Slavic) powerful
princess. The feminine form of
Vladyslav.
Valeskah

Valley (English) from the valley.
Valea, Valeah, Valee, Valei, Valeigh,
Valey, Vali, Valia, Valiah, Vallea,
Valleah, Vallee, Vallei, Valleigh,
Valli, Vallia, Valliah, Vallie, Vally,
Valy, Valya, Valyah

Valli (Latin) strength. A form of
Valerie, strong; brave; healthy.
(O/Eng) from the valley.
Valea, Valeah, Valee, Valei, Valeigh,
Valey, Vali, Valia, Valiah, Vallea,
Valleah, Vallee, Vallei, Valleigh,
Valley, Vallia, Valliah, Vallie, Vally,
Valy, Valya, Valyah

Vallia (Spanish) powerful protector.
Valia, Valiah, Valliah, Vallya,
Vallyah

Vallonia (Latin) acorn.
Valloniah, Vallonya, Vallonyah,
Valona, Valonah, Valoniah,
Valonya, Valonyah

Valma (Welsh) may flower.
(Ger) protector. (Fin) battle.
Valmah, Valmai (Wel), Valmar,
Valmara, Valmarah

Valonia (Latin) strong, brave,
courageous one who is alone.
(O/Eng) from the lonely valley.
Lonia, Loniah, Vallonia, Valloniah,
Vallonya, Vallonyah, Valoniah,
Valione, Valionee, Valioney,
Valioni, Valionia, Valioniah,
Valionie, Valiony, Valionya,
Valionyah, Valyona, Valyonah,
Valyonia, Valyoniah, Valyony,
Valyonya, Valyonyah

Valonu (Latin) belonging to the
valley.
Valona, Valonah, Valone

Valora (Latin) brave; strong;
courageous.
Valorah, Valore, Valoree, Valorey,
Valori, Valoria, Valoriah, Valory,
Valorya, Valoryah, Valorye

Valua (Latin/English) desired;
important.
Valuah, Value

Vana (Polynesian) sea urchin.
Vanah, Vanna, Vannah

Vanaja (Hindi) daughter from the
forest.
Vanaia, Vanaiah, Vanajah, Vanya,
Vanyah

Vanalika (Hindi) sunflower.
Vanalikah, Vanalyka, Vanalykah

Vanda (Teutonic) stem.
(Ger) wander. A form of Wanda.
Vandah

Vandani (Hindi) honourable.
Vandanee, Vandaney, Vandani,
Vandanie, Vandany

Vanessa (Greek) butterfly.
Vanassa, Vanesa, Vanesha, Vaneshia,
Vanesia, Vanesse, Vanessee,
Vanessia, Vanessica, Vanetta,
Vaneza,Vania, Vaniah,Vaneice,
Vaniessa, Vanija, Vanika, Vanisa,
Vaniss, Vanissa, Vanisse, Vanissee,
Vanita, Vanna, Vannah, Vannessa,
Vannesse,Vannessee, Vannia,
Vanniah, Vannysa, Vannysah,
Vannyssa, Vannyssah, Vanysa,
Vanysah, Vanyssa, Vanyssah

Vanetta (Dutch) little one of
nobility; belonging to or from.
The feminine form of Van.
Vaneta, Vanetah, Vanete, Vanett,
Vanettah, Vanette

Vani (Hindi) voice.
Vanee, Vaney, Vanie, Vany

V

Vania (Hebrew) God is gracious. The feminine form of Ivan.
Vanea, Vaneah, Vaniah, Vannea, Vanneah, Vannia, Vanniah, Vannie, Vannya, Vannyah, Vanya, Vanyah

Vanilla (Latin/English) sweetly scented; the vanilla bean plant.
Vanila, Vanilah, Vanillah, Vanyla, Vanylah, Vanylla, Vanyllah

Vanity (English) vain.
Vanita, Vanitah, Vanitee, Vanitey, Vaniti, Vanitie, Vanittee, Vanittey, Vanitti, Vanittie, Vanitty, Vanyti, Vanytia, Vanytie, Vanyty

Vanja (Scandinavian) God is gracious.
Vanjah, Vanya

Vanka (Russian/Hebrew) graceful. The Russian form of Ann/e.
Vancan Vancka, Vankah, Vankia, Vankiah, Vankya, Vankyah

Vanna (English) high.
Vana, Vanah, Vania, Vaniah, Vannah, Vannia, Vanniah, Vannya, Vannyah, Vanya, Vanyah

Vanni (Italian/Hebrew) graceful. The Italian form of Ann/e.
Vanea, Vanee, Vaney, Vani, Vania, Vaniah, Vanie, Vanna, Vannah, Vanne, Vannee, Vanney, Vannie, Vanny, Vany

Vanora (Celtic) white wave.
Vanorah, Vanorea, Vanoree, Vanorey, Vanori, Vanoria, Vanoriah, Vanorie, Vanory, Vanorya, Vanoryah, Vevay

Vantrice (Greek) from the harvest.
Vantricia, Vantriciah, Vantricya, Vantricyah, Vantrise, Vantrisia, Vantrisiah, Vantrisya, Vantrisyah, Vantrysia, Vantrysiah, Vantrysya, Vantrysyah

Vanya (Russian/Hebrew) graceful. A form of Ann/e.
Vania, Vaniah, Vanja, Vannia, Vanniah, Vannja, Vannya, Vannyah, Vanyah

Vara (Norse) cautious.
Varah, Varia, Variah

Varana (Hindi) river.
Varanah, Varanna, Varannah

Varda/Vardina/Vardis (Hebrew/ Arabic) rose.
Vardia, Vardiah, Vardin, Vardinah, Vardine, Vardinia, Vardiniah, Vardyce, Vardyn, Vardyna, Vardynah, Vardyne, Vardys, Vardysa, Vardyse

Varina/Varine (Russian) stranger. (O/Eng) thorn. A form of Barbara.
Varinah, Varyna, Varynah, Varyne

Varsha (Hindi) rain.
Varshah

Varvara (Latin) stranger. (O/Eng) thorn. A form of Barbara.
Vara, Varah, Varneka, Vardice, Vardina, Vardine, Vardis, Vardissa, Vardisse, Vardit, Vardita, Vardyta, Vardytah

Vasanta (Sanskrit) born at spring time.
Vasantah, Vasante

Vashti (Persian) very beautiful.
Vashtee, Vashtie, Vashty

Vassy (Cornish/Persian) most beautiful.
Vashti, Vasi, Vasie, Vassee, Vassey, Vassi, Vassie, Vasy

Veanna (American/Hebrew) graceful. A form of Anna.
Veeana, Veeanah, Veeann, Veanna, Veeannah, Veeanne, Veena, Veenah

Veda (Sanskrit) wisdom; who has great sacred understanding.
Vedah

Vedavati (Sanskrit) vocal; loud.
Vedavatee, Vedavatey, Vedavaty

Vedette (Old French) guardian; protector.
Vedet, Vedeta, Vedetah, Vedete, Vedett, Vedetta, Vedettah

Vedis (Teutonic) sacred forest spirit.
Vediss, Vedissa, Vedisse, Vedys, Vedyss, Vedyssa, Vedysse

Veera (Hindi) strength.
Veara, Vearah, Veerah, Vira, Virah, Vyra, Vyrah

Vefa (Bavarian/Welsh) white wave. A form of Guinevere.
Vefah, Vefeli (Illy)

Vefeli (Illyrian) fair-haired.
Vefelia, Vefelie, Vefely

Vega (Arabic) falling star. A constellation.
Vegah

Vegena (Hawaiian) feminine.
Vegeen, Vegeena, Vegeene, Vegenah, Vegin, Vegina, Vegine, Vegyn, Vegyna, Vegynah, Vegyne

Vehka (Bulgarian) great glory.
Vehkah

Vekoslava (Slavic) eternal glory.
Velislava

Vela (Latin) star; a constellation in the Milky Way.
Velah, Vella, Vellah

Velda (German) open field.
Veldah

Veleda (Teutonic) wisdom.
Velda, Veldah, Veleda

Velika (Slavic) great wisdom.
Velikah, Velyka, Velykah

Velinda (African American/Latin/Greek) gentle. (Lat) sweet like honey. A combination of Mel/Linda, sweet; beautiful.
Velindah, Velynda, Velyndah

Veliya (Slavic) great.
Veliyah

Vellamo (Finnish) rocking motion.
Velamo

Velma (German) determined guardian; wilful. The short form of Wilhelmina. A feminine form of William.
Valma, Valmah, Valmara, Valmarah, Vellma, Vellmah, Vellmara, Vellmarah, Vilma, Vilmah, Vilmara, Vilmarah, Vylma, Vylmah, Vylmara, Vylmarah

Velvet (Middle English) velvety; soft, gentle; strength; determination. (Lat) fleece.
Velveta, Velvetah, Velvete, Velvett, Velvetta, Velvettah, Velvette, Velvina, Velvinah, Velvit, Velvor (USA), Velvyt

Venecia (Italian) from Venice in Italy.
Vanecia, Veneciah, Venetia, Veneise, Venesa, Venesha, Venesher, Venessa, Venesse, Venessia, Venetia, Venetta, Venette, Venezia, Venice, Venicia, Veniece, Veniesa, Venise, Venisha, Venishia, Venita, Venitia, Veniza, Venize, Vennesa, Vennice, Vennisa, Vennise, Vonita, Vonitia, Vonizia, Vonizya, Vonysia, Vonysiah, Vonysya, Vonysyah

Venedict (Russian) one who brings joy.
Venedicta, Venedycta

Venetia (Latin) kind; merciful. The Celtic form of Beatrice, she brings joy and happiness.
Venda, Veneta, Venetiah, Venita, Vinetia, Vinetiah, Vinita, Vinitah, Vynita, Vynitah, Vynyta, Vynytah

Venice (Italian) (Geographical) a city in Italy.
Veneece, Venyce

Ventura (Latin) brave in the face of danger. (Span) fortunate; lucky.
Venturah, Venture

Venus (Latin) goddess of love and beauty.
Venisa, Venita, Venusa, Venussa, Venys, Vinita, Vynita, Vynys, Vynyta

Vera (Russian) faithful; loyal. (Lat) true.
Veradis, Verah, Verena, Verene, Verenia, Vereniah, Verina, Verine, Verla, Verra (Slav), Vjera, Vyra, Vyrah

Veradis (Latin) faithful.
Veradissa, Veradisse, Veradys, Veradysa, Veradyss, Veradyssa

Verbena (Latin) sacred branch.
Verbeen, Verbeena, Verbeene, Verben, Verbene, Verbin, Verbina, Verbine, Verbyn, Verbyna, Verbyne

Verda (Persian) rose. (Lat) fresh.
Verdah

Verdad (Spanish) truthful.
Verdada

Verdi (Latin) green like springtime.
Verda, Verdah, Verdea, Verdee, Verdey, Verdi, Verdie, Verdy, Verne, Vernique, Vernita, Vernona, Virida, Viridis, Virdisa, Virdisah, Virdys, Virdysa, Virdysah, Vyrdis, Vyrdisa, Vyrdisah, Vyrdys, Vyrdysa, Vyrdysah

Verdiana (Latin) truth is gracious; gacious green springtime. A combination of Verdi/Anna.
Verdian, Verdiane, Verdiann, Verdianna, Verdianne, Verdyan, Verdyana, Verdyane, Verdyann, Verdyanna, Verdyanne, Virdian, Virdiana, Virdiane, Virdiann, Virdianna, Virdianne, Vyrdian, Vyrdiana, Vyrdiane, Vyrdyan, Vyrdyana, Vyrdyane, Vyrdyann, Vyrdyanna, Vyrdyanne

Verena/Verene (Swiss) possessor of sacred wisdom. (Lat) true. (O/Ger) defender.
Vera, Verna, Veradis, Verean, Vereana, Vereane, Vereen, Vereena, Vereene, Verenah, Verene, Verina, Verine, Verinka, Verita, Verity, Verla, Verochka, Veronica, Veryn, Veryna, Veryne, Virna, Virnah, Vyrna, Vyrnah

Verger (Latin/English) carer of the church interior.
Vergera

Verina (Latin) faithful.
Varyn, Varyna, Varyne, Vera, Verah, Veria, Veriah, Verin, Verine, Verya, Veryah, Veryn, Veryna, Veryne

Verita/Verity/Verona (Italian) truthful.
Verita, Veritah, Vertitea, Veritee, Veritey, Veriti, Veritie, Verla, Verlah, Veronah, Verone, Veryta, Verytah, Verytea, Verytee, Verytey, Veryti, Verytie, Veryty

Verna (Latin) spring like; flowery. (O/Fren) alder tree. The feminine form of Vernon.
Verasha, Verka, Verla, Vermona, Vermonah, Vermone, Vermonia, Vermoniah, Vermonie, Vernah, Verne, Verneta, Vernese, Vernesha, Verneshia, Vernessa, Vernetia,

Vernia, Verniah, Vernice, Vernise,
Vernisha, Vernisheia, Vernita,
Vernitia, Verda, Verena, Vernis,
Verusya, Viera, Vierah, Vierna,
Viernah, Viridia, Virna, Virnah,
Virnella, Virnelle, Vyrna, Vyrnah,
Vyrnel, Vyrnela, Vyrnele, Vyrnella,
Vyrnelle, Vyrnessa, Vyrnessah,
Vyrnesse

Vernice (Latin/Greek) strong and
brave like a bear; warrior. The
feminine form of Bernie.
Vernica, Vernicah, Vernicca,
Verniccah, Verniqua, Vernique,
Vernyca, Vernycah, Vernycca,
Vernyccah, Vernyqua, Vernyque

Veronica (Latin) truthful; true to
image; like her mother.
Ronica, Ronicah, Ronika, Ronikah,
Roniqua, Roniquah, Ronique,
Ronnica, Ronnika, Ronnikah,
Varnonica, Varonicca, Varoniccah,
Vera, Veraniqua, Veraniquah,
Veranique, Verenice, Verhonica,
Verinica, Verohnica, Verona,
Veronic, Veronice, Veronicka,
Veronika, Veronike (Ger), Veroniky,
Veroniqua, Veroniquah, Veronique
(Fren),Veronna, Veronne,
Veronnica, Veruszhka, Vironica,
Vironicah, Vironicca, Vironiccah,
Vironika, Vironiqua, Vironiquah,
Vironique, Vronica, Vronicah,
Vronika, Vroniqua, Vroniquah,
Vronique, Vyronica, Vyronicah,
Vyronicca, Vyroniccah, Vyronika,
Vyronikah, Vyroniqua,
Vyronyquah, Vyronyque
Veruszhka, Vironica, Vironicah,
Vironika, Vironiqua, Vironique,
Vronica, Vronicah, Vronika,
Vroniqua, Vronique

Verrani (Sri Lankan) persistent.
Veeranee, Veeraney, Veeranie,
Veerany

Vervain (Old English) sacred.
Verbena, Vervayn

Vespera (Latin) evening star.
Versperah

Vest (Sicilian) goddess of fire; the
Latin goddess of the home.
Vestah, Vestea, Vestee, Vestey

Vestah (Latin/Greek/Persian) star.
Vesta, Vestar

Veta (Slavic/Latin) holy; sacred to
God. A form of Elizabeth.
Veeta, Vetah, Vita, Vitah, Vitta,
Vyta, Vytah, Vytta, Vyttah

Veva/Vevay (Illyrian) white wave. A
short form of Guinevere.
Vevah, Vevae, Vevai, Vevay (Celt)

Vevetta/Vevette (French/Welsh)
white wave; fair-haired.
Vevet, Veveta, Vevete, Vevett

Vevila (Irish) harmonious.
Vevilla, Vevillia, Vevilliah, Vevyla,
Vevylah, Vevyle, Vevyll, Vevylla,
Vevyllah, Vevylle

Vevina (Gaelic) sweet lady.
Vevin, Vevinah, Vevine, Vevyn,
Vevyna, Vevynah, Vevyne

Vi (Latin/French) little violet. The
short form of names starting with
'Vi' e.g. Viola.
Vy

Vianca (Spanish/Italian) white. A
form of Bianca.
Vianeca, Vianica, Vianka, Vyaneca,
Vyanica, Vyanka

Vianna/Vianne (Old French/
Hebrew/Latin) graceful violet
flower.
Viana, Vianah, Viann, Viannah,
Vyan, Vyana, Vyanah, Vyane,
Vyanna, Vyannah, Vyanne

Vica (Hungarian/Hebrew) life. A form of Eve.
Vicah, Vicka, Vickah, Vika, Vikah, Vyca, Vycah, Vycka, Vyckah, Vyka, Vykah

Vicki/Vicky (Latin) victory. The short form of Victoria.
Viccee, Viccey, Vicke, Vickee, Vickey, Vickia, Vickiah, Vickiana, Vickie, Vickilyn, Vickilyna, Vickilyne, Vickkee, Vickkey, Vickki, Vickkie, Vickky, Vicky, Vika, Vikah, Vikia, Vikka, Vikki, Vikkia, Vikie, Vikkee, Vikkey, Vikki, Vikkie, Vikky, Viky, Vycke, Vyckee, Vyckey, Vycki, Vyckie, Vycky, Vykki, Vykkie, Vykkie, Vykky, Vyky

Victoria (Latin) victory.
Victoire (Fren), Victorean, Victoreana, Victoreane, Victoreen, Victoreena, Victoreene, Victorina, Victorinah, Victorine, Victoryn, Victoryna, Victorynah, Victoryne, Viktoria, Viktoriah, Viktorya, Viktoryah, Vitoria (Span), Vitoriah, Vitorie (Fren), Vittoria (Ital), Vittoriah, Vittorya, Vittoryah, Vyctoria, Vyctoriah, Vyctorina, Vyctorine, Vyctoryn, Vyctoryna, Vyctorynh, Vyctoryne, Vyktorin, Vyktorina, Vyktorynah, Vyktorine, Vyktoryn, Vyktoryna, Vyktorynah, Vyktoryne

Vida (Hebrew) beloved. The feminine form of David.
Vidah, Vyda, Vydah

Vidal (Latin) life.
Vital, Vydal, Vytal

Vidonia (Portugese) vine branch.
Vidoniah, Vidonya, Vidonyah, Vydonia, Vydoniah, Vydonya, Vydonyah

Vienna (Hebrew/Latin) graceful. (Geographical) the capital of Austria.
Veena, Veenah, Vena, Venah, Venia, Venna, Vennah, Vennia, Viana, Vianah, Viannah, Vienetta, Vienette, Vienne, Vina, Vinah, Vyana, Vyanah, Vyanna

Vigilia (Latin) awake; alert.
Vigilia, Vigiliah, Vijilis, Vijiliah, Vygilia, Vygyliah, Vyjilia, Vyjiliah

Vigilu (Latin) alert.
Vigula, Vygilu, Vygylu

Vignette (French) little vine.
Vignet, Vigneta, Vignete, Vignett, Vignetta, Vygnet, Vygneta, Vygnete, Vygnett, Vygnetta, Vygnette

Vija (Latvian) garland (wreath of flowers).
Vyja

Vika (Latin/Polynesian) victory.
Vikah, Vikka, Vikkah, Vyka, Vykah, Vykka, Vykkah

Vila (Latin) dweller in the country house.
Vilah, Villa, Villah, Vyla, Vylah, Vylla, Vyllah

Vilhelmina/Vilhelmine (German) determined guardian; wilful. A short form of Wilhelmina. A feminine form of William.
Velma, Vilhalmine (Swed), Vilma, Vilmah, Vilmara, Vilmarah, Vylhelmina, Vylhelmine

Villette (French) little dweller from the country estate.
Vilet, Vileta, Viletah, Vilete, Vilett, Viletta, Vilettah, Vilette, Villet, Villeta, Villetah, Villett, Villetta, Vylet, Vyleta, Vyletah, Vylete, Vylett, Vyletta, Vylettah, Vylette, Vyllet, Vylleta, Vylletah, Vyllette

V

Vilma (Dutch) wilful.
(Russ) protecting guardian.
Vilmah, Vilmar, Vilmara, Vilmarah, Vylma, Vylmah

Vina (Spanish) vineyard. (Scott) beloved. The feminine form of David.
Vinah Vinna, Vinnah, Vyna, Vynah, Vynna, Vynnah

Vincentia/Vincenza/Vincenzia (Italian/Latin) victory. The feminine form of Vincent.
Vincensa, Vincensah, Vincensia, Vincensiah, Vincenta, Vincentah, Vincenza, Vincenzah, Vincenziah, Vyncenzia, Vyncenziah, Vyncenzya, Vyncenzyah

Vine (Old French) worker from the vineyard.
Viner, Vyne

Vinia (Latin) grapes; wine.
Viniah, Vinviann, Vinianna, Vinianne, Vynia, Vyniah, Vyniann, Vynianna, Vynianne, Vynya, Vynyah, Vynyann, Vynyanna, Vynnyanne

Vinita (Spanish) vineyard.
Vineet, Vineeta, Vineete, Vinetta, Vinette, Vinitha, Vinta, Vintah, Vinti, Vintia, Vintiah, Vynetta, Vynette, Vynita, Vynyta, Vynytta, Vynytte

Vinna (Spanish) from the vine.
Vinni, Vinnia, Vinniah, Vinnie, Vinny, Vynna, Vynnah

Viola/Violanie/Violante (Latin) the violet flower; violet colour. (Ital) stringed musical instrument; singer.
Eolande, Iolande, Iolanthe, Jolanda, Jolande, Veigel, Viola (Ital/Span/Port), Violah, Violain, Violaina, Violane, Violanee, Violaney, Violani, Violania, Violanta, Violante (Span), Violany, Viole, Violeta, Violete, Violetta, Violette, Vyoila, Vyoilah, Vyola, Vyolah, Vyolani, Vyolania, Vyolanie, Vyolany, Vyolanya, Vyolet, Vyoleta, Vyolete, Vyolett, Vyoletta, Vyolette, Yolanda, Yolande, Yolane, Yolanthe

Violet/Violetta (Latin/Old French) the violet flower; violet colour; little violet flower.
Eolande, Iolande, Iolanthe, Jolanda, Jolande, Veigel, Viola (Ital/Span/Port), Violante, Violatta (Ital), Viole, Violet, Violeta, Violetah, Violete, Violett, Violetta, Virginia, Virginie (Fren), Voletta, Violet, Vyoleta, Vyoletah, Vyolete, Vyolett, Vyoletta, Vyolette, Yolanda, Yolande, Yolane, Yolanthe

Vira (Spanish/Teutonic/Latin) blond-haired. (Ger) closed. (Span) elf.
Virah, Vyra, Vyrah

Virgilia (Latin) one who carries a staff.
Virgilea, Virgileah, Vigilee, Virgileigh, Virgili, Virgilie, Virgily, Virgilya, Virjil, Virjilea, Virjilieah, Virjilee, Virjileigh, Virjiley, Virjili, Virjilie, Virjily, Vyrgilia, Vyrgiliah, Vyrgylya, Vyrgylyah

Virginia (Latin) purity.
Virgeen, Virgeena, Virgeenah, Virgeenee, Virgeenia, Virgeeniah, Virgene, Virginie (Fren/Dut), Virjinea, Virjineah, Virjinee, Virjinia, Virjiniah, Vyrginia, Vyrgyniah, Vyrgynya, Vyrgynyah

Viridis (Italian) green. (Lat) fresh; blooming like a flower.
Viridiss, Viridissa, Viridys, Viridyss, Viridyssa, Vyridis, Vyridiss, Vyridissa, Vyridys, Vyridyss, Vyridyssa

Virtue (Latin) purity.
Vertue, Virtu, Vyrtu, Vyrtue

Visolela (African) imagination.
Visolelah, Vysolela

Vita/Vital (Latin) full of life. The
short form of Davita, beloved.
Vida, Vidah, Vidal, Vitalian,
Vitaliana, Vitalianah, Vitaliane,
Vyta, Vytah

Vittoria (Italian) victory.
Vitoria, Vitoriah, Vittoriah,
Vittorya, Vytoria, Vytoriah,
Vyttoria, Vyttoriah

Viv/Viva (Latin) full of life;
springtime. The short form of
Vivien.
Vivah, Vive, Viveca (Scand),
Vivecah, Viveka, Vyv, Vyva, Vyvah

Vivian (Latin) full of life.
Vevay, Viveca, Vivia, Viviann,
Vivianna (Ital), Viviannah,
Vivianne, Viviem, Vivien, Vivienne,
Vivyan, Vivyanne, Vyan, Vyvyann,
Vyvyanna, Vyvyanne

Vixen (Latin) female fox.
Vyxen

Vjera (Russian) faith.
Vjerah

Vlasta (Slavic) powerful princess;
glorious chief. The feminine form
of Vladyslav.
Vlastah

Voila (French) behold.
Voilah, Voyla, Voylah

Volante (Italian) flying; soaring.
Volanta, Volantah

Voleta (Old French) flowing veil.
Volet, Volett, Voletta, Volette,
Volita, Volitt, Volitta, Volitte,
Volyta, Volytah, Volyte, Volytt,
Volytta, Volyttah, Volytte

Vonda (Irish/Hebrew) one who is
admired. The Irish form of Joanna/
Siobhain, God is gracious.
Vondah

Vondra (Slavic) brave; courageous.
Vonda, Vondah, Vondrah, Vondrea

Vonna/Vonny (French) archer.
(Scand) yew wood. A form of
Yvonne.
Vona, Vonah, Vonia, Voniah,
Vonnah, Vonni, Vonnia, Vonniah,
Vonnie, Vonny, Vonnya, Vony,
Vonya

Vontricia (French/Latin) noble
archer.
Vontrece, Vontrese, Vontrice,
Vontriece, Vonricha, Vontrichia,
Vontricia, Vontrisha, Vontrishia,
Vontrycia, Vontryciah, Vontrycya,
Vontrycyah

Vorsila (Greek) little bear. A form of
Ursula.
Vorsilla, Vorsula, Vorsulah,
Vorsulla, Vorsyla

Vovo (Tongan) delicious.

Vread (Irish/Latin) pearl. A form of
Margaret.
Vreada, Vreadah

Vreneli (German) truthful; true to
image; like her mother. A form of
Veronica.
Vrenelee, Vreneley, Vrenelie,
Vrenely

Vrida (Spanish) green.
Vridah, Vryda, Vrydah

Vulpine (Latin/English) fox-like.
Vulpina, Vulpinah, Vulpyna,
Vulpynah, Vulpyne

Vye (Frisian) wisdom.
Vi, Vie, Vy

Vyoma (Hindi) sky.
Vioma, Viomah, Vyomah

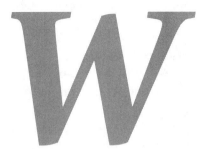

Wadd (Arabic) beloved.
Wad

Wahalla (Old Norse) immortal.
Valhalla, Walhalla

Wahkuna (Native American) wood of arrows.
Wahkunah

Waida (German) warrior.
Waidah, Wayda, Waydah

Waikiki (Hawaiian) stream from which water gushes.
Waikikee, Waikikie, Waikiky

Wainani (Hawaiian) beautiful water.
Wainanee, Wainanie, Wainany

Waja (Arabic) noble.
Wajah

Wakana (Japanese) plant.
Wakanah

Wakanda (Dakota) magic power.
Wakandah

Wakeisha (Swahili) life. (Arab) woman.
Wakeishah, Wakeishia, Wakesha, Wakeshia, Wakesia, Wakesiah, Wakeysha, Wakeyshah, Wakeyshia, Wakeyshiah, Wakeyshya, Wakeyshyah

Wakenda (Old Norse) to waken.
Wakendah

Walad (Arabic) newborn child.
Waladah, Walida, Walidah, Walyda, Walydah

Walanika (Hawaiian) true to image. A form of Veronica.
Walanikah, Walanyka, Walanykah

Walda (German) famous; powerful. The feminine form of Waldo, ruler.
Waldah, Waldina, Waldine, Walida, Walidah, Wallda, Walldah, Waldyna, Waldyne, Welda, Weldah, Wellda, Welldah

Waleria (Polish/Latin) strong; brave; healthy. (Eng) from the valley. A form of Valerie.
Waleriah, Walerya, Waleryah, Walleria, Walleriah, Wallerya, Walleryah

Walker (English) walker; cloth.
Wallker

Wallis (English) Welsh one; stranger. The feminine form of Wallace.
Walice, Walise, Wallisa, Wallise, Wallys, Wallysa, Wallyse

Wanaao (Hawaiian) dawn.

Wanda (German) wanderer.
Vanda, Vandah, Wahnda, Wandah, Wandely, Wandi, Wandie, Wandis, Wandisa, Wandise, Wandja, Wandy, Wandzia, Wannda, Wanndah, Wonda, Wondah, Wonnda, Wonndah

Wandy (German) wandering.
Wandea, Wandee, Wandey, Wandi, Wandie, Wandis, Wandisa, Wandisah, Wandissa, Wandissah, Wandisse, Wandys, Wandysa, Wandysah, Wandyss, Wandyssa, Wandyssah

W

Waneta (Native American) charger, a horse that rides into battle. A form of Juanita, God is gracious.
Waneata, Waneatah, Waneeta, Waneetah, Waneita, Waneitah, Wanetah, Wanete, Wanita, Wanitah, Wanite, Wanneata, Wanneatah, Wanneeta, Wanneetah, Wanneita, Wanneitah, Wanneta, Wannetah, Wannete, Wannetta, Wannette, Waunita, Wonnita, Wonnitah, Wonnitta, Wonnitte, Wonnytta, Wonnytte, Wonyta, Wonytah, Wonyte, Wonytta, Wonyttah, Wonytte

Wanika (Hawaiian/Spanish) God is gracious. A form of Juanita.
Waneeka, Wanikah, Wanyka, Wanykah

Wannetta (Old English) little pale one.
Waneata, Waneatah, Waneeta, Waneetah, Waneita, Waneitah, Waneta, Wanetah, Wanete, Wanita, Wanitah, Wanite, Wanneata, Wanneatah, Wanneeta, Wanneetah, Wanneita, Wanneitah, Wanneta, Wannetah, Wannete, Wannette, Waunita, Wonnita, Wonnitah, Wonnitta, Wonnitte, Wonnytta, Wonnytte, Wonyta, Wonytah, Wonyte, Wonytta, Wonyttah, Wonytte

Wapeka (Old Norse) weapon used for protection.
Wapekah

Wapin (Native American) dawn.

Waratah (Australian Aboriginal) red flowering tree.
Waratah, Warrata, Warratah

Warda (Teutonic) guardian; protector. The feminine form of Ward.
Wardah

Warooka (Australian Aboriginal) parrot with beautiful feathers.
Warookah

Washi (Japanese) eagle.
Washee, Washie, Washy

Washta (Sioux) good.

Wasila (English) good; healthy.
Wasila, Wasilla, Waylsa, Wasylah, Wasylla, Wasyllah

Wattan (Japanese) home land.
Watan

Wauna (Moquelumnan) snow goose.
Waunakee, Waunah

Wava (Slavic/Latin) stranger. A form of Barbara.
Wavah, Wavia, Waviah, Wavya, Wavyah

Waynette (English) little maker of wagons.
Wainet, Waineta, Wainetah, Wainete, Wainetta, Wainettah, Wainette, Waynel, Waynela, Waynelah, Waynell, Waynella, Waynelle

Waynoka (Cheyenne) water that is clean.
Wainoka, Wainokah, Waynokah

Weayaya (Sioux) sun setting.
Weayaia

Weeko (Dakota) pretty girl.
Weiko, Weyko

Wenda (Welsh) white-skinned. A form of Wendy.
Wendah, Wendaina, Wendainah, Wendaine, Wendalin, Wendalina, Wendalinah, Wendaline, Wendayn, Wendayna, Wendalynah, Wendayne

Wendelle (English) wanderer.
Wendalina, Wendalinah, Wendaline, Wendall, Wendalla,

Wendallah, Wendalle, Wendalyn,
Wendalyna, Wendalynah,
Wendalyne, Wendelin, Wendelina,
Wendelynah, Wendeline,
Wendelyn, Wendelyna,
Wendeynah, Wendelyne

Wendy (Welsh) white-skinned. The
feminine form of Wendelle.
Wendea, Wendee, Wendey, Wendi,
Wendia, Wendiah, Wendie,
Wendya, Wendyah, Wendye

Wera (Polish/Latin) truthful.
Werah

Weronika (Polish/Latin) true image.
A form of Veronica.
Weronica, Weronicah, Weronicka,
Weronickah, Weronikah, Weronike,
Weronikra, Weroniqua,
Weroniquah, Weronique,
Weronyca, Weronycah, Weronycka,
Weronyka, Weronykah,
Weronyqua, Weronyquah,
Weronyque

Wesisa (Musoga) foolish.
Weisash, Wesisah, Wesysa, Wesysah

Weslea (English) from the westerly
meadow. The feminine form of
Wesley.
Wesla, Weslah, Wesleah, Weslee,
Weslei, Wesleigh, Wesley, Wesli,
Weslia, Wesliah, Weslie, Wesly,
Weslya, Weslyah

Whaley (Old English) belonging to
the whale meadow.
Whalea, Whaleah, Whalee, Whalei,
Whaleigh, Whali, Whalia, Whaliah,
Whalie, Whaly, Whalya, Whalyah

Whitley (English) from the white
meadow.
Whitlea, Whitleah, Whitlee,
Whitlei, Whitleigh, Whitli, Whitlia,
Whitliah, Whitlie, Whitly, Whitlya,
Whitlyah, Whytlea, Whytleah,

Whytlee, Whytlei, Whytleigh,
Whytley, Whytli, Whytlia,
Whytliah, Whylie, Whytly, Whytlya,
Whytlyah

Whitney (English) from the clear
white water.
Whitnee, Whitni, Wnitnie, Whitny,
Whytnee, Whytney, Whytni,
Whytnie, Whytny

Whoopi (English) happy.
Whoopee, Whoopey, Whoopie,
Whoopy

Wicahpi (Sioux) star
Wicahpee

Wicktoria (Polish/Latin) victory. A
form of Victoria.
Wicktoriah, Wicktorja, Wiktoria,
Wiktoriah, Wiktorja, Wycktoria,
Wycktoriah, Wycktorja, Wyktoria,
Wyktoriah, Wyktorja

Windy (English) strong breeze.
Windea, Windee, Windi, Windie,
Wyndea, Wyndee, Wyndey, Wyndi,
Wyndie, Wyndy

Wikolia (Hawaiian) victory. A form
of Victoria.
Wikoliah, Wikolya, Wikolyah

Wila (Hawaiian) faithful.
Wilah, Willa, Willah, Wyla, Wylah,
Wylla, Wyllah

Wilda (English) untamed.
Wildah, Wilder, Wylda, Wyldah,
Wylder

Wileen (English/German)
determined guardian.
Wilean, Wileana, Wileanah,
Wileane, Wileena, Wileenah,
Wileene, Wilin, Wilina, Wilinah,
Wiline, Wilyn, Wilyna, Wilynah,
Wilyne, Wylean, Wyleana,
Wyleanah, Wyleane, Wyleen,
Wyleena, Wyleenah, Wyleene,

Wileen cont.
Wylin, Wylina, Wylinah, Wyline,
Wylyn, Wylyna, Wylynah, Wylyne

Wilhelmina (German) little
determined guardian.
Vilhelmina, Vilhelmine, Wilean,
Wileana, Wileanah, Wileane,
Wileen, Wileena, Wileenah,
Wileene, Wilhelmine, Willamina,
Willaminah, Willamine,
Willemina, Willeminah,
Willemine, Willetta, Willette,
Williamina, Williamine, Willmina,
Willmine, Wilma, Wilmah,
Wimina, Wimine, Winnie,
Wylhelmin, Wylhelmina,
Wylhelminah, Wylhelmine,
Wylhelmyn, Wylhelmyna,
Wylhelmynah, Wylhelmyne,
Wyllhelmin, Wyllhelmina,
Wyllhelmine, Wyllhelmyn,
Wyllhelmyna, Wyllhelmynah,
Wyllhelmyne

Wilikinia (Hawaiian/Latin) purity. A
form of Virginia.
Wilkiniah

Willa (German) determined
guardian.
Wila, Wilabel, Wilabela, Wilabele,
Wilah (Dut), Willabel, Willabela,
Willabele, Willabell, Willabella,
Willah, Wyla, Wylabel, Wylabela,
Wylabele, Wylabell, Wylabella,
Wylabella, Wylabelle, Wylla,
Wyllah, Wyllabel, Wyllabella,
Wyllabelle

Willabelle (German/French)
beautiful, wilful one. The
feminine form of William.
Wila, Wilabel, Wilabela, Wilabele,
Wilah, Willabel, Willabela,
Willabele, Willabell, Willabella,
Willabelle, Wyla, Wylabel,
Wylabela, Wylabele, Wylabell,
Wylabella, Wylabella, Wylabelle,

Wylla, Wyllah, Wyllabel,
Wyllabella, Wyllabelle

Willee (English/Welsh) wilful one
from the meadow. The feminine
short form of Willy/William.
Wilea, Wileah, Wilee, Wilei,
Wileigh, Wiley, Wili, Wilie, Willea,
Willeah, Willei, Willeigh, Willi,
Willie, Willy, Wily

Willmot (Teutonic) mountain of the
wilful one.
Willmott, Wilmot, Wilmott,
Wyllmot, Wylmot

Willow (English) willow tree.
Willo, Wyllo, Wyllow, Wylo,
Wylow

Wilma (German) determined
guardian. The short form of
Wilhelmina.
Wilmah, Wylma, Wylmah

Wilona (German) resolute guardian.
(Dut) wilful.
Vilma, Vilmah, Vylma, Vylmah,
Wilma, Wilmah, Wilonah, Wilone,
Wylona, Wylone, Wylonah

Wilva (Teutonic) determined.
Wilvah, Wilvar, Wylva, Wylvah

Win (German/Welsh) white-
skinned.
Winn, Wyn, Wynn, Wynne

Winda (Swahili) hunter.
Windah, Wynda, Wyndah

Winema (Native American) woman
chief.
Winemah, Wynema, Wynemah

Winifred (German) peaceful;
friendly.
Winafred, Winefred, Winefrid,
Winefride, Winfreda, Winfrieda,
Winiefrida, Winifrid, Winifrida,
Winifryd, Winifryda, Winnafred,
Winnafreda, Winnifred,

Winnifreda, Winnifrid, Winnifrida, Wynafred, Wynafreda, Wynafrid, Wynafrida, Wynefred, Wynefreda, Wynefryd

Winna (African) friend.
Winnah, Wyna, Wynah, Wynna, Wynnah

Winnie (English) peaceful; friendly. The short form of names starting with 'Win' e.g. Winifred.
Winee, Winey, Wini, Winie, Winnee, Winney, Winni, Winny, Winy, Wyn, Wynee, Wyney, Wyni, Wynie, Wynnee, Wynney, Wynni, Wynnie, Wynny, Wyny

Winnipeg (Native Canadian) muddy water.
Winipeg, Wynipeg, Wynnipeg

Winola (Teutonic) gracious, generous friend.
Winolah, Wynola, Wynolah

Winona (Lakota) first-born daughter.
Wanona, Wanonah, Wenona, Wenonah, Winonah, Wynona, Wynonah

Winter (English) born during winter time.
Winta, Wintah, Wynta, Wyntah, Wynter

Wira (Polish/Latin) blond-haired. (Ger) closed.
Wirah, Wyra, Wyrah

Wisconsin (Algonquian) long river.
Wisconsyn

Wisia (Polish/Latin) victory. A form of Victoria.
Wicia, Wiciah, Wikta, Wisiah, Wysia, Wysiah, Wysya, Wysyah

Woorak (Australian Aboriginal) honeysuckle.
Wooraka

Worsola (Bohemian) little she-bear. A form of Ursula.
Worsolah, Worsula, Worsulah

Wrena/Wrena (Old English) the wren bird.
Wrenah, Wrenda, Wrendah, Wrenee, Wrenie, Wrenn, Wrenna, Wrennah, Wreny

Wyanet/Wyaneta (Native American) her beauty is legendary.
Wianet, Wianeta, Wianete, Wianett, Wianetta, Wianette, Waianita, Waianitta, Wyaneta, Wyanete, Wyanett, Wyanetta, Wyanette, Wyanita

Wynne (Celtic) fair-haired.
Win, Winetta, Winette, Winn, Winne, Wyn, Wyna, Wyne, Wynet, Wyneta, Wynetah, Wynete, Wynett, Wynetta, Wynettah, Wynette, Wynne

Wyoming (Algonquian) broad plains. (Geographical) a state in America.
Wyoh, Wyomia, Wyomiah, Wyomya, Wyomyah

Wyuna (Australian Aboriginal) clear water.
Wyunah

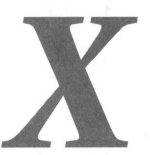

Xana (Greek) golden-haired; blond.
Xanna, Xanne, Xantha, Xanthia, Xanthippe, Zanna, Zanne, Zantha, Zanthia, Zanthippe

Xandi (Greek) defender of humankind. A form of Sandy.
Sabdea, Sandee, Sandey, Sandi, Sandie, Sandy, Xandea, Xandee, Xandey, Xandi, Xandie, Xandy, Zandea, Zandee, Zandey, Zandi, Zandie, Zandy

Xandra (Greek/Spanish) defender of humankind. A form of Sandra.
Xandrah, Xandria, Xandriah, Xandrya, Xandryah, Zandra, Zandrah, Zandria, Zandriah, Zandrya, Zandryah

Xanthia (Greek) yellow-haired; blond.
Xanthiah, Zanthia, Zanthiah

Xanthis (Latin) golden-haired; blond.
Xanthos, Xanthius, Xanthyus

Xantippi (Greek) light coloured horse.
Xantippie, Zanthippie, Zantippie

Xara (Hebrew) princess. A form of Sara.
Sahra, Sahrah, Sara, Sarah, Sarra, Sarrah, Xarah, Xarra, Xarrah, Zahra, Zahrah, Zarah, Zarra, Zarrah

Xaveria (Aramaic) bright.
Xaveree, Xaverey, Xaverie, Xavery, Zaveree, Zaverey, Zaveri, Zaveria, Zaveriah, Zaverie, Zavery

Xaviera (Arabic) bright; brilliant; splendid. (Span) owner of the new house. The feminine form of Xavier.
Xavierah, Xaviere, Xavyera, Xavyerah, Xavyere, Zaviera, Zavierah, Zaviere, Zavyera, Zavyerah

Xayvion (African American) new home.
Zayvion

Xela (French) from the mountain home.
Xelah, Xella, Xellah, Zela, Zelah, Zella, Zellah

Xen (Japanese) religious.
Xena, Xenah, Zen, Zena, Zenah

Xena (Greek) welcomed.
Xene, Xenia, Ximena, Xina, Xinah, Xyna, Xynah, Zena, Zenah, Zenia, Zeniah, Zina, Zinah, Zyna, Zynah

Xenia (Greek) hospitable; guest.
Cena, Cenah, Sena, Senah, Xeena, Xeenia, Xeeniah, Xena, Xenah, Xene, Xeniah, Xenya, Xenyah, Ximena, Xiomara, Xyna, Xynah, Zeena, Zeenia, Zena, Zenia, Zeniah, Zenya, Zenyah, Zina, Zinah, Zyna, Zynah

Xenosa (Greek) stranger.
Xenos, Xenosah, Zenos, Zenosa, Zenosah

Xerena (Latin) tranquil. A form of Serena.
Seren, Serena, Serenah, Serene, Xeren, Xerenah, Xerene, Zerena, Zerenah, Zirena, Zirenah, Zyrena, Zyrenah

X

Xiang (Chinese) fragrant.
Xeang, Xeeang, Xyang, Zeang,
Zeeang, Ziang, Zyang

Ximena (Spanish) heroine.
(Heb) listening. The Spanish
feminine form of Simon.
Simena, Simenah, Simona,
Simonah, Simone, Symena,
Symenah, Symona, Symonah,
Ximenah, Ximona, Ximonah,
Ximone, Xymena, Xymenah,
Xymona, Xymonah, Zimena,
Zimenah, Zimene, Zimona,
Zimonah, Zimone, Zymena,
Zymenah, Zymona, Zymonah

Xina (English) little.
(Grk) welcomed.
Xeena, Xeenah, Xinah, Xyna,
Xynah, Zeena, Zeenah, Zina,
Zinah, Zyna, Zynah

Xirena (Greek) alluring; Siren. A
form of Sirena.
Sireena, Sireenah, Siren, Sirena,
Sirenah, Sirene, Sirina, Sirinah,
Syren, Syrena, Syrenah, Syrene,
Xireena, Xireenah, Xirenah, Xirene,
Xirina, Xirinah, Xyren, Xyrena,
Xyrenah, Xyrene, Xyrina, Xyrinah,
Xyryna, Xyrynah, Zireena,
Zireenah, Zirina, Zirinah, Ziryna,
Zirynah, Zyreena, Zyreenah,
Zyrina, Zyrinah, Zyryna, Zyrynah

Xiu-Mei (Chinese) beautiful plum.

Xuan (Vietnamese) spring.
Xuana, Zuan, Zuanah

Xuxa (Brazilian/Hebrew) lily.
Xuxah

Xya (Latin) trembling. (Lat) grain.
(Ital) aunt. A form of Zia.
Xia, Zia, Ziah, Zya, Zyah

Xyleena (Greek) from the forest.
Xilean, Xileana, Xileanah, Xileane,
Xileen, Xileena, Xileenah, Xileene,

Xilin, Xilina, Xilinah, Xiline, Xilyn,
Xylina, Xilynah, Xilyne, Xylean,
Xyleana, Xyleanah, Xyleane,
Xyleen, Xyleenah, Xyleene, Xylin,
Xylina, Xylinah, Xyline, Xylyn,
Xylyna, Xylynah, Xylyne

Xylia (Greek) from the forest.
Xilia, Xiliah, Xilina, Xylya, Xylyah,
Xylina, Xylinah, Xylyna, Xylynah,
Zilia, Ziliah, Zilina, Zilinah, Zylia,
Zyliah, Zylina, Zylinah, Zylyna,
Zylynah

Xylina (Greek) from the forest.
Xylin, Xylinah, Xyline, Xylyn,
Xylyna, Xylynah, Xylyne, Zilin,
Zilina, Zilinah, Zilyna, Zilynah,
Zylin, Zylina, Zylinah, Zylyn,
Zylyna, Zylynah

Xylona (Greek) from the forest.
Xilon, Xilona, Xilonah, Xilone,
Xilonia, Xiloniah, Xylon, Xylonah,
Xylone, Xylonia, Xyloniah,
Xylonya, Xylonyah

Xylophia (Greek) lover of the forest.
Xilophia, Xilophiah, Xylophiah,
Xylophila, Xylophilah, Zilophia,
Zilophiah, Zylophia, Zylophiah

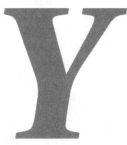

Yaa (Ghanian) born on a Thursday.
Ya

Yaara (Hebrew) honey; honeycomb.
Yara

Yachi (Japanese) lucky.

Yachne (Hebrew) hospitable.
Yachnee

Yael (Hebrew) mountain goat.
Yaela, Yaele, Yaell, Yaella, Yaelle

Yaffa (Hebrew) lovely.
Yaffah

Yagoona (Australian Aboriginal)
today.
Yagoonah

Yaki (Japanese) snow.

Yakira (Hebrew) precious.
Yakirah, Yakyra, Yakyrah

Yalanda (Greek) violet flower;
purple. A form of Yolanda.
Yalandah, Yolande, Yolando, Ylana,
Ylanah, Ylanda

Yalena (Greek/Russian) shining
light. A form of Helen.
Yalana, Yalanah, Yalane, Yaleana,
Yaleanah, Yaleane, Yaleena,
Yaleenah, Yaleene, Yalina, Yalinah,
Yaline, Yalyna, Yalynah, Yalyne,
Yelana, Yelanah, Yelane, Yeleana,
Yeleanah, Yeleane, Yeleena,
Yeleena, Yeleenah, Yeleene, Yelina,
Yelinah, Yeline, Yelyna, Yelynah,

Yelyne, Yileana, Yileanah, Yileane,
Yileena, Yileenah, Yileene, Yilina,
Yilinah, Yiline, Yilyna, Yilynah,
Yilyne

Yalika (Native American) flowers of
spring.
Yalyka

Yaluta (Native American) talking
woman.
Yalutah

Yamary (Hebrew) wished-for child;
star of the sea; bitter. A form of
Mary.
Yamairee, Yamairey, Yamairi,
Yamairie, Yamairy, Yamaree,
Yamarey, Yamari, Yamaria,
Yamariah, Yamaris, Yamarissa,
Yamarisse, Yamarya, Yamaryah,
Yamayra, Yamayrah

Yamelia (German) hard-working;
industrious. A form of Amelia.
Yameliah, Yamila, Yamile, Yamilla,
Yamille, Yamelya, Yamelyah,
Yamilya, Yamilyah

Yamilla (Slavic) merchant; trader.
Yamil, Yamila, Yamile, Yamill,
Yamille, Yamyl, Yamyla, Yamyle,
Yamyll, Yamylla, Yamylle

Yaminah (Arabic) right; proper.
Yamina, Yamyna, Yamynah

Yamini (Hindi) night time.
Yaminia, Yaminiah

Yamka (Hopi) blossom; flower.
Yamkah

Yamuna (Hindi) sacred river.
Yamunah

Yana (Slavic/Hebrew) God is
gracious.
Ana, Anah, Yanae, Yanah, Yanet,
Yanetam Yanethm Yanik, Yanika,
Yanina, Yaninah, Yanis, Yanisha,
Yanitza, Yanixia, Yanna, Yannah,

Yannica, Yannick, Yannicka,
Yannika, Yannina, Yannyca,
Yannyck, Yannycka, Yannyka,
Yannyna

Yanaba (Navajo) brave.
Yanabah

Yanaha (Navajo) one who confronts
her enemy.
Yanahah

Yang (Chinese) sun.

Yani (Australian Aboriginal)
peaceful.
Yanee, Yaney, Yania, Yaniah, Yanie,
Yannee, Yanney, Yanni, Yannie,
Yanny, Yany

Yara/Yarna (Australian Aboriginal)
bird of the sea; seagull.
Yarah, Yarnah, Yarra, Yarrah

Yaralla (Australian Aboriginal)
camping area.
Yara, Yarala, Yaralah, Yarallah

Yardena (Hebrew) descended.
Yardenah

Yardeniya (Hebrew) garden of God.

Yarina (Slavic/Greek) peaceful.
Yarinah, Yarine, Yaryna, Yarynah,
Yaryne

Yarkona (Hebrew) green.
Yarkonah

Yarmilla (Slavic) trader.
Yarmila, Yarmilah, Yarmillah,
Yarmille, Yarmyla, Yarmylah,
Yarmylla, Yarmyllah, Yarmylle

Yarra (Australian Aboriginal) fast.
Yara, Yarah

Yashna (Hindi) prayer.
Yashnah

Yashodhana (Hindi) famous;
prosperous.

Yasmine (Arabic) (Botanical) the
jasmine flower.
Jasmin, Jasmina, Jasminah,
Jasmine, Jazmin, Jazmina,
Jazminah, Jazmine, Yaslin, Yaslyn,
Yasmeen, Yasmeen, Yasmeena,
Yasmeenah, Yasmin, Yasmina,
Yasminah,Yasmyn, Yasmyna,
Yasmynah, Yasmyne, Yazmin,
Yazmina, Yazminah, Yazmine,
Yazmyn, Yazmyna, Yazmynah,
Yazmyne

Yasu (Japanese) tranquil.
Yazoo

Yatva (Hebrew) good.
Yatvah

Ye (French/Greek) kind; good. A
form of Agatha.

Yedda (English) singer.
Yeda, Yedah, Yeddah

Yedida (Hebrew) dearest, most
beloved friend.
Yedidah, Yedyda, Yedydah

Yehudit (Hebrew) praised. A form
of Judith.
Yudit, Yudita, Yudyta, Yudytah,
Yuta

Yei (Japanese) flourishing.

Yeira (Hebrew) light.
Yeirah, Yeyra, Yeyrah

Yelena (Latin) lily blossom; shining
light. A form of Helena.
Yelana, Yelanah, Yelane, Yelenah

Yelenah (Russian/Latin) shining
light. A form of Elena/Helena.
Elaina, Elan, Elana, Elanah, Elane,
Ellain, Ellaina, Ellainah, Ellaine,
Ellayna, Ellayne, Ellen, Ellena,
Yelain, Yelaina, Yelainah, Yelaine,
Yelana, Yelanah, Yelane, Yellaina,
Yellaine, Yellayna, Yellaynah,
Yelenah, Yellena, Yellenah, Yellene

Yelisabeta (Russian/Hebrew) holy and sacred to God. A form of Elizabeth.
Yelizaveta

Yemena (Arabic) from Yemen.
Yemina, Yeminah, Yemyna, Yemyah

Yemina (Hebrew) little dove.
Jemima, Jemimah, Jemina, Jeminah, Jemyna, Jemynah, Yemima, Yemimah, Yeminah, Yemynah

Yen (Chinese) yearning; desired.
Yeni, Yenie, Yenih, Yenny

Yenene (Native American) shaman; medicine woman.
Yenena, Yenenah, Yenina, Yeninah, Yenyna, Yenynah, Yenyne

Yenta (Hebrew) home ruler.
Yentah

Yeo (Korean) mild.
Yee

Yepa (Native American) snow girl.
Yepah, Yeppa, Yeppah

Yera (Australian Aboriginal) joyful.
Yerah, Yerra, Yerrah

Yesenia (Latin) flower.
Yecenia, Yeseniah, Yesenya, Yesenyah, Yessenia, Yesseniah, Yessenya, Yessenyah

Yeshara (Hebrew) direct.
Yesharah

Yeshisha (Hebrew) old.
Yeshysha

Yesima (Hebrew) strength of the right hand.
Yesimah, Yessima, Yessimah, Yessyma, Yessymah

Yessica (Hebrew) wealthy. A form of Jessica.
Jesica, Jesicka, Jesika, Jessicam Jessicka, Jessika, Yesica, Yesicah, Yesicka, Yesickah, Yesika, Yesikah, Yessica, Yessicah, Yessicka, Yessickah, Yessika, Yessikah, Yessena, Yessenah, Yessenia, Yesseniah, Yessenya, Yessenyah

Yetta (Old English) ruler of the house. The feminine form of Henry.
Yeta, Yette

Yeva (Ukrainian/Greek) good news bringer. A form of Eve, life.
Yevah

Yevgenia (Russian/Greek) noble; well born. A form of Eugenia. A feminine form of Eugene.
Yevgena, Yevgeniah, Yevgenya, Yevgenyah, Yevgina, Yevginah, Yevgyna, Yevgynah

Ygerne (Celtic) graceful. A form of Igraine.
Igraine

Yiesha (Arabic) woman. (Afri/Swah) life. A form of Aisha.
Iesha, Liesha, Yieshah

Yilla (Australian Aboriginal) cicada.
Yila, Yilah, Yillah

Yin (Chinese) silver.

Yirki (Australian Aboriginal) evening star.
Yirkee, Yirkie, Yirky

Ynes (Spanish/Greek) purity. A form of Agnes.
Ynesita, Ynez

Yoi (Japanese) born in the evening.
Yoy

Yoki (Hopi) blue bird.
Yokee, Yokie, Yoky

Yoko (Japanese) positive woman.

Y

Yola (Greek) the violet flower;
purple. A short form of Yolanda.
Yolah, Yolee, Yoli, Yolie, Yoly

Yolanda (Greek) the violet flower;
purple.
Eolande, Ioland, Iolande, Iolantha,
Iolanthe (Grk), Yolanda, Yolande
(Fren), Yolane, Yolantha, Yolanthe

Yolota (Native American) goodbye
to spring.
Yolotah

Yoluta (Native American) flower of
summer; seed.
Yolutah

Yon (Burmese) rabbit. (Kor) lotus
flower.
Yona, Yonah, Yonna, Yonnah

Yone (Japanese) wealth; rice.
Yonee, Yoney, Yoni, Yonie, Yony

Yoni/Yonina/Yonita (Hebrew) dove,
the bird of peace.
Jona, Jonah, Jonati, Jonatia,
Jonatiah, Jonina, Joninah, Jonyna,
Jonynah, Jonyta, Jonytah, Yona,
Yonah, Yonati, Yonatia, Yonatiah,
Yonee, Yoney, Yoni, Yonie, Yonina,
Yoninah, Yonita, Yonitah, Yony,
Yonyna, Yonynah, Yonyta, Yonytah

Yoola (Australian Aboriginal) hill.
Yoolah

Yoomee (Coos) star.
Yoome

Yoorana (Australian Aboriginal)
loving.
Yooranah

Yootha (English/Spanish) mountain
dweller.
Uta, Utah, Yutta

Yordana (Basque) descended.
Yordanah, Yordanna, Yordannah

Yori (Japanese) reliable.
Yoriko, Yoriyo

Yosepha (Hebrew/French) God will
increase; God has added a child.
A feminine form of Joseph.
Yosefa, Yosifa, Yosyfa, Yuseffa

Yoshe (Japanese) lovely.
Yoshee

Yoshi (Japanese) quiet; respected.
Yoshee, Yoshey, Yoshie, Yoshy

Yoshiko (Japanese) good.
Yoshyko

Yovela (Hebrew) happiness.
Yovelah, Yovella, Yovelle

Ysabel (Spanish) dedicated to God.
A form of Isabelle.
Isabel, Isabell, Isabella, Isabelle,
Ysabela, Ysabelah, Ysabell,
Ysabella, Ysabelle, Ysbel, Ysbela,
Ysbele, Ysbella, Ysbelle, Ysobel,
Ysobela, Ysobele, Ysobell, Ysobella,
Ysobelle

Ysanne (Spanish/Hebrew) dedicated
to God. A form of Isabelle.
Ysanda, Ysande, Ysann, Ysanna,
Ysannah

Yseult (Irish) light-skinned.
Yseulte, Ysolt

Yu (Chinese) jade stone.

Yuana (Spanish) God is gracious.
Yuan, Yuanah, Yuanna, Yuannah

Yudelle (English) prosperous. A
form of Udele.
Yudela, Yudelah, Yudele, Yudella,
Yudellah, Yudelia, Yudeliah,
Yudelya, Yudelyah

Yudita (Russian/Hebrew) praised.
Yuditah, Yuditta, Yudyta, Yudytah,
Yudytta, Yudyttah

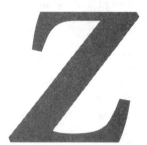

Yuki (Japanese) snow; lucky.
Yukee, Yukey, Yukie, Yukiko, Yuky

Yula (Russian) young.
Yulah

Yulan (Chinese) jade orchid.
Ulan

Yulene (Basque/Latin) youthful. A form of Julia.
Yulean, Yuleana, Yuleanah, Yuleane, Yuleen, Yuleena, Yuleenah, Yuleene, Yulena, Yulenah

Yulia (Russian/Latin) youthful. A form of Julia.
Yula, Yulah, Yulenka, Yuliah, Yulinka, Yulya, Yulyah, Yulynka, Yulka, Yulya

Yumiko (Japanese) arrow child.
Yumyko

Yuri (Japanese) lily.
Yuriko, Yuriyo, Yury

Yuriko (Japanese) child of the lilies.
Yuryko

Yusra (Arabic) wealthy.

Yvanna (Slavic) God is gracious. A form of Ivana.
Yvan, Yvana, Yvanah, Yvannah,Yvania, Yvannia, Yvanniah, Yavannya, Yavannyah, Yavanya, Yavanyah

Yvette (French) young archer. The feminine form of Yves.
Evet, Evetta, Evette, Yevetta, Yevette, Yvet, Yvett, Yvette

Yvonne (French) archer. The feminine form of Yves.
Eve, Evette, Evon, Evone, Evonn, Evonna, Evonne, Ivon, Ivone, Ivonn, Ivonne

Zabrina (English) boundary. (Heb) seventh daughter; promise. A form of Sabrina.
Zabreana, Zabreanah, Zabreane, Zabreena, Zabreenah, Zabreenia, Zabreeniah, Zabrinah, Zabrinia, Zabriniah, Zabrinna, Zabrinnah, Zabrinnia, Zabrinniah, Zabryna, Zabrynah, Zabrynia, Zabryniah, Zabrynya, Zabrynyah

Zacharie (Hebrew) God remembers.
Zacara, Zacarah, Zacaree, Zacarey, Zacari, Zacaria, Zacariah, Zaccaree, Zaccarey, Zaccareaus, Zaccari, Zacchaea, Zachoia, Zachola, Zackeisha, Zackery, Zakaria, Zakariah, Zakary, Zakarya, Zakaryah, Zakir, Zakira, Zakiya, Zakiyah, Zechari, Zecharie, Zechary

Zada (Arabic) lucky.
Sada, Zaida, Zayda

Zafina (Arabic) triumph.
Zafinah, Zafyna, Zafynah

Zafirah (Arabic) victory; success.
Zafira, Zafire, Zafyra, Zafyrah, Zafyre

Zahar (Hebrew) dawn.
Zahara, Zaher, Zahera, Zahir Zahira, Zahirah, Zahyr, Zahyra, Zahyrah

Zahara (African) flower.
Sahara, Saharah, Zaharah

Z

Zahavah (Hebrew) gold.
Zachava, Zachavah, Zechava,
Zechavah, Zehava, Zehavah,
Zehavi, Zehavia, Zehaviah, Zehavit,
Zahavya, Zehavyah, Zeheva,
Zehuva

Zahira (Arabic) bright.
Zahirah, Zahyra, Zahyrah

Zahra (Arabic) white. (Afr/Swah)
flower. (Heb) princess. A form of
Sara.
Sahra, Zahera, Zaherah, Zahira,
Zahrah, Zajirah

Zaida (Arabic) good fortune;
growth; hunter.
Sada, Saida, Sayda, Zada, Zayda

Zaidee (Arabic) wealthy.
Saidea, Saidee, Saidey, Saidi,
Saidie, Saidy, Zaidea, Zaidee,
Zaidey, Zaidi, Zaidie, Zaidy,
Zaydea, Zaydee, Zaydi, Zaydie,
Zaydy

Zainab (Arabic) mother of the poor.
Zaina, Zainah, Zayna, Zaynab,
Zaynah

Zaira (Arabic) dawn. (Ir) princess. A
form of Sara.
Sair, Sar, Sara, Sareena, Sarina,
Sarinah, Sarine, Zair, Zairah, Zara,
Zareena, Zarina, Zarinah, Zarine,
Zayra, Zayrah

Zakah (Hebrew) purity.
Zackz, Zackah, Zaka

Zakelina (Russian) God remembers.
A feminine form of Zack.
Zakeleana, Zakeleanah, Zakeleane,
Zakeleen, Zakeleena, Zakelleene,
Zakelin, Zakelinah, Zakeline,
Zakelyn, Zakelyna, Zakelynah,
Zakelyne

Zakia (Swahili) intelligent.
(Arab) purity.
Zakiah, Zakya, Zakyah

Zakiya (Swahili) purity.
Zakia, Zakiah, Zakiyah, Zakiyya
(Hin), Zakiyyah, Zakya, Zakyah,
Zakyya, Zakyyah

Zali (Hebrew/Polish) princess. A
form of Sara.
Zalea, Zaleah, Zalee, Zalei, Zaleigh,
Zaley, Zalia, Zaliah, Zalie, Zaly,
Zalya, Zalyah

Zalika (Swahili) well born.
Salika, Salikah, Zalik, Zalikah,
Zalyka, Zalykah, Zuleika

Zaltana (Native American) high
mountain.
Zaltanah

Zan (Chinese) praised.

Zana (Persian) woman.
San, Sanah, Zan, Zanah

Zandra (Greek) defender of
humankind. A form of Sandra. A
feminine form of Alexander.
Sandra, Sandrah, Zandrah, Zandri,
Zandria, Zandriah, Zandrie,
Zandirah, Zandry, Zandrya,
Zandryah

Zaneta (Hebrew) with the grace of
God.
Saneta, Sanetah, Sanete, Sanett,
Sanetta, Sanette, Zaneata, Zaneatah,
Zaneeta, Zaneetah, Zanetah, Zanete,
Zanett, Zanetta, Zanettah, Zanette,
Zanita, Zanitah, Zanyta, Zanytah

Zanna (Spanish) God is gracious. A
form of Jane. The English form of
Susanna, graceful lily.
Zana, Zanah, Zanella, Zanelle,
Zanetta, Zanette, Zannah,
Zannetta, Zannette, Zannia,
Zanniah, Zannya, Zannyah

Zanta (Latvian) bright.
Santa, Santah, Zantah

Zara (Arabic) dawning brightness;
easterly; princess. A form of Sara.
Sahra, Sara, Sarah, Zahra, Zarah
(Heb)

Zarifa (Arabic) success.
Zarifah, Zaryfa, Zaryfah

Zarina (Hindi) gold.
Zareana, Zareanah, Zareena,
Zareenah, Zarinah, Zaryna,
Zarynah

Zarita (Hebrew) princess. A form of
Sara.
Zareata, Zareatah, Zareate, Zareeta,
Zareetah, Zareete, Zaritah, Zarite,
Zaritta, Zaritte, Zaryt, Zaryta,
Zarytah, Zaryte

Zarzia (Hebrew) hard-working;
industrious.
Sarzia, Sarziah, Serzia, Serziah,
Zarziah, Zarzya, Zarzyah, Zeriza,
Zerziah, Zezya, Zezyah

Zasha (Russian) defender of
humankind. A form of
Sasha/Alexandra.
Zascha, Zashenka, Zashka, Zasho

Zatkelina (Russian/Hebrew) God
remembers. A feminine form of
Zack.
Zacelin, Zacelina, Zacelinah,
Zaceline, Zacelyn, Zacelyna,
Zacelynah, Zacelyne, Zackelin,
Zackelina, Zackelinah, Zackeline,
Zackelyn, Zackelyna, Zackelynah,
Zackelyne, Zakelin, Zakeline,
Zakelyn, Zakelyna, Zakelynah,
Zakelyne

Zaviera (Spanish/Arabic) bright.
(Basq) new house owner.
Zavera, Zaverah, Zavira, Zavirah

Zawadi (Swahili) olive.
Zawadea, Zawadee, Zawadie,
Zawady

Zawati (Swahili) gift.
Zawatia, Zawatiah, Zawaty,
Zawatya, Zawatyah

Zayit (Hebrew) olive.
Zayita

Zaynab (Arabic) plant.
Zainah

Zaza (Hebrew) golden; moving
swiftly.
Saza, Zazah, Zehavi, Zehavit, Zazu

Zdena (Greek) follower of Dionysos
(god of wine).
Zdenah

Zea (Latin) grain.
Sea, Seah, Sia, Siah, Zeah, Zia,
Ziah, Zya, Zyah

Zeborah (African
American/Hebrew) honey bee. A
form of Deborah.
Zebora

Zeffa (Portuguese) rose.
Zefa, Zefah, Zeffah

Zefiryn (Polish) west wind goddess.
Zefirin, Zefirina, Zefirinah,
Zefiryna, Zefirynah, Zefyrin,
Zefyrina, Zefyrinah, Zefyryn,
Zefyryna, Zefyrynah

Zehara (Hebrew) light.
Zeharah

Zehava (Hebrew) golden; brilliant.
Sehara, Sehari, Sehava, Sehavit,
Sehuva, Sohar, Soheret, Zehara,
Zehari, Zehavi, Zehavia, Zehaviah,
Zehavit, Zehavya, Zehavyah,
Zehuva, Zohar, Zoheret

Zehira (Hebrew) protected;
guarded.
Sehira, Sehirah, Zehirah, Zehyra,
Zehyrah

Zeita (Portuguese) rose.
Zeta, Zetah, Zettah

Zelda (Yiddish/Teutonic) grey-
haired.
Zeldah

Zelene (English) sunshine.
Zeleen, Zeleena, Zeleenah, Zelena,
Zelenah, Zelina, Zeline, Zelyn,
Zelyna, Zelyne

Zelenka (Slavic) little innocent one.
Selen, Selenka, Selenkah, Zelen,
Zelenk, Zelenkah

Zelia (Greek) enthusiastic.
(Span) sunshine.
Selia, Seliah, Selya, Selyah, Zeliah,
Zelya, Zelyah

Zelizi (Basque/Latin) feminine. The
Irish form of Cecilia, unseeing.
Zelizia, Zelziah, Zelzya, Zelzyah

Zelkova (Russian) elm tree.
Selkova, Selkovah, Zelkovah

Zella (Hebrew) shelter.
Sela, Selah, Sella, Sellah, Zela,
Zelah, Zellah

Zelmah (Turkish) safe; protected.
Selma, Selmah, Zelma

Zemira (Hebrew) song.
Semir, Semira, Semirah, Semyr,
Semyra, Semyrah, Zemir, Zemirah,
Zemyr, Zemyra, Zemyrah, Zimira,
Zimirah, Zymira, Zymirah,
Zymyra, Zymyrah

Zen (Chinese) purity. A religious
belief. A form of Zhen.
Zena, Zenah, Zenn, Zenna,
Zennah, Zhen, Zhena, Zhenah,
Zhenn, Zhenna, Zhennah

Zena (Persian) woman. (Grk) guest.
Sena, Senah, Senia, Seniah, Senya,
Senyah, Xena, Xenah, Xihna,
Xihnah, Xina, Xinah, Xyhna,
Xyhnah, Xyna, Xynah, Zenah,
Zenia, Zeniah, Zenya, Zenyah,
Zihna, Zihnah, Zina, Zinah, Zyhna,
Zyhnah, Zyna, Zynah

Zenaida (Greek) wild dove.
Zenaidah, Zenayda, Zenaydah

Zenaide (Greek) daughter of Zeus;
the living; bright sky.
Zenaida, Zenayda, Zenayde,
Zenochika

Zenanda (Persian) queen.
Senanda, Xenanda

Zenda (Persian) sacred; feminine.
Senda, Sendah, Zendah

Zenevieva (Russian) white wave. A
form of Genevieve.
Zeneviev, Zenevievah

Zenia (Greek) enthusiastic guest.
Senia, Seniah, Senya, Senyah,
Xenia, Xeniah, Xenya, Xenyah,
Zeniah, Zenya, Zenyah

Zenobia (Greek) given life by Zeus;
the living; bright sky.
Sena, Senaida, Senda, Senia,
Senobe, Senobia, Senobie, Senovia,
Sizi, Zenobia, Xenobiah, Xenobya,
Xenobyah, Zena, Zenaida, Zenda,
Zenna, Zenia, Zenobe, Zenobiah,
Zenobie (Fren), Zenobya,
Zenobyah, Zenovia, Zizi, Zyzy

Zephaniah (Hebrew) the Lord has
hidden.
Sephanee, Sephaney, Sephani,
Sephania, Sephaniah, Sephanie,
Sephany, Zephania, Zephaniah,
Zephanee, Zephaney, Zephani,
Zephanie, Zephany, Zephanyah

Z

Zephira (Hebrew) morning; dawn.
Seffira, Seffire, Sephir, Sephire,
Zeffir, Zeffira, Zeffire, Zephir,
Zephirah, Zephyra, Zephyrah

Zephrine (English) breeze.
Sephrin, Sephrina, Sephrine,
Zephrean, Zephreana, Zephreanah,
Zephreane, Zephreen, Zephreena,
Zephreenah, Zephreene, Zephrin,
Zephrina, Zephrinah, Zephryn,
Zephryna, Zephrynah, Zephryne

Zephyr (Greek) west wind.
Sephir, Sephyr, Zephir

Zera (Latin) seeds.
Sera, Serah, Zerah

Zerdali (Turkish) wild apricot.
Zerdalia, Zeradaly, Zeradalya

Zeresh (Hebrew) golden.
Zeresha, Zereshah

Zerlina (Hebrew/Latin) beautiful
dawn.
Serlin, Serlinda, Serlina, Serlinah,
Serline, Serlyn, Serlyna, Serlynah,
Serlynda, Serlyne, Zerlea, Zerlean,
Zerleana, Zerleanah, Zerleane,
Zerlee, Zerleen, Zerleena,
Zerleenah, Zerleene, Zerlinah,
Zerline, Zelinda, Zerlyn, Zerlyna,
Zerlynah, Zerlinda, Zerlynda,
Zerlyne, Zorina, Zorinah, Zoryna,
Zorynah

Zerrin (Turkish) golden.
Zerran, Zerren, Zerron, Zerryn

Zeta (Hebrew) olive.
Seta, Sita, Syta, Xeta, Xetah, Xita,
Xitah, Xyta, Xytah, Zayit, Zetana,
Zetta, Zita, Zitah, Zyta, Zytah

Zeva (Greek) sword. (Heb) wolf.
Seva, Sevah, Zevah, Zevia, Zeviah,
Zevya, Zevyah

Zevida (Hebrew) gift.
Sevida, Sevuda, Zevuda, Zevyda

Zhen (Chinese) purity.
Zen, Zenn, Zhena, Zhenah.
Zhenna, Zhennah

Zia (Hebrew) trembling. (Lat) grain.
(Ital) aunt.
Sea, Seah, Sia, Siah, Sya, Syah, Xia,
Xiah, Xya, Xyah, Zea, Zeah, Ziah,
Zya, Zyah

Zigana (Hungarian) gypsy.
Ziganah, Zigane, Zygana, Zyganah

Zihna (Hopi) spinner of tops.
Xihna, Xihnah, Xyhna, Xyhnah,
Zihnah, Zyhna, Zyhnah

Zila (Hebrew) shade.
Sila, Silah, Silla, Sillah, Zilah, Zilla,
Zillah, Zyla, Zylah, Zylla, Zyllah

Zilia (Italian) white wave. A form of
Genevieve.
Xilia, Xiliah, Xilya, Xilyah, Xylia,
Xyliah, Xylya, Xylyah, Ziliah, Zilya,
Zilyah, Zylia, Zyliah, Zylya, Zylyah

Zillah (Hebrew) shadow.
Sila, Silah, Silla, Sillah, Zila, Zilah,
Zilla, Zillah, Zyla, Zylah, Zylla,
Zyllah

Zilpah (Hebrew) sprinkling.
Silpa, Silpah, Xilpa, Xilpah, Xylpa,
Xylpah, Zylpa, Zylpah

Zilya (Russian/Greek) harvester. A
form of Teresa.
Xilya, Xilyah, Xylya, Xylyah, Zilyah,
Zylya, Zylyah

Zimra (Hebrew) branch; song of
praise.
Samoka, Samira, Samora, Samyra,
Semira, Semora, Semyra, Simria,
Simrriah, Xamira, Xamirah,
Ximara, Ximarah, Ximra, Ximrah,
Xymra, Xymrah, Zamira, Zamoka,
Zamora, Zamyra, Zemira, Zemora,
Zemyra, Zimria, Zimrriah, Zymria,
Zymriah, Zymrya, Zymryah

Z

Zina (African) name.
(Heb) abundant; plenty.
Sena, Senah, Senia, Seniah, Senya,
Senyah, Xena, Xenah, Xihna,
Xihnah, Xina, Xinah, Xyhna,
Xyhnah, Xyna, Xynah, Zenah,
Zenia, Zeniah, Zenya, Zenyah,
Zihna, Zihnah, Zina, Zinah, Zyhna,
Zyhnah, Zyna, Zynah

Zinerva (Italian) fair-haired.
Xinerva, Xinervah, Xynerva,
Xynervah, Zinervah, Zynerva,
Zynervah

Zinnia (Latin) the zinnia flower.
Sinia, Siniah, Sinnia, Sinniah,
Xinia, Xiniah, Xinya, Xinyah,
Xynia, Xyniah, Xynya, Xynyah,
Zinia, Ziniah, Zinniah, Zinya,
Zinyah, Zynia, Zyniah, Zynya

Zippora (Hebrew) beautiful little
bird.
Cipora, Ciporah, Cippora,
Cipporah, Sipora, Siporah,
Sippora, Sipporah, Zipora,
Ziporah, Zipporah, Zypora,
Zyporah, Zyppora, Zypporah

Ziracuny (Kiowa) water stealer.
Zyracuny

Zita (Spanish) little rose. (Ir)
enticing; intriguing. (Lat) hope.
Sita, Siath, Xita, Xitah, Xyta, Xytah,
Zitah, Zyta, Zytah

Zitkala (Sioux) bird.
Zitkalah, Zytkala, Zytkalah

Ziva (Hebrew) shining bright; light.
The Slavic goddess of light.
Siva, Sivah, Syva, Syvah, Zivit,
Zyva, Zyvah

Zizi (Russian) father's ornament.
Zsi Zsi, ZyZy

Zlatka (Slavic) gold.
Zlatkah

Zocha (Polish/Greek) wisdom.
Zochah

Zoe (Greek) life.
Soe, Soee, Soia, Soiah, Zoa, Zoah,
Zoee, Zoey, Zoela, Zoeta, Zoi, Zoia
(Russ), Zoiah, Zolida, Zolita, Zoy,
Zoya, Zoyah, Zoye, Ziva, Zyva

Zofia (Slavic/Greek) wisdom. A
form of Sophia.
Zofee, Zofey, Zofi, Zofiah, Zofie,
Zofy, Zofka, Zophee, Zophey,
Zophi, Zophia, Zophiah, Zophya,
Zophyah, Zsofia, Zsofiah, Zsofie,
Zsofy, Zsophee, Zsophey, Zsophi,
Zsophia, Zsophiah, Zsophie,
Zsophy

Zohar (Hebrew) brilliant; shining.
Zohara, Zoharah, Zohera, Zoheret

Zohra (Arabic) blossom.
Sohra, Sohrah, Zohrah

Zohreh (Persian) happy.
Zahreh, Zohra, Zohrah

Zoia (Russian) life.
Zoe, Zoee, Zoey, Zoi, Zoiah, Zoya,
Zoyah

Zolah (Italian) mound of earth;
ball.
Sola, Solah, Zola

Zona (Greek) girdle.
Sona, Sonah, Zonah

Zondra (Greek) defender of
humankind. A form of Sandra.
Zohndra, Zohndria, Zohndriah,
Zohndrya, Zohndryah, Zondrah,
Zondria, Zondriah, Zondrya,
Zondryah

Zophie (Bohemian) wisdom. A
form of Sophie.
Sofee, Sofey, Sofi, Sofie, Sofy,
Sophee, Sophey, Sophi, Sophia
(Grk), Sophiah, Sophie (Grk),
Sophy, Zofee, Zofey, Zofi, Zofia,

Z

Zophie cont.
Zofiah, Zofie, Zofy, Zofya, Zofyah,
Zophee, Zophey, Zophi, Zophia,
Zophiah, Zophy, Zophya,
Zophyah, Zsophee, Zsophey,
Zsophi, Zsofia, Zsofiah, Zsofie,
Zsofya, Zsofyah, Zsophee, Zsophey,
Zsophi, Zsophia (Hung),
Zsophiah, Zsophie, Zsophy,
Zsophya, Zsophyah

Zora (Slavic) beautiful aurora;
dawn; morning star.
Aura, Aurah, Aurea, Aureah, Auria,
Auriah, Aurya, Auryah, Sora, Sorah,
Sorana, Sorane, Sorin, Sorina,
Sorine, Soryna, Soryne, Zorah,
Zorana, Zorane, Zorin, Zorina,
Zorine, Zoryna, Zoryne, Zyra

Zorina (Slavic) gold.
Zorana, Zoranah, Zorean, Zoreana,
Zoreanah, Zoreane, Zoreen,
Zoreena, Zoreenah, Zoreene,
Zorinah, Zorine, Zorna, Zornah,
Zoryn, Zoryna, Zorynah, Zoryne

Zosa (Swiss) lily. A form of Susan.
Zosah, Zoza, Zozah, Zozel (Swis)

Zosima (Greek) lively, wealthy
woman.
Sosima, Sosimah, Sosyma,
Zosimah, Zosyma, Zosymah

Zoya (Slavic/Greek) life. A form of
Zoe.
Zoia, Zoiah, Zoiia, Zoiiah, Zoyara,
Zoyarah, Zoyechka, Zoyenka,
Zoyah, Zoyya, Zoyyah

Zsa Zsa (Hungarian/Hebrew) lily. A
form of Susan.
Zsa

Zsuzsan (Hungarian) lily. A form of
Susan.
Zsa, Zsa Zsa, Zsuska, Zsuzsa,
Zsuzsana, Zsuzsanah, Zsuzsane,

Zsuzsann, Zsuzsanna (Pol),
Zsuzsannah, Zsuzsanne, Zsuzsi,
Zsuzsika, Zsuzska

Zudora (Sanskrit) hard-working;
industrious.
Zudorah

Zuette (French) yew; little bow
bearer.
Ivet, Iveta, Ivetah, Ivete, Ivett,
Ivetta, Ivettah, Ivette, Suet, Sueta,
Suetah, Suete, Suett, Suetta,
Suettah, Suette, Zuet, Zueta,
Zuetah, Zuete, Zuetta, Zuettah

Zuleika (Persian) bright; pretty;
brilliant. (Arab) peace.
Suleika, Suelia, Sueliah, Zuelia,
Zueliah, Zuelya, Zuelyah

Zulema (Hebrew/Arabic) peace.
Sulema, Sulima, Zulemah, Zulima,
Zulyma

Zurafa (Arabic) lovely.
Ziraf, Zirafa, Zuruf, Zurufa

Zuri (Swahili) beautiful.
(Basq) white complexioned.
Zuree, Zurey, Zuria, Zuriah, Zurie,
Zury, Zurya, Zuryah

Zusa (Slavic/Polish/Hebrew) lily. A
form of Susan.
Zusah, Zuza, Zuzah, Zuzana,
Zuzane, Zuzanka, Zuzia, Zuziah,
Zuzka, Zuzu

Zverda (Slavic) star.
Zverdana

Zwetlana (Russian) star.
Swetlana

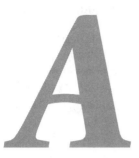

Aaron (Hebrew) enlightened. (Arab) messenger.
Aahron, Aaran, Aaren, Aareon, Aarin, Aaronn, Aarron, Aarronn, Asryn, Aarynn, Aeran, Aharon, Ahran, Ahren, Aranne, Arek, Aren, Ari, Arin, Aron, Aronek, Arron, Arryn, Aryn

Abadi (Arabic) eternal; lasting.

Abasi (Swahili) stern.
Abasee, Abasey, Abasie, Abasy

Abba (Aramaic) father. (Heb) addressed to God.
Aba, Abad, Abbas, Abbe, Abbey, Abbie, Abboid, Abbot, Abbott, Abby

Abban (Latin) white.
Abbana, Abben, Abbena, Abbin, Abbina, Abbine, Abbon, Abbona

Abbas (Arabic) Muhammed's uncle; stern.
Abba

Abbey (Hebrew) father rejoiced. A form of Abe, father of the multitudes.
Abbee, Abbi, Abbie, Abby, Abee, Abey, Abi, Abie, Aby

Abbot (Old English) father of the abbey.
Abad (Span), Abba, Abad (Span), Abbe (Fren), Abboid (Gaelic), Abbott (Anglo-Sax), Abby, Abot, Abott (Fren)

Abdul (Arabic) servant of Allah.
Abdal, Abdala, Abdel, Abdela, Abdula, Abdulah, Abdulla, Abdullah

Abe (Hebrew) father of the multitudes. A short form of Abraham.
Abbe, Abbee, Abbey, Abbi, Abbie, Abby, Abee, Abey, Abi, Abie, Aby

Abel (Hebrew) breath; son.
Ab, Abb, Abbe, Abbey, Abbi, Abbie, Abby, Abe, Abebt, Abelard, Abeles, Abell, Abey, Abi, Abie, Able, Ablius, Awel, Hevel, Nab

Abelard (Old German) one who is born of firm, high nobility; ambitious one.
Abelarde

Abernethy (Scottish/Gaelic) mouth or beginning of a river.
Abernethi, Abernathie

Abi (Turkish) elder brother.
Abbe, Abbee, Abbey, Abbi, Abbie, Abby, Abe, Abee, Abey, Abie, Aby

Abiah (Hebrew) God is my father.
Abia, Abiel, Abija, Abijah, Abisha, Abishi, Abishal, Aviya, Aviyah, Avyya, Avyyah

Abias (Hebrew) one who serves the Lord.
Abyas

Abidan (Hebrew) father of judgment.
Abiden, Abidin, Abidon, Abydan, Abyden, Abydin, Abydon, Abydyn

Abie (Arabic) servant.
Abbe, Abbee, Abbey, Abbi, Abbie, Abby, Abdie, Abdiel, Abe, Abee, Abey, Abie, Aby

Abir (Hebrew) strength.
Abyr

Abisha (Hebrew) gift of God.
Abija, Abijah, Abisha, Abishai,
Abishal, Abysha, Abyshah

Abishur (Hebrew) my father's
glance.
Abyshur

Abner (Hebrew) divine father of
light.
Avner, Ebner

Abraham (Hebrew) father of the
multitudes.
Abrahamo, Abrahan (Span),
Abrahin (Span), Abrahem, Abramo
(Ital), Abran, Abraomas (Lith),
Alibaba, Avraham, Avram, Avrom,
Avrum, Habreham, Ibrahim

Abram (Hebrew) son of the highly
praised father.
Abrama, Abramah, Abramo (Ital),
Avram, Avrom, Bram (Dut),
Brama, Bramah

Absalom (Hebrew) father of peace.
Absolam, Absolom, Solam, Solom,
Solomon

Abu (Arabic) father.

Acar (Turkish) bright.
Accerlee, Accerleigh, Accerley,
Ackerlea, Ackerlee, Ackerleigh,
Ackerli, Ackerlie, Acklea, Acklee,
Ackleigh, Ackley, Ackli, Acklie,
Ackly, Akerlea, Akerlee, Akerleigh,
Akerli, Akerlie, Akerly

Ace (Latin) unity; one.

Achilles (Greek) without lips.
Achil, Achill, Achille, Achilleus,
Achyl, Achyll, Achylle, Achylleus

Acim (Hebrew) the Lord will judge.
Achim, Achym, Akim, Akym

Ackerley (English) from the
meadow of oak trees.
Ackerlea, Ackerleah, Ackerlee,
Ackerleigh, Ackerli, Ackerlie,
Ackerly, Akerlea, Akerleah, Akerlee,
Akerley, Akerli, Akerlie, Akerly

Ackley (Middle English) dweller at
the oak tree.
Acklea, Ackleah, Acklee, Ackleigh,
Ackli, Acklie, Ackly, Aklea, Akleah,
Aklee, Akleigh, Akley, Akli, Aklie,
Akly

Acton (Old English) belonging to
the town with oak trees.
Actan, Acten, Actin, Actun, Actyn

Adahy (Cherokee) in the oak tree
woods.
Adahi

Adair (Scottish/Gaelic) dweller by
the oak tree.
Adare, Adaire, Adayr, Adayre,
Addair, Addaire, Addar, Addare,
Addayr, Addyre

Adalard (Old German) noble; brave.
Adalarde, Adelard, Adelarde

Adalric (German) noble ruler.
Adelric, Adelrich, Adelrick, Adelrik,
Alderyc, Adelryck, Adelryk

Adam (Hebrew) of the red earth.
Adamo (Ital), Adams, Adamson,
Adan (Span), Adao (Port), Adas
(Port), Addam, Addison, Addos,
Addoson, Adekin, Adem, Adham,
(Irish/Scott), Adim, Adinet, Ado
(Est), Adom, Adomas (Lith),
Adym, Edam, Edem, Edim, Edom,
Edynm

Adamanan (Irish) little Adam; of
the red earth.
Adam

Adan (Arabic) one who brings pleasure.
Aden, Adin, Adon, Adun, Adyn

Adar (Hebrew) dark; cloudy.
Addair, Addar, Addare, Adin, Adino, Adna, Ard

Addison (Old English) descended from Adam; of the red earth.
Addis

Ade (Yoruba) royal.
Ad

Adel (Old German) noble.
Addel, Adell

Adelhard (German) noble; resolute.
Adelhart

Aden (Irish) fiery.
Adan, Adin, Adon, Adyn, Aidan, Aiden, Aidin, Aidon, Aidun, Aidyn, Aydan, Ayden, Aydin, Aydon, Aydyn

Ader (Hebrew) flock.
Adder

Adham (Arabic) black.

Adiel (Hebrew) ornament of the Lord.
Addiel

Adil (Arabic) wise; just.
Adeel, Adeele, Adill, Adyl, Adyll

Adilo (German) noble.
Addilo

Adin (Hebrew) voluptuous; beautiful. The masculine form of Adina.
Addin, Addyn, Adyn

Adiv (Hebrew) pleasant; gentle.
Adeev, Adev

Adlai (Hebrew) refuge of God. (Arab) to justify.
Addlai, Addlay, Adlay

Adler (Old German) eagle.
Addla, Addlah, Addlar, Addler, Adlar

Adley (Hebrew) righteous; just.
Adlea, Adleah, Adlee, Adleigh, Adli, Adlie, Adly

Adnan (Arabic) pleasant.
Adnane

Adney (Old English) dweller at the noble one's island.
Adnee, Adni, Adnie, Adny

Adolf/Adolphus (Old German) noble, fierce wolf; hero.
Adof, Addof, Addoff, Addofo (Span/Ital), Adolfius, Adolfo (Span/Lat), Adolfus, Adolph (Ger), Adolphe, Adolphius, Adolpho, Adolphus (Fren), Adolphu (Swed), Adolphus, Aethelwulf, Atofu (W/Sam), Dolf, Dolph, Dolphus

Adom (Akan) God will help.

Adon (Hebrew) belonging to the Lord.
Adonie (A/Abor), Adonis (Heb), Adonys

Adoni (Australian Aboriginal) sunset; dusk.
Adonee, Adoney, Adonie, Adony

Adonis (Hebrew) lord. (Grk) handsome.
Adonai, Adonay, Adonise, Adonys, Adonyse

Adri (Pakistani) rock.
Adree, Adrey, Adrie, Adry

Adrian (Latin) dark; mysterious; from the Adriatic Sea. A masculine form of Adriana.
Adriano (Ital/Span), Adrianus, Adrien (Fren), Adrin, Adryan, Adryen, Adryn, Arje (Dut), Arne, Arrian, Hadrian, Hadrien, Hadrion, Hadryan, Hadryen, Hadryin

Adriel (Hebrew) of God's Kingdom.
Adrial, Adriall, Adriell, Adryel,
Adryell

Adwin (Ghanian) creative.
Adwyn

Aegir (Old Norse) a sea god.
Aegyr

Aeneas (Greek) praised.
Angus, Aonghus, Eneas, Enne,
Oenghus, Oengus, Oneas

Afa (Tongan) hurricane.
Afah

Afram (African) Ghanaian river.

Afton (English) (Geographical)
from Afton in England.
Aftan, Aften, Aftin, Aftyn

Agastya (Sanskrit) one who moves
mountains.
Agastia, Agastiah, Agastyah

Agatho (Greek) good.
Agath, Agathe

Agostino (Italian) anguished;
misery.
Agostine, Agostyne

Agrey (Latin) open field.
Aggray, Agray, Agray

Agrippa (Latin) born with the feet
first.
Agripa, Agripah, Agrippah, Agrypa,
Agrypah, Agryppa, Agryppah

Agu (Ibo) leopard.

Agustin (Latin) highly praised.
Agustine, Agustyn, Agustyne,
Augustin, Augustine, Augustyn,
Augustyne

Ahab (Hebrew) uncle.

Ahdik (Native American) deer;
caribou.
Ahdic, Ahdick, Ahdyc, Ahdyck,
Ahdyk

Ahearn (Scottish) lord of the
horses. (Eng) the heron bird.
Ahearne, Aherin, Ahern, Aherne,
Aheron, Aheryn, Hearn, Hearne,
Hern, Herne

Ahmad (Arabic) praised; comfort.
Ahmad, Amadi, Amed

Ahrens (Old German) powerful
eagle.
Ahren

Ahu (Tongan) smoke.

Aidan (Irish/Gaelic) little fiery one.
Adan, Aiden, Aidon, Aidyn,
Aidwin, Aidwyn, Aydan, Ayden,
Aydin, Aydon, Aydyn, Edan, Eden,
Edin, Edyn

Aikane (Polynesian) friendly.
Aikan, Aykan, Aykane

Aiken (Old English) made of oak.
of the red earth

Aimery (German) hard-working
leader.
Aimeree, Aimerey, Aimeri, Aimeric,
Aimerie, Ameree, Amerey, Ameri,
Americ, Amerie, Aymeree, Aymerey,
Aymeri, Aymerie, Aymery

Aimon (French) house.
Aymon

Ain (Scottish) belonging to oneself.
The short form of names
beginning with 'Ain' e.g. Ainsley.
Ains, Ayn, Ayns

Aindrea (Irish) strong, brave,
courageous one. A form of
Andrew.
Aindrea, Aindreas, Andrea,
Andreas, Ayndrea, Ayndreas

Ainsley (Old English) from the
meadow clearing.
Ainslea, Ainsleah, Ainslee, Ainslei,
Ainsleigh, Ainsli, Ainslie, Ainsly,

A

Aynslea, Aynsleah, Aynslee,
Aynsley, Aynsli, Aynslie, Aynsly

Aisi (Tongan) ice.
Aisy

Ajala (Yoruba) pot maker.
Ajalah

Ajax (Greek) eagle.
Ajacks

Ajay (Punjabi) victorious.
A.J. Ajae, Ajai, Ajaye, Ajaz, Jae, Jai,
Jay, Jaye

Akama (Austalian Aboriginal)
whale.
Akam, Akamah

Akar (Turkish) stream.
Akara, Akare

Akash (Hindi) sky.
Akasha, Akashah

Akbar (Arabic) great.
Akbara, Akbare

Akecheta (Lakota) warrior.
Akechetah

Akelina (Russian) eagle.
Akelin, Akelinah, Akeline, Aquila,
Aquilah

Akemi (Japanese) dawning.
Akemee, Akemie, Akemy

Akeno (Japanese) morning; from
the shining field.
Keno

Akil (Arabic) intelligent.
Akile, Akyl, Akyle

Akim (Hebrew) God will establish.
Achim, Ackeem, Ackim, Ackime,
Ackym, Ackyme, Ahkiem, Ahkieme,
Ahkyem, Ahkyeme, Akeam, Akee,
Akeem, Akiem, Akima, Akimah,
Arkeem, Arkeeme, Arkym, Arkyme

Akins (Yoruba) brave.
Akin, Akyn, Akyns, Atkin, Atkins,
Atkyn, Atkyns

Akio (Japanese) bright.
Akyo

Akira (Japanese) intelligence.
Akihito, Akio, Akirah, Akiyo,
Akyra, Akyrah

Akiyama (Japanese) autumn; fall.
Akima, Akimah, Akyama,
Akyamah, Arkeem, Arkeeme

Akma (Australian Aboriginal) fresh
water.
Akmah, Akmara

Akmal (Arabic) perfection.
Ackmal

Aksel (German) tiny oak tree.
Aksell

Akule (Native American) he looks
up.
Akul

Al (English) handsome. The short
form of names starting with 'Al'
e.g. Alan.

Aladdin (Arabic) Allah's servant.
Aladdan, Aladden, Aladdyn,
Aladan, Aladen, Aladin, Aladyn

Alair (Irish) happy.
Alaire, Alayr, Alayre

Alaire (French) joy.
Alair, Alayr, Alayre

Alam (Arabic) universe.
Alame

Alan (Irish/Gaelic) handsome; fair;
bright; happy.
Ailan, Ailin (Irish), Alaen, Alaene,
Alain (Fren), Alaine, Aland,
Alando, Alane, Alano (Ital),
Alanus, Alwawn, Alein, Aleine,
Allena, Aleyn, Aleyne, Allan,

Alan cont.
Allane, Allayn, Allayne, Allen,
Allene, Alleyn, Alleyne, Allin,
Alline, Allwyn, Allyn, Allyne,
Allun, Allune, Allyn, Allyne, Alun,
Alunalyn, Alune, Alyn, Alyne

Alard (Old German) hard; noble.
Alarde

Alaric (Old German) wolf ruler;
fierce; hard, noble, supreme ruler
of all.
Airik (Swed), Alarich, Alarick,
Alarico (Span), Alarik, Alaryc,
Alaryck, Alaryk, Ulrie, Ulrich

Alba (Australian Aboriginal) wind.
Albah

Alberic (German) clever, wise ruler.
Alberi, Alberich, Alberyc, Alberyck,
Alberyk, Auberi, Auberon, Aubrey,
Aubry, Avery, Oberon

Albern (German) noble;
courageous.
Alberne, Alburn, Alburne

Albert (German) noble; industrious;
bright; famous.
Adalbert, Adel, Adelbert, Adell, Albe,
Alberti, Albertino (Ital), Alberto
(Ital/Span), Albertus, Albi, Albrecht
(Ger), Albret (Fren), Albyrt, Albyrte,
Aubert, Bertal, Bertel, Delbert,
Elbert, Elvert, Ethelbert, Halbert,
Imbert, Olbracht, Ulbricht

Albie (German/French) noble;
bright. The short form of names
starting with 'Albi' e.g. Albion.
Albee, Albey, Albie, Alby

Albin (Latin) white.
Alba, Alban (Ir), Alben, Albene,
Albin, Albino, Albion, Albon,
Albun, Albyn, Aloin

Albion (Celtic) white cliffs.
Albyon, Allbion, Allbyon

Alcander (Greek) defender of
humankind. A form of Alexander.
Allcander

Alcott (Old English) dweller from
the old cottage.
Alcot, Alscot, Alscott

Aldan/Alden (Old English) wise,
old friend; helmet.
Aldin, Aldon, Aldyn

Alder (Old English) the alder tree.
Aldar, Aldare, Aldir, Aldyr

Alderidge (Old English) from the
alder ridge.
Alderige, Aldrige, Aldrydge, Aldryge

Aldis (Old French) from the old
house.
Aldis, Aldiss, Aldous, Aldus, Aldys

Aldo (Old German) old; wise.
Alda, Aldous, Alter

Aldous (Old German) old; wise.
(O/Eng) from the old house.
Aldan, Alden, Aldin, Aldon, Aldis,
Aldo, Aldos, Aldren, Alous,
Aldwin, Aldwyn,, Aldys, Ealder,
Elden, Elder, Eldon, Eldor, Eltis,
Elton

Aldred (Old English) old, wise
counsel.
Alldred

Aldrich (Old German) old, wise
powerful ruler.
Aldric, Aldrige, Alric, Alrich, Alrick,
Aldryc, Aldryck, Aldryk, Audric
(Fren), Eldric, Eldrige

Aldwin (English) old friend.
Aldwan, Aldwen, Aldwon, Aldwyn,
Eldwin, Eldwyn

Alec/Alex/Alexis (Greek) defender of
humankind. The short form of
Alexander.
Alec, Aleck, Alecko, Aleik (Russ),

A

Aleizo, Alejo (Span), Alek, Alekko, Aleko, Alexi, Alexio (Port), Alexis (Grk), Alexx, Alexys, Alezio, Alezios, Alezius, Alic, Alick, Alik, Alika, Alikka, Aliko, Alixx, Allix, Allixx, Allyx, Allyxx, Alyc, Alyck, Alyk, Alyko, Ellec, Elleck, Ellic, Ellick

Alem (Arabic) wisdom.
Alim, Alym

Aleric (German) ruler of all.
Alerick, Alerik, Alleric, Alleryc, Alleryck, Allyrk

Aleron (Latin) wing.
Aleronn

Alexander (Greek) defender of humankind.
Alcander, Alecander, Alecsander, Alecksander, Alecxander, Aleckxander, Aleister, Alejandro (Span), Aleksajender (Slav), Aleksander (Dan/Nor/Russ), Aleksandr (Russ), Aleksei, Aleksy, Aleczi, Alessander, Alessandre (Russ), Alexandre (Fren), Alexius, Alezios, Alezius, Alisander, Alisandre, Alisaunder, Alixsander, Alixander, Alixxander, Alixxzander, Alixzander, Alyxxsander, Alyxxander, Alexxzander, Alexzander

Alford (Old English) wise counsellor from the old ford.
Allford

Alfred (Old English) old counsellor; wise judge.
Aelfric, Ailfrid, Alfeo, Alfredas (Lith), Alfric, Alfrick, Alfrid, Alfried (Ger), Alfris, Alfryd, Alured, Auveray, Avere, Avery, Elfric, Elfrick, Elfrid, Fred

Alger (Old German) noble spearman.
Aelgar, Algar, Algor, Elgar, Eylga

Algernon (Old French) one who has a beard or moustache.
Aelgernon

Algis (German) spear.
Algiss

Ali (Arabic) highly praised; great.
Aly

Alim (Arabic) all knowing; wisdom.
Alem, Alym

Allambee (Australian Aboriginal) quiet place.
Alambee, Alambey, Alambi, Alambie, Alamby, Allambey, Allambi, Allambie, Allamby

Allard (Old English) brave; noble; determined.
Alard (Fren)

Allison (Old English/Old German) Alice's son; son of the little, truthful one.
Allisan, Allisen, Allisun, Allisyn, Allysan, Allysen, Allyson, Allysun, Allysyn

Allistair (Greek) the avenger.
Alasdair, Alastair, Alastor, Alistair, Alister, Allister, Allistir, Alsandair (Ir), Alystair, Alystyr, Alystyre

Allunga (Australian Aboriginal) sun.
Allungah, Alunga, Alungah

Almeric (Old German) powerful ruler.
Amauric, Amaurick, Amaurik, Amaury, Amauryc, Amauryck, Amauryk, Ameri, Americk, Amerik, Amery, Ameryc, Ameryck, Ameryk

Almo (Old English) noble; famous.
Allmo

A

Almon (Hebrew) widower.
Alman, Almen, Almin, Almyn

Alon (Hebrew) oak; strength.
Alonn, Allon, Allonza, Allonzo
(O/Ger), Alonza, Alonzo (O/Ger)

Alonzo (Old German) noble.
Allon, Allonza, Allonzo, Alon,
Alonz, Alonza, Alonzah, Alonze

Aloysius (Old German) famous,
glorious warrior of battle.
Alaois, Alois (Hung), Aloisia,
Aloisio, Aloisy, Aloys

Alpha (Greek) first-born.
Alfa, Alfah, Alfia, Alfiah, Alfya,
Alfyah, Alphah, Alphia, Alphiah,
Alphya, Alphyah

Alpheus (Greek) a river god.
Alfeus, Alpheous

Alphonse (Old German) noble;
eager to do battle.
Alfons, Alfonso (Ital), Alfonzo,
Alford, Alonso, Alonzo (Span),
Alphonsine, Alphonso, Alphonsus

Alphonse/Alphonso (Spanish)
ready; noble.
Alfonce, Alfonco, Alfonse,
Alphonce, Alphonco, Alphonso

Alpin (Scottish) high mountains;
blond/fair-haired.
Alpine, Alpyn, Alpyne

Alpinolo (Italian) old friend.
Alpin, Alpyn, Alpynolo

Alric (Old German) all powerful.
Alrich, Alrick, Alrik

Alroy (Old English) red-haired.
Alroi

Alston (Old English) from the
noble one's town; temple stone.
Alstan, Alsten, Alstin, Alstun,
Alstyn

Altair (Greek) star. (Arab) eagle
flying.
Altayr, Altarye

Alter (German) elder; senior.
Altar, Altor

Altman (Old German) wise; old.
Altmen

Alton (Old English) dweller from
the old town.
Altown

Alva (Latin) blond/fair-haired.
(Heb) praised highly.
Alvah, Alvan

Alvan (Hebrew) tall.
Alven, Alvin, Alvon, Alvun, Alvyn

Alvar (Hebrew) sin; justice.
Alva, Alvah

Alvaro (German/Spanish) speaker
of truth.
Alvar

Alvern (Latin) spring.
Alverne

Alvin (Old German) beloved; wise
friend to all.
Alban, Albin, Albon, Aloin, Aluin
(Fren), Aluino (Span), Alvan,
Alven, Alwin (Ger), Alwyn

Alvis (Old Norse) all-wise friend.
(O/Ger) loved by all.
Aloin, Aluin, Aluino, Alva, Alvan,
Alwin, Alwyn, Elvin, Elvis

Alwan (Welsh) harmonious.
Alwen, Alwin, Alwon, Alwun,
Alwyn

Alwyn (Old English) noble, old,
wise, reliable friend.
Aluin, Aluino, Alvan, Alvin, Alvyn,
Alwan, Alwen, Alwin, Alwyn,
Eldan, Elden, Eldin, Eldon, Edwin,
Eldwyn, Eldwynn

Amadeus (Latin) beloved of God.
Amadeo (Span), Amadis, Amado,
Amando

Amal (Hebrew) industrious.
(Arab) hope.
Amahl

Amama (Polynesian) open-mouthed
one.
Amamah

Aman (Indonesian) security.
Amana

Amar (Punjabi) immortal.
(Arab) builder.
Amari, Amrio, Amarios, Amaris,
Amarjit, Ammar, Ammer

Amaroo (Australian Aboriginal)
beautiful place.
Amaro

Amasa (Hebrew) bearer of burdens.
Amasah

Amat (Indonesian) observation.
Amatt

Amato (French) loved.
Amat

Ambert (Old German) shining,
bright light.
Amber

Ambler (English) stable keeper.
Ambla, Amblah, Amblar

Ambrose (Greek) divine; immortal.
Ambrois, Ambroise (Fren),
Ambrogio (Ital), Ambroisius
(Dut/Ger/Swed)Ambros (Irish),
Ambrosio (Span), Ambrosios
(Grk), Ambrossij (Russ),
Ambrossye, Ambrosye, Ambrotos,
Ambroz (Boh), Ambrozij (Pol),
Ambrzio

Amerigo (Italian) hard-working.
Amerygo

Amery (Old French) ruling worker.
Amerie, Aymeree, Aymerey, Aymeri,
Aymeric, Aymerick, Aymerie,
Aymerik, Aymery, Aymeryc,
Aymeryck, Aymeryk

Ames (French) friend.
Amess

Amfrid (German) ancestral peace.
Amfred, Amfryd

Ami (Hebrew) my people.
(Lat) beloved friend.
Amiel, Amiram, Amy

Amico (Italian) friend to all.
Amic, Amick, Amicko, Amik,
Amiko, Amyc, Amyck, Amycko,
Amyk, Amyko

Amiel (Hebrew) lord of my people.
Amiell, Amyel, Amyell

Amik (Native American) beaver.
Amike

Amin (Hebrew) trustworthy; loyal.
Amen, Ammen, Amnon, Amor,
Amyn, Amynn

Amir (Arabic) prince.
Amyr

Amit (Punjabi) unfriendly.
(Arab) highly praised.
Amita, Amitan, Amreet, Amrit,
Amrita, Amritan, Amryt, Amryta,
Amrytan

Ammon (Egyptian) hidden.
Amon, Amond, Amun

Amon (Hebrew) faithful;
trustworthy.
Aman, Amen, Amin, Amman,
Ammen, Ammin, Ammon,
Ammyn, Amyn

Amory (Old German) famous,
divine ruler. (Lat) love.
Ameree, Amerey, Ameri, Amerie,
Amery, Ammeree, Ammerey,

Amory cont.
Ammeri, Ammerie, Ammery,
Ammoree, Ammorey, Ammori,
Ammorie, Ammory, Amoree,
Amorey, Amori, Amorie

Amos (Hebrew) born by God.
Amous

Amoz (Hebrew) fast, vigorous one.
Amozz

Amr (Arabic) life.
Am

Amram (Hebrew) nation of might.
Amarien, Amran, Amren, Amryn

Amund (Scandinavian) divine
protector; guardian.
Amond, Amondo, Amundo

An (Chinese/Vietnamese) peace.
Ana, Anah

Ana (Tongan) cave.
Anah

Anada (Sanskrit) blessed.
Anadah

Analo (German) ancestral.

Anan (Hebrew) cloud.
Anane

Anand (Hindi) bliss.
Ananda, Anandah, Anant, Ananth

Anastasius (Greek) resurrection;
springtime. The masculine form
of Anastasia.
Anastas, Anastase, Anastasio
(Span), Anastatius, Anastice,
Anastagio, Anastasios, Anastasij
(Russ), Anastasl, Anastasi,
Anastazij, Anastazy (Pol), Nastagio

Anatole (Greek) eastern.
Anatol, Anatolia, Anatoliah,
Anatolio (Span), Antoly, Antal,
Anatolie, Anatolis

Anbiorn (Old Norse) bear; eagle.
Anbjorn

Ancel (Latin) servant.
Ancelin, Ancelot, Ansela, Ansell,
Ansellus, Ansila, Ansyl

Anchali (Taos) painter.
Anchalee, Anchaley, Anchalie,
Anchaly

Ancher (Greek) anchor.
Anchor

Andre (French/Hebrew) strong;
brave; courageous. A form of
Andrew.
Andas, Andar, Anders (Grk),
Andra, Andrae, Andrecito, Andree,
Andrei, Andrie, Aundre

Andrew (Greek) strong; brave;
courageous.
Aindreas (Gae), Analo, Anderewe,
Anders, Andersen, Anderson,
Andias (Slav), Andonis, Andor,
Andras (Est/Hung), Andre (Fren),
Andrea, Andreas (Dut/Ger), Andrei
(Russ), Andreian (Russ), Andrej
(Slav), Andreja (Serb), Andrejeen
(Slav), Andrejek (Slav), Andrewe,
Andronicus (Grk), Andronycus,
Andru, Andruw

Andy (Greek) strong; brave;
courageous. The short form of
Andrew.
Ande, Andee, Andey, Andi, Andie

Anga (Tongan) nature; shark.
Angah

Angel/Angelo (English) angel;
messenger of God.
Angel, Angell, Angello, Angelos,
Angelous, Angiolo, Anglico, Aniello,
Anjel, Anjell, Anjello, Anjelo

Angus (Scottish/Gaelic) the only choice. (Celt) chosen; possesses strength.
Ennis

Anh (Vietnamese) safety; peace.

Anil (Hindi) god of wind.
Aneal, Aneel, Anel, Aniel, Aniello, Anielo, Anyl, Anyll

Anker (Danish/Greek) strong; brave; courageous. A form of Andrew.
Ankor, Ankur

Anlon (Celtic) great champion.
Anlone

Annan (Celtic) from the stream.
Annen, Annin, Annon, Annun, Annyn

Anno (Hebrew) graceful. The masculine form of Ann.
Ano

An-nur (Arabic) light.
Annur

Anoke (Native American) actor.
Anokee, Anokey, Anoki, Anokie, Anoky

Ansel (Old French) under God's protection.
Ansell, Anselino, Anselyno

Anselm (Old German) warrior possessing divine protection.
Anse, Ansel, Anselme, Anselmi (Ital), Anselmo (Span/Port), Ansheim (Ger)

Ansley (Old English/Hebrew) graceful meadow.
Andlea, Ansleah, Anslee, Ansleigh, Ansli, Anslie, Ansly

Anson (Old English/Hebrew) Ann's son; son of the graceful one. The masculine form of Ann.
Ansan, Ansen, Ansin, Ansyn

Antares (Greek) a star.

Anthe (Greek) strong; brave; courageous. A form of Andrew.
Anthey, Anthi, Anthie, Anthy, Anti, Antty, Anty

Anthony (Latin) priceless.
Anfonee, Anfoney, Anfoni, Anfonie, Anfony, Antain, Antaine, Antal, Antek, Antanas, Ante, Antholin, Anthonee, Anthoney, Anthoni, Anthonie, Antin, Anto, Antoin (Irish), Antoine (Fren), Anton (Ger/Swed/Russ), Antone, Antonee, Antoney, Antoni (Pol), Antonie, Antonij (Russ), Antonija, Antonin, Antonina, Antonio (Ital/Span/Port), Antonius (Lat), Antons, Antony (Ital), Hanto

Antti (Finnish/Greek) strong; brave; courageous. A form of Andrew.
Anthey, Anthi, Anthie, Anthy, Anti, Antty, Anty

Anwar (Arabic) ray of light.
Anward

Anwell (Welsh) dearest.
Anwel, Anwil, Anwill, Anwyl, Anwyll

Apiatan (Kiowa) wooden lance.

Apollo (Greek) sunlight
Apolinario, Apolinaro, Apolo, Apolonio, Appollo, Appolo, Appolonio

Apurta (Australian Aboriginal) stone.
Apurtah

Aquila (Latin) eagle.
Aquil, Aquill, Aquilla, Aquyl, Aquyla, Aquyll, Aquylla

Ara (Latin) altar.
Arah

Arafat (Arabic) mountain of recognition.
Ara

Araldo (Spanish/Scandinavian) ruler of the army.
Haraldo

Aram (Hebrew) highly praised; height.
Ara, Arem, Arim, Arum, Arym

Aran (Thai) forest.
Arane

Arawa (Maori) shark.
Arawah

Archard (French) sacred; powerful. (O/Eng) archer.
Archar, Archer, Archor

Archer (Old English) bow; archer.
Archar, Archard, Archor

Archibald/Archie (Old German) very brave; bold; valuable.
Archaimbaud (Ger), Archambaud, Archambault (Fren), Arche, Archee, Archey, Archibaldes, Archibales (Lith), Archi, Archibaldo (Ital), Archy, Archybald, Archybalde, Archybaldes, Archybauld, Archybaulde

Archimedes (Greek) brilliant.
Archim, Archymedes

Ardai (Celtic) high valour; brave; warrior.
Ardae, Ardal, Arday

Ardell (Latin) eager.
Ardall, Ardall, Ardel

Arden (Latin) ablaze. (O/Eng) dwelling place.
Ardan, Ardent, Ardin, Ardint, Ardyn, Ardynt

Ardley (Old English/Latin) from the fiery meadow; from the ardent one's meadow.
Ardlea, Ardlea, Ardlee, Ardleigh, Ardli, Ardlie, Ardly

Ardmore (Latin) intense desire; ardent.
Ardmoar, Ardmoare, Ardmoor, Ardmoore, Ardmor

Ardon (Hebrew) bronze.
Ardan, Arden, Ardin, Ardun, Ardyn

Aren (Danish) eagle ruler.
Aaran, Aaren, Aarin, Aaron, Aaryn, Aran, Arin, Aron, Aryn

Aretino (Italian) virtuous; purity.
Aretin, Aretine, Artyn, Artyno

Argus (Greek) bright-eyed; vigilant.
Arguss

Argyle (Gaelic) from Ireland.
Argile, Argiles, Argyles

Ari (Hebrew) strong, worthy lion.
Aree, Arey, Arie, Ary

Aric (Old English) ruler.
Aaric, Aarick, Aarik, Arick, Arik, Aryc, Aryck, Aryk

Ariel (Hebrew) God's lion.
Airal, Arel, Areli, Ariele, Ariell, Arielle, Ario, Aryeh, Aryel, Aryell, Aryl, Aryll, Arylle

Aries (Latin) ram; war-like one.
Arees, Aryes

Arif (Arabic) all-knowing.
Areef, Aryf

Ariki (Maori) first-born child. (Poly) chief.
Aricki, Arikee, Arikey, Arikie, Ariky

Arion (Greek) magic horse.
Arian, Arien, Ariona, Arionah, Aryon, Aryona, Aryonah

A

Aristides (Greek) descendant of the brilliant one.
Aristede, Aristedes, Aristide, Arisztid, Arysrides, Arystydes

Aristo (Greek) brilliant.
Aristophanes, Aristotle, Arysto, Arystotle

Aristotle (Greek) brilliant thinker.
Aristotal, Aristotel, Aristotol, Aristott, Aristotyl, Arystotte

Arjuna (Sanskrit) white.
Arjun, Arjunah

Arkady (Russian/German) bold.
Arkadee, Arkadey, Arkadi, Arkadie

Arkell (Old Norse) eagle cauldron.
Arkel

Arkin (Norwegian) son of the eternal king.
Aricin, Arkeen, Arkyn

Arledge (English) from the ledge of the hares.
Arlege, Arlidge, Arlledge, Arllege

Arlen (Irish/Gaelic) promise.
Arlan, Arland, Arlin, Arlon, Arlyn

Arlo (Latin/Greek) strong, brave, courageous one. A form of Andrew.
Arlow

Arlyn (Old German) adventure at the waterfall pool.
Arland, Arlin, Arlind, Arlynd

Arman (Hebrew) castle.
Armani, Armanie, Armany, Armen, Armin, Armon, Armyyn

Armand (Old German/Greek) strong, brave, courageous army.
Arman, Armando, Armin, Armon, Armond

Armany (Hungarian) cunning; sly.
Armanee, Armaney, Armani, Armanie

Arminius (Latin) chief.
Arminyus, Armynius, Armynyus

Armon (Hebrew) castle.
Armond, Armondo

Armourel (Gaelic) dweller by the sea.
Armourell

Armstrong (Old English) strong armed.
Armstron, Armstronge

Arnan (Hebrew) joyful; happy; quick.
Arnane

Arne/Arnie (Old German) eagle. The short form of Arnold, strong; powerful like an eagle.
Arnee, Arney, Arni, Arnie, Arno, Arnot, Arnott, Arnotte, Arny

Arnette (English) little ruling eagle.
Arnat, Arnatt, Arnet, Arnett, Arnot, Arnott

Arnfinn (Old Norse) white.
Arnfin, Arnfyn, Arnfynn

Arnold (Old German) strong; powerful like an eagle.
Ahnald, Ahnaldo, Ahneld, Ahneldo, Ahnold, Ahnoldo, Ahrelds, Ahrent, Arend, Arman, Armand, Armant, Arnal, Arnald, Arnalde, Arnaldo (Span), Arnall, Arnelle, Arnaud (Fren), Arnaude, Arnaut, Arndt, Arnel, Arnele, Arnell, Arnelle, Arnes, Arness, Arnet, Arnett, Arnhold (O/Ger), Arnie, Arno (Ger), Arnolda, Arnoldah, Arnoldas, Arnolde, Arnoldo (Ital), Arnol, Arnoll, Arnolt, Arnot, Arnott, Arnoud, Arold, Arnyld

Arnon (Hebrew) river rushing.
Arnan, Arnen, Arnin, Arnyn

Arod (Hebrew) fast; rapidly moving.

Aron (Hebrew) enlightened singing.
Aaran, Aarin, Aaron, Aaryn,
Aharon, Ahron, Arend, Ari, Arin,
Arnie, Arny, Aron, Arrin, Arron,
Arryn, Erin, Haroun

Aroon (Thai) dawn.
Aroone

Arran (Scottish) island dweller.
Aran, Aren, Arin, Aron, Arren,
Arrin, Arron, Arryn, Aryn

Arrio (Spanish) war-like.
Ario, Arryo, Aryo

Arsenio (Greek) masculine.
Arsen, Arsene, Arseneo, Arsenius,
Arseny, Arsenyo, Arsinio, Arsinyo,
Arsynio, Arsynyo

Arsha (Persian) venerable; old;
great.
Arshah

Art (English) rock. (Ir) noble one
from the lofty hill. (Scott/Wel)
bear. (Ice) follower of Thor;
thunder. The short form of
Arthur, noble strength.
Arte

Artamenes/Artemis (Persian)
intelligent.
Artameenes, Artwmene

Arthur (Celtic) noble strength.
(Scott/Wel) bear.
Artai (Scott), Artemas, Atremin,
Artemus, Arther, Arthyr, Artur
(Port/Ger), Arturo (Ital/Span),
Artus (Fren), Aurthur, Arto (Finn),
Artius, Artor, Artorioos (Grk),
Atorus

Arun (Cambodian/Hindi) sun.
Aruns

Arundel (English) from the eagle
valley.
Arundle

Arva (Latin) from the coastal area.
(Dan) eagle.
Arvah

Arvad (Hebrew) wandering.
(Eng) friend.
Arved, Arvid, Arvind, Arvinder,
Arvyd, Arvydas

Arval (Latin) from the cultured land.
Arvel, Arvil, Arvol, Arvyl

Arve (Norwegian) heir.
Arv

Arvin (Old German) friend to the
people.
Arvan, Arven, Arvon, Arvyn, Arwan,
Arwen, Arwin, Arwon, Arwyn

Aryeh (Hebrew) lion.
Arye

Asa (Hebrew) healer. (Jap) born in
the morning.
Asah

Asad (Arabic) lion.
Asaad, Asad, Asid, Assad, Azad

Asadel (Arabic) prosperous.
Asadour, Asadul, Asadyl, Asael

Asaph (Hebrew) gathering.
Asaf

Asarel (Hebrew) God has bound.
Asarell

Asbjorn (Norse) divine bear.
Bjorn

Asbrand (Norse) divine sword.
Asbran, Asbrando, Asbrandt

Ascott (Old English) dweller at the
cottage in the east.
Ascot

A

Asenath (Egyptian) dedicated to God.
Asenaf

Asgard (Norse) divine guardian.
Asgar

Ash (English) ash tree. The short form of Ashley.

Ashburn (Old English) dweller at the ash-tree stream.
Ashbern, Ashberne, Ashbirn, Ashbirne, Ashborn, Ashborne, Ashbourn, Ashbourne, Ashburne, Ashbyrn, Ashbyrne

Ashburton (Old English) from the burnt ash-tree town.
Ashbert, Ashberton, Ashbirt, Ashbirton, Ashburt, Ashbyrt, Ashbyrton

Ashby (Scandinavian) by the ash trees.
Ashbee, Ashbey, Ashbi, Ashbie

Asher (Hebrew) happy, blessed.
Asha, Ashah, Ashar, Asherman

Ashford (Old English) from the ash-tree ford.
Ashforde

Ashley (Old English) from the ash-tree meadow.
Ashlea, Ashleah, Ashlee, Ashleigh, Ashli, Ashlie, Ashlin, Ashly

Ashon (Swahili) seventh-born child.
Ashan, Ashen, Ashin, Ashyn

Ashton (Old English) dweller at the ash-tree town.
Ashtan, Ashten, Ashtin, Ashtown, Aston, Astown, Ashtyn

Ashur (Hebrew) black.
Asher, Ashir, Ashyr

Ashwin (Hindi) star.
Ashwan, Ashwen, Ashwon, Ashwyn

Asiel (Hebrew) created by God.
Asyel

Asim (Arabic) protector; guardian.
Asym

Asker (Turkish) warrior.
Aske

Aslak (Norse) divine sport.

Asmunder (Old Norse) divine hand.
Asmund, Asmundo

Astley (Greek) star-lit field.
Asterlea, Asterleah, Asterlee, Asterleigh, Asterley, Asterli, Asterlie, Asterly, Astlea, Astleah, Astlee, Astleigh, Astli, Astlie, Astly

Aston (Old English) from the easterly town.
Ashton, Ashtown, Astan, Asten, Astin, Aston, Astown, Astyn

Asvard (Norse) divine, powerful guardian; protector.
Asvardo

Asvor (Norse) discreet.
Asvar, Asver, Asvir, Asvyr

Aswad (Arabic) black.
Aswald

Ata (Fanti) twin.
Atah

Atalik (Hungarian) like his father.
Atalyk

Atamai (Maori) knowing all. (Tong) intellect.
Atama, Atamay

Atarah (Hebrew) crown.
Atara

Athan (Greek) immortal.
Ateef, Atek (Pol), Atef, Athen, Athens, Athin, Athins, Athon, Athons, Athyn, Athyns

Athelstan (Old English) reliable; noble; stone.
Athalstan, Athilstan, Athol (Scott), Atholstan, Athylstan

Atherton (Old English) dweller at the stream town.
Athaton, Atheton, Atholton

Athol (Scottish/Gaelic) from Ireland.
Affol, Affolton, Athal, Athalton, Athel, Athelton, Athil, Athilton, Atholton, Athyl, Athyton

Ati (Maori) clan; family.
Atee, Atey, Atie, Aty

Atid (Thai) sun.
Atyd

Atif (Arabic) caring.
Atyf

Atiu (Polynesian) the eldest.

Atkins (Old English) at the relations' place.
Akin, Akins, Akyn, Akyns, Atkin, Atkyn, Atkyns

Atley (English) at the meadow.
Atlea, Atleah, Atlee, Atleigh, Atli, Atlie, Atly, Attlea, Attleah, Attlee, Attleigh, Attley, Attli, Attlie, Attly

Atofu (Western Samoan) noble, fierce wolf; hero. A form of Adolf.

Attila (Greek) father.
Attilah, Attilio, Attyla, Attylah, Atou

Attlee (Old English) at the woods in the meadow.
Atlea, Atleah, Atlee, Atleigh, Atley, Atli, Atlie, Atly, Attlea, Attleah, Attleigh, Attley, Attli, Attlie, Attly

Atwater (English) at the edge of the water.
Attwater

Atwell (English) at the edge of the well.
Attwel, Atwel, Atwell

Atwood (English) at the wood.
Attwood

Atworth (English) at the farm.
Attworth

Auberon (Old German) king of the fairies. A form of Oberon.
Oberon

Aubin/Auburn (French) reddish/brown-haired.
Abern, Aberne, Abirn, Abirne, Aburn, Aburne, Abyrn, Abyrne, Auban, Auben, Aubern, Auberne, Aubin (Fren), Aubirn, Aubirne, Aubun, Auburne, Aubyn, Aubyrn, Aubryne, Aurburn, Aurburne

Aubrey (Old French) reddish/brown-haired; powerful, wise leader.
Alberik, Auberon, Aubree, Aubri, Aubrie, Aubry, Avery, Oberon

Auden (English) old friend.
Audan, Audin, Audon, Audyn

Audie (German) noble; strong.
Audee, Audey, Audi, Audiel, Audley, Audy

Audon (French) rich; old.
Audan, Audelon, Auden, Audin, Audyn

Audric (English) wise ruler.
Audri, Audrick, Audrik, Audryc, Audryck, Audryk

Audun (Scandinavian) deserted space. (O/Eng) old friend.
Audan, Audel, Auden, Audin, Audley, Audon, Audyn

Auguste (Latin) majestic; royal; worthy of honour.
Agosto, Aguistin, Agusteen,

A

Agustein, Agusteyne, Agustin,
Agustine, Agustyn, Agustyne,
Augusteen, Augustein, Augusteyn,
Augusteyne, Augustin, Augustine,
Augusto, Augustus, Augustyn,
Augustyne, Austen, Austin, Auston,
Austyn

Augustus (Latin) majestic; royal;
worthy of honour.
Agustas, Agustin, Agustus, Agustys,
August, Auguste (Fren), Augustin,
Augustinas (Lith), Augustine,
Augustino (Lat), Augusto,
Augustyne (Pol), Austen, Austin,
Auston, Avgust (Russ)

Aukai (Hawaiian) seafarer; sailor.
Aukay

Aurek (Polish) golden-haired.
Aurec

Aurelian (Latin) golden dawn.
Aurel, Aurelio, Aurelius, Aurelyan,
Aurelyus

Aurick (German) protecting ruler.
Auric, Aurik, Auryc, Auryck, Auryk

Austin (Latin) little but majestic.
Austan, Austen, Auston, Austyn

Avel (Russian) breath.
Avell

Avent (French) born during Advent.
Advent, Aventin, Aventino,
Aventyno

Averall (Middle English) born in
April.
Averal, Averel, Averey, Avery

Avi (Hebrew) my father.
Avie, Avy

Aviv (Hebrew) youthful; spring
time.
Avyv

Avlar (German) old army.
Avler, Avlor, Avlyr

Avram (Hebrew) father of the
multitudes.
Arram, Avraham, Avrom, Avrum,
Avrym

Awan (Native American) somebody.
Awen, Awin, Awon, Awun, Awyn

Awwal (Arabic) first born.
Awal

Axel (Norse/Old German) father of
peace.
Axil, Axl, Axyl

Aydin (Turkish) intelligence.
Aidan, Aiden, Aidin, Aidon, Aidyn,
Aydan, Ayden, Aydon, Aydyn

Ayer (Old French) heir; son.
Aier

Ayinde (Yoruba) given praise.

Aylmer (Old English) noble; famous.
Ailmer

Aylward (Old English) noble
guardian.
Ailward

Aylwin (Old English) noble friend.
Ailwan, Ailwen, Ailwin, Aileon,
Ailwyn, Alwan, Alwen, Alwin,
Alwon, Alwyn, Aylwan, Aylwen,
Aylwon, Alwyn

Aymil (Greek) industrious.
Aimil, Aimyl, Aymyl

Aymon (French) mighty, wise
protector.
Aiman, Aimen, Aimin, Aimon,
Aimyn, Ayman, Aymen, Aymin,
Aymyn

Azad (Turkish) freedom.
Asad, Azad, Azzad

Azariah (Hebrew) God aids and
blesses.
Azaria

Azeem (Arabic) defender.
Aseem, Asim, Azzeem

Azel (Hebrew) noble.
Azal, Azil, Azol, Azyl

Azi (Nigerian) youth.
Azee, Azie, Azy

Azik (Russian/Hebrew) laughter;
God smiles. A form of Isaac.
Azyk

Azim (Arabic) great.
Aziz, Azizz, Azym

Aziz (Swahili) precious.
Aziz

Azuriah (Hebrew) aided by God.
Azaria, Azariah, Azryel, Azuria,
Azurya, Azuryah

Azzan (Hebrew) great strength.
Azza, Azzah

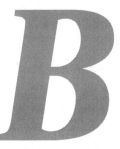

Baasu (Hindi) prosperous.
Basu

Babar (Hindi) lion.

Badar (Arabic) full moon.
Badr, Badru

Baden (German) to bathe.
Badan, Bade, Badin, Badon, Badyn,
Bagan

Badhur (Arabic) born at the full
moon.
Badhir

Badrick (Old English) axe ruler.
Badric, Badrik, Badryc, Badryck,
Badryk

Baez (Welsh) boar.

Baha (Arabic) brilliant.

Bahir (Arabic) dazzling; bright.
Bahur

Bahram (Persian) ancient king.
Bairam

Bailey (Old French) bailiff; sherriff's
officer. (Mid/Eng) from the outer
castle wall meadow.
Bail, Baili, Bailie, Bailea, Baileah,
Bailee, Baileigh, Baili, Bailie,
Baillea, Bailleah, Baillee, Bailleigh,
Bailley, Bailli, Baillie, Bailly, Baily,
Baylea, Bayleah, Baylee, Bayleigh,
Bayli, Baylie, Bayly, Beylea,
Beyleah, Beylee, Beyleigh, Beyley,
Beyli, Beylie, Beyly

Bain (Irish) fair-haired.
Baenbridge, Baenebridge,
Bainbridge, Baine, Bainebridge,
Bayn, Baynbridge, Bayne,
Baynebridge

Bainbridge (Old English) bridge
over white water.
Baenbridge, Baenebridge,
Bainebridge, Baynbridge,
Baynebridge

Baird (Irish/Gaelic) singer of
ballads.
Bairde, Bard, Barde, Bayrd, Bayrde

Bais (Arabic) awake.
Bays

Bakari (Swahili) promise of
nobility.
Bakarie, Bakary

Baker (Old English) baker of bread.
Bakker

Bakr (Arabic) camel.

Bal (Gypsy) hair. (Per) war council.

Bala (Hindi) child.

Balbo (Latin) indistinct speaker.
Bailby (Fren), Balbi (Ital), Balbie,
Balby

Baldemar (Teutonic) famous; bold;
prince.
Baldur (Nrs), Baldmar, Baldmare,
Baumer (Fren)

Balder (Old English) bold army
leader.
Alder, Baudier (Fren), Baulder

Baldric (Teutonic) bold; princely;
powerful ruler.
Baldri, Baldrick, Baldrik, Baldryc,
Baldryck, Baldryk, Baudrey, Baudri

Baldwin (Teutonic) bold protector;
friend.
Aldwin, Aldwyn, Baden, Baldewin,
Baldewyn, Baldovino (Ital),
Balduin (Ger/Swed/Dan),
Baldwyn, Baudoin (Fren),
Baudouin, Bawden, Bealdwine,
Bodkin, Bowder

Balfour (Scottish) from the village
pasture.
Balfor, Balfore

Balin (Hindi) mighty warrior from
the stream.
Baline, Balyn, Balyne

Balint (Hungarian) healthy; strong.
(Lat) one who dances.
Balynt

Ballard (German) brave; strong.
Balard, Balerd, Ballerd

Balsys (Lithuanian) war council.
Balsis

Banan (Celtic) white.
Banen, Banin, Banon, Banquo
(Celt), Banyn

Bancroft (Middle English) from the
small bean pasture.
Banbank, Banney

Bandi (Hungarian/Greek) strong;
brave; courageous. A form of
Andrew.
Bandee, Bandey, Bandie, Bandy

Bandit (English) bushranger.
Banditt, Bandyt, Bandytt

Bane (Hawaiian/Hebrew) son of the
farmer. A form of Bartholomew.
Baen, Baene, Bain, Baine, Ban,
Bayn, Bayne

Banner (English/Scottish) sign
bearer.
Banna, Bannah, Bannar, Bannor

Banning (Irish/Gaelic) little blond,
fair-haired one. (O/Eng) son of
the slayer.
Baning

Bao (Chinese) treasure.

Bapp (Australian Aboriginal)
bluegum tree.
Bap

Baptist (Greek) to baptise.
Badezon, Baptista, Baptiste,
Baptysta (Pol), Battista

Baradine (Australian Aboriginal)
red wallaby (small kangaroo).
Baradin, Baradyn, Baradyne

Barak (Hebrew) flash of light;
lightning.
Barrack, Baruch

Baram (Hebrew) son of the people.
Barem, Barim, Barom, Barym

Baran (Russian) ram.
Baren, Barin, Baron, Barran, Barren, Barrin, Barron, Barryn, Baryn

Barasa (Kikuyu) meeting area.
Barasah

Barclay (Old English) from the clay meadow with the birch trees.
Barclae, Barclaey, Barclai, Barclaie, Barcklae, Barcklaey, Barcklai, Barcklaie, Barkclay, Bartlea, Bartleah, Bartlee, Bartleigh, Bartley, Bartli, Bartlie, Bartly, Berkelea, Berkeleah, Berkelee, Berkeleigh, Berkeley, Berkeli, Berkelie, Berkely, Berklea, Berkleah, Berklee, Berkley, Berkli, Berklie, Berkley

Bard (Irish/Gaelic) poet.
Baird (Scott), Bairde, Barde (Fren), Bardoul (Fren), Bardoul (Fren), Bayrd, Bayrde

Barden (Old English) from the valley where barley is grown; from the poet's valley.
Baedan, Baede, Baeden, Baedin, Baedon, Baedyn, Baird, Bairdan, Bairden, Bairdin, Bairdon, Bairdyn, Bardan, Barden, Bardon, Bardyn, Bayrdan, Bayrden, Bayrdin, Bayrdon, Bayrdyn, Bordan, Borden, Bordin, Bordon, Bordyn

Bardin (Australian Aboriginal) ironbark tree.
Bardan, Barden, Bardin, Bardon, Bardyn

Bardo (German) giant. (Aust/Abor) light or water.
Bardot

Bardolf (Teutonic) bright, fierce wolf. (O/Eng) axe wolf.
Bardell, Bardolfe, Bardolph, Bardolphe

Bardrick (Teutonic) axe ruler.
Bardric, Bardrik, Bardryck, Bardryk

Barend (Dutch) strong bear.
Barand

Baringa (Australian Aboriginal) light.
Baringah

Barker (Old English) birch tree.
Barkker, Barklea, Barkleah, Barklee, Barkleigh, Barkley, Barkli, Barklie, Barkly

Barlow (Old English) dweller at the low barley hill; dweller at the bare hill.
Barloe, Barlowe

Barnabas (Hebrew/Greek) son of prophecy.
Barna (Ital), Barnaba (Ital), Barnabe (Fren), Barnabie, Barnaby, Barnebas, Barnebus (Span), Barnibas, Barnibus, Barnybas, Barnybus, Bernabe, Burnabas, Burnaby

Barnard (English/German) brave bear.
Barnard (Fren), Barnet, Barnett, Barnhard, Barnhardo, Barnhart, Bearnard (Scott), Berents (Lett), Bernad, Bernadek, Bernaldim, Bernaldo (Ital), Bernadyn, Bernard (Ital/Span), Berneen (Irish), Berngard (Russ), Bernhard (Ger/Swed), Bernhart (Dut), Burnard

Barnes (English) brave bear; barn worker.

Barnett (English) leader of honourable birth.
Barnet, Barnete, Barnette

Barney (Old English) dweller from the barn.
Barnee, Barni, Barnie, Barny

Barnum (Old English) from the noble person's stone house.

Baron (Old English) noble person. (Heb) son of Aaron; son of the enlightened one.
Baran, Baren, Barin, Baron, Baryn, Barran, Barren, Barrin, Barron, Barryn, Beron

Barr (Old English) gateway. (Ger) bear.
Bar, Barre

Barra (Irish) fair-haired.
Bara, Barah, Barrah

Barret (Teutonic) strong; mighty like a bear.
Baret, Barett, Barit, Baritt, Barrhet, Barrhett, Barrit, Barritt, Baryt, Barytt

Barric (English) from the grain farm.
Barrick, Barrik, Baryc, Baryck, Baryk, Beric, Berrick, Berrik, Beryc, Beryck, Beryk

Barrington (English/French) from the fenced town.
Barington

Barris (Old Welsh) son of Harris; son of the army ruler
Baris, Barrys, Barys

Barry (Irish) spear; marks-person.
Baree, Barey, Barett, Bari (Fren), Barie, Barnard, Barnet, Barnett, Barra, Barree, Barrey, Barri, Barrie, Barrington, Barris, Barrymore, Bary, Bearach

Bart (Hebrew) son. The short form of Bartholomew, son of the farmer.
Barte

Bartholomew (Hebrew) son of the farmer.
Baremo, Barholomee, Bartek (Pol), Bartel (Ger), Barthel (Ger), Barthelemy (Fren), Barteleleus (Swed), Bartelmes (Dut), Barteo

(Illy), Barth, Barthel, Barthelemi (Fren), Barthelemy, Barthol, Bartholdy (Ger), Bartholomacus (Lat/Ger), Bartholome (Fren), Bartholomu, Bartholomy

Bartley (Old English) from the barley meadow.
Bart, Bartlea, Bartleah, Bartlee, Bartleigh, Bartlet, Bartlett, Bartli, Bartlie, Bartly, Beartlaiah (Ir)

Barton (Old English) from the barley town.
Bartan, Barten, Bartin, Bartyn

Bartram (English) glorious raven.
Barthram, Bertram

Baruti (Botswana) one who teaches.

Barwon (Australian Aboriginal) magpie (black-and-white bird).

Basam (Arabic) smiling.
Basem, Basim, Bassam, Bassem, Bassim

Basil (Greek) royal; majestic; basil herb.
Basile (Fren), Basilio (Ital/Span/Port), Basilius (Dut/Ger/Swed), Basino, Bazel (Dut), Bazyli (Poly), Vasilis, Vassilij, Vassili, Vassily

Basir (Arabic) seer; psychic.
Basyr

Bassett (English) little one.
Baset, Basett, Basset

Bastien (German/Greek) venerable; old; great. (Lat) revered. A form of Sebastian, honoured above all others.
Baste, Bastiane, Bastyan, Bastyane

Bat (English) son of the farmer. A form of Bartholomew.
Bato

Baul (Gypsy) wind.

Baum (German) tree.
Baume

Bavol (Gypsy) wind; air.
Baval, Bavel, Bavil, Bavyl, Beval,
Bevel, Bevil, Bevyl

Baxter (Old English) baker of
bread.

Bay (Vietnamese) seventh-born son.
(Fren) chestnut; brown. (Eng) to
howl.
Bae, Bai, Baye

Bayard (Old French)
reddish/brown-haired.
Baeyard, Baiyard, Baylen

Beacan (Irish) small.
Beacen, Becan, Becen

Beacher (Old English) dweller at
the birch tree.
Beecher

Beagan (Irish) little one.
Beegan

Beal (English/French) handsome. A
form of Beau.
Beale, Beal, Beall, Bealle, Beil, Beill,
Beille, Beyl, Beyll, Beyelle

Beaman (Old English) bee keeper.
Beamen, Beeman, Beemen

Beamer (Old English) trumpet
player.
Beemer

Beamon (Irish) good.
Beemon

Bear (English) grizzly bear.

Bearach (Irish) spear-like one.

Beasley (Old English) from the
meadow where peas are grown;
from the bee keeper's meadow.
Beaslea, Beasleah, Beaslee, Beasleigh,

Beasli, Beaslie, Beasly, Peaslea,
Peasleah, Peaslee, Peasleigh, Peasley,
Peasli, Peaslie, Peasly

Beattie (Irish/Gaelic) one who
grants blessings.
Beatie, Beatti, Beatty, Beeti, Beetie,
Beety

Beau (Old French) handsome.
Bo

Beaufort (French) from the
handsome fort.
Bofort

Beaumont (French) handsome
mountain.
Bomont

Beauregard (French) handsome
guard.
Beaureguard, Boregard, Boreguard

Beaver (English) beaver.
Beever

Bebe (Spanish) baby.

Becan (Irish) little.
Becen, Becin, Becon, Becyn

Becher (Hebrew) first-born child.
Beacher, Beecher

Beck (Old Norse) from the small
stream.

Bedaws (Welsh) birch tree.

Bede (Middle English) prayer.

Bedir (Turkish) full moon.
Bedire, Bedyr, Bedyre

Bedivere (Welsh) hero of the birch
tree meadow.
Bedver, Bedwin, Bedwyn

Beegan (Irish) little.
Beagan

Bejay (French/English) handsome
jay bird.
Beajae, Beajai, Beajay, Beejae,

Beejai, Beejay, Beejaye, B.J.

Bela (French) handsome.
(Slav) white. (Hung) bright.
Belah, Beldon

Beldan (French/English) dweller
from the handsome valley.
Beldan, Belden, Beldin, Beldon,
Beldyn, Belidan, Baliden, Balidin,
Balidon, Balidyn, Belldan, Bellden,
Belldin, Belldon, Belldyn

Beli (Welsh) brightness.
Belee, Beley, Belie, Bely

Bell (French) handsome.
(Eng) ringer of bells.
Bel

Bellamy (Old French) handsome;
fair-haired friend.
Belami, Belamie, Belamy

Bello (African) Islam helper.
Belo

Belmiro (Portuguese) handsome.
Belmirow, Belmyro, Belmyrow

Belveder (Italian) beautiful to look
at.
Belvedear, Belvedere, Belvidere,
Belvydear, Belvydere

Bem (Tiv) peace.
Behm

Bemidii (Ojibwa) from the river
near the lake.
Bemidi

Bemus (Latin) platform.
Bemis

Ben (Hebrew) son. The short form
of Benjamin.
Benn

Bendall (Old English) from the
corner where beans are grown.
Bendal

Benedict (Latin) blessed.
Banet, Banko, Baruch, Benayt,
Bendic, Bendick, Bendict, Bendik
(Nrs), Bendikkas (Lith), Bendix,
Benedetto (Ital), Benedic,
Benedick, Benedictas (Lith),
Benedicto (Span), Benedik,
Benedikt (Ger), Benediktas,
Benedit (Illy), Benedix (Ger),
Benedyc, Benedyck, Benedyct,
Benedyk, Benek (Hung)

Ben-Hur (Hebrew) son of Hur;
purity.
Ben-Hir

Benign (French) kind-hearted.
Benigne

Benito (Italian/Latin) blessed.
Benedo, Benino, Bennito, Benno,
Beno, Benyto, Betto

Benjamin (Hebrew) favourite son.
Banjaman, Banjamen, Banjamin,
Banjamyn, Beathan (Scott),
Bengaman, Bengamen, Bengamin,
Bengamon, Bengamyn, Bengee,
Bengey, Bengi, Bengie, Bengy,
Beniamino (Ital), Benjaman,
Benjamen, Benjamon, Benjamyn,
Benjee, Benjey, Benji, Benjie, Benjy,
Bennjaman, Bennjamen,
Bennjamin, Bennjamon,
Bennjamyn, Benson, Binyamin
(Arab)

Benji (Hebrew) favourite son. The
short form of Benjamin.
Bengee, Bengey, Bengi, Bengie,
Bengy, Benjee, Benjey, Benjie,
Bennjee, Bennjey, Bennji, Bennjie,
Bennjy, Benjy

Benjiro (Japanese) one who enjoys
peace.

Bennes (Czech) blessed.

Bennet (French) little blessed one.
Benet, Benett, Benit, Benitt,

Bennet cont.
Bennet, Bennett, Bensan, Bensen,
Bensin, Benoit, Benoitt, Benson,
Bensyn, Benyt, Benytt

Benny (Hebrew) son. The short
form of names beginning with
'Ben' e.g. Benjamin.
Ben, Bene, Benee, Beney, Beni,
Benie, Benn, Benne, Bennee,
Benney, Benni, Bennie, Benno,
Beno, Beny

Beno (Mwera) member of the band.
(Heb) son.

Benoit (French) blessed. A form of
Benedict.
Benoit, Benoyt, Benoytt

Benoni (Hebrew) sorrow.
Benonee, Benoney, Benonie,
Benony

Benson (Hebrew) son of Benjamin.
son of the favourite son.
Bennsan, Bennsen, Bennsin,
Bennson, Bennsyn, Bensan,
Bensen, Bensin, Bensyn

Bentley (Old English) from the
grassy moor.
Bentlea, Bentleah, Bentlee,
Bentleigh, Bentli, Bentlie, Bently

Benton (English) dweller from the
moor town.
Bentan, Benten, Bentin, Bentyn

Benzi (Hebrew) son of Zion; son of
the sign.
Benzee, Benzey, Benzie, Bezny

Beppe (Italian/Hebrew) God will
increase; God has added a child.
A form of Joseph.
Bepe, Pepe, Peppe

Ber (Old Norse) dweller.
Berlin, Berlyn

Berach (Irish) looking straight at
the mark.
Berac, Berack, Berak, Birac, Birack,
Birak, Burac, Burack, Burak, Byrac,
Byrack, Byrak

Berdy (Russian) clever.
Berdee, Berdey, Berdi, Berdie, Berdy

Bered (Hebrew) sprinkle.
Beared

Berenger (Teutonic) bear spear.
Beringer, Berynger

Beresford (Old English) from the
barley ford; from the ford near
the berries.
Beresforde

Berg (German) from the mountain
or hill.
Bergen, Berger, Bergin, Borg, Borga,
Borge, Bourke, Burke

Bergen (French) shepherd. (O/Ger)
place on the hill.
Bergan, Berger, Bergin, Bergon,
Bergyn

Bergren (Scandinavian) mountain
stream.
Berggren, Bergin

Berk (Turkish) rugged one.
Berc, Berck

Berkeley (Old English/Irish)
meadow where birch trees grow.
Barclae, Barclai, Barclay, Barklea,
Barkleah, Barklee, Barkleigh,
Barkley, Barkli, Barklie, Barkly,
Berklay, Berklea, Berkleah, Berklee,
Berkleigh, Berkley, Berkli, Berklie,
Berkly

Berl (German) wine servant.
(Eng) tree with a knot.
Berle, Burl, Burle

Berlyn (German) son of Berl; son of the wine servant. (Eng) tree with a knot by the pool.
Berl, Berle, Berlea, Berleah, Berlee, Berleigh, Berley, Berlin, Burlin, Burlyn

Bernal (German) strong like a bear.
Bernaid, Bernaldo, Bernel, Bernhald, Bernhold, Bernold, Burnal, Burnel

Bern/Bernard/Bernie (Teutonic) strong and brave like a bear; warrior.
Barnard (Fren), Barnee, Barnet, Barnett, Barney, Barni, Barnie, Barny, Bearnard (Scott), Berents (Lett), Bern (Teu), Bernad, Bernadek, Bernaldim, Bernaldo (Ital), Bernadyn, Bernard (Ital/Span), Berne, Bernee, Berneen (Ir), Berngard (Russ), Bernhard (Ger/Swed), Bernhart (Dut), Berni, Bernie, Burnard, Burnee, Burney, Burni, Burnie, Burny

Bernstein (German) amber stone.
Bernsteen, Bernsteyn, Bernsteyne

Berrigan (Australian Aboriginal) wattle (a tree with small fluffy flowers).

Berry (Old English) berry, small fruit.
Berri, Berrie

Bersh (Gypsy) young one.
Besh

Bert (Old English) bright; shining; illustrious. The short form of names ending in 'Bert' e.g. Albert.
Birt, Burt, Byrt

Berthold (Teutonic) bright ruler.
Bertin, Berthoud (Fren), Bertoide, Bertoldi (Ital), Bertold, Bertolt, Bertuccio (Ital), Burthold, Burtholde

Bertil (Scandinavian) bright.
Bertyl, Birtil, Birtyl, Burtil, Burtyl, Byrtil, Byrtyl

Bertin (Spanish) special friend.
Bertan, Berten, Berton, Bertyn, Burtan, Burten, Burtin, Burton, Burtyn

Berto (Spanish/German) noble; industrious; bright; famous. A form of Alberto, noble, industrious, bright, famous one.
Burto

Berton (Old English) from the brilliant one's town.
Berten, Burton

Bertram (Teutonic) bright, shining, famous raven.
Bartok, Bartram, Beltran (Span), Bertramus, Bertran, Bertrand (Fren), Bertrando (Ital), Bertrem

Bertrand (German) bright shield.
Bertran, Bertrando, Bertranno, Burtrand

Berwick (Old English) from the barley farm.
Berwic, Berwik, Berwyc, Berwyck, Berwyk

Berwin (English) powerful son; harvester friend; bear friend.
Berwin, Berwyn, Berwynn, Berwynne

Bethlem (Hungarian) house of bread.
Bethlam

Betram (Teutonic) bright raven.
Bartram, Bertrand, Bertrando, Bertram, Bertrem, Bertrym

Beval (English) windy.
Bevel, Bevil, Bevyl

Bevan (English) son of Evan; son of the well-born one. (Wel) glorious raven; son of the warrior. (Celt) young archer.
Beavan, Beaven, Beven, Bevin, Bevon, Bevyn

Beverly (Old English) from the beaver stream meadow.
Beverlea, Beverleah, Beverlee, Beverleigh, Beverley, Beverli, Beverlie

Bevis (Old French) fair view. (O/Eng) oxen.
Beavis, Beavys, Bevys, Beuves, Eudes

Beynon (Welsh) reliable.
Beinon

Bhima (Sanskrit) mighty; strong.
Bhama

Bickel (German) pick axe.
Bikel

Bickford (Old English) from the pick-axe maker's ford.
Bickforde, Bikford, Bycford, Byckford, Bykford

Bigtha (Persian) gift of God.

Bijan (Persian) ancient hero.
Bihjan, Bijann, Byjan

Bilal (Arabic) the chosen one.
Bila, Billal

Bill (German) wilful one. The short form of William.
Bil

Billy (German)/English wilful one. The short form of William.
Bil, Bilea, Bileah, Bilee, Bileigh, Biley, Bili, Bilie, Bill, Billea, Billeah, Billee, Billey, Billi, Billie, Bily

Bilyana (Australian Aboriginal) wedge-tailed eagle.
Bilyan, Bilyanah

Binah (Hebrew) understanding; wise.
Bina, Byna, Bynah

Bindus (Lettish) blessed.
Bindis, Bindys

Bing (Teutonic) clearing with a hollow. The short form of names starting with or containing 'Bing' e.g. Bingley.
Byng

Bingham (German) one who lives by the bridge.
Bing, Bingam

Binh (Vietnamese) peace.
Bin

Bink (English) dweller by the sloping bank.
Binkentios, Binki, Binkie, Binko, Binky

Birch (Old English) birch tree.
Birk

Birger (Norwegian) rescuer.
Berger

Birin (Australian Aboriginal) cliff.
Biriyn, Byrin, Byryn

Birkey (Old English) birch tree.
Berkee, Berkey, Berki, Berkie, Berky, Birkee, Birki, Birkie, Birky

Birkitt (English) from the birch-tree coast.
Biret, Birit, Burket, Burkett, Burkitt

Birley (Old English) from the birch-tree meadow.
Berlea, Berleah, Berlee, Berleigh, Berley, Berli, Berlie, Berly, Birlea, Birleah, Birlee, Birleigh, Birlie, Birly

Birney (Old English) dweller on the birch-tree island.
Bernee, Berney, Berni, Bernie, Berny, Birnee, Birney, Birni, Birnie,

Birny, Burnee, Burney, Burni,
Burnie, Burney, Burny

Birtle (Old English) from the birch-tree hill with the birds.

Bishop (English) bishop.

Bjorn (Norse/Swedish) bear.
Bjorne

Blackburn (Scottish) from the black stream. (Eng) from the burnt field.
Blackbern, Blackberne, Blackburne

Blade (Old English) prosperity; glory; sword. (Ir) lean.
Blaid, Blaide, Blane, Blaney, Blayd, Blayde, Blayne

Bladud (Welsh) belonging to the fierce wolf tribe.

Blagden (Old English) from the dark valley.

Blaggost (Slavic) good; welcomed.
Blagost

Blagorod (Illyrian) good birth.

Blaine (Irish/Gaelic) slender. (O/Eng) flame.
Blain, Blane, Blaney, Blayn, Blayne (Ir)

Blair (Irish/Gaelic) from the marsh on the plain.
(Scot) field of battle.
Blaire

Blaise (English) burning flames.
Balas (Hung), Balds (Hung), Blais, Blas (Span), Blase, Blasien (Ger), Blasias, Blasio, Blasius (Swed), Biagio (Ital), Blayse, Blayze, Blaze (Fren)

Blake (Old English) dark hair/complexion.
Blaec, Blaek, Blaik, Blaike, Blayk, Blayke

Blakeley (Old English) from the black meadow.
Blakelea, Blakeleah, Blakelee, Blakeleigh, Blakeleigh, Balkeli, Blakelie, Blakely

Blanco (Spanish) white.
Blanko

Bland (Latin) mild; gentle.
Blande

Blandford (Old English) where the grey-haired one crosses the ford.
Blandforde

Blase (Greek) one who stammers.
Balas (Hung), Balds (Hung), Blais, Blaise, Blas (Span), Blasien (Ger), Blasias, Blasio, Blasius (Swed), Biagio (Ital), Blayse, Blayze, Blaze, Blazej (Czech)

Blaxland (Old English) from the black land.

Bleddian (Welsh) little fierce; hero wolf.
Bleddin, Bledian, Bledin, Bledyn

Bledig (Welsh) fierce wolf.
Bledri

Blenda (German) amazing one.
Blendah

Bliss (Old English) bringer of joy; happiness.
Blis, Blys, Blyss

Blumenthal (German) from the flowery valley.

Blundel (Old French) blond-haired.
Blundell, Blundelle, Blunden

Bly (Native American) high.
Bli, Bligh, Bly

Blythe (Old English) cheerful; gentle.
Blith, Blithe, Blyth

Bo (Chinese) precious.
Beau

Boaz (Hebrew) swift; fast; strong; the Lord is strength.
Bo

Bob/Bobby (English) famous; brilliant. The short form of Robert.
Bobb, Bobbee, Bobbey, Bobbi, Bobbie, Bobee, Bobek (Czech), Bobey, Bobi, Bobie, Boby

Bobo (Ghanian) born on a Tuesday.

Bodaway (Native American) maker of fire.

Boden (Scandinavian) shelter. (O/Fren) messenger.
Bodene, Bodine, Bodyn

Bodil (Norse) dominant warrior.
Bodyl

Bodnar (Danish) lead warrior in battle.
Bodna

Bodo (German) leader.

Bodua (Akan) tail of an animal.
Boduah

Bodulf (Danish) fierce wolf leader.

Bogart (Old French) strong bow. (Dan) archer.
Bo, Bogar, Bogey, Bogie

Bogdan (Slavic) God's gift.
Bogden, Bogdin, Bogdon, Bogdyn

Bogo (German) bow.

Bogomil (Slavic) receives God's love and praise.
Bogo, Bogomile, Bogomyl

Bogoslav (Slavic) receives God's glory.
Bogo

Bohdan (Ukrainian) proud ruler.
Bogdan, Bogdashka, Bohdon

Bohumir (Czech) God is great.

Boldisar (Hungarian) member of the war council.
Boldyslav

Boleslav (Slavic) greatest glory.
Boleslaw (Pol)

Bolton (Old English) from the bold one's manor town.
Boltan, Bolten, Boltin, Boltyn

Bomani (Malawian) strong warrior.
Boman, Bomany

Bon (Latin) good.
Bono

Bonar (Old French) courteous; gentle; kind.
Bonnar, Bonner

Bonaro (Italian/Spanish) good friend.
Bon, Bona, Bonah, Bonar

Bonaventure (Italian) good adventure.
Boaventura (Port)

Bond (English) one who tills the soil.

Boniface (Italian) handsome face. (Lat) good doer.
Bonifacio (Ital/Span), Bonifacius (Ger/Swed/Dut)

Bono (Latin) good.
Bon, Bonus

Booker (Old English) book reader.
Bookker

Boone (Old French) blood blessing.
Boon

Booral (Australian Aboriginal) large.
Boral

B

Booth (Old Norse/English) shelter; hut.
Boothe, Bothe

Bor (Gypsy) from the row of hedges.

Borak (Arabic) lightning; flash of light.
Borac, Borack, Borak

Borden (Old English) from the valley of the boars.
Bordan, Bordin, Bordon, Bordyn

Borg (Old Norse) from the settlement area. (Scan) from the castle.
Borge

Boris (Russian) warrior.
(Slav) stranger; unknown.
Borka, Borys

Borka (Russian) warrior.
Borkah, Borkinka

Bornani (Malawian) warrior.

Borr (Swedish) young.
Bor

Boryslaw (Polish) glorious battle.

Boseda (Nigerian) born on a Sunday.
Bosedah

Bosley (Old English) from the boar meadow with the trees.
Boslea, Bosleah, Boslee, Bosleigh, Bosli, Boslie, Bosly

Boston (Old English) from the boar town.
Bostan, Bosten, Bostin, Bostyn

Boswell (Old English) from the boar enclosure by the stream.
Boswel, Bozwel, Bozwell

Bosworth (Old English) from the boar enclosure.
Bozworth

Botan (Japanese) long-lived.
Boten, Botin, Boton, Botyn

Botolf (Old English) fierce wolf.
Botolph

Bour (African) rock.

Bourey (Cambodian) county.
Bouree

Bourne (Old English) from the stream.
Born, Borne, Bourn

Boutros (Arabic/Greek) rock. A form of Peter.
Boutro

Bowen (Old English) son of Owen; son of the well-born one.
(Gae) little, victorious one.
Bohan, Bohann, Bohannon, Bowan, Bowden, Bowin, Bowon, Bowyn, Bowynn

Bowie (Irish) blond-haired.
Bowee, Bowey, Bowi, Bowy

Bowle (Gypsy) snail.
Bowel, Bowl

Bowyer (Old English) maker of bows.
Bowier

Boy (English) young man.
Boi

Boyce (French) one who lives near the forest.
Boice, Boise, Boyse

Boyd (Scottish/Gaelic) blond-haired.
Boydan, Boyde, Boyden, Boydin, Boydon, Boydyn

Boyne (Irish/Gaelic) white cow.
Boin, Boine, Boyn

Boynton (Irish/Gaelic) from the white-cow river town.
Bointon, Bointown, Boyntown

Brad/Bradley (Old English) from the broad meadow. (Scott) clearing in the woods.
Bradd, Braddlea, Braddleah, Braddlee, Braddleigh, Braddley, Braddli, Braddlie, Braddly, Bradlea, Bradleah, Bradlee, Bradleigh, Bradli, Bradlie, Bradly

Bradburn (Old English) from the broad stream.
Bradbern, Bradberne, Bradborn, Bradborne, Bradbourn, Bradbourne, Braddborn, Braddborne, Braddbourn, Braddbourne

Braden (Old English) from the broad valley. (Ir) salmon.
Bradan, Brade, Bradie, Bradin, Bradon, Bradun, Bradyn

Bradford (Old English) from the broad ford.
Braddford, Bradforde

Bradman (Old English) broad man.
Bradmen, Bradmin, Bradmon, Bradmyn

Bradon (English) from the broad valley.
Bradan, Braden, Bradin, Bradon, Bradyn, Braean, Braeden, Braedin, Braedon, Braedyn, Braidan, Braiden, Braidin, Braidon, Braidyn, Braydan, Brayden, Braydin, Braydon, Braydyn

Bradshaw (Old English) from the broad shore.
Braddshaw, Braddshore, Bradshore

Bradwell (Old English) from the broad stream.
Braddwel, Braddwell, Bradwel

Brady (Irish/Gaelic) spirited one from the long island. (Eng) broad one.
Bradie, Bradan, Bradyn, Brae, Braedan, Braedee, Braedey, Braedi,

Braedie, Braedy, Braiden, Braidie, Braidey

Brae (Scottish) hill.
Braey, Brai, Bray (O/Eng)

Brage (Old Norse) a god in Norse mythology.
Bragg, Braggo

Bragi (Scandinavian) poet.
Brage

Braham (Hindi) creator.
Braheem, Braheim, Brahiem, Brahima, Brahimah, Brahm

Brainard (Old English) fierce, bold raven.
Bainard, Baynard, Braynard

Brajan (Illyrian) brother.
Brayjan

Bram (Hebrew) father of the multitudes. The short form of names starting with 'Bram' e.g. Bramwell.
Bramston, Bramwel, Bramwele, Bramwell, Bramwen, Bramwin, Bramwyn

Bramwell (Old English) from the bramble-bush stream.
Bramwel, Bramwele, Bramwen, Bramwin, Bramwyn

Bran (Celtic) raven.
Brand, Brande, Brando, Brann

Branch (Latin) tree branch.
Bran

Brand (Old English) torch; beacon. The short form of names starting with 'Brand' e.g. Brandon.
Bran, Brande, Brando

Brandan (Irish/Gaelic) youthful; bold; brave. (Celt) raven.
Branden, Brandin, Brandon, Brandyn

Branden (English) beacon in the valley.
Brandan, Brandin, Brandon, Brandyn

Brander (Old Norse) torch; sword.
Brandar, Brandir, Brandor

Brando (Old English/Celtic) raven.
Brandan, Branden, Brandin, Brandon, Brandyn, Brannan, Brannen, Brannin, Brannon, Brannyn

Brandon (Old English/Celtic) raven.
Brandan, Branden, Brandin, Brandyn, Brannan, Brannen, Brannin, Brannon

Brandt (English) proud raven.
Brand

Brandy (Dutch) brandy; wine.
Brandee, Brandey, Brandi, Brandie

Brannon (Irish/English) from the beacon hill.
Branan, Branen, Brannan, Brannen, Brannin, Brannyn, Bransin, Brantson

Branson (English) son of Brandon; son of the raven.
Bransan, Bransen, Bransin, Bransyn, Brantson

Brant (Old English) torch.
Brandt, Brantlee, Brantleigh, Brantley, Brantan, Branten, Brantin, Branton

Branwell (Celtic) raven from the stream.
Branwel, Branwele

Brasil (Irish) war.
Brasill, Brasyl, Brasyll, Brazyl, Brazyll

Bravac (Slavic) wild boar.
Bravack, Bravak, Bravoc, Bravock, Bravok

Brawley (Old English) from the hill meadow.
Brawlea, Brawleah, Brawlee, Brawleigh, Brawli, Brawlie, Brawly

Braxton (English) from Brock's town; from the badger's town.
Braxtan, Braxten, Braxtin, Braxtyn

Brazil (Celtic) strength.
Brazill, Brazille, Brazyl, Brazyll, Brazylle

Breck (Irish) freckled.
Brec, Breik (Gae), Brek

Brede (Scandinavian) iceberg.
Bred

Breese (Old English) son of Rhys; son of the ardent, enthusiastic one.
Brease, Breaz, Breaze, Breez, Breeze

Brencis (Latvian/Latin) crowned with laurel leaves.
Brencys

Brendan (Celtic) little raven. (Ir) sword.
Brandan, Branden, Brandin, Brandon, Brandyn, Brannan, Brannen, Brannin, Brannon, Brenden, Brendin, Brendon, Brendyn, Breendan, Brennden, Brenndin, Brenndon, Brenndyn

Brennan (Irish/Gaelic) sip; taste of water.
Brenan, Brenen, Brennen, Brennin, Brennon, Brennun, Brennyn

Brent (English) from the burnt field on the steep hill. The short form of Brenton.
Brentan, Brenten, Brentin, Brenton, Brentun, Brentyn

Brenton (Old English) from the town on the steep hill.
Brentan, Brenten, Brentin, Brentown, Brentun, Brentyn

Brett (Celtic) from Britain.
Bret, Bretan, Breten, Bretin,
Brettan, Bretten, Brettin, Bretton,
Brettun, Brettyn, Bretyn, Britt,
Brittain, Brittan, Britten, Brittin,
Britton, Brittun, Brittyn

Brewster (English) ale maker;
brewer of beer.
Brewstar, Brewstarr, Brewstir,
Brewstor

Brian (Irish) hill. (Celt) strong;
honourable.
Braiano (Ital), Briant, Brien, Brient,
Brion, Bryan, Bryant, Bryon, Bryce
(Scott/Gae), Brycen, Brydan,
Bryden, Brydon, Rian, Rien, Rion,
Ryan, Ryin, Ryon

Brice/Bryce (Scottish/Gaelic/Welsh)
ambitious; quick-minded. (Celt)
son of Rhys; son of the ardent,
enthusiastic one.
Bricen, Brise, Brisen, Brison,
Brycen, Bryse, Brysen

Brick (English) bridge; stone
building material.
Bric, Brik, Bryc, Bryck, Bryk

Bridgely (English) from the
meadow near the bridge.
Bridgelea, Bridgeleah, Bridgelee,
Bridgelei, Bridgeleigh, Bridgeley,
Bridgeli, Bridgelie

Bridger (Old English) builder of
bridges.
Bridgar, Bridge, Bridges, Bridgir,
Bridgor

Brighton (English) (Geographical)
from Brighton in England; from
the sunny town.

Bringham (Old English) dweller by
the enclosed bridge homestead.
Bringhem, Bringholm

Brinley (English) burnt wood in the
meadow.
Brinlea, Brinleah, Brinlee, Brinlei,
Brinleigh, Brinli, Brinlie, Brinly,
Brynlea, Brynleah, Brynlee, Brynley,
Brynlei, Brynleigh, Brynli, Brynlie,
Brynly

Brishan (Gypsy) born in the rain.
Brishen, Brishin, Brishon, Bryshan,
Bryshin, Bryshon, Bryshyn

Brit (Scottish) from Britain.
Britain, Briton, Britt, Brittain,
Brittan, Britten, Britton, Brittyn,
Brityce, Brytyn

Brock (Old English) badger.
Broc, Brocas, Brockman, Brockway,
Brocton, Brok, Broxton, Broxtown

Brod (English) broad. The short
form of Broderick, renowned
ruler.
Brodi, Brodie, Brody

Broder (Scandinavian) brother.
Brodee, Brodey, Brodi, Brodie,
Brody

Broderick (Welsh) son of Roderick;
son of the renowned ruler.
(Scan) brother.
Brodaric, Brodarick, Brodarik,
Broderic, Broderik, Broderyc,
Broderyck, Broderyk

Brodie (Scandinavian) brother.
(Scott) second-born son.
(Ir/Gae) canal builder.
Brodee, Broden, Brodey, Brodi,
Brodie

Brodny (Slavic) from the place by
the stream.
Brodnee, Brodney, Brodni, Brodnie

Bromley (Old English) dweller in
the meadow.
Bromlea, Bromleah, Bromlee,

Bromleigh, Bromli, Bromlie,
Bromly

Brone (Celtic) sorrowful one.
Bron, Broney, Broni, Bronie, Brony

Bronislav (Slavic) glorious one;
weapon.
Bronyslav

Bronson (Old English) brown's
son; son of the brown/reddish-
complexioned one.
Bronsan, Bronsen, Bronsin,
Bronsun, Bronsyn

Brook (Old English) dweller from
the stream.
Brooc, Brooclin, Brooclyn,
Broocklin, Broocklyn, Brooke,
Brookes, Brooklin, Brooklyn,
Brooks, Broox

Brooks (English) brook's son; son
of the dweller from the stream.
Brooc, Brooclin, Brooclyn,
Broocklin, Broocklyn, Brook,
Brooke, Brookes, Brooklin,
Brooklyn, Broox

Brougher (Old English) dweller at
the tower fortress.
Brough

Broughton (Old English) from the
tower fortress town.
Brough, Broughtan, Broughten,
Broughtin, Broughtown

Brown (Middle English)
brown/reddish-complexioned.
Browne

Bruce (Old English) dweller at the
dense shrubs.
Brooce, Broose, Bruse

Bruno (Teutonic/Italian/Portugese)
brown-haired.
Braun (Ger)

Brunon (Polish) brown.
Brunen, Brunin, Brunun, Brunyn

Brutus (Latin) liberator of Rome.
Brootus, Brutas, Brutis, Brutiss,
Brutos, Brutoss, Brutuss

Bryant (Irish) strong; honourable.
A form of Bryan.
Briant, Brient, Bryent

Brychan (Welsh) freckled.
Brichan, Brynach

Bryden (English) (Geographical)
from Bryden in England; from
the hill in the valley.
Briden

Bryn (Welsh) mountain.
(Lat) boundary line.
Brin, Brinn, Brynn

Brynmor (Welsh) large hill.
(Eng) hill in the moors
Brinmor, Brinmore, Brynmore

Bryon (English) twisting vine; bear.
(Ger) cottage.
Brian, Brion

Bryson (Welsh) Bryce's son; son of
the ambitious, quick-minded one.
Brison

Bu (Vietnamese) leader.

Bubba (American) mate; friend.
Buba, Bubah, Bubbah

Buchanan (Scottish/Gaelic) house
of the clergy.
Buchannan, Buchanen, Bukanon

Buck (Old English) male deer;
buck. The short form of Buckley.
Buc, Buk

Buckley (Old English) dweller at
the buck/deer meadow.
Bucklea, Buckleah, Bucklee,
Buckleigh, Buckli, Bucklie, Buckly,
Buclea, Bucleah, Buclee, Bucleigh,

B

Buckley cont.
Bucley, Bucli, Buclie, Bucly, Buklee, Bukleigh, Bukley, Bukli, Buklie, Bukly

Buddy (Old English) messenger; friend.
Bud, Budd, Budde, Buddee, Buddey, Buddi, Buddie, Buddy, Budi, Budie, Budo, Budy

Buell (German) dweller at the hill.
Buel

Buford (English) from the ford near the cattle.
Burford

Bundy (Old English) freedom.
Bundee, Bundey, Bundi, Bundie

Bunyan (Australian Aboriginal) place where pigeons live.
Bunyen, Bunyin, Bunyon, Bunyyn

Burac (Slavic) storm; tempest.
Burack, Burak

Burbank (Old English) dweller at the castle slope.
Berbanc, Berbanck, Berbank, Burbanc, Burbanck

Burch (Middle English) birch tree. The short form of Burchard.
Berch, Berche, Birch, Birche, Byrch, Byrche

Burchard (Old English) powerful, strong castle.
fortress

Burden (Old English) birch-tree valley.
Berdan, Berden, Berdin, Berdon, Berdyn, Birdan, Birden, Birdin, Birdon, Birdyn, Burdan, Burdin, Burdon, Burdun, Burdyn

Burdett (Old French) little shield.
Berdet, Berdett, Berdette, Burdet, Burdette

Burford (Old English) from the birch-tree ford.
Berford, Berforde, Birford, Birforde, Burforde, Byrford, Byrforde

Burgess (Old English) dweller in the birch trees.
Bergess, Birgess, Byrgess

Burian (Ukrainian) dweller near the weeds.
Berian, Beriane, Beryan, Beryane, Birian, Biriane, Biryan, Biryane, Buriane, Byrian, Byriane, Byryan, Byryane

Burke (Old English) dweller from the birch-tree manor on the hill.
Berc, Berk, Berke, Bertkett, Berkette, Birk, Birke, Bourke, Burk, Burkett, Byrk, Byrke

Burkett (Old French) from the little stronghold.
Berket, Berkette, Birket, Birkett, Burket, Burkette, Byrket, Byrkett

Burl (Old English) wine servant. (Eng) tree with a knot.
Bearl, Bearle, Berl, Berlton, Birl, Birle, Burle, Burlea, Burleah, Burlee, Burleigh, Burley, Burli, Burlie, Burly, Burnell, Burnett, Burnette, Byrl, Byrle

Burleigh (Old English) clearing at the manor with knotted tree trunks.
Berlea, Berleah, Berlee, Berleigh, Berley, Berli, Berlie, Berly, Birlea, Birleah, Birlee, Birleigh, Birley, Birli, Birlie, Birly, Burlea, Burleah, Burlee, Burley, Burli, Burlie, Burly

Burley (Old English) dweller at the castle meadow.
Berlea, Berleah, Berlee, Berleigh, Berley, Berli, Berlie, Berly, Birlea, Birleah, Birlee, Birleigh, Birley, Birli, Birlie, Birly, Burlea, Burleah,

B

Burlee, Burleigh, Burli, Burlie,
Burly

Burnaby (Old Norse) from the
warrior's estate.
Barnabee, Barnabey, Barnabi,
Barnabie, Barnaby, Bernabee,
Bernabey, Bernabi, Beranbie,
Bernaby, Birnabee, Birnabey,
Birnabi, Birnabie, Birnaby,
Burnabee, Burnabey, Burnabi,
Burnabie, Byrnabi, Byrnabie,
Byrnaby

Burne (Old English) from the
stream.
Bern, Berne, Bourn, Bourne, Burn,
Byrn, Byrne

Burnell (Old French) little brown-
haired one.
Bernall, Bernalle, Bernel, Bernell,
Bernelle, Birnel, Birnell, Birnelle,
Burnele, Burnelle, Byrnel, Byrnell,
Byrnelle

Burnett (English) burnt nettle.
Bernet, Bernett, Birnet, Birnett,
Burnet

Burney (Old English) dweller at the
burnt stream island.
Bernee, Berney, Berni, Bernie,
Berny, Birnee, Birney, Birni, Birnie,
Birny, Burnee, Burnie, Burny,
Byrnee, Byrney, Byrni, Byrnie, Byrny

Burns (Scottish) from the stream.
Bern, Berne, Bernes, Birn, Birne,
Birnes, Burn, Burne, Burnes, Byrn,
Byrne, Byrnes, Byrns

Burr (English) prickly coat.
(Swed) youthful.
Bur, Burral, Burrel, Burril, Burrol,
Burryl

Burril (Australian Aboriginal)
wallaby (small kangaroo).
Bural, Burel, Buril, Burol, Buryl,
Burral, Burrel, Burrol, Burryl

Burris (English) from the birch-tree
town.
Buris, Buriss, Burys, Buryss

Burt (Old English) bright. The short
form of Burton, bright, famous
town.
Bert, Birt, Byrt

Burton (Old English) bright,
famous town.
Bertan, Berten, Bertin, Berton,
Bertyn, Birtan, Birten, Birtin,
Birton, Birtyn, Burtan, Burten,
Burtin, Burtyn, Byrtan, Byrten,
Bytin, Byton, Byrtyn

Busby (Scottish/Old Norse) dweller
at the village thicket.
Busbee, Busbey, Busbi, Busbie,
Busby, Buzbi, Buzbie, Buzby

Bushrod (Old Danish) shrub; bush.

Buster (English) raider.
Busta, Bustar

Butcher (English/American) butcher.
Butch

Butler (French) head servant.
Butlar, Butlor, Buttlar, Buttler,
Buttlor

Buzz (English) noisy; busy.

Byford (Old English) dweller by the
river ford.
Biford, Biforde, Byforde

Byram (Aramaic) celebration.
Biram

Byrd (Old English) bird-like.
Berd, Bird

Byrger (Danish) guardian warrior.
Berger, Birger, Burger

Byrne (Celtic) dweller from the
field in the summit.
Bern, Berne, Bernes, Burn, Burne,
Burnes, Byrn, Byrnes

C

Byron (Old French) bear strength. (Old/Eng) from the country estate.
Biran, Biren, Birin, Biron, Byran, Byren

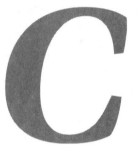

Cable (Old English) rope maker.
Cabe, Kabe, Kable

Cadal (Celtic) warrior.
Cadall, Kadal, Kadall

Cadby (Old Norse/Old English) dweller by the warrior's estate.
Cadbee, Cadbey, Cadbi, Cadbie

Caddoc (Welsh) warrior; keen for battle.
Cadock, Cadok

Cade (Welsh) battle warrior.
Caid, Cayd

Cadell (Celtic) battle in the valley.
Cade, Cadel, Caden, Caidel, Caidell, Caydel, Caydell, Cayden

Cadfan (Welsh) high battle.
Caedfan, Caidfan, Caydfan

Cadfer (Welsh) lord of battle.
Caedfer, Caidfer, Caydfer

Cadman (Celtic) warrior.
Cadmen, Caedman, Caidman, Caydman

Cadmar (Celtic) brave warrior.
Cadmer, Cadmir, Caedmar, Caidmar, Caydmar

Caelan (Irish/Gaelic) powerful in battle.
Caelen, Caelin, Caelon, Caelyn, Cailan, Cailen, Cailin, Cailon, Cailyn, Calan, Calcalin, Cale, Callan, Callen, Callin, Caylan, Caylen, Caylin, Caylon, Caylyn

Caesar (Latin) imperial; long-haired.
Caesare, Caesario, Caesarius (Swed/Dan), Casar (Ger), Casare (Ital), Cesar (Fren/Span/Port), Kaiser, Saecer, Saeser, Tsar

Caffer (Celtic) protection for the head in battle; helmet.
Caffer

Cahil (Turkish) young; naive.
Cahill, Kahil, Kahill, Kahyl, Kahyll

Cahir (Celtic) warrior.
Cahyr, Kahir, Kahyr

Cai (Welsh/Latin) happy.
Cae, Caio, Caius, Caw, Cay, Kae, Kai, Kay

Cain (Hebrew) possession; spear. (Gae) tribute.
Caen, Caene, Cainan, Caine, Caineth, Cayn, Cayne, Cayneth, Kain, Kayn, Kayne

Cairn (Welsh) landmark piled with stones.
Cairne, Cairnes, Carn, Carne, Carnes, Cayrn, Cayrne, Cayrnes

Cairo (Arabic) (Geographical) the capital of Egypt.
Cayro, Kairo, Kayro

Caislav (Slavic) glory; victory; honour.
Cayslav, Kaislav, Kayslav

C

Calder (English/Scottish) from the rough water stream with the stones.
Cale

Caldwell (Old English) dweller by the old stream.
Caldwel, Kaldwel, Kaldwell

Cale (Hebrew) faithful.
Cael, Caell, Cail, Caill, Calle, Cayl, Cayll, Kael, Kaell, Kail, Kaill, Kale, Kayl, Kayll

Caleb (Hebrew/Arabic) faithful, bold, victorious dog.
Caelab, Cailab, Calab, Cale, Caley, Caylab, Cayleb, Kaylab, Kaleb

Caley (Irish/Old English) slender one from the meadow.
Calea, Caleah, Calee, Caleigh, Caley, Cali, Calie, Callea, Calleah, Callee, Calleigh, Calley, Calli, Callie, Cally, Caly, Kalea, Kaleah, Kalee, Kaleigh, Kaley, Kali, Kalie, Kaly

Calhoun (Irish) hero warrior of the forest.
Calhoon, Colhoun, Colquhoun, Kalhoon, Kalhoun

Callaghan (Irish) conflicted.
Calaghan, Calahan, Callahan, Kalaghan, Kallaghan, Kallahan

Callagun (Australian Aboriginal) blue fig.
Calagun, Kalagun, Kallagun

Callan (Australian Aboriginal) the sparrow-hawk bird.
Calan, Calen, Calin, Callen, Callin, Callon, Callyn, Calon, Calyn, Kalan, Kalen, Kalin, Kallan, Kallen, Kallin, Kallon, Kallyn, Kalin, Kalon, Kalyn

Callis (Latin) goblet or cup; chalice.
Calliss, Callys, Callyss, Kallis, Kalliss, Kallys, Kallyss

Callum (Scottish/Gaelic) follower of St Columb; gentle. (Ir) dove; peace.
Calam, Calem, Calim, Callam, Callem, Callim, Calum, Callym, Colm, Colum, Kallum, Kalum

Calvert (Old English) cowboy; herder of calves.
Calbert, Calburt, Kalbert, Kalvert

Calvin (Latin) bald one.
Caiv, Calvan, Calven, Calvino (Ital/Span), Calvon, Calvun, Calvyn, Kalvan, Kalven, Kalvin, Kalvon, Kalvun, Kalvyn

Cam (Gypsy) loved. The short form of Cameron, crooked, bent nose.
Kam

Camden (Irish) dweller in the winding, windy valley.
Camdan, Camdin, Camdon, Camdyn, Kamdan, Kamden, Kamdin, Kamdon, Kamdyn

Cameron (Scottish/Gaelic) crooked, bent nose. (Kurd) happy.
Camar, Camaron, Cameran, Camerson, Camiren, Camiron, Camron (Scott), Cameran, Camerin, Camran, Camrin, Camron, Cameryn, Kameran, Kameren, Kamerin, Kameron, Kameryn

Camilo (Tongan/French) ceremonial attendant. (Lat) born in freedom.
Camiel, Camillo, Camilow, Camillus, Kamillo, Kamillow, Kamilo (Tong), Kamyllo, Kamylo

Camlo (Gypsy) lovely.
Camlow, Kamlo, Kamlow

Campbell (Scottish/Gaelic) crooked, bent mouth. (Fren) from the beautiful, bright field.
Cambel, Cambell, Camp, Kambel, Kambell, Kamp, Kampbell

Canada (Iroquois) cabin. (Geographical) the country.
Canadah, Kanada, Kanadah

Candide (French) white.
Candid, Candida, Candide (Fren), Candido (Lat), Candonino, Kandida, Kandide, Kandido

Canice (Celtic) handsome.
Canyce, Kanice, Kanyce

Cannon (French) church official; cannon; gun shooter.
Canan, Canen, Canin, Cannan, Cannen, Cannin, Cannyn, Canon

Cantrell (Latin) singer.
Cantrel

Canute (Scandinavian) knot. (Lat) white-haired/complexioned. (O/Nrs) race.
Cnut, Cnute, Kanut, Kanute, Knud, Knut (Scan), Knute

Cappi (Gypsy/Italian) prosperity; luck; good fortune; profit.
Cappee, Cappey, Cappie, Cappy, Kappee, Kappey, Kappi, Kappie, Kappy

Car (Irish) from the castle.
Carr, Kar, Karr

Caradoc (Welsh) friend.
Caractacus, Caradawg, Carartacos, Carthae, Carthage, Karadoc

Carden (Old French) one who combs out wool fibres; a card.
Cardan, Cardin, Cardon, Cardyn

Cardew (Old Welsh) black foot.
Carew

Carey (Greek) pure. (Wel) from the castle on the rocky island.
Care, Caree, Carre, Carrey, Carry, Cary

Carl (Old German) strong; courageous. A form of Charles.
Cael, Cahal, Carlan, Carlew, Carlin, Carlos (Span), Carlo (Ital), Karl, Karlan, Karlew, Karlin, Karlo, Karlos

Carleton (Old English) from the town of Charles; from the strong, courageous town.
Carlton, Karleton, Karlton

Carlin (Irish) little champion. (O/Eng) strong, courageous one from the pool.
Carlan, Carlen, Carley, Carli, Carlie, Carling, Carlino, Carlon, Carly, Karlan, Karlen, Karlin, Karlon, Karlyn

Carlo/Carlos (Italian) strong; courageous. A form of Charles.
Carolo, Carlos (Span/Ital), Charlo, Chalos, Karlo, Karlos

Carlton (Old English) from Carl's/Charles' town; from the strong, courageous town.
Carlen, Carlin, Carlisle, Carlson, Charl, Charlton, Karlen, Karlin, Karlisle, Karlson, Kharl, Kharlton

Carlyle (Celtic) dweller at the strengthened castle. (Eng) from Carl's island; from the strong, courageous island.
Carlisle, Carlysle, Karlisle, Karlyle

Carmen (Arabic) vineyard of the Lord.
Carmeli, Carmelo (Heb), Carmen, Carmi, Carmiel, Carmine, Carmyn, Carmyne, Karmel, Karmeli, Karmi, Karmiel

Carmelo (Hebrew) fruitful orchid.
Carmel (Arab), Karmel, Karmelo,
Karmilo

Carmichael (Scottish) friend of St
Michael. (Ir) from the castle of St
Michael.
Karmichael

Carmine (Latin) song; red.
Carman, Carmen, Carmon,
Karmine

Carnell (English) one who defends
the castle.
Carnel, Karnel, Karnell

Carney (Irish) victorious warrior.
Carnee, Carney, Carnie, Karnee,
Karney, Karni, Karnie, Karny

Carol/Carollan (German/Hebrew)
strong; courageous; farmer;
graceful. (Eng) joyful Christmas
song.
Karollan

Carr (Scandinavian/Norse) from the
marsh.
Car, Carson, Carsten, Carvel, Kar,
Karr, Karson, Karsten, Karvel, Kerr,
Kerwin

Carrick (Gaelic) from the rocky
headland; cliff.
Carric, Carrik, Carrington, Karric,
Karrick, Karrington

Carroll (German) strong;
courageous. (Eng) joyful
Christmas song. (Celt) champion
warrior.
Carol, Carrol, Karrol, Karroll

Carson (English/Scottish) son of
the marsh dweller.
Carsan, Carse, Carsen, Carsin,
Karsan, Karsen, Karsin, Karson,
Karsyn

Carswell (Old English) dweller at
the watercress stream.
Carswel, Carswold, Karswel,
Karswell, Karswold

Carter (Old English) cart maker and
driver.
Cart, Cartar, Cartor, Kart, Kartar,
Karter, Kartor

Cartland (Scottish/English) from
the island; from the cart builder's
land.
Cartlan, Kartlan, Kartland

Cartwright (English) cart maker.
Cartright

Carvel (Manx) song. (Fren) from
the wood carver's village.
Carvell, Carvelle, Karvel, Karvell,
Karvelle

Carver (English) one who carves
wood; sculptor.
Carvar, Carvir, Carvor, Kavar, Kaver,
Kavir, Kavor

Cary (Celtic) loving; from the castle.
Caree, Carey, Cari, Carie, Caree,
Carrey, Carri, Carrie, Carry, Karee,
Karey, Kari, Karie, Karree, Karrey,
Karri, Karrie, Karry, Kary

Casey (Irish) brave, aggressive
warrior.
Casee, Casi, Casie, Cassee, Cassey,
Cassi, Cassie, Casy, Caswell, Casy,
Cayse, Caysewell, Cazzee, Cazzey,
Cazzi, Cazzie, Cazzy, Kasee, Kasey,
Kasi, Kasie, Kassee, Kassey, Kassi,
Kassie, Kassy, Kasy, Kazee, Kazey,
Kazzee, Kazzey, Kazzi, Kazzie,
Kazzy, Kazy

Cash (Latin) vain. (Eng) wealth;
money.
Cashe

C

Cashel (Irish) fortified, strengthened castle wall.
Cashell, Kashel, Kashell

Cashlin (Celtic) from the little castle by the stream.
Cashlind, Cashlyn, Cashlynd, Kashlin, Kashlind, Kashlyn

Casimir (Polish) peace is announced.
Casimiro (Span), Cazimir, Cazimier, Kashis, Kashmir, Kasimir (Ger/Slav), Kazimier, Kazimerz, Karmer

Caslav (Slavic) honour; glory.
Castilav, Kaslav

Casper (Persian) guardian of the treasure.
Caspar, Caspir, Gappe, Gaso, Gaspar, Gasparas, Gaspard, Gaspardo, Jaspar, Jasper, Josper, Kaspar, Kasparas, Kaspe, Kasper, Kaspers, Kaspir, Kuanoi

Cassidy (Irish) clever; curly-haired.
Cassian, Cassidee, Cassidey, Cassidi, Cassidie, Cassion (Ital), Casius, Caskey, Kassidee, Kassidey, Kassidi, Kassidie, Kassidy, Kassion, Kasius, Kaskey

Cassie (Greek) prophet. (Ir) clever, curly-haired one. The short form of names starting with 'Cass' e.g. Cassidy.
Casi, Casie, Cassi, Cassy, Casy, Cazi, Cazie, Cazy

Cassius (Latin) vain.
Caskey, Casius, Cassio (Ital), Cazzius, Kaskey, Kasius, Kassio, Kassius, Kazzius

Castimir (Slavic) peace; honour.
Kastimir

Castle (Latin) from the castle.
Cassle, Castal, Castel

Castor (Latin) beaver. (O/Eng) castle attendant.
Castar, Caster, Castir, Castor, Kastar, Kaster, Kastir, Kastor, Kastyr

Catalin (Irish) magical wizard. The masculine form of Caitlin, pure pool.
Caitalin, Kaitalin, Katalin

Cater (English) one who caters for parties.
Cat, Cate, Catee, Catey, Cati, Catie, Caty

Cathal (Celtic) mighty; wise in the eye of battle. A masculine form of Cathy, purity.
Cathel, Cathol, Kathal, Kathel, Kathol

Cathbert (Old English) bright; famous.
Courtenay (Fren), Courtland, Courtlandt, Courtney, Cudbert, Cudbright, Cumbert, Curcio, Curtell, Cuthbrid, Curtys

Cathmor (Irish/Gaelic) great warrior. (O/Eng) from the pure moor. A masculine form of Cathy, purity.
Cathmore, Cathmoor, Cathmoore, Cathmore, Kathmor, Kathmore, Kathmoor, Kathmoore

Cato (Latin) cautious wisdom.
Caton, Kato, Katon

Cavanaugh (Irish) handsome.
Cavan, Caven, Cavin, Cavon, Kavan, Kaven, Kavin, Kavon, Kavanaugh

Cavell (Old French) little; active. (O/Eng) from the cave valley.
Cavel, Kavel, Kavell

Cavill (Old English) from the field of jackdaw (bird).
Cavil, Caville, Kavil, Kavill, Kaville

C

Cawley (Scottish/Old Norse) ancestral relic; ancient. (O/Eng) from the cow meadow.
Calea, Cawleah, Cawlee, Cawleigh, Cawli, Cawlie, Cawly, Kawlee, Kawleigh, Kawley, Kawli, Kawlie, Kawly

Cecil (Latin) unseeing. The masculine form of Cecelia.
Cacilius (Dut), Caecilianus, Caecilius, Cecile, Cesilio, Cecilus, Cescis, Cecyl, Kilian, Seisyllt, Sitsylit

Cedomil (Slavic) child of love.
Cedomilo

Cedric (Welsh) gift; splendour. (O/Eng) war chief.
Cadadoc, Caddaric, Cedric, Cedrick, Ceredic, Cerdic, Cedro, Cidro, Sedric, Sedrick

Cedro (Spanish) cedar; juniper tree.
Cedro

Celerino (Latin) faster.
Celerin

Celestine (Greek/French/Latin) little moon; little heavenly one.
Celestino (Ital), Celestyn (Pol), Selestin, Selestine, Selestino, Selestyn

Cemal (Arabic) handsome.
Cemal

Cephas (Aramaic) stone.
Cephus

Cerdic (Welsh) beloved.
Caradoc, Caradog, Ceredig, Ceretic

Cerek (Polish) lord.
Cerik

Ceri (Welsh) loved.
Seri

Cesar (Latin) imperial; long-haired.
Caesar, Casar, Cesare, Cesareo, Cesario, Cesaro, Ceser, Cesir, Cesor

Ceslav (Illyrian) honour; glory.
Cestislav

Chace (English) hunter.
Chaice, Chaise, Chase, Chayce, Chayse

Chad (Old English) from the warrior's estate. The short form of Chadwick.
Ceadd, Chaad, Chadd, Chaddi, Chaddie, Chaddy, Chadleigh, Chadler, Chadley, Chadlin, Chadlino, Chadlyn, Chadlyno, Chadman, Chadmen, Chado, Chadron, Chady

Chadrick (German) mighty warrior.
Chaderic, Chaderick, Chaderik, Chadrick, Chadrik, Chadryc, Chadryck, Chadryk

Chadwick (Old English) from the mighty warrior's estate.
Chadwic, Chadwik, Chadwyc, Chadwyck, Chadwyk

Chago (Spanish) replacer. A form of James.
Chango, Chanti

Chahaya (Indonesian) light.
Chahayah

Chaim (Hebrew) life.
Chai, Chaimek, Chaym, Chayme, Haim, Khaim

Chalmer (Scottish) head of the house.
Chalmers, Chalmr, Chamar, Chamarr

Champion (Latin) flat and open area. (Eng) the best.
Champyon

Chan (Sanskrit) shining bright.
Chann, Channo, Chano, Chayo

Chanan (Hebrew) cloud.
Chanan, Chanen, Chanin,
Channan, Channen, Channin,
Channon, Channyn, Chanon,
Chanyn

Chance (Middle English) good
fortune; luck.
Chanc, Chancey, Chancy, Chanse,
Chansy, Chants, Chants, Chanz,
Chaunce, Chauncey, Chauncy

Chancellor (Latin) keeper of
records; keys. (M/Eng) merchant
or trader.
Chance, Chancelen, Chancelor

Chander (Hindi) moon.
Chand, Chandan, Chandani,
Chandanie, Chandany, Chandara,
Chanaravth, Chandon, Chandonn

Chandler (Old French) candle
maker.
Chandlah, Chandlan

Chandra (Sanskrit) moon.
Chandrah, Chandria, Chandriah,
Chandrya, Chandryah

Chane (Swahili) dependable; plant.
Chaen, Chaene, Chain, Chaine,
Chayn, Chayne

Channing (Old French) high church
official. (Lat) singer. (Eng)
young, fierce wolf.
Chana, Chanen, Chanin, Chaning,
Chanon, Channen, Channin,
Channon, Channyn, Chanyn

Chante (French) singer.
Chant, Chanta, Chantae, Chantah,
Chantha, Chanthar, Chantra,
Chantrah, Chanty, Shanta,
Shantae, Shantah

Chanti (Hispanic) replacer.
Chantee, Chantey, Chantie, Chanty

Chapman (Old English) merchant;
trades person.
Chapmann, Chapmen, Chapmin,
Chapmyn

Chapple (Old French) of the chapel.
Chapal, Chapel, Chapell, Chaple

Charles (Old German/French)
strong; courageous.
Alcuin, Carel, Cahil (Ir), Carl
(Ger/Swed), Carleton, Carlie,
Carling, Carlisle, Carlo (Ital),
Carlos (Span), Carlson, Carlton,
Carly, Carlyle, Carol, Caroll,
Carolle, Carolus, Carrol, Cary,
Carry, Caryl, Cathal, Chad,
Chaddie, Chaddy, Char, Charlet,
Karolius, Karol, Karole, Karoll,
Karoley, Karoly, Siarl, Tearlach
(Scott)

Charlie (German/English) strong,
courageous one from the
meadow.
Charlea, Charleah, Charlee,
Charleigh, Charley, Charli, Charly

Charlton (Old English) from
Charles' town; from the strong,
courageous town.
Carleton, Carlton, Charleton

Charro (Spanish) rider of horses.
Charo

Chase (French) hunter.
Chaice, Chaise, Chasen, Chasin,
Chason, Chass, Chasse, Chasyn,
Chayce, Chayse, Chuck

Chaska (Sioux) first-born son.
Chaskah

Chatham (Old English) from the
warrior's cottage.
Chathem, Chathom, Chathim,
Chatym

C

Chauncey (Old French) chance; luck; fortune.
Chancellor, Chaunce, Chauncee, Chauncer, Chaunci, Chauncie, Chauncy

Chayton (Lakota) falcon.
Chaiton

Chaz (German/English) strong; courageous. A form of Charles.
Chas, Chazwick, Chazz

Chen (Chinese) vast; great.
Chan

Chencho (Spanish/Latin) crown of laurel leaves; victory. A form of Lawrence.
Chanco

Cheney (Old French) belonging to the oak-grove forest.
Chenee, Cheni, Chenie, Cheny, Chesnee, Chesney, Chesni, Chesnie, Cheyney

Cheng (Chinese) correct; righteous.
Chen

Chepe (Spanish) God will increase; God has added a child. A form of Joseph.
Cepito

Cherokee (Native American) people of the cave country; people with a different speech. A tribal name.
Cherokey, Cheroki, Cherokie, Cheroky

Cherubino (Italian) little cherub; angel.
Cherub, Cherubin, Cherubyno

Chesmu (Native American) abrasive; rough.
Chesmue

Chester (Old English) dweller at the fortified camp.
Castar, Caster, Castor, Chesleigh, Chesley, Cheslie, Chestan, Chesten, Chestin, Cheston

Chet (English) (Geographical) from Rochester in England.
Chett

Chetwin (Old English) belonging to the cottage with the winding path; from a friend's cottage.
Chatwin, Chatwyn, Chetwyn

Chevalier/Chevy (French) knight.
Chevalyer, Chevee, Chevey, Chevi, Chevie, Chevrolet

Cheyenne (Native American) name of a great Native American nation. (O/Fren/Hebrew) graceful oak tree.
Cheienne

Cheyne (Scottish) oak hearted; strength.
Sheyne

Chi (Nigerian) guardian angel. (Chin) young.
Chee

Chico (Spanish) young boy. The short form of Francisco, freedom.
Chiko (Jap)

Chiel (Old English) youth.
Chal, Chelovik

Chik (Gypsy) of the earth.
Chic (Span), Chyc, Chyk

Chike (Ibo) the power of God.
Chik, Chyk, Chyke

Chiko (Japanese) arrow; promise.
Chico (Span), Chyko

Chill (English) cold.
Chil, Chyl, Chyll

Chilo (Latin) freedom.
Chylo

Chilton (Old English) the children's spring town.
Chilt, Chiltown, Chylt, Chylton

Chim (German) God will judge. (Viet) bird.
Chym

Chintoo (Australian Aboriginal) sun.
Yindi, Uuna, Tonahleah

Chinua (Ibo) the blessing of God.
Chino, Chinou, Chinuah, Chynua, Chynuah

Chioke (Ibo) gift of God.
Chyoke

Chip (Native American) short form of a Native American tribe known as Chippewas.
Chipman, Chipmen, Chipp, Chipper, Chippeu, Chippewa, Chippewas, Chyp, Chypman, Chypmen, Chypp, Chypper, Chyppeu

Chippia (Australian Aboriginal) duck.
Chipia, Chipiah, Chippiah, Chippya, Chippyah, Chipya, Chipyah, Chypia, Chypiah, Chyppia, Chyppiah, Chyppya, Chyppyah, Chypya, Chypyah

Chiram (Hebrew) high; noble.
Chyram

Chitto (Creek) brave.

Chitty (German) cub or pup; youngster.
Chitee, Chitey, Chiti, Chitie, Chittee, Chittey, Chitti, Chittie, Chity, Chytee, Chytey, Chyti, Chytie, Chyttee, Chyttey, Chytti, Chyttie, Chytty, Chyty

Chris (Greek) Christ bearer. The short form of Christopher.
Chriss, Chrys, Chryss, Cris, Criss, Khris, Khriss, Kris, Kriss, Khrys, Khryss

Christian (Latin/Greek) follower of Christ.
Crestien (Fren), Chestra, Chestien, Chetien, Christiaan, Christiano (Ital/Span), Christos, Cristan, Cristen, Cristian, Cristien, Cristiene, Cristin, Cristyn, Crystian, Crystien, Crystyn, Karstan, Karsten, Karstin, Karston, Kerestal, Kerstan, Kerste, Khristan, Khristian, Khrystan, Khrystian, Krisat, Kristian, Krystan, Krystian

Christmas (English) born at Christmas time.
Chrystamas

Christoff (Russian) Christ bearer. A form of Christopher.
Christof, Christoph, Chrisstof, Chrisstoff, Chrisstoph, Khristof, Khristoff, Khristoph, Khrystof, Khrystoff, Khrystoph, Kristof, Kristoff, Kristoph, Krystof, Krystoff, Krystoph

Christopher (Greek) Christ bearer.
Chrisstof, Christo, Christobal, Christof (Ger/Russ), Christofer (Dut), Christoffer (Dan), Christoph, Christoforo, Christophe (Fren), Christophor, Christophoro, Christophorus (Grk), Christphur, Christos, Christovac (Port), Christovao, Cristofano, Cristo, Cristoforo (Ital), Cristogal, Cristopal (Span), Cristos, Crysteffer, Crysteffor, Gilchrist, Gristouolo, Khristofer, Khristoffer, Khristopher, Khrystofer, Khrystoffer, Khrystopher, Kina, Kristagis, Kristal, Kristo, Kristobel, Kristof, Kristoff, Kristofer, Kristofor (Swed), Kristopais, Kristopas,

C

Kristopher, Krystof, Krystofer,
Krystopher, Krysztof, Xit

Chrysander (Greek) golden.
Chrisander, Chrisandor,
Chrisandre, Chrysandor,
Chrysandre

Chrysanthus (Greek) golden flower.
Chrisanthias, Chrisanthyas,
Chrisanthus, Chrysanthias,
Chrisanthius, Chrysanthus,
Crisanthas, Crisanthias, Crisanthus,
Crysanthas, Crysanthias,
Crysanthus

Chucho (Hebrew) God will help. A
form of Jesus.

Chuck (American/English/German)
strong; courageous. A form of
Charles.
Chuckee, Chuckey, Chucki,
Chuckie, Chucky, Chuk, Chuki,
Chukie, Chuky

Chui (Swahili) leopard.

Chul (Korean) firmness.

Chuminga (Spanish/Latin) of the
Lord. A form of Dominic.
Chumin, Chumingah

Chumo (Spanish/Greek) twin. A
form of Thomas.

Chung (Chinese) intelligent.

Churchill (Old English) dweller at
the church hill.
Churchil, Churchyl, Churchyll

Cian (Irish/Gaelic) ancient.
Celin, Cianan, Cyan, Kian, Kyan

Cicero (Latin/Italian) chick pea.
Ciceron, Cicerone, Ciceroni, Ciro,
Cyrano, Cyro

Cid (Spanish) lord; master.
Cidd, Cyd, Cydd, Sid, Sidd, Syd,
Sydd

Cirrillo (Italian/Greek) lord.
Cirilio, Cirilio, Ciro, Cyrillo,
Cyrilo, Cryryllo, Cyrylo

Cisco (Spanish/Latin) freedom.
Cisca, Cysco

Clancy (Gaelic) belonging to the
family. (Ir) red-haired.
Clance, Clancee, Clancey, Clancie,
Clanse, Clansee, Clansey, Clansi,
Clansie, Clansy

Clarence (Latin) illustrious;
shining; famous.
Clair, Claire, Clairis, Claral,
Clarance, Clare, Clarin, Clarince,
Claron, Claronce, Claryn, Clarynce

Clark (Old French) learned scholar.
Clarke, Clarkson, Claxton

Clarkson (Old French) Clark's son;
son of the scholar.
Clarkeson, Claxton

Claude (Latin) weak.
Claud, Claudian, Claudianus,
Claudis, Claudio (Ital/Span),
Claudios, Claudius (Ger/Dut),
Claus, Clawd, Clawde, Clawed,
Cludell, Glade, Klaade, Klaud,
Klaude, Klaudij, Klaudio, Klaudius,
Klawd, Klawde

Claus (German/Greek) victory of
the people. A form of Nicholas.
Claas, Claes, Clause, Klaus, Klause

Clay (Old English) from the clay or
earth.
Clae, Claeborn, Claeborne,
Claebourn, Claebourne, Claeburn,
Claeburn, Clai, Claiborn,
Claiborne, Claiburn, Claiburne,
Claybourn, Claybourne, Clayburn,
Clayburne, Clayd, Cle, Clea, Clee

Claybourne (Old English) born of
clay or earth.
Clae, Claeborn, Claeborne,

Claybourne cont.
Claebourn, Claebourne, Claeburn,
Claeburn, Clai, Claiborn,
Claiborne, Claiburn, Claiburne,
Clay, Claybourn, Clayburn,
Clayburne, Clayd

Clayton (English) town built on clay.
Claeton, Claiton

Cleanth (Old English) pure; clean.
Clenth

Cleary (Irish/Gaelic) scholar;
knowledge.
Clearey, Cleari, Clearie

Cleavon (Old English) from the
cliff.
Cleavan, Cleaven, Cleaver, Cleavin,
Cleavlan, Cleavland, Cleavyn,
Clevan, Cleven, Clever, Clevin,
Cleveland, Clevon, Clevyn

Cledwyn (Welsh) blessed sword
friend.
Cledwin

Clement (Latin) mild; gentle.
Clemence (Fren), Clemens (Dan),
Clement (Fren), Clemente
(Ital/Span), Clementius (Dut),
Clemento (Ital), Clemon,
Clemmon, Clemmons, Kalman,
Kalmen, Kaloymous, Keleman,
Klemans, Klemen, Klemens (Ger),
Klement, Klemet, Klemin,
Klemonte, Kliementas, Klimt,
Klyment, Klymint, Klymynt

Cleon (Greek) famous.
Cleophus, Clio, Kleon

Cletus (Greek) illustrious; hard-
working.
Cleo, Cleon, Cleytus

Cleveland (Old English) from the
cliffed land.
Cleavlan, Cleavland, Cleon,
Cleven, Clevon

Cliff (Old English) from the cliff.
Clif, Cliffe, Clyf, Clyff, Clyffe, Clyfe

Clifford (Old English) from the
ford at the side of the cliff.
Cliffith, Clifton, Clyfford, Clyffton,
Clyford, Clyfton

Clifton (Old English) belonging to
the town near the cliff.
Cliffton, Clyffton, Clyfton

Clint/Clinton (English) from the
town on the hill. The short form
of Clinton.
Clindon, Clintan, Clinten, Clintin,
Clintwood, Clyndon, Clynt,
Clyntan, Clynten, Clyntin,
Clynton, Clyntwood

Clive (Old English) from the cliff.
Cleave, Cleavant, Cleavon, Cleeve,
Cleiv, Cleive, Cleveland, Clevland,
Cleyv, Cleyve, Clifford, Clifton,
Cliv, Clyv, Clyve

Clovis (Old German) famous
warrior.
Clodoveo (Span), Clovys

Cloyce (Middle English)
obstruction.
Clice, Cloice, Cloise, Cloyd, Cloyse

Clunies (Scottish/Gaelic) meadow
resting place.
Clunee, Clunees, Cluney, Cluneys,
Cluni, Clunie, Cluny

Clure (Latin) good fame.
Clur

Clyde (Scottish/Gaelic) high, rocky
area of land. (Ir) heard from afar.
Clide, Clydel, Clydell, Clyd

Clydri (Welsh) famous ruler.
Clidri, Clidry, Clydry

Cobham (Old English) from the
homestead near the river bend.
Cobbham

C

Coburn (Old English) where the streams meet.
Cobern, Coberne, Cobirn, Cobirne, Cobourn, Cobourne, Coburne, Coburnes, Cobyrn, Cobyrne, Cobbyrnes

Coby (Hebrew) replacer. The form of Jacob.
Cobe, Cobee, Cobey, Cobi, Cobie

Cochise (Apache) warrior; wood.
Cochyse

Coco (Spanish) coconut.
Coko, Koko

Cody (Old English) cushion; pillow. (Ir/Gae) helpful.
Codee, Codey, Codi, Codie

Coffie (Ewe) born on a Friday.
Cofi, Cofie

Coile (Gaelic) battle follower.
Coil, Coile, Coyle

Cola (Italian) victory of the people. A form of Nicholas.
Colah, Colar, Colas, Kola, Kolah, Kolas

Colbert (English) outstanding, brilliant sailor. (Fren) clearing through the mountains; valley.
Calbert, Calburt, Calvert, Colburt, Colvert, Culbert, Culvert

Colbrand (English) black sword; coal sword.
Brando, Colbran, Colbrando, Colbrandt, Colbrant

Colby (English) by the coal town; dark-haired.
Colbee, Colbert, Colbey, Colbi, Colbie

Cole (Celtic) promise. (M/Eng) coal.
Coal, Coale, Col, Colby, Coleman, Colier, Colman, Colson, Colton, Colville, Colvin

Coleman (English) charcoal worker.
Colemann, Colman, Colmann

Colin (Irish/Gaelic) young child. (Ir) peaceful dove. (O/Eng) from the coal pool.
Cailean, Colan, Collan, Cole, Colen, Collen, Collie, Collin, Collino, Collins, Colon, Collyn, Colyn, Nicolin (Fren/Grk)

Colley (Old English) black-haired one from the meadow.
Colea, Colee, Coleigh, Coley, Coli, Colie, Collea, Colleah, Collee, Colleigh, Colli, Collie, Collier, Colly, Coly

Collier (English) coal merchant; trader.
Colier, Colis, Collyer, Colyer

Collins (Greek) Colin's son; son from the coal pool. (Ir) holly.
Colin, Colins, Collin, Collyn, Collyns, Colyn, Colyns

Colson (English) Col's son; son of coal.
Colsan, Colsen, Colsin, Colsyn

Colt (English) frisky, young horse.
Colter, Coltrane, Coulter, Kolt, Kolter

Colter (English) herder of colts or horses.
Colt

Colton (English) from the black coal town.
Coltan, Colten, Coltin, Coltyn, Koltan, Kolten, Koltin, Kolton, Koltyn

Columba (Latin) dove.
Cailean (Scott), Coim, Colmicille, Colan, Colum, Columb, Columbah, Columbia (Lat), Columbias, Columbas, Columbus, Colym, Culva

Colwyn (Welsh) hazel grove.
(O/Eng) coal friend.
Colwin, Colwyne, Colwynn,
Colwynne

Coman (Arabic) noble. (Ir) bent.
Camen, Comin, Comyn

Compton (Old English) town in the
valley.
Comptom, Comton

Comyn (Irish) crooked.
Comin

Conal (Irish) high; mighty.
Conel, Conell, Conelle, Connal,
Connall, Connel, Connell,
Connelle, O'Conal, O'Conall,
O'Conel, O'Conell, O'Conelle

Conan (Celtic) wisdom; intelligence.
Conal, Conant, Conlan, Connal,
Conor, Kinan, Konan, Kynan

Coniah (Hebrew) gift sent from God.
Conia, Conya, Conyah

Conlan (Irish) hero.
Conland, Conlin, Conlon, Conlyn

Conn (Celtic) high.

Connor (Celtic) one with high will
and desire.
Conar, Coner, Connar, Conner,
Connaire, O'Conar, O'Coner,
O'Connar, O'Conner, O'Connor,
O'Conor

Conrad (Old German) bold, wise
counsel.
Coenraad (Dut), Cheudler (Swiss),
Conrade (Ital/Span), Conrado,
Conroy, Corradino (Ital), Currado
(Ital), Cort, Curt, Koeraad (Dut),
Konrad (Swed/Ger), Konradin,
Konratij, Kort (Ger), Kunad,
Kunds, Kunel, Kunrat, Kunsch, Kurt
(Ger), Quenes

Conroy (Irish) wisdom.
(Celt) persistent.
Conroi

Constant (Latin) steadfast; constant.
Constante

Constantine (Latin) little steadfast,
constant one.
Considine, Constain, Constance,
Constancio (Port), Constane,
Constant, Constantin
(Ger/Dan/Fren), Constantino
(Ital/Span), Constantinos,
Constantinus, Costin, Costino,
Curt, Custance, Kastaden,
Konstani, Konstantin (Swed),
Konstantine, Konstanty,
Konstantyn, Konstantyne

Conway (Welsh) holy water.
(Ir) hound from the plains.
Conwai

Cooba (Australian Aboriginal) black
bee.
Coobah

Cook (English) chef.
Cooki, Cookie, Cooky

Cooper (Old English) barrel maker.
Couper, Keupper, Kooper, Kuepper

Corbett (Old English) raven.
Corbet, Corbey, Corbin, Corwan,
Corwin, Corwyn, Corwyne,
Corwynne, Cory, Korbet, Korbett,
Korbin

Corbin (Old French) raven; dark-
haired.
Corban, Corben, Corbet, Corbett,
Corbyn, Corvin, Korban, Korben,
Korbin, Korbob, Korbyn

Cordell (Old French) little rope
marker from the valley.
Cordale, Cordel

C

Cordero (Spanish) little lamb.
Cordaro, Cordeal, Cordeara,
Cordearo, Cordeiro, Cordeiro,
Cordera, Corderal, Corderall,
Corderro, Corrderio, Coorderyo

Core (English) the chosen one.
Coree, Corey, Cori, Corie, Coree,
Correy, Corry, Curey, Currey, Curry

Corey/Cory (Irish) from the hollow;
head protection; helmet used for
battle.
Coree, Cori, Corie, Corki, Corkie,
Corky, Corree, Correy, Corri,
Corrick, Corrie, Corry, Cory, Koree,
Korey, Kori, Korie, Korree, Korrey,
Korri, Korrie, Korry, Kory

Corin (Greek) youthful.
Coran, Coren, Corine, Corron,
Corun, Coryn, Koran, Koren,
Korin, Koron, Koryn

Cormac (Gaelic) chariot racer.
(Grk) tree trunk.
Core, Corey, Cormack, Cormick,
MacCormack

Cormag (Scottish) raven.

Cornelius (Latin) horn colour; horn
blower; cornell tree.
Cornall, Corneille (Fren), Cornel,
Cornelio (Port/Span/Ital), Cornelis
(Dut), Cornell, Cornellus, Kornal,
Kornel, Kornelius, Korneliusz,
Kostelius, Neal, Neel, Neil, Neilus,
Neyl, Neylus

Cornwallis (English)
(Geographical) from Cornwall.
Cornwalis

Corowa (Australian Aboriginal)
rocky river.
Corowah

Corrigan (Irish) spear carrier.
Corigan, Corogan, Corrigon,

Corrigun, Corrogan, Corrogun,
Korrigan, Korrigun

Corrin (Irish) spear user.
Corin, Coren, Corren, Coryn,
Corryn, Koran, Koren, Korin,
Koron, Koryn

Cort (Old German/Old Norse) bold
court attendant.
Cortlan, Cortland, Court,
Courtenay (Fren), Courtlan,
Courtland, Courtney, Kort, Kortlan,
Kortland, Kourt, Kourtney

Cortez (Spanish) courteous.
Kortez

Corwin (Gaelic) from beyond the
hill. (O/Eng) friend of the heart.
Corwyn, Corwyne, Corwynn,
Korwin, Korwyn, Korwynn

Corydan (Irish/Hebrew) head
protection; helmet. (Ir) from the
hollow; God is my judge. A
combination of Cory/Dan.
Coridan, Coriden, Coridon,
Coridyn, Coryden, Corydin,
Corydon (Grk), Corydyn, Koridan,
Koriden, Koridin, Koridon,
Koridyn, Korydan, Koryden,
Korydin, Korydin, Korydon,
Korydyn

Cosgrove (Irish) from the cow
grove.

Cosmo (Greek) universal harmony.
Cosma, Cosmah, Cosmas (Grk),
Cosme (Fren), Cosimo (Ital/Span),
Cosmo (Grk), Cosmos, Kauzma,
Kosmas, Kosmo, Kosmos

Costa (Greek) little, constant,
steadfast one. The short form of
Constantine.
Costah, Costandinos,
Constantinos, Costas, Costes

Coty (French) from the slope.
Cotee, Cotey, Coti, Cotie, Cottee,
Cottey, Cotti, Cottie, Cotty

Count (Old French) companion;
friend; noble.
Counte, Countee

Courtenay (Old French) short-
nosed. (O/Eng) of the court.
Cortney, Courtney, Kortney,
Kourtney

Courtland (Old English) dweller at
the court land.
Cortlan, Cortland, Courtlan,
Kortlan, Kortland, Kourtlan,
Kourtland

Courtney (Old French) one who
lives near the farmstead.
Cortney, Courtenay (Fren),
Courtnay, Kortney, Kourtney

Covell (Old English) dweller at the
cave slope.
Covel

Covey (Old English) from the cove.
Covi, Covie, Covy

Covington (Old English) town with
a cove.
Covyngton

Cowan (Australian Aboriginal) from
the cow land. (M/Eng) hooded
robe. (Ir) hillside hollow.
Coe, Cowen, Cowin, Cowyn,
Cowle

Coy (Latin) shy; sweet; modest.
Coi, Coye

Coyan (French) modest.
Coian, Coin, Coine, Coyn, Coyne

Coyle (Irish) leader in the battle.
Coil, Coile

Craddock (Welsh) beloved.
Craddoc, Craddoch, Cradoc,
Cradock, Cradoch

Craig (Scottish) from the rock.
Craeg, Craege, Craegg, Crag,
Craige, Craigg, Crayg, Crayge,
Craygg, Creag, Creage, Creagh,
Creaghe, Crieg, Criege, Criegg,
Creyg, Creyge, Creygg, Kraig, Krayg

Cramer (Old English) to fill.
Crammer, Kramer, Krammer

Crandell (Old English) belonging
to the valley of the cranes.
Crandel

Crane (Old English) the crane bird.
Crain, Craine, Crandal, Crandall,
Crandel, Crandell, Crayn, Crayne

Cranley (Old English) from the
meadow of the cranes.
Cranlea, Cranleah, Cranlee,
Cranleigh, Cranli, Cranlie, Cranly

Cranog (Welsh) the heron, wading
bird with grey and white
plumage.
Kranog

Cranston (Old English) belonging
to the town of the cranes.
Crainston, Craynston

Crawford (Old English) from the
crow ford.
Craw, Crow, Crowford

Creed (Latin/English) one who
believes; kin.
Creedan, Creedance, Creeden,
Creedence, Creedin, Creedyn

Creek (English) from the small
stream; Native American tribal
name.

Creighton (English) from the town
close to the rocks.
Craighton, Crayton, Creighm,
Creight, Creighto, Creightow,
Creightown, Crichton, Crichtyn

C

Cremer (Middle English) merchant; trader.
Creamer, Kreamer, Kremer

Creon (Greek) prince; ruler.
Kreon

Crepin (French/Latin) curly-haired. A form of Crispin.
Crepyn

Cresswell (Old English) stream where cress grows.
Cresswel, Creswel, Creswell

Crevan (Irish) fox.
Creven, Crevin, Crevon, Crevyn

Crichton (Welsh) belonging to the hill-top town.
Creight, Creighton, Crighton, Cryghton

Crieghton (Middle English) dweller at the creek town.
Crayton, Creight, Crichton, Cryghton

Crisiant (Welsh) crystal.
Crisient, Crisyant, Crysiant, Crysyant, Krisiant, Krisient, Krysient, Krysyent

Crispin (Latin) curly-haired.
Crepin, Cresianus, Crispian, Crispinian, Crispino (Ital), Crispinianus, Crispinus, Crispo (Span), Crispus (Ger), Crispyn, Cryspyn, Krispijn (Dut), Krispin, Kryspyn

Croft (Old English) small pasture.
Crighton, Crite, Crofton, Kroft

Crofton (Irish) from the small pasture town with cottages.
Krofton

Cromwell (Old English) dweller at the winding stream.
Cromwel, Cromwill, Cromwyl, Cromwyll

Cronan (Irish) dark-brown-haired or complexioned. (Grk) companion; friend.
Kronan

Crosby (Old Norse) from the village with a cross. (O/Eng) dweller by the town crossing.
Crosbee, Crosbey, Crosbi, Crosbie

Crosley (Old English) belonging to the cross meadow.
Croslea, Crosleah, Croslee, Crosleigh, Crosli, Croslie, Crosly

Crowell (Old English) town crier.
Crawel, Crawell, Crowel, Crowil, Crowill, Crowyl, Crowyll

Cruz (Portuguese/Spanish) cross.
Cross, Cruzz, Kruz, Kruzz

Cullen (Old French) colony. (Ir) handsome.
Culen, Cullan, Culley, Cullin, Culyn

Culley (Irish/Gaelic) forest.
Culea, Culeah, Culee, Culey, Culi, Culie, Cullea, Culleah, Cullee, Culleigh, Culli, Cullie, Cully, Culy

Culver (Old English) dove of peace.
Colvar, Colver, Culvar

Cunningham (Irish) village with the milk pails.
Cunning

Curran (Irish) dagger; hero.
Curren, Currin, Curron

Curroon (Australian Aboriginal) fog on top of a mountain.

Currumbin (Australian Aboriginal) pine tree.
Currumbyn

Curruto (Spanish/French) courteous. (Lat) from the enclosure.
Curcio

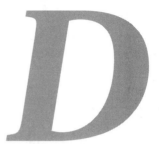

Curt (English) courtier; attendant at the court.
Court, Courtis, Courtys, Curtis, Curtys, Kurt, Kurtis

Curtis (Old French) courteous. (Lat) belonging to the courtyard.
Courtis, Curcio, Curt, Curtiss, Curtys, Curtyss, Kurtis, Kurtiss, Kurtys, Kurtyss

Cuthbert (English) brilliant.
Cuthberte, Cuthburt

Cutler (Old French) knife maker.
Cutlar, Cutlir, Cutlor, Kutler

Cuyler (Irish) chapel.
Cuiler

Cy (Persian) sun; throne. The short form of Cyrus.
Ci

Cynan (Welsh) chief.
Cinan, Cinen, Cinin, Cinon, Cinyn, Cynin, Cynon, Cynyn

Cyprian (Latin) from Cyprus.
Cipriano (Span), Cyprianus, Cyprien (Fren), Cyprrian

Cyr (French) Sunday's child; born on Sunday.
Cyrano, Cyriack, Syriack

Cyrano (Greek) from Cyrene.
Cirano

Cyril (Greek) lordly ruler.
Ciril (Illy), Cirill, Cirille, Cirillo (Ital), Cirilo (Span), Ciro, Cyriack, Cyril, Cyrill (Ger/Fren), Cyrille, Cyrillus, Cyro, Cyrrils (Port), Cyrus, Cyryl (Pol), Girigel, Girioel, Gwril, Keereel, Kiril, Kyril, Kyrillos, Kyryl, Syriack, Vashka

Cyrus (Persian) sun; throne.
Ciro, Cyrie, Cyro, Kyros

Dabi (Basque/Hebrew) beloved. A form of David.
Dabee, Dabey, Dabie, Daby

Dabir (Arabic) tutor.
Dabar, Daber, Dabor, Dabyr

Dace (English/French) of nobility.
Dacee, Dacey, Daci, Dacie, Dacio, Dacy, Daic, Daice, Dayc, Dayce

Dacey (Irish/Gaelic) southerner.
Dacee, Daci, Dacie, Dacy, Daice, Daicee, Daicey, Daici, Daicie, Daicy, Dayce, Daycee, Dacycey, Dayci, Daycie, Daycy

Dada (Yoruba) curly-haired.
Dadah, Dadi

Daegan (Irish/Gaelic) black-haired.
Daegen, Daegin, Daegon, Daegyn, Dagan, Daigan, Daigen, Daigin, Daigin, Daigyn. Daygan, Daygen, Daygin, Daygon, Daygyn

Daegel (English) (Geographical) from Daegel in England.
Daigel, Daygel

Dafydd (Welsh/Hebrew) beloved. A form of David.
Dafid, Dafidd, Dafyd

Dagan (Eastern Semitic) little fish.
Dagen, Dagin, Dagon, Dagyn

Dagda (Irish/Gaelic) good spirit.
Dagdah

D

Dago (Spanish) day.
Darg (Ice), Tag, Tajo

Dagwood (Old English) from the bright one's forest; daggerwood.

Dahy (Irish) swift moving.
Daiy

Dai (Japanese) large.
Dae, Dai, Daie, Daye

Dakarai (Shona) happy.
Dakara

Dakota (Native American) friend.
Dakotah

Daksh (Hindi) efficient.
Dakshi

Dal (Scandinavian) from the valley.
Dail, Daile, Dale, Dayl, Dayle

Dalal (Sanskrit) broker.

Dalbert (Old English) pride.
Dalbirt, Dalburt, Dalbyrt, Delbert, Delbirt, Delburt, Delbyrt

Dale (Old English) from the valley.
Adale, Dael, Dail, Dal, Daley

Dallan (Irish) unseeing.
Daelan, Daelen, Daelin, Dailan, Dailen, Dailin, Dalan, Dalain, Dallen, Dallin, Dallyn, Dalyn

Dallas (Scottish) from the waterfall valley.
Dallis, Dallus, Dallys

Dalman (Australian Aboriginal) from the place of plenty.
Dallman, Dallmen, Dallmin, Dallmon, Dallmyn, Dalmen, Dalmin, Dalmon, Dalmyn

Dalphin (French) dolphin.
Dalphine, Dalphyn, Dalphyne, Dolphin, Dolphine, Dolphyn, Dolphyne

Dalston (English) from Dale's town; from the valley town.
Dalis, Dallas, Dallen, Dallin, Dallon, Dallston, Dallyn

Dalton (Old English) from the town in the valley.
Dalltan, Dallten, Dalltin, Dallton, Dalltyn, Daltan, Dalten, Daltin, Daltyn

Dalziel (Scottish) from the small field.
Dalzil, Dalzyel, Dalzyl

Damario (Spanish) gentle.
Damaryo, Demario, Demaryo

Damek (Slavic)/(Hebrew) of the red earth. A form of Adam.
Adamek, Damik, Damyk

Damian (Greek) tamer.
Damien (Fren), Damiano (Ital), Damiao (Port), Damion (Grk), Damionos (Grk), Damyan, Damyen, Damyin, Damyon, Damyyn

Damon (Greek) one who tames; constant. (Lat) spirit.
Daemian, Daemien, Daemiin, Daemion, Daemiyn, Daimian, Daimien, Daimiin, Daimion, Daimiyn, Damas, Damian (Ger), Damiano (Ital), Damien (Fren), Damion, Damiyn, Daymian, Daymien, Daymiin, Daymion, Daymiyn

Dan (Hebrew) God is my judge.
Dann

Dana (Irish) fire. (O/Eng) bright day; from Denmark.
Daha, Dahanah, Danah, Danne

Dancel (Dutch) God is my judge.
Dansel, Dansil, Dansyl

D

Dandin (Hindi) holy.
Dandan, Danden, Dandon, Dandyn

Dandre (French/Greek) strong; brave; courageous. A form of Andre/Andrew.
D'Andre, Dandrae, Dandras, Dandray, Dandrea

Dane (Danish) from Denmark.
Daen, Daene, Dain, Daine, Dayn, Dayne

Danforth (English/Hebrew) God is my judge.

Daniel (Hebrew) God is my judge.
Dancel, Dancil, Dane, Daneel (Dut), Danelo, Danielle (Fren), Daniil (Rus), Danil, Danila (Slav), Danilo, Danjels (Lett), Dannal, Dannel (Swiss), Dannil, Dannol, Danyel, Danyell, Danyil, Danyill, Danyl, Danyll, Tanel, Taniel, Tanyel, Tanyell

Danior (Gypsy) born with teeth.
Danyor

Danladi (Hausa) born on a Sunday.
Danladee, Danladey, Danladie, Danlady

Dannon (English/American) gathering in the meadow.
Daenan, Daenen, Dainon, Danaan, Danen, Dannan, Dannen, Dannin, Danno (Jap), Dannon, Dannyn, Danon, Danyn

Danny (Hebrew/English) God is my judge. A short form of names starting with 'Dan' e.g. Daniel.
Danee, Daney, Dani, Danie, Dannee, Danney, Danni, Dannie, Danno, Dano, Dany

Dante (Italian/Spanish) enduring. A form of Durante.
Dantae, Dantee

Danyon (Old English/Hebrew) God is my judge.
Danion

Dar (Hebrew) pearl.
Darr

Dara (Cambodian) star.
Darah

Darby (Irish) freedom. (Scan) from the deer estate.
Darbe, Darbee, Darbey, Darbi, Darbie, Derbe, Derbee, Derbey, Derbi, Derbie, Derby

Darcy (Irish) dark-haired. (Fren) fortress.
Darce, Darcee, Darcey, Darci, Darcie, D'Arcy, D'arcy, Darse, Darsee, Darsey, Darsi, Darsie, Darsy

Dareh (Persian) wealthy.
Dare

Darel (Australian Aboriginal) blue sky.
Daral, Daril, Darol, Darral, Darrel, Darril, Darrol, Darryl, Daryl

Daren (Nigerian) born at night.
Daran, Darin, Daron, Daryn

Darence (Irish) great. A form of Darren, gift. (Eng) rocky hill.
Darance, Darrance, Darrence

Darile (Australian Aboriginal) rosella parrot.
Darel, Darele, Daryl, Daryle

Darin (Greek) gift.
Darian, Darien, Dario (Span), Darion (Span), Darrian, Darrin, Darryn, Daryn, Daryo (Span), Dayrin, Dayrinn, Dearin, Dharin, Dharyn

Dario (Spanish) wealthy.
Darion, Daryo

D

Darius (Persian) ruler.
(Grk) wealthy.
Dairus, Darieus, Dario, Darrios,
Darioush, Darrias, Darrious,
Darris, Darrius, Darrus, Darus,
Daryos, Daryus, Derius, Derieus,
Derio, Derrious, Derris, Derrius,
Derryus, Deryus

Darkon (Old English) dark one.
Darkan, Darken, Darkin, Darkun,
Darkyn

Darnell (English) hidden.
Darnel, Darnele, Darnelle

Darren (Irish/Gaelic/Australian/New
Zealand) gift.
Daran, Daren, Darian, Darien,
Darin, Darion, Daron (Ir), Darran,
Darrian, Darrick (Ger), Darrien,
Darrin, Darryn, Darun, Daryn,
Darran, Darrin, Darrion (Ir),
Darron, Darrun, Darryn, Deran,
Deren, Derin, Deron, Derun,
Derran, Derran, Derrian, Derrin,
Derron, Derrun, Derryn, Deryn

Darrie (Irish) red-haired one.
Dari, Darie, Darry, Dary

Darryl/Darrel/Daryl (French) little
darling from the oak-tree grove. A
form of Darren, gift.
Dahril, Daral, Darall, Daralle,
Darel, Darele, Darell, Darelle,
Daril, Darile, Darill, Darille,
Darral, Darrel, Darril, Darryl,
Darryl, Daryl, Daryle, Deril, Derol,
Derril, Derryl, Deryl, Deryle,
Deryll, Derylle

Darshan (Hindi) God.
Darshen, Darshin, Darshon,
Darshyn

Darton (English) from the deer
town.
Dartal, Dartan, Dartei, Dartrel,
Darten, Dartin, Dartyn

Darvell (English/French) from the
town of eagles.
Darvel, Darvele, Darvelle, Darvil,
Darvile, Darvill, Darville, Darvyl,
Darvyle

Darvin (French/Old English)
beloved, dearest, famous sea
friend.
Darvan, Darven, Darvon, Darvyn

Darwin (Old English) beloved,
dearest friend.
Darwen, Darwyn, Derwen, Derwin,
Derwyn

Dasan (Pomo) bird-clan leader;
chief.
Dasen, Dasin, Dason, Dasyn

Daudi (Swahili) loved one.
Dawud

David (Hebrew) beloved.
Dabit, Daeved, Daevid, Daevyd,
Daibiah (Scott), Daived, Daivid,
Daivyd, Dako, Datsch, Dauld
(Swa),Daveon, Davidas, Davidd,
Davidde (Ital), Davide (Fren),
Davidos, Davidos, Davidus, Daviel,
Daviot, Davood (Arab), Davyd,
Davydd, Davyde, Davydas (Lith),
Davydos, Davydus, Davyn, Dawed
(Pol), Dawfydd, Dawudd (Arab),
Deinion (O/Wel), Deved, Devid,
Devidd, Devidde, Devyd, Devydd,
Devydde, Devod, Devodd, Toveli,
Taffi, Taffie, Taffy, Tafi, Tafie, Tafy

Davin (Scandinavian) bright, happy
person from Finland.
Davan, Daven, Davon, Davyn

Davis (English) son of David; son
of the beloved.
Davidson, Davies, Davison, Davys,
Davyson, Dawsan, Dawsen,
Dawsin, Dawson, Dayson, Dayton

Davorin (Slavic) of the war God, Davor.
Davoran, Davoren, Davoron, Davoryn

Dawit (Hebrew) beloved. A form of David.
Dawyt

Dawson (English) David's son; son of the beloved.
Dawsan, Dawsen, Dawsin, Dawsyn

Dax (French/English) water.

Dayan (Hebrew) judge. (O/Eng) day's end.
Daean, Daian

Daylon (African American) the day is long.
Daelon, Dailon

Dayne (Scandinavian) from Denmark.
Daen, Daene, Dain, Daine, Dane, Dain, Daine, Dayn

Dayton (English) from the sunny town.
Daeton, Daiton

De (Chinese) virtuous.

Deacon (Greek/English) dusty, hard-working servant.
Deakin, Deicon, Dekel, Dekle, Deycon

Dean (Old English) one who lives in the valley.
Deam, Deame, Deane, Deen, Deene, Deme, Dene, Dino (Ital/Span), Dyn, Dyne

Deandre (French/Greek) strong, brave, courageous one from the valley. (Lat) divine. The combination of Dean/Andre.
Deenandre, Deiandre, Dayandre

Deangelo (Italian/Greek) angel; messenger of God.
Dangelo, Danglo, Deaenglo, Deanglo, Diangelo, Diangello, Dyangello, Dyangelo

Dearborn (English) born near the stream with the deer.
Dearborne, Dearbourn, Dearbourne, Deerborn, Deerborne, Deerbourn, Deerbourne

Decarlos (Spanish/English) strong; courageous. A form of Charles.
Dacarlo, Dacarlos, Decarlo, Dicarlo, Daycarlo

Decha (Thai) strength.
Dech, Dechah

Decimus (Latin) tenth-born child.
Decymus

Declan (Irish) praying.
Daclan, Diclan, Dyclan

Dedrick (German) the people's ruler.
Deadric, Deardick, Dederic, Dederick, Dederik, Dedryc, Dedryck, Dedryk, Dedryk, Diedri, Diedrick, Diedrik, Dietrich, Detric, Detrick, Detrik

Deemer (Old English) judge.
Deamer, Deimer, Deymer

Deems (English) the judge's child.
Deam, Deama, Deim, Deima, Deym, Deyms

Defrain (Australian Aboriginal) mountains.
Derain, Derayn, Derayne

Dejuan (Spanish/Hebrew) God is gracious. A form of John.
Dejan, Dejon, Dejun, Dewan, Dewaun, Dewon, Dijaun, Dwon

Dekel (Hebrew/Arabic) palm tree.
Dekal, Dekil, Dekyl

D

Del (French) of the (used as a prefix to other names). (O/Eng) from the wood hollow.
Dell

Delaney (French/Irish) of the elder-tree grove.
Delan, Delain, Delainey, Delaini, Delanie, Delano (Fren), Delany

Delano (Old French) of the night. (Lat) alder grove.

Delbert (English) noble; bright.
Dalbert, Dalbirt, Dalburt, Dalbyrt, Delbirt, Delburt, Delbyrt

Delfino (Latin) dolphin.
Delfin, Delfine, Delfyn, Delfyne, Delfyno, Delphin, Delphine, Delphino, Delphyn, Delphyne, Delphyne

Deli (Chinese) virtuous.
Deshi

Dell (English) of the small valley; wood hollow.
Del

Dellinger (Scandinavian) from the day-time spring.

Delmar (Latin/Old French) of the sea.
Delmer

Delmon (English/French) of the mountain.
Dalman, Dalmen, Dalmin, Dalmon, Dalmyn, Delman, Delmen, Delmin, Demond, Delmyn

Delroy (French) of the king.
Dalroi, Dalroy, Delroi

Delsin (Native American) truthful.
Delsan, Delsen, Delson, Delsyn

Delton (English) of the valley town.
Daltan, Dalten, Daltin, Dalton, Daltyn, Deltan, Delten, Deltin, Deltown, Deltyn

Delvin (English) Godly friend.
Dalvin, Dalvyn, Delvyn

Dema (Russian) calmness.
Demah

Deman (Dutch) the man.
Demann

Dembe (Luganda) peace.
Damba

Demetrios (Greek) covering of earth; of Demeter, goddess of fertility. The masculine form of Demetria.
Demetre (Fren), Demetri, Demetrio (Ital), Demetrius, Demetryus, Dimiter, Dimitrij, Dimitrije, Dimitry, Dmitar, Dmitri (Russ), Dymetree, Dymetrey, Dymetri, Dymytrie, Dymetrias, Dymetrius, Dymetriys, Dymetryas, Dymetryus

Demos (Greek) people.
Demas, Demosthenes, Demous

Demothi (Native American) talks while walking.
Demoth

Dempsey (Irish) proud.
Dempsi, Dempsie, Dempsy

Dempster (Old English) judge.
Dempstar

Denby (Old English) by the valley.
Danbi, Danbie, Danby, Denbey, Denbi, Denbie

Denell (African American/Hebrew) God is my judge. A masculine form of Danielle.
Denel

Denham (Old English) from the valley homestead.
Denhem

Denis/Dennis (Greek) follower of Dionysos, the god of wine; celebration.
Danas, Dannis, Dannys, Denas, Denes, Denet, Dennas, Dennet, Dennett, Dennison, Denny, Dennys, Dienes, Dion, Dionigi (Ital), Dionigio (Ital), Dionigo, Dionis (Span), Dionisio (Ital/Span), Dionissy (Rus), Dionizas (Lith), Dionizy (Pol), Dionysio (Port), Dionysios, Dionysus (Ger), Divis (Boh), Dynas, Dynes, Dyness, Dynis, Dyniss, Dynys, Dynyss, Tafi, Tafie, Taffi, Taffie, Taffy, Tafy, Teenis, Tenis, Trents, Zdenek

Denley (English) from the meadow in the valley.
Denlea, Denleah, Denlee, Denli, Denlie, Denly

Denman (Old English) from the valley.
Denmen

Dennison (English) son of Denis; son of the follower of Dionysus, the god of wine; celebration.
Denison, Dennyson, Denyson

Denny (Greek) follower of Dionysus, the god of wine; celebration.
Deni, Denie, Denni, Dennie, Deny

Denton (English) of the valley town.
Dentown

Denvor (Old English) from the valley village.
Denver

Denzel (Cornish) high; from the stronghold in the valley.
Denzal, Denzall, Denzalle, Denzell, Denzelle, Denzil, Denzill, Denzille, Denzyl, Denzyll, Denzylle

Denzo (Japanese) discretion.
Denzio, Denzyo

Dequan (Comanche) fragrant; sweet smelling.
Dequanah

Derek (Teutonic) gifted ruler of the people.
Darec, Dareck, Darek, Daric, Darick, Darric, Darrick, Darryc, Darryck, Darryk, Derec, Dereck, Deric, Derick, Derik, Derrec, Derreck, Derrek, Derric, Derrick, Derrik, Deryc, Deryck, Deryk, Derryc, Derryck, Derryk, Diederich (Ger), Dirc, Dirck, Dirk, Dyrc, Dyrck, Dyrk, Dyrrc, Dyrrck, Dyrrk, Dyrryc, Dyrryck, Dyrryk, Dyryc, Dyryck, Dyryk

Dermot (Irish) freedom.
Dermott, Dermont, Diarmid, Diarmit

Deron (Hebrew) bird.
Daaron, Daron, Darone, Darron, Dayron, Dereon, Deronn, Deronne, Derrin, Derrion, Derron, Derronn, Derronne, Derryn, Deryn, Diron, Duron, Durron, Dyron

Deror (Hebrew) freedom lover.
Derori, Derorie, Derory

Derrilin (Australian Aboriginal) falling stars.
Derilin, Derylin, Derylyn

Derry (Irish) red-haired.
Deri, Derie, Derri, Derrie, Dery

Derryn (Welsh) little bird.
Alderin, Alderyn, Derran, Derren, Derrin, Derron, Derrun, Deryn

D

Derward (English) keeper of the deer.
Derwood, Dirward, Dirwood, Durward, Durwood, Dyrward, Dyrwood

Derwin (Welsh) dear friend.
Dervin, Dervon, Dervyn, Dervyne, Derwyn, Derwyne, Durwin, Durwyn, Durwyne

Derwood (English) from the deer wood.
Derward, Durward, Durwood

Deshawn (Hebrew/African American) God is gracious. A form of Shaun.
Dasean, Dashaun, Dashwn, Desean, Deshaun, Deshaune, Deshauwn, Deshawan, D'Sean, D'Shaun, D'Shawn, Dusean, Dushaun, Dushawn, Dysean, Dyshaun, Dyshawn, Dyshon, Dyshone, Dyshyn, Dyshyne

Desi (Latin) yearning.
Dezi

Desiderio (Spanish) desired.
Desideryo

Desmond (Irish/Gaelic) from South Munster.
Desmund, Dezmond, Dezmund

Destin (French) fate. The masculine form of Destiny.
Destan, Desten, Destine, Deston, Destun, Destyn

Deutsch (German) from Germany.
Deutch

Deven (Hindi) for God.
Deaven, Deiven, Diven, Dyven

Devin/Devon (Irish) poet. (Lat) perfection. (O/Eng) from Devonshire; people of the deep valley.
Deavan, Deaven, Deavin, Deavon, Deavyn, Devan, Deven, Devon, Devun, Devyn

Devine (Latin) divine. (Ir) ox.
Devyn, Devyne

Devlin (Irish) fierce; brave.
Devlan, Devland, Devlen, Devlend, Devlind, Devlyn, Devlynd

Dewei (Chinese) highly virtuous.
Dewey

Dewey (English) morning dew.
Dewi, Dewie, Dewy, Duey, Duie

Dewitt (Flemish) blond-haired.
Dewit, Dewyt, Dewytt, Dwight

Dexter (Latin) dexterous; skilful, right-handed.
Dexta, Dextar, Dextor, Dextur

Diamond (Greek/English) diamond; precious.
Dymond

Dian (Indonesian) candle.
Dyan

Didier (French) desired. The masculine form of Desiree.
Didyer

Diego (Spanish/Hebrew) replacer. A form of James.
Iago, Diaz, Jago

Dieter (German) the people's army.
Deyter, Diehardt (Teut), Deirhard, Dihard, Dihardt, Dyehard, Dyehardt, Dyhard, Dyhardt

Dietman (Teutonic) man of the people.
Dyetman

Dietrich (Teutonic) wealthy; powerful.
Detric, Detrich, Didhrikr, Didric, Didrick, Didschis (Let), Diedric, Diedrich, Diedrik (Dut), Dierk

Dietrich cont.
(Dut), Dieterico (Ital), Dietl, Dietz, Dippolt, Ditrik, Dyterych

Digby (Old Norse) from the farm by the ditch.
Digbe, Digbee, Digbey, Digbi, Digbie

Diggory (Cornish) almost lost. (O/Eng) digger.
Diggori, Diggorie, Digori, Digorie, Digory

Dilgon (Australian Aboriginal) like the moon.
Dylgon

Dillon (French) like a lion. (Ir) faithful.
Dilan, Dilen, Dillan, Dillen, Dilon, Dillyn, Dilyn, Dylan, Dylen, Dyllan, Dyllen, Dyllin, Dyllon, Dyllyn, Dylyn

Dilwyn (Welsh) from the place with the shady trees.
Dillwin, Dillwyn, Dilwin, Dilwyn

Dima (Russian) famous prince; form of Vladimir.
Dimah, Dimka, Dimkah, Dyma, Dymah

Dimiter/Dimitri (Greek) covering of earth; of Demeter, goddess of fertility.
Demetra, Demetri, Demitri, Dhimitrios, Dimitra, Dimetri, Dimetric, Dimetrie, Dimetrios, Dimetrius, Dimetrus, Dimitr, Dimitricus, Dimitrij (Rus), Dimitrije (Illy), Dimitris, Dimitrios, Dimitrius, Dimitry, Dymiter, Dymitri, Dymitr, Dymitry, Dymyter

Dinh (Vietnamese) peace.
Din, Dyn, Dynh

Dinko (Slavic) born on Sunday.
Dincko, Dyncko, Dynko

Dino (Italian/Spanish) from the valley. A form of Dean.
Diandre, Dinos (Grk), Dionte, Diondre, Dondre, Dyno, Dynos, Dynot

Dinsmore (Irish) from the fortress hill.
Dinmoar, Dinmoor, Dinmoore, Dinmor, Dinmore, Dinsmoor, Dinsmoore, Dynmoar, Dynmoor, Dynmoore, Dynmor, Dynmore

Diomedes (Greek) belonging to Media.
Dyomedes

Dion (Greek) god of wine; celebration. A short form of Dionysus.
Deon, Dio, Dione, Dionigi, Dionis, Dionn, Dionne, Dionta, Diontae, Dionte, Diontai, Diontray, Dyon, Dyone

Dionysus (Greek) god of wine; celebration.
Dion, Dionesios, Dionicio, Dionisios, Dionusios, Dionysios, Dionysius, Dyonisios, Dyonisus, Dyomysus, Dunixi

Dirk (German) wealthy. The German form of Theodore. A form of Derek, gifted ruler of the people.
Derc, Derck, Derk, Dirc, Dirck, Dirke, Dyrc, Dyrk

Dix (German) blessed.
Dixx

Dixon (English) son of the rich, powerful ruler. A form of Richard.
Dixan, Dixen, Dixin, Dixyn, Dyxan, Dyxen, Dyxin, Dyxon, Dyxyn

Doane (Irish) poem. (O/Eng) from down the hill. (Eng/Heb) graceful deer.
Doan

Dobry (Polish) good one.
Dobri, Dobrie

Dohasan (Kiowa) cliff.

Doherty (Irish) harm.
Docherty, Dougherty, Douherty

Dolan (Irish) dark; bold.
Dollan

Dolph (German) noble, fierce wolf.
Dolf, Dolff, Dolffe, Dolfe, Dolphe, Dolphus (Teut), Dulph, Dulphe

Dom (Latin) of the Lord. The short form of Dominic.
Domm

Domenic (Latin) of the Lord.
Domenick, Domenik, Dominic, Dominick (Lat), Dominik, Domingo, Dominique (Fren), Domokos (Hung), Domenyc, Domenyck, Domenyk

Domingo (Spanish) born on a Sunday.
Domyngo

Don (Celtic/English/American/Australian/New Zealand) little ruler. The short form of names starting with 'Don' e.g. Donald.
Donn

Donahue (Gaelic) brown-haired warrior.
Donahu, Donahugh, Donehue, Donohoe, Donohu, Donohue, Donohugh

Donald (Celtic) ruler of the world.
Domnal, Domnall, Donal (Ir), Donalds, Donel, Doneld, Donil, Donild, Donyl, Donyld

Donatien (French) gift.
Donathan, Donathon, Donato (Ital), Donatyen

Donato (Spanish/Italian) gift from God.
Doneto

Donegal (Irish) fort of foreigners.
Donigal, Donygal

Donkor (Akan) humble.
Donko

Donnell (Irish) brave, dark-haired one.
Doneal, Donel, Donell, Donelle, Donelly, Doniel, Donielle, Donnel, Donnelle, Donniel, Donnyl, Donyl

Donny (Irish/Scottish) proud ruler. The short form of names starting with 'Don' e.g. Donald.
Donee, Doney, Doni, Donie, Donnee, Donney, Donni, Donnie, Dony

Donovan (Celtic) dark-haired warrior.
Donavan, Donaven, Donavin, Donavyn, Donevan, Donevin, Donevon, Donyvon

Dooley (Irish) dark hero.
Doolea, Dooleah, Dooleigh, Dooli, Doolie, Dooly

Dor (Hebrew) generation.

Dorak (Australian Aboriginal) lively.
Dorek, Dorik, Doryk

Doran (Irish) stranger. (Grk) gift.
Doren, Dorin, Doron, Dorran, Dorren, Dorrin, Dorron, Dorryn, Doryn

Dore (Celtic) stream.
Dor

Dorian (Greek) gift.
Doran, Dorien, Dorran, Dorrance, Dorren, Dorrin, Dorryn, Doryn

Dorrell (Scottish) the keeper of the king's door.
Dorrel, Dorrelle, Durel, Durell, Durelle

Dory (French) golden.
Doree, Dorey, Dori, Dorie

Dotan (Hebrew) law.
Dothan

Doug (Gaelic/Irish) dark stranger from the dark-blue stream. A short form of Douglas.
Douge, Dougee, Dougey, Dougi, Dougie, Dougy, Dug, Dugee, Dugey, Dugi, Dugie, Dugy

Dougal (Gaelic/Irish) dark stranger from the dark-blue stream. A short form of Douglas.
Doogal, Doogall, Dougall, Dougie, Douglass, Dugald, Duglass

Douglas (Gaelic/Irish) dark stranger from the dark-blue stream.
Douglass, Duglass

Dov (Hebrew) bear. (Eng) dove, bird of peace. The Hebrew form of David, beloved.
Dove, Dovi, Dovid, Dovidas, Dowld

Dover (Hebrew) water; speaker.
Dova, Dovah, Dove, Dovor

Doyle (Irish) dark stranger.
Doial, Doiale, Doiall, Doil, Doile, Dotal, Dotel, Doyal, Doyel, Doyele, Doyell, Doyelle

Dragan (Slavic) dear.
Dragen, Dragin, Dragon, Dragyn

Dragoslav (Slavic) dear glory.

Drake (Old English) dragon; male duck.
Draek, Drago (Ital), Draik, Draike, Drayk, Drayke

Draper (English) fabric or curtain maker.
Draeper, Draiper, Drayper

Dreng (Norwegian) brave friend.

Drew (Gaelic) strong, brave, courageous one. The short form of Andrew.
Drewe, Dru, Drue

Driscoll (Irish) one who interprets.
Driscol, Driscole, Dryscol, Dryscoll, Dryscolle

Drover (Australian) sheep or cattle herder.
Drova, Drovah, Drove, Drovir, Drovor, Drovyr

Drummond (Scottish) from the mountain of the Druids.
Drummund, Drumond, Drumund

Drury (English/French) beloved.
Druree, Drurey, Druri, Drurie

Dryden (English) from the dry valley.
Dridan, Driden, Dridin, Dridyn, Drydan, Drydin, Drydon, Drydyn

Duane/Dwayne (Irish) dark one.
Dewain, Dewan, Dewane, DeWayne, Dewayne, Duane, Dwain, Dwaine, Dwayn, DWayne (Gae)

Duarte (Portuguese) prosperous guardian. The Portuguese form of Edward, wealthy guardian.
Duart

Dubham (Celtic) black.
Dubhem, Dubhim, Dubhom, Dubhym

D

Dubric (Old English) black ruler.
Dubrick, Dubrik, Dubryc, Dubryck,
Dubryk

Duc (Vietnamese) moral.
Duoc, Duy

Dudley (Old English) from the
meadow.
Dudlea, Dudleah, Dudlee,
Dudleigh, Dudli, Dudlie, Dudly

Dudon (Italian) given from God.
Dudan, Duden, Dudin, Dudun,
Dudyn

Duer (Scottish) hero.

Duff (Gaelic) black-haired.
Duf

Dugan (Gaelic) dark-haired.
Doogan, Doogen Dougan,
Dougen, Douggan, Douggen,
Dugen

Duke (Old French) leader.
Duk

Dukker (Gypsy) teller of fortunes.
Duker

Dulani (Ngoni) cutter.
Dulanee, Dulaney, Dulanie,
Dulany

Duman (Turkish) mist.
Dumen, Dumin, Dumon, Dumyn

Dumont (French) of the mountains.
Duemont

Duncan (Old English) brown-haired
warrior.
Doncan, Dunkan

Dunham (Old English) from the
brown homestead.
Dunhem

Dunley (Old English) from the
brown, hilly meadow.
Dunlea, Dunleah, Dunlee,
Dunleigh, Dunli, Dunlie, Dunly

Dunlop (Old English) from the
brown, mud hill.
Dunlope

Dunmore (Old English) from the
brown moor fort.
Dumoar, Dunmoor, Dunmoore,
Dunmor

Dunn (Scottish) brown-haired.
Dun, Dunne

Dunstan (Old English) from the
brown hill stone.
Dunsten, Dunstin, Dunston,
Dunstyn

Dunton (English) from the brown
hill town.
Duntan, Dunten, Duntin, Duntyn

Dural (Australian Aboriginal) hollow
from where smoke is rising.
Durel, Duril, Duryl

Durant (Latin) enduring.
Dant, Dante, Duran, Durance,
Durand, Durante, Durontae,
Durrant

Durbin (Latin/Gaelic) city dweller.
Durban, Durben, Derbon, Derbun,
Durbyn

Dureau (French) strength.
Durea

Durril (Gypsy) gooseberry.
Duril, Durryl, Durryll, Duryl

Durward (Old English) keeper of
the door.
Derward, Durwood

Dusan (Czech) spirited.
Dusen, Dusin, Duson, Dusyn

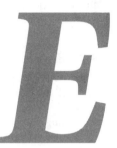

Dustin (Teutonic/Old English) warrior.
Dustan, Dusten, Duston, Dustyn

Dusty (English) covered in dust. The short form of Dustin, warrior.
Dustee, Dustey, Dusti, Dustie

Duval (French) of the valley.
Duvall, Duveuil, Duvyl

Dwade (English) dark-haired traveller.
Dwaid, Dwaide, Dwayd, Dwayde

Dwight (Gaelic) white. (Scand) valiant.
Dwhite, Dwite, Dwyte

Dyami (Native American) eagle soaring.
Dyani

Dyer (English) dyer of fabric.
Dier

Dylan (Celtic) from the sea.
Dilan, Dilen, Dilin, Dillan, Dillen, Dillin, Dillon, Dillyn, Dilyn, Dylane, Dylen, Dylin, Dyllan, Dylon, Dylyn

Dymock (Old Welsh) pig sty.
Dimock

Dyre (Danish) dear.
Dire

Ea (Irish/German) brilliant; famous.
Eah

Eachan (Irish) works with horses.
Eachen, Eachin, Eachon, Eachyn, Egan, Egen, Egin, Egon, Egyn

Eamon (Irish/English) wealthy protector.
Eaman, Eamen, Eamin, Eamman, Eammen, Eammin, Eammon, Eammun, Emmyn, Eamun, Eamyn, Eiman, Eimen, Eimin, Eimon, Eimyn, Etman, Eymen, Eymin, Eymon, Eymyn

Ean (English/Scottish) God is gracious. A form of Ian.
Eaen, Eann, Eion, Eon, Eonn, Eyan, Eyen, Eyon, Eyyn, Ian

Earl (Irish) promise. (Eng) noble one.
Airle, Earld, Earle, Earli, Earlie, Earlson, Early, Eorl, Erral, Errel, Erril, Errol, Erryl, Eryl

Earnest (English) sincere.
Earneste, Earnesto, Eirnest, Eranest, Ernest, Erneste, Ernist, Ernyst, Eyrnest

Earvin (English) friend of the sea. A form of Irving.
Earving, Ervin, Erving, Ervyn, Ervyng

Easter (Hebrew) born at Easter time.

Easton (English) from the eastern town.
Eason, Eastan, Easten, Eastin, Eastyn

Eaton (English) from the estate town by the river.
Eatton, Eton, Eyton

Ebal (Hebrew) naked.
Ebale

Eben (Hebrew) rock.
Eban, Ebenn, Ebin, Ebon, Ebyn

Ebenezer (Hebrew) stone foundation.
Ebbaneza, Eben, Ebeneezer, Ebeneser, Ebenezar, Evanezer, Eveneser, Ibenezer

Eber (Hebrew) overcomes problems.

Eberhard (German) courageous boar.
Eberhardt, Evard, Everard, Everardo, Everart, Everhardt, Everhart

Ebilo (German) hardy boar.
Ebbo, Ebert, Ebylo

Ebner (English/Hebrew) father of light.
Abnar, Abner, Abnor, Ebnar, Ebnir, Ebnor, Ebnyr

Ebo (Fanti) born on a Tuesday.
Ebot

Eborico (Spanish) wild boar king.
Eboryco

Ebrulf (Teutonic) wild, fierce wolf.

Eccelino (Italian) like his father.
Eccelyno

Eckhardt (German) firm; formidable.
Eckart, Eckhard

Ed (English) success. The short form of names starting with 'Ed' e.g. Edgar.
Edd, Eddi, Eddie, Eddy, Edi, Edie, Edy

Edan (Celtic) fire.
Eadan, Eaden, Eadin, Eadon, Eadyn, Edin, Edon, Edun, Edyn

Edel (German) noble.
Adel, Edelmar, Edelweiss

Edelmar (Old English) noble; famous.

Eden (Hebrew) pleasure.
Eadan, Eaden, Eadin, Eadon, Eadyn, Edan, Edin, Edon, Edun, Edyn

Eder (Hebrew) flock.
Edar, Edir, Edor, Edyr

Edgar (English) successful spear thrower.
Edek, Edgaras (Lith), Edgard (Fren), Edgardo (Ital), Edgars, Edger, Edgir, Edgor, Edgy

Edin (Irish/Scottish) God is gracious. A form of John.
Eadan, Eaden, Eadin, Eadon, Eadyn, Edan, Eden, Edon, Edun, Edyn

Edison (English) Edward's son; son of the wealthy friend.
Eddisen, Eddison, Eddisyn, Eddyson, Edisen, Edysen, Edyson

Edmond (English) wealthy protector.
Eaman, Eamen, Eamon, Edman, Edmen, Edmon, Edmonde, Edmondo (Span/Ital/Port), Edmonson, Edmun, Edmund, Edmundo (Ital/Port), Edmunds, Edmynd, Esmon, Esmond

Edred (Old English) rich, happy counsel.
Edredd

Edrei (Hebrew) strong leader.
Edrey

Edric (English) wealthy ruler.
Eddric, Eddrick, Eddrik, Eddryc, Eddryck, Eddryk, Ederic, Ederick, Ederik, Ederyc, Ederyck, Ederyk, Edrice, Edreece, Edreese, Edrice, Edrick, Edrik, Edris, Edryc, Edryck, Edryk, Edrys

Edsel (English) from the rich one's house; deep thinker.
Edsell

Edson (English) Edison's son; son of the wealthy friend.
Eddson

Edur (Basque) snow.
Edure

Edwald (Old English) wealthy ruler.
Edwarldo

Edward (English) wealthy ruling guardian.
Edic, Edick, Edik, Edko, Edoardo (Ital), Edorta (Bas), Edouard (Fren), Eduard (Ger/Dut), Eduardo (Span), Edus, Edvard (Swed/Dan), Edvardo, Edwardo, Edwards, Edvard, Edvood, Edzio, Ekewaka, Etzio, Ewart

Edwin (English) wealthy friend.
Eadwin, Eadwinn, Edik, Edlin, Eduino, Edwinn, Edwyn, Edwynn

Eehu (Australian Aboriginal) rain.

Efrain (Hebrew) fruitful.
Efraine, Efrayn, Efrayne, Efren, Efrim, Efrin, Efrum, Efryn

Egan (Irish) fiery.
Egann, Egen, Egin, Egon, Egyn

Egbert (English) bright sword.
Egbirt, Egburt, Egbyrt

Egede (Danish/Norwegian/Greek) young goat. A form of Giles, carrier of the shield.
Eged, Egide (Fren), Egidio (Ital), Egidus (Dut)

Egerton (English) from Edgar's town; from the town of the successful spearer.
Edgarton, Edgartown, Egerton, Ergeryn, Egeton

Egil (Norwegian) awe-inspiring.
Egils (Nrs), Egyl, Eigel, Eygel

Eginhard (German) powerful sword.
Eginhardt, Einhard, Einhardt, Egynhard, Egynhardt

Egmont (Old English) top of the mountain.
Egmount

Egon (German) formidable.
Egan, Egen, Egin, Egun, Egyn

Egor (Russian/Greek) farmer. A form of George.
Igor, Yegor

Ehren (German) honourable.
Eren

Ehud (Hebrew) praised; union.

Eiddwen (Welsh) fond and faithful.
Eiddweyn, Eidwin, Eidwyn, Eyddwen, Eyddwyn

Eikki (Finnish) ever-powerful.
Eiki

Eilif (Norse) living forever.
Eileif

Einar (Scandinavian) individual. (Nors) warrior chief.
Eimar (Ir), Ejar, Inar

Einfeld (Scandinavian/German) individual field.
Seinfeld

Eion (Irish/English/Scottish) God is gracious. A form of Ian.
Ean, Eann, Ein, Eon, Eyon, Ian

Eirig (Welsh) happy.
Eyrig

Eiros (Welsh) bright.
Eros, Eyros

Eisak (Russian) laughter.
Eysak

Eisenbart (Greek) bright iron.
Eysenbart

Eisonbolt (Teutonic/Greek) iron prince.
Eysonbolt

Ekon (Nigerian) strength.
Ek, Kon, Koni, Konie, Kony

Elam (Hebrew) highland.
Elame

Elan (Native American) friendly. (Heb) tree.
Elann

Elbert (German/French/English) noble; bright. A form of Albert.
Elbirt, Elburt, Elbyrt

Elden (English) wise, old friend; helmet. A form of Alden.
Eldan, Eldin, Eldon, Eldun, Eldyn

Elder (English) elder-tree dweller; senior.
Aldar, Alder, Aldir, Aldor, Aldyr, Eldar, Eldir, Eldor, Eldyr

Eldorado (Spanish) gilded; covered with gold. (O/Ger) wise one.

Eldred (English) old, wise counsel. A form of Aldred.
Eldrid, Eldred, Eldryd

Eldridge (English) old, wise, powerful ruler. A form of Aldrich.
Eldred, Eldredge, Eldrege, Elderydg, Elderydge, Eldrid, Eldrige, Elric, Elrick, Elrik

Eldwin (Old English) old friend.
Eldwen, Eldwyn

Eleazar (Hebrew) God helps.
Elasar, Elasaro, Elazar, Elazaro, Eleasar, Eliasar, Eliazar, Elieser, Eliezer, Elizar, Elizard, Elizardo

Elek (Hungarian/Greek) defender of humankind. A form of Alec.
Elec, Eleck, Elic, Elick, Elik, Elyc, Elyck, Elyk

Elfyn (Welsh) elf friend.
Elfin

Elger (German) noble spearer.
Elgar, Elgir, Elgor, Elgiy

Elgin (English) noble; white.
Elgan, Elgen, Elgon, Elgyn

Eli (Hebrew) uplifting. The short form of Elijah, the Lord is my God.
Elay, Elian, Elie, Elien, Elier, Elion, Eloi, Eloy, Ely, Elyan, Elyen, Elyin, Elyon, Elyn

Elia (Zuni) to lift.
Eliah, Eliya, Elya, Elyah

Elias (Greek/Hebrew) uplifting. A form of Elijah.
Elia, Eliah, Eliasz, Elice, Ellice, Ellis, Elyas

Elijah (Hebrew) the Lord is my God.
Elia, Eliah, Elias (Grk), Elija, Elijuo, Elishjsha, Eliya, Eliyahu, Ellija, Ellijah, Ellis, Ellija, Ellyjah, Ellys, Elys

Elika (Hawaiian/Greek) wealthy. A form of Rick.
Elyka

Elisha (Hebrew) God is my salvation.
Elijsha, Elisee, Eliseo, Elish, Elisher, Elishia, Elishua, Elishuah, Elysha, Elyshja, Elysha

Elizur (Hebrew) God is my rock.
Elyzur

Eljon (Syrian) going up.

Elk (American) large deer.
Elke

Elkan (Hebrew) God is jealous.
Elkana, Elkanah, Elkin, Elkins, Elkyn, Elkyns

Elki (Moquelumnan) hanging over the top.
Elkie, Elky

Ellard (German) sacred; brave.
Alard, Allard, Elard, Ellerd

Ellery (English) from the elder-tree island.
Elari, Elarie, Ellari, Ellarie, Ellary, Ellary, Elleri, Ellerie, Ellery, Elery

Elliot (Hebrew) the Lord is my God.
Eliot, Eliott, Eliud, Elliott, Ellyot, Ellyott, Elyot, Elyott

Ellis (Hebrew) the Lord is my God. (O/Eng) noble.
Elis, Ellison, Ellys, Ellyson, Elys, Elyson

Elman (German) elm tree.
Elmen

Elmer (English) noble; famous.
Almer, Aylmar, Aylmer, Elmar, Ulmer

Elmo (Greek) amiable; friendly.

Elmore (Old English) elm-tree moor dweller.
Ellmoar, Ellmoor, Ellmoore, Ellmor, Ellmore, Elmoar, Elmoor, Elmoore

Elonzo (Spanish/German) noble; famous.
Alonz, Alonzo, Elonz

Eloy (Latin) chosen.
Eloi

Elrad (Hebrew) God rules.
Ellrad, Elradd

Elroy (Latin) royal.
Elroi, Elroye

Elsdon (Old English) from the noble one's hill.
Elsden, Elsdin, Elsdyn

Elson (Old English) Ellis' son; the noble one's son. The Lord is my God.
Ellson

Elston (Old English) from Ellis' town; from the noble one's town.
Ellston

Elsu (Native American) soaring, swooping falcon.

Elsworth (Old English) from Ellis' estate; from the noble one's estate.
Ellsworth

Elton (English) from the old town.
Eltan, Elten, Eltin, Eltyn

Elvern (Latin) spring. A form of Alvern.
Elverne, Elvirn, Elvirne, Elvyrn, Elvyrne

Elvin (English) elf friend.
Elvyn, Elwin, Elwyn, Elwynn

E

Elvio (Spanish) blond-haired.
Elvyo

Elvis (Old Norse) elf friend.
Elviss, Elvys, Elvyss

Elvy (Old English) elf warrior.
Elvi, Elvie

Elwell (Old English) from the old stream.
Elwel

Elwin (English) friend of the elves.
Elvain, Elvyn, Elwen, Elwyn

Elwood (Old English) from the old forest.
Ellwood

Emerson (Old English) Emery's son; son of the industrious ruler.

Emery (Teutonic) industrious, hard-working ruler.
Amerigo (Ital), Emeree, Emeri (Fren), Emerie, Emmeree, Emmeri, Emmerie, Emmerich (Ger), Emmery, Emmori, Emmorie, Emmory, Emory

Emil/Emile/Emilio (Gothic/German) hard-working. (Lat) compliment giver.
Amiel, Amile, Emiel, Emile (Fren/Ger), Emiliano (Ital/Span), Emilio (Span), Emille, Emyl, Emyll, Emylle, Emlyn (Wel)

Emlyn (Welsh) waterfall.
Emlin

Emmanuel (Hebrew) God is with us.
Eman (Czech), Emanual, Emanuel, Emanuele (Ital), Emanuell, Emek, Emmaneuol, Emmanle, Emmanueal, Emmanuele, Emmanuil, Manuel (Span), Emanuel (Ger), Imanual, Imanuel, Imanuele, Immanuel, Immanuele, Manuel

Emmett (Teutonic) hard-working; strong. (O/Eng) ant.
Emmet, Emmit, Emmitt, Emmot, Emmott, Emmyt, Emmytt, Emyt, Emytt

Emre (Turkish) brother.

Emrick (German) hard-working ruler.
Emric, Emrik, Emryc, Emryck, Emryk

Emry (Welsh) honourable.
Emree, Emrey, Emri, Emrie, Emyr

Enan (Welsh) hammer.
Enen, Enin, Enon, Enyn

Enapay (Lakota) to give a brave appearance.
Enapai

Enda (Irish) bird.
Endah

Endor (Hebrew) the fountain of youth; adorable. The masculine form of Endora.

Endre (Greek) strong; brave; courageous. A form of Andre.
Ender, Endres (Ger)

Endrikas (Lithuanian/German) ruler of the house. A form of Henry.
Endrika, Endryka, Endrykas

Eneas (Irish/Greek) praised. A form of Aeneas.

Eneco (Latin) fiery. A form of Ignatius.

Engelbert (German) bright angel.
Engelburt, Englebert, Englebirt, Engleburt, Englebirt, Ingelbert, Ingelburt, Inglebert, Inglburt

Enli (Dene) dog over there.
Enly

Ennis (Greek) mine; ninth-born child. (Celt) island.
Ennys, Enis, Enys

Enoch (Hebrew) dedicated.
Enoc, Enock, Enok

Enos (Hebrew) man.
Enosh

Enric (Romanian/German) ruler of the house. A form of Henry.
Enrica, Enricah, Enrick, Enrico (Ital), Enrigue, Enrik, Enrika, Enrikah, Enrikos (Grk), Enriq, Enrique (Span), Enriquez, Enrrique, Enryc, Enryck, Enryk, Enryka, Enrykah

Enright (Irish) the attacker's son.
Enrit, Enrite, Enryght, Enryte

Ensor (Old English) from the blessed bank.
Ensar, Enser, Ensir, Ensyr

Enver (Turkish) bright; handsome.

Enyeto (Native American) walking like a bear.
Enieto

Enz (Swiss/Latin) crown of laurel leaves; victory. A short form of Lawrence.
Enzo

Enzi (Swahili) powerful.
Enzie, Enzy

Enzo (Italian) ruler of the house. A form of Henry.
Enzio

Eran (Hebrew) vigilant.
Eren, Erin, Eron, Eryn

Erbert (German) glorious warrior.
Ebert, Erberto (Ital), Erbirt, Erbirto, Erburt, Erburto, Erbyrt, Erbyrto

Ercole (Italian) great gift.
Ercoal, Ercol

Erebus (Greek) dark-haired.

Erhard (German) strong; resolute.
Erhardt, Erhart

Eric (Scandinavian) ruler. (O/Eng) brave ruler.
Ehric, Ehrich, Elika, Enrich, Enrick, Erek (Scand), Eric, Erich (Czech/Ger), Erick, Erica, Ericah, Erich, Erick, Erickson, Erico, Ericson, Erik (Scand), Eriks (Scand), Erikson, Erikur (Ice), Erric, Errick, Errik, Eryc, Eryk

Eriha (New Zealand Maori) God.
Eryha

Erin (Irish) peace. (Celt) from Ireland.
Eran, Eren, Erine, Erinn, Erino, Eron, Eryn, Erynn

Erland (English) from the noble one's land.
Earlan, Earland, Erlan, Erlen, Erlend

Erling (English) the noble one's son.
Erlin

Ermanno (German) warrior.
Erman, Ermano (Span), Ermin

Ermo (Italian) friendly.
Ermot

Ernan (Irish) experienced.
Ernen, Ernin, Ernon, Ernyn

Ernest/Ernie (English) sincere.
Earnre, Earnee, Earnest, Earni, Earnie, Earny, Ernee, Erneste (Fren), Ernestino, Ernesto (Span), Ernests (Lett), Ernestus (Dut), Erneszt (Hung), Erney, Erni, Ernie, Erno (Hung), Ernst (Ger), Erny

Ernijo (Hungarian/Greek) peace.
Earnijo

Erol (Turkish) strong; courageous.
Eroll

Errando (Basque) bold.
Erando

Errol (Latin) wanderer.
Erel, Erell, Eril, Erill, Erol, Erold, Errel, Errell, Erril, Errill, Erroll, Erryl, Erryll, Eryl, Eryll

Erroman (Basque) from Rome.
Eroman

Erskine (Scottish) from the high cliff. (Eng) from Ireland.
Ersin, Erskin, Erskyn, Erskyne

Eruera (New Zealand Maori) wealthy ruling guardian. A form of Edward.
Eruerah

Ervin (English) sea friend.
Earvan, Earven, Earvin, Earvon, Earvyn, Ervan, Erven, Ervine, Ervon, Ervyn, Ervyne, Erwan, Erwinek, Erwin, Erwinn, Erwyn, Erwynn

Esau (Hebrew) rough-haired.
Esaw

Esbern (Danish) holy bear.
Esberne, Esbirn, Esbirne, Esburn, Esburne, Esbirn, Esbyrne

Eskil (Norwegian) vessel of God.
Eskyl

Esko (Finnish) leader.

Esmond (Old English) gracious protection; shelter.
Esmon, Esmun, Esmund

Espen (Danish) bear.
Espan, Espin, Espon, Espyn

Essien (Ochi) sixth-born child.
Esien

Este (Italian) from the east.
Estes

Esteban (Spanish/Greek) crowned. A form of Stephen.
Estabon, Estebe (Bas), Estefan, Estephan, Estevan, Estevao (Span), Esteven, Estevez, Estiven, Estyvan, Estyven, Estyvin, Estyvon, Estyvyn, Etienne (Fren), Etyven

Ethan (Hebrew) strength; steadfast; reliable.
Eatha, Eathen, Eathin, Eathon, Eathyn, Efan, Efen, Effan, Effen, Effin, Effon, Effyn, Efin, Efon, Efyn, Eithan, Eithen, Eithin, Eithon, Eithyn, Ethen, Ethin, Ethon, Ethyn, Eythan, Eythen, Eythin, Eython, Eythyn

Ethel (Old English) noble.
Ethal, Ethil, Ethol, Ethelred, Ethyl

Etienne (French/Greek) crowned. A form of Stephen.
Etiene

Ettore (Italian/Greek) reliable; steadfast.
Etore

Etu (Native American) sunny.
Eetu

Euan (Scottish) sunny.
Ewan, Ewen, Ewin, Ewon, Ewyn, Euen, Euin, Euron, Euryn

Euclid (Greek) true glory.
Euclyd

Eudo (Teutonic) youngster.
Eu

Eugene (Greek) noble; well born.
Eugeen, Eugeene, Eugen-Ger), Eugenio (Ital/Span/Port), Eugenios, Eugenius (Dut), Eujean, Eujeane, Eujeen, Eujein, Eujeyn, Evgeny (Rus/Grk), Ezven (Czech), Gene

Eureka (Greek) found.
Eurekah

Euroa (Australian Aboriginal) joy.
Euroah

Eurwyn (Welsh) gold; fair-haired.
Eurwen, Eurwin

Eustace (Greek) abundant corn.
Eustacee, Eustache (Fren),
Eustachio (Ital), Eustachy (Pol),
Eustaquio (Span), Eustathios
(Grk), Eustis, Eustazio (Ital),
Eustasius-Ger), Eustquio (Span),
Eustatius (Dut), Stacey, Stacy

Evagelos (Greek) strong; brave;
courageous. A form of Andrew.
Evaggelos, Evangelo, Evangelos

Evan (Welsh) well born.
Bowen, Even, Evin, Evon, Evun,
Evyn, Ewan, Ewen, Owain, Owen,
Yvain, Ywaine

Evander (Greek) evangelist;
preacher.
Evandar

Evelyn (Hebrew) from the pool of
life.
Evelin

Everard (Old English) strong; brave
like a boar.
Eberhard (Ger), Eberhardt,
Everarado (Ital), Evered, Everett,
Everhardt, Everhart (Dut), Evraud
(Fren)

Everett (English) mighty like a boar.
Eber, Everard, Evered, Everet,
Everhard, Everhardt, Everhet,
Everhett, Everit, Everitt, Everyt,
Everyte, Everytt, Everytte, Evraud,
Evre, Evryt, Evryte, Evrytt, Evrytte,
Eward, Ewardo, Ewart, Ret, Rett,
Rhet, Rhett

Everley (Old English) from Evan's
meadow; from the well-born
one's meadow.
Evanlea, Evanleah, Evanlee,
Evanleigh, Evanli, Evanlie, Evanly,
Evenlea, Evenleah, Evenlee,
Evenleigh, Evenli, Evenlie, Evenly

Everton (English) from the well-
born one's town.

Evgeny (Russian/Greek) noble; well
born. A form of Eugene.
Evgenij, Evgenyi

Ewald (Old English) always
powerful.
Evald, Evold, Ewold

Ewan (Welsh) God is gracious. A
form of John.
Eoghan, Eoin, Evan, Even, Evin,
Evon, Evun, Evyn, Ewen, Ewin,
Ewon, Ewyn, Owen, Owin, Owyn

Ewert (Old English) herder of ewes.
Ewirt

Ewing (English) law friend.
Ewin, Ewyn, Ewyng

Exelby (Old Norse) divine cauldron.
Exelbi

Eyar (Norse) island warrior.
Eiar

Eydis (Norse) island fairy.
Eidis

Eyota (Native American) great.
Eiota, Eyotah

Eystein (Norse) from the island
stone.
Einstein, Einsteyn, Eynstein,
Eynsteyn

Eyvar (Norse) island of prudence.
Eivar

Ezekiel (Hebrew) strength of God.
Ezechiel, Ezeck, Ezeeckel, Ezekeial,
Ezekial, Ezell, Ezequiel, Eziaka,
Eziakah, Eziechiele, Eziequel, Zeke

Ezra (Hebrew) helper.
Esdras, Esra, Esdras, Esra, Esrah, Ezer, Ezera, Ezerah, Ezrah

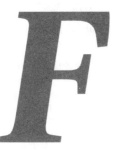

Fa (Chinese) the beginning.
Fai

Faas (Scandinavian) one who gives wise counsel.
Fas

Fabian (Latin) prosperous bean grower.
Faba, Fabag, Fabar, Fabean, Faber (Ger), Fabia, Fabiano (Ital), Fabien (Fren), Fabijan (Slav), Fabio (Ital), Fabir, Fabius (Lat), Fabiusz (Pol), Fabor, Fabyan (Ital), Fabyous, Fabyr

Fabron (French) little blacksmith.
Fabre (Fren), Fabra, Fabriano, Fabrizio (Ital), Fabroni (Ital), Fabryn

Fadey (Ukrainian/Russian/Greek/Hebrew) courageous; bold. A short form of Thaddeus, praising God.
Faday, Faddel, Faddey, Faddi, Faddie, Faddy, Fadeyka, Fadi, Fadie, Fady

Fadi (Arabic) the redeemer.
Fadee, Fadey, Fadie, Fady

Fadil (Arabic) generous.
Fadal, Fadel, Fadyl

Fagan (Irish/Gaelic) little fire.
Faegan, Faegen, Faegin, Faegon, Faegyn, Fagen, Fagin, Fagon, Fagyn, Faigan, Faigen, Faigin, Faion, Faigyn, Faygan, Faygen, Fayfin, Faygon, Fagyn

Fahd (Arabic) the lynx cat.
Fahad

Fahey (Old English) joyful; happy.
Fahay, Faiey, Fayey

Fairfax (Old English) light, blond-haired.
Fayrfax

Faisal (Arabic) decisive.
Faisel, Faisil, Faizal, Fasel, Fasil, Faysal, Fayzal, Fayzel

Fakhir (Arabic) excellence.
Fahkri, Fahkry

Falco (Latin) falcon trainer.
Falcon, Falcko, Falckon, Falconn, Falconner, Falconnor, Faulco, Faulconer, Faulconner, Faulconnor, Faulknre

Falkner (Old English) falconer.
Falcon, Faulkner, Fowler

Fane (English) joyful; from the bull/sheep meadow.
Fain, Faine, Faines, Fains, Fanes, Fayn, Fayne

Faraji (Swahili) consolation.
Farajy

Faramond (Teutonic) protected traveller.
Farman, Farmannus, Farrimond, Phareman

Farid (Arabic) duty; unique.
Farad, Fared, Farod, Faryd

F

Faris (Arabic) horse rider.
Faress, Fariss, Farrys, Farys

Farlane (Old English) from the far lane.
Farlaen, Farlaene, Farlain, Farlaine, Farlayn, Farlayne

Farley (Old English) from the far meadow.
Fairlea, Fairleah, Fairlee, Fairleigh, Fairley, Farlay, Farlea, Farleah, Farlee, Farleigh, Farli, Farlie, Farly

Farnell (English) hill covered with ferns.
Farnal, Farnald, Farnalde, Farnall, Farnalle, Farnel, Farneld, Farnell, Farnelle, Fernal, Fernald, Fernalde, Fernall, Fernalle, Furnal, Furnald, Furnalde, Furnall, Furnalle, Furnel, Furneld, Furnell, Furnelle, Fyrnel, Fyrnele, Fyrnell, Fyrnelle

Farnham (Old English) from the cottage with the field of ferns.
Farnam, Farnem, Farnhem

Farnley (English) from the fern meadow.
Farnlea, Farleah, Farnlee, Farnleigh, Farnli, Farnlie, Farnly, Fernlea, Fernleah, Fernlee, Fernleigh, Fernley, Fernli, Fernlie, Fernly

Faroh (Latin) ruler.
Faro, Farro, Farrow, Pharo, Pharoh

Farouk (Arabic) one who knows wrong from right.
Farook, Faroukh

Farquhar (Gaelic) friendly.
Farquar, Farquarson, Farquharson

Farr (English) traveller.
Faer, Far, Farran, Farren, Farrin, Farring, Farrington, Farron, Farrun, Farryn

Farrar (Old English) farrier; blacksmith.
Farar, Farer, Farrel, Farrell, Farrer, Farris, Ferris, Ferrol

Farrell (Celtic/Irish) hero.
Faral, Farel, Faril, Farol, Farral, Farrel, Farrel, Farryl, Faryl, Ferrel, Ferrell, Ferril, Ferryl

Farrow (English) little piglet.
Farow

Farruca (Spanish) freedom; from France. (O/Eng) honest. A form of Frank.
Farruka, Faruca, Farucah, Frascuelo, Furrucah

Faste (Norwegian) firm.
Fast

Fate (Latin) destiny.
Faet, Fait, Fayt, Fayette

Fath (Arabic) victorious.

Fatin (Arabic) clever one.
Fatine, Fatyn, Fatyne

Faust (Latin) fortunate.
Faust, Fauste, Faustice, Faustin, Faustine, Faustino (Ital), Faustis, Faustise, Fausto (Ital), Faustos, Faustow, Faustus, Faustyce, Faustyn (Pol), Faustus, Faustys

Favian (Latin) understanding.
Favien, Favion, Favyon

Faxi (Norse) hair.
Faxee, Faxey, Faxie, Faxy

Faxon (German) long-haired.
Faxan, Faxen, Faxin, Faxyn

Fay (Irish/Gaelic) raven.
Fae, Fah, Fai, Fayard, Fayette

Fazio (Italian) good worker.
Fazyo

F

Fazl (Arabic) abundance.
Faisal, Faisel

Fearghas (Scottish) strength.
Feargus, Fergus, Ferguss

Featherstone (English) from the
feather stone.

Fedlim (Irish) good.
Fedlym

Fedor (Russian) gift of God. The
Russian form of Theodore.
Feador, Fedore, Feedore, Fidor,
Fidore, Fydor, Fydore

Fehin (Irish) little raven.
Fechin

Feivel (Yiddish) God will aid.
Feyvel

Feke (Tongan) octopus.

Felicius (Latin) happy.
Felicyus, Felycius, Felycyus

Felimy (Irish) forever good.
Felymy

Felipe (Spanish) one who loves
horses.
Feeleep (Russ), Felep, Felipinho
(Port), Philip, Phillip, Phylip,
Phyllip

Feliz (Latin) fortunate.
Felic, Felice (Ital), Felicio, Felike,
Feliks (Pol), Feliksa (Lith), Felis,
Felizio, Fellcio, Filix, Filyx, Fylix,
Fylyx, Phelix, Phelyx

Felton (English) from the field
town.
Feltan, Felten, Feltin, Feltun, Feltyn

Feng-Shui (Chinese) wind and
water.

Fenton (English) from the marsh
town.
Fentan, Fenten, Fentin, Fentun,
Fentyn

Feodor (Slavic/Greek) gift of God. A
form of Theodore.
Feaodor, Feaodore, Fedar, Fedinka,
Fedor, Fedya, Feeodor, Feeodore,
Fiodor, Fiodore, Fyodor, Fyodore

Feoras (Greek) smooth rock.
Feora, Feorah

Ferd (German) horse.
Ferde, Ferdi, Ferdie, Ferdy

Ferdinand (Teutonic) adventurer;
peace maker. (Goth) life
adventure. The feminine form of
Fernanda.
Ferdinan, Ferdinando (Ital),
Ferdinandus (Lith), Ferdynand,
Ferdynando, Fergus (Ir), Fernando
(Span), Ferrand, Ferrante (Fren),
Ferrando, Ferynand (Pol),
Ferynando (Span/Ger), Hernan,
Hernando (Span)

Ferenc (Hungarian) freedom; from
France. (O/Eng) honest. A form
of Francis.
Feren, Ferke, Ferko

Fergal (Irish) strength.
Firgal, Fyrgal

Fergus (Irish) strength. (Celt)
choice.
Fearghas, Fearghus, Feargus,
Ferghas, Ferghus, Ferguson,
Fergusson, Firgus, Firgusen,
Firguson, Furgus, Furgusen,
Furguson, Fyrgus, Fyrgusen,
Fyrguson

Fermac (Irish) brightness.
Fearmac, Fermack, Fermak

Fermin (Spanish) firm strength.
Feridon, Firman (Fren), Firmin,
Firmyn, Furman, Furmin, Furmyn,
Fyrman, Fyrmen, Frymin, Fyrmyn

Fernando (Spanish/German)
adventurous.
Ferdinando, Ferdnando, Fernand,
Fernandez

Feroz (Persian) fortunate.
Firoz, Fyroz

Ferran (Arabic) baker.
Feran, Feren, Ferin, Feron, Ferren,
Ferrin, Ferron, Ferryn, Feryn

Ferrand (Old French) grey-haired.
(O/Ger) adventurer.
Faran, Farand, Farran, Farrand,
Farrando, Farrant, Feran, Ferand,
Ferran, Ferrant

Ferrars (Latin) iron.
Ferrar

Ferrell (Irish) hero.
Ferel, Ferell, Ferrel

Ferris (Irish/Gaelic) stone; rock. A
form of Peter. (Ir) choice.
Farice, Farrice, Farris, Feris, Ferrice,
Ferrise, Ferryce, Ferryse, Ferryss

Festus (Latin) happy.
Festys

Fiacre (Celtic) eagle.
Fiach, Fiak, Fiakryusz, Fyacre

Fico (Spanish/German) peaceful
ruler.
Ficko, Fiko, Fyco, Fycko, Fyko

Fidel (Latin) faithful.
Fidele (Fren), Fidelio (Ital),
Fidelinsz, Fildes, Fydal, Fydel,
Fydil, Fydyl

Fielding (English) from the fields.
Fielder

Fife (Scottish) (Geographical) from
Fife in Scotland.
Fif, Fyf, Fyfe

Fillbert (English) brilliant.
Filbert, Filberte (Fren), Filberti,
Filberto (Ital/Span), Filbirt,
Filbirte, Fillbert, Fillberte, Fillbirt,
Fillbirte, Fylbert, Fylberte, Fyllbert,
Fyllberte, Fyllbirt, Fyllbirte,
Fyllbyrt, Fyllbyrte, Philbert,
Philberti, Philberto, Phylbert

Filmer (Old English) famous.
Fillmore, Filmore, Fyllmer,
Fyllmore, Fylmer, Fylmore

Filmore (Old English) more
famous.
Fillmore, Filmore, Fyllmore,
Fylmore

Filya (Russian) one who loves
horses. A form of Phillip.
Filyah, Fylya, Fylyah

Finbar (Celtic) fair-haired, blond
chief.
Finnbar, Fynbar, Fynbarr

Findlay (Celtic/Gaelic) fair-haired,
blond warrior.
Findlea, Findleah, Findlee,
Findleigh, Findley, Finlay (Ir),
Finlea, Finleah, Finlee, Finleigh,
Finnlay, Finnlea, Finnleah, Finnlee,
Finnleigh, Finnley, Fyndlay,
Fyndlea, Fyndleah, Fyndlee,
Fyndleigh, Fyndley, Fynlay, Fynlea,
Fynleah, Fynlee, Fynleigh, Fynley,
Fynndlay, Fynndlea, Fynndleah,
Fynndlee, Fynndleigh, Fynndley,
Fynnlay, Fynnlea, Fynnleah,
Fynnlee, Fynnleigh, Fynnley

Fineas (Irish/Hebrew) oracle.
(Egypt) dark-skinned.
Finea, Fynea, Fyneas

Fingal (Celtic) fair warrior.
Finngal, Fyngal, Fynngal

Finian (Celtic) fair-haired, blond
child.
Finan, Fineen, Finien, Finyan,
Fynian, Fynyan, Phinean, Phinian,
Phinyan, Phynian, Phynyan

F

Fink (German) the finch bird.
Finke, Fynk, Fynke

Finlay (Irish) blond-haired.
Findlay (Celt), Findlea, Findleah,
Findlee, Findleigh, Findley, Finlea,
Finleah, Finlee, Finleigh, Finnlay,
Finnlea, Finnleah, Finnlee,
Finnleigh, Finnley, Fyndlay,
Fyndlea, Fyndleah, Fyndlee,
Fyndleigh, Fyndley, Fynlay, Fynlea,
Fynleah, Fynlee, Fynleigh, Fynley,
Fynndlay, Fynndlea, Fynndleah,
Fynndlee, Fynndleigh, Fynndley,
Fynnlay, Fynnlea, Fynnleah,
Fynnlee, Fynnleigh, Fynnley

Finn (Irish/Gaelic) blond-haired,
fair-complexioned. (O/Ger) from
Finland.
Eifion, Fin, Finan, Finbar, Finbarr,
Finian (Celt), Finnegan, Finnian,
Fion, Fyn, Fynn

Finnegan (Irish) light-
complexioned.
Finegan, Fineghan, Finneghan,
Fynbegan, Fyneghan, Fynnegan,
Fynneghan

Fintan (Irish) from Finland; from
Finn's town.
Finten, Fintin, Finton, Fintyn,
Fyntan, Fynten, Fyntin, Fynton,
Fyntyn

Fiorello (Latin) little flower.
Fiorellea, Fiorelleah, Fiorelleigh,
Fiorelley, Fiorelli, Fiorellie, Fiorelly,
Fyorellea, Fyorelleah, Fyorellee,
Fyorelleigh, Fyorelley, Fyorelli,
Fyorellie, Fyorello, Fyorelly

Firas (Arabic) persistent.
Fira, Firah, Fyra, Fyrah, Fyras

Firman (French) strength.
Feridon, Firmen, Firmyn, Furman,
Furmin, Furmyn, Fyrman, Fyrmen,
Frymin, Fyrmyn

Firth (English) from the woodlands.
Fyrth

Fischel (Yiddish) one who loves
horses. A form of Phillip.
Fyschel

Fiske (English) fish.
Fisk, Fysk, Fyske

Fitch (English) weasel.
Fytch

Fitz (Old English) son. The short
form of names beginning with
'Fitz' e.g. Fiztgerald.
Fits, Fyts, Fytz

Fitzgerald (Old English) son of
Gerald; son of the brave spear
carrier.
Fitsgerald, Fitzgeraldo, Fystgerald,
Fytsgeraldo, Fytzgerald,
Fytzgeraldo, Gerald, Geraldo

Fitzhugh (Old English) son of
Hugh; son of the intelligent one.
Fitshu, Fitshue, Fitshugh, Fitzhu,
Fitzhue, Fytshu, Fytzhue, Fytzhugh

Fitzpatrick (Old English) Patrick's
son; son of the noble one.
Fitspatric, Fitspatrik, Fitzpatric,
Fitzpatrik, Fytspatric, Fytspatrick,
Fytspatrik, Fytzpatric, Fytzpatrick,
Fytzpatrik

Fitzroy (French) son of Roy; son of
the king.
Fitsroi, Fitsroy, Fitzroi, Fytsroi,
Fytsroy, Fytzroi, Fytzroy

Flann (Celtic) blood red; red-
haired.
Flan, Flanan, Flanen, Flanin,
Flannan, Flannen, Flannin,
Flannon, Flannyn, Flanon, Flanyn

Flavian (Latin) fair; blond-haired.
Flavias, Flavio (Ital) Flavius (Lat),
Flavyan, Flawian (Pol), Flawyan

Flavio (Italian) blond.
Flabio, Flabious, Flavio, Flavious,
Flavius, Flavyo

Fleet (Scandinavian) channel.
Fleat

Fleming (Old English) from the
lowlands; Dutch one.
Flemming, Flemmyng, Flemyng

Fletcher (Old French) arrow maker.
Flecher

Flint (Old English) rock.
Flinte, Flynt, Flynte

Flip (Spanish) one who loves
horses. A form of Phillip.
Flipp, Flyp, Flypp

Floranz (Latin) flowering.
Floranzo (Ital), Florence, Florenz,
Florenzo (Ital)

Florent (French) flowering.
Fiorenci, Florencio, Florentin,
Florentine, Florentino, Florentyn,
Florentyne, Florentyno, Florentz,
Florenzo, Florinio, Florino,
Floryno, Florynt, Florynte

Florian (Latin) flowering.
Floenc, Florence, Fiorelli, Fiorello,
Florent, Florentino, Florents,
Florentz, Florenz, Florenzo,
Florien, Florion, Floryan, Floryant,
Floryante

Florus (Latin) flower.
Florius, Floryus

Floyd (Old English) grey-haired.
Floid, Floyde, Lloyd, Loyd, Loyde

Flurry (English) flourishing;
flowering.
Fluri, Flurie, Flurri, Flurrie, Flury

Flynn (Irish/Gaelic) son of the red-
haired one; son of Finn.
Flin, Flinn, Flyn

Fokai (Tongan) chameleon.

Fokisi (Tongan) fox.

Folke (German) guardian of the
people.
Folk, Folkman

Foluke (Yoruba) given to God.

Foma (Russian/Bulgarian) twin.
Fomah

Fonda (Latin) deep.
Fondah, Fondar

Fonso (German/Italian) ready;
noble. A form of Alphonse.
Fonzo

Fontaine (French) fountain.
Fontain, Fontayn, Fontayne,
Fountain (Lat), Fountaine,
Fountayn, Fountayne

Fonu (Tongan) turtle.

Fonzie (German/Italian/Spanish)
noble; ready to do battle. A form
of Alphonse.
Fonsee, Fonsey, Fonsi, Fonsie,
Fonsy, Fonzee, Fonzey, Fonzi, Fonzy

Forbes (Irish/Gaelic) wealthy owner
of fields. (Scott) headstrong.
Forbs

Ford (Old English) from the
shallow river crossing.
Forde

Fordel (Gypsy) forgiven.
Fordal, Fordele, Fordell, Fordelle,
Fordil, Fordile

Fordon (Teutonic) destroyer.
Fordan, Forden, Fordin, Fordyn

Forester/Forrest (Old French)
dweller in the forest.
Forest, Forreste (Fren), Forrester,
Forster, Foster

Fortino (Italian) fortunate.
Fortin, Fortine, Fortyn, Fortyne

Fortney (Old English) strong fort.
Fortnum

Fortune (Old French) lucky.
Fortunato (Lat), Fortunio (Ital)

Foster (Old English) guardian of
the forest.
Forest, Forester, Forestor, Forrest,
Forrester, Forrestor, Forster

Fountain (Latin) from the spring.
Fontain, Fontaine (Fren), Fontayn,
Fontayne, Fountaine, Fountayn,
Fountayne

Fowler (Old English) wild fowl
trapper.
Falconer, Falkner

Fox (Old English) fox.
Foxx

Foy (Middle Dutch) parting feast for
a journey.
Foi

Francis (Latin) freedom.
Chico, Ferenc (Hung), Ferencz,
Ferko, Franas (Lith), Franc (Slav),
France, Francesco (Ital), Franchot
(Fren), Francilo (Span), Francisco
(Span/Port), Francisek (Boh),
Francisganinho, Franciskus (Ger),
Franciszek (Pol), Francois, Francy,
Francys, Frane (Yugo), Frantik,
Frantyc, Frantyck, Frantyk, Franz,
Franzen, Franzisk, Frasco,
Frasquito, Paco, Pacorro, Panchito,
Pancho, Paquito, Phrankiscos
(Grk), Prancas, Ranssu, Spranzio

Frank (Latin) freedom. (O/Eng)
honest. The short form of
Franklin.
Franc

Franklin (Old English) from the
honest, free one's stream.
Francklin, Francklyn, Franklin,
Franklyn

Fraser (Old French) strawberry.
(O/Eng) curly-haired.
Frasier, Frazer, Frazier, Frazyer

Frayne (Old French) ash tree. (Eng)
stranger.
Frain, Fraine, Frean, Freane, Freen,
Freene, Frein, Freine, Freyn, Freyne

Fred (Teutonic) old cousellor; wise
judge. The short form of names
beginning with 'Fred' or
containing 'fred' e.g. Frederick,
Alfred.
Fredd, Freddi, Freddie, Freddo,
Freddy, Fredi, Fredie, Fredo (Span),
Fredson, Fredy

Frederick (Teutonic) king of peace.
Eric, Erich, Erick, Erik, Fadrique,
Farruco, Federico, Federigo,
Fedrick, Fedrik, Feidrik, Fidrich,
Fledrik, Frederic (Fren), Frederico
(Span/Port), Frederigo (Ital),
Frederik (Dan/Dut/Slav),
Frederikos (Grk), Fredric, Fredrick,
Fredrik (Swed), Fredson, Freerik
(Dut), Frek, Frid, Frideric,
Friderick, Friderik, Fridko, Fridli,
Fridrich, Fryderic, Fryderick,
Fryderyk (Pol), Frydric, Frydrich,
Frydrick, Frydrik, Priczus, Pridriks,
Rietu, Sprizzio, Wettrikki, Wridiks,
Wridyks, Wrydriks

Fredson (Old English) son of Fred;
son of the old counsellor; wise
judge.
Freddson, Friddson, Fridson

Freeborn (Old English) child of
freedom.
Free, Freborn

Freeman (Old French) free man.
Freedman, Freeland, Freemon

Freidank (German) free thinker.
Freidan, Freydan, Freydank

Fremantle (Old French) cold cloak.
Fremantel, Fremantell, Fremantl

Fremont (Teutonic) guardian of freedom; noble protector.
Fremonte

Frewin (English) free, noble friend.
Freewan, Freewen, Frewan, Frewen, Frewon, Frewyn

Frey (English) noble. The masculine form of Freya, a goddess of love.
Frai, Fray, Frei

Frick (English) bold.
Fric, Friq, Frique, Frik, Fryc, Fryck, Fryk, Fryq, Fryque

Fridmar (German) famous peace.
Frydmar

Fridmund (German) peaceful protector.
Frimond, Frymond, Frymund

Fridolf (Old English) peaceful wolf.
Freydolf, Freydolph, Freydolphe, Freydulph, Freydulphe, Fridolf, Fridolph, Fridolphe, Fridulf, Frydolph, Frydolphe, Frydulf

Fridrad (German) peace council.
Frydrad

Friedmann (German) peace loving.
Friedman, Fryedman, Fryedmann

Fritz (German) peaceful ruler.
Fritson, Fritt, Fritzchen, Fritzl, Frytson, Frytzon

Frode (Norwegian) wisdom.
Frod

Frowin (German) free friend.
Frowyn

Fry (Old Norse) child.
Frye, Fryer

Fudo (Japanese) god of fire and wisdom.

Fuhai (Chinese) happiness as plentiful as the Eastern Sea.

Fulbright (Teutonic) very bright.
Fulbert, Fulbirt, Fulburt, Fulbyrt, Philbert, Philbirt, Philburt, Philbyrt, Phylbert, Phylbirt, Phylburt, Phylbyrt

Fulk (Teutonic) kin; relation.
Fawk, Fawke, Foke, Foker, Fokke, Fokker, Folke (Nrs), Folker (Ger), Folkvard (Nor), Fouchier, Foulquie, Fowk, Fowke, Fulco, Fulke, Volguard

Fuller (Old English) clothing presser.
Fuler

Fulton (English) from the field near the town; dweller at the muddy enclosure.
Faulton, Folton

Funsan (Malawian) ask.

Funsoni (Ngoni) asked-for.
Funsony

Fushen (Chinese) god of happiness.

Fuzzy (German) curly-haired.
Fuzzi, Fuzzie

Fynn (Ghanian) river.
Fin, Finn, Fyn

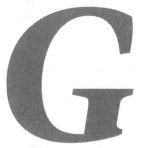

Gabe/Gabriel (Hebrew) strength of God. The short form of the name of the Archangel, Gabriel.
Gab, Gabby, Gabe, Gabel, Gabela (Swiss), Gabelah, Gabell, Gabirol, Gabor (Hung), Gabriele, Gabrielius (Balt), Gabriello (Ital), Gabryel (Pol), Gabryele, Gabryell, Gabryelle, Gaby, Gavril (Russ), Gavrilla, Gavryl, Gavryle, Gavryll, Gavrylle, Jibrail (Arab), Jibri (Arab), Jivrail

Gad (Arabic) lucky.
Gadi, Gadie, Gady

Gadiel (Hebrew) God is my fortune.
Gadman, Gadyel

Gael (Irish) Gaelic.
Gaelic

Gage (French) promise.
Gaig, Gaige, Gayg, Gayge

Gaia (Greek) earth.
Gaiah, Gaya, Gayah

Gair (Irish) small.
Gaer, Gayr, Gearr, Geir, Geirr

Galahad (Welsh) hawk; from Gilead. A biblical name.

Galbraith (Irish) a Scottish person living in Ireland.
Galbrayth

Gale (Old English) happy.
Gael, Gail, Gayl

Galegina (Cherokee) stag.

Galen (Old English) happy.
Galan, Galin, Galon, Galyn

Galeran (French) healthy ruler.
Galerano (Ital)

Galileo (Italian/Celtic) male bird.
Galyleo

Gallagher (Celtic) helper who is eager.

Galloway (Irish) from the highway near the gallows.
Gallwai, Gallway, Gallowai, Galwai, Galway

Galt (Norwegian) from the high ground.

Galton (English) from the rented land in the town.
Galtan, Galten, Galtin, Galtyn

Galvin (Irish) bright; sparrow.
Galvan, Galven, Galvon, Galvyn

Gamal (Arabic) camel. A form of Jamal, beautiful.
Gamall, Gamil

Gamba (Zimbabwean) warrior.
Gambah

Gamble (Norse/Scandinavian) elder. (Eng) one who bets; gambler.
Gambal, Gambel, Gambil, Gambil, Gambyl

Gamliel (Hebrew) God is my reward.
Gamliell

Gamlyn (Old Norse) little elder.
Gamlin

Gan (Chinese) adventurous. (Viet) close by.

Ganan (Australian Aboriginal) west.
Ganen, Ganin, Ganon, Ganyn

Gandhi (Sanskrit) great.
Gandhee

Gandolf (German) fierce wolf.
Gandolfo

Gannon (Irish) light skin.
Ganan, Ganen, Ganin, Gannan,
Gannen, Gannin, Gannon,
Gannyn. Ganon, Ganyn

Ganya (Zulu) clever.
Gania, Ganiah, Ganyah

Garai (Zimbabwean) settler.
Garae, Garay

Garbhan (Irish) small, tough child.
Garban

Garcia (Spanish/Teutonic) brave
spear carrier. A form of Gerald.
Garcias, Garcillasso, Garsias
(Span), Garcya, Garcyah, Garcyas,
Garsya, Garsyah, Garsyas

Gard (Norse) dwelling place.
Garde, Guard

Gardiner (Old English) garden
worker.
Gardnar, Gardner, Gardnor,
Gardyner

Garek (Polish/English) successful
spear thrower. A form of Edgar.
Garak, Garik, Garok, Garyk

Gareth (Welsh) gentle; old.
Garef, Gareff, Garif, Gariff, Garith,
Garyf, Garyff, Garyth

Garfield (Old English) from the
spear or triangular-shaped field.
Garfyeld

Gariana (Hindi) yell.
Garianah, Garyana, Garyanah

Garibaldo (Italian) prince of war.
Garibald, Garybald, Garybaldo

Garland (English) from the battle
ground. (O/Fren) wreath of
flowers.
Garlan, Garlande

Garman (Welsh) from Germany.
Garmen, German, Germin,
Germon, Germyn

Garner (English) to gather.
(Fren) army guard.
Garna, Garnar, Garnir, Garnor,
Garnyr

Garnet (Middle English) dark red;
precious gem.
Garnett, Garnier

Garnock (Welsh) alder-tree river
dweller.
Garnoc, Garnok

Garrad (English/Irish) brave spear
thrower.
Gared, Garrard, Garred, Garrod,
Garryd, Gerred, Jared

Garrett (Old English/Teutonic) hard
spear thrower.
Garet, Garett, Garit, Garret, Garrit,
Garritt, Garryt, Garrytt, Garyt,
Garytt

Garrick (German) mighty spear
ruler.
Garic, Garick, Garik, Garric, Garrik,
Garryc, Garryck, Garryk, Garyc,
Garyck, Garyk

Garrie (Australian Aboriginal) emu
(large flightless bird, ostrich-
like); sleepy.
Gari, Garie, Garri, Garry, Gary

Garrin (English/German) mighty
with a spear.
Garan, Garen, Garin, Garon,
Garran, Garren, Garron, Garryn,
Garyn

Garrison (Old English) Gary's son; son of the spear carrier. (Fren) troops stationed at the fort.
Garison, Garryson, Garyson

Garth (Scandinavian) from the enclosure. (Old/Eng) spear carrier.
Garthe

Garton (English) from the spear town; triangle-shaped town.
Gartown

Garve (Gaelic) from the rough place.
Garvee, Garvey, Garvi, Garvie, Garvy

Garvey (Irish) peace.
Garvee, Garvi, Garbie, Garvy

Garvin (German) friend who is in trouble.
Garvan, Garven, Garvon, Garvyn, Garwan, Garwen, Garwin, Garwon, Garwyn

Garwood (English) from the forest with the fur trees.

Gary (English) spear carrier.
Garee, Garey, Gari, Garie, Garree, Garrey, Garri, Garrie, Garry

Gascoyne (Old French) (Geographical) from Gascony in France.
Gascoin, Gascoine

Gaso/Gaspar (Illyrian/Persian) guardian of the treasure. A form of Casper.
Gasparas (Lith), Gaspard (Fren), Gaspar (Ital), Gaspare (Ital), Gaspardo (Ital), Gasper, Jaspar, Jasper

Gaston (English) from the gas town. (Fren) from Gascony in France.
Gascon, Gastan, Gasten, Gastin, Gastyn

Gatier (French/Teutonic) powerful warrior. A form of Walter.
Galtero, Gatyer, Gaulterio, Gaultier, Gaultiero, Gauthier (Fren)

Gauta/Gaute (Norwegian) great. Goth (East German people originally from Scandinavia).
Gaut, Gauntah, Gaunte

Gautulf (Swedish) gothic wolf (East German people originally from Scandinavia).
Gautolf

Gavin (Welsh/German) hawk.
Gavan, Gaven, Gavon, Gavun, Gavyn

Gavra (Slavic) hero of God.
Gavrah, Gavriil (Russ), Gavril

Gavrie (Russian) belonging to God.
Gabril, Gavri, Gavry, Ganya

Gavriel (Hebrew) strength of God. A form of the name of the Archangel, Gabriel.
Ganya, Gavrel, Gavril (Russ), Gavrilo (Ital), Gavrilushka, Gavryel, Gavryele, Gavryell, Gavryelle

Gawain (Welsh) hawk. A form of Gavin.
Gauvain, Gavan, Gaven, Gavin, Gavon, Gavyn, Gawayn, Gawayne, Gawen, Gawne

Gawath (Welsh) hawk of battle.

Gayadi (Australian Aboriginal) platypus, native Australian mammal.
Gaiadi

Gaylord (Old French) high-spirited.
(O/Eng) happy Lord.
Gaelor, Gaelord, Gailard, Gailor,
Gailord, Gayler, Gaylor

Gaynor (Irish) the fair-skinned
one's son.
Gaenor, Gainor

Gazza (Australian/English) spear
carrier. A form of Gary.
Gaza

Geary (Middle English) changes.
Gearee, Gearey, Geari, Gearie

Geb (Egyptian) earth.

Gellies (Dutch) maker of war.
Gellyes

Gemalli (Hebrew) rider of camels.
Gemali

Gemini (Latin) twins.
Geminy

Gene (Russian/Greek) noble; well
born. A form of Eugene.
Gena (Russ), Genek

Gennaro (Italian) born in January.
Genaro

Geno/Gino (Italian/Hebrew) God is
gracious. A form of John.
Genio, Gyno, Jeno, Jino, Jyno

Gent (Italian/English) gentle; kind.
Gental, Gentel, Gentile (Ital/Eng),
Gentle, Gentyl, Gentyle

Gently (Irish/English) snow.
Genti, Gentie

Geoff/Geoffrey (English) gentle;
kind; God's peace. The English
form of Godfrey, divine peace.
Gef, Geff, Geffree, Geffrey, Geffri,
Geffrie, Geffry, Geof, Geoff,
Geoffroi (Fren), Geofredo (Ital),
Giotto (Ital), Jef, Jeffm Jefferee,

Jefferey, Jefferi, Jefferie, Jeffery,
Jeofree, Jeofrey, Jeoffree, Jeoffrey

George (Greek) farmer.
Djuro (Slav), Egor (Russ), Egorka
(Russ), Gayeirges, Gayorgee,
Georg (Dan/Ger/Swed), Georgas
(Scott), Georges (Fren), Georij,
Georgio (Ital), Georgios (Grk),
Georgit, Georgius, Georgiz, Gergel
(Bav), Gheorghe (Rom), Gjorghic
(Illy), Giorghic, Giorgio (Ital),
Gjuraj (Illy), Gjuro (Illy), Gorej
(Slav), Gorgel, Hori (Poly), Jiri,
Jorg, Jorge, Jurgen, Jurgi (Russ),
Jugis, Jurica, Jurn, Jurnica, Jurria,
Seiorse, Yiorgis, Yrjo, Yuri

Geraint (Welsh) elder.
Geraynt

Gerald/Gerard (Teutonic) brave
spear carrier.
Gearalt (Ir), Gebhard (Ger),
Gebhardine (Ger), Gebhardt (Ger),
Geerd (Fris), Gellert (Hung),
Gerard (Ger), Gerardo (Span),
Geraud (Fren), Gerel (Fris),
Gerhard (Ger), Gerhardt (Ger),
Gero (Hung), Gerold (Ger),
Gerrard, Gerrit (Euro), Gerryt,
Geryld

Gerber (German) tanner of leather.

Geremia (Italian/Hebrew) chosen
by God. A form of Jeremiah.
Geremya

Gerlach (Scandinavian) spear
thrower.

Germain (French) from Germany.
Germaine, Germayn, Germayne,
Jermain, Jermaine, Jermayn,
Jermayne

Geronimo (Spanish/Latin) sacred
name of God. A form of Jerome.
Geronymo

Gershom (Hebrew) exiled.
Gersh, Gersham

Gervase (Teutonic) honourable.
Garvas, Garvase, Gerivas, Gervais,
Gervas, Gervasio (Span), Gervasy,
Gerwazy

Gerwyn (Welsh) fair love.
Gerwen, Gerwin

Gesar (Tibetan) from the lotus
temple.

Geshem (Hebrew) rain.

Gesio (Portuguese/Hebrew) God
will help. A form of Jesus.
Gesyo

Gethin (Welsh) dark-skinned.
Gethyn

Geysa (Hungarian) chief.
Geisa, Geza

Ghazi (Arabic) conquering.

Ghilchrist (Irish) God's servant.
Ghylchrist, Gilchrist, Gilcrist

Gi (Korean) brave.

Gia (Vietnamese) family.
Giah, Gya, Gyah

Giacinto (Portuguese/Spanish)
hyacinth; purple. A form of
Jacinto.
Giacintho, Gyacinto, Gyacynto

Giacomo (Italian/Hebrew) replacer.
A form of Jacob.
Gyacomo

Gian (Italian) God is gracious. A
form of John.
Gianetto, Giann, Giannes, Gianni,
Giannis, Giannos, Ghian, Ghyan,
Gyan

Giancarlo (Italian/Hebrew) God's
gracious, strong, courageous one.
A form of John/Charles.
Giancarlos, Gyancarlo

Gibor (Hebrew) strength.
Gibbor

Gibson (Old English) Gilbert's son;
son of the trusted, promised one.
Gibbson

Gideon (Hebrew) destroyer; great
warrior.
Gydeon

Gifford (Teutonic) bold giver.
Gifferd, Gyfford, Gyford

Gig (English) carriage which is
horse-drawn.

Gil (Greek) shield carrier. (Heb)
happy. The short form of names
starting with 'Gil' e.g. Gilbert.
Gill, Gyl, Gyll

Gilad (Arabic) hump on a camel;
from Giladi in Saudi Arabia.
Giladi, Giladie, Gilead, Gylad,
Gylead

Gilamu (Basque/Old English)
wilful. A form of William.
Gylamu

Gilbert (Old English/German) trust;
promise. (Heb) joy.
Gilibeirt (Ir), Gilberto (Ital),
Gilleabert (Scott), Gillbert,
Gillburt, Gilburt, Gilburto,
Giselbert (Ger), Gylbert, Gylbirt,
Gylburt, Gylbyrt

Gilby (Scandinavian) from the
estate of the hostage. (Ir) blond-
haired.
Gilbee, Gilbey, Gilbi, Gilbie,
Gillbee, Gillbey, Gillbi, Gillbie,
Gillby, Gylbee, Gylbey, Gylbi,
Gylbie, Gyllbee, Gyllbey, Gyllbi,
Gyllbie, Gyllby, Gylby

G

Gildea (Irish) God's servant.
Gildee, Gildey, Gildi, Gildie, Gildy

Gilen (German/Basque) illustrious promise.
Gilenn, Gylen

Giles (Greek) carrier of the shield.
Egide (Fren), Egidio (Ital), Egidius (Dut), Gide, Gilles (Fren), Gyles, Gylles

Gillean (Scottish) Saint John's servant.
Gillan, Gillen, Gillian, Gillyan

Gillespie (Irish) son of the bishop's servant.
Gillis, Gyllespie, Gyllespy

Gillet (French) Gilbert's son; son of the trusted one.
Gilet, Gilett, Gilette, Gillit, Gylet, Gylett, Gylit, Gylitt, Gylyt, Gylytt

Gillie (Gypsy) song.

Gilmer (Old English) famous host.
Gilmar, Gilmor, Gilmore, Gylmar, Gylmer, Gylmor, Gylmore

Gilmore (Irish) devoted one from the moor.
Gillmoor, Gillmoore, Gillmor, Gillmore, Gilmor, Gilmmor, Gilmoore, Gilmour, Gylmoor, Gylmoore, Gylmor, Gylmore,

Gilon (Hebrew) circle.
Gylon

Gilroy (Irish) devoted to the king.
Gilderoi, Gilderoy, Gildrai, Gildray, Gildroi, Gildroy, Gillroi, Gillroy, Gyllroi, Gyllroy, Gilroi, Gylroy

Gilus (Scandinavian) shield.

Ginger (Old English) red-haired; ginger spice.
Gynger

Gionah (Italian/Hebrew) dove. A form of Jonah.
Giona, Gyona, Gyonah

Giosia (Italian/Hebrew) God is my salvation. A form of Joshua.
Giosiah, Giosya, Gyosef, Gyosefa, Gyoseff, Gyoseffa, Gyosia, Gyosya, Gyosyah

Giovanni (Italian/Hebrew) God is gracious. A form of John.
Geovanni, Gian (Ital), Gianni (Ital), Giannino, Giovannie, Giovanno, Giavanny, Giovany, Giovanathon, Giovonni, Giovonnie, Giovonny, Gyovani, Gyovanie, Gyovany

Gipsy (English) wanderer.
Gipson, Gypson, Gypsy

Girra (Australian Aboriginal) creek.
Girrah, Gyrra, Gyrrah

Girvin (Irish) little; rough.
Girvyn, Gyrvyn

Gitano (Spanish) gypsy; wanderer.
Gytano

Giulio (Italian/Latin) youthful. A form of Jules.
Gyulio, Gyulyo

Giustino (Italian/Latin) righteous; just. A form of Justin.
Giusto (Ital), Giustyno, Gyustino, Gyusto, Gyustyno

Given (Old English/Puritan) one who is given.
Givan, Givin, Givon, Givyn

Givon (Hebrew) hill.
Givan, Given, Givun, Givyn, Gyvon

Gjosta (Swedish) God's staff; stick.
Gjostah

Gladstone (English) from the boundary stone at the happy one's estate.
Gladston

Gladus (Welsh) unseeing.
Gladius

Gladwin (English) happy.
Gladwen, Gladwenn, Gladwinn, Gladwyn, Gladwynn

Glanville (English) from the oak-tree village.
Glanvil, Glanvill, Glanvyl, Glanvyll, Glanvylle

Glasson (English/Scottish) son of the glass blower. (Scot) son from Glasgow; green hollow.
Glason, Glassan, Glassen, Glassin, Glassyn

Glaukos (Greek) sea-green colour.
Gla, Glau

Glen (Scottish) from the valley.
Glean, Glenn, Glennis, Glennon, Glenon, Glenton, Glyn (Wel), Glynn

Glendon (Scottish) from the valley fortress.
Glendan, Glenden, Glendin, Glendun, Glendyn, Glenn, Glenndan, Glennden, Glenndin, Glenndon, Glenndun, Glenndyn, Glyn (Wel), Glyndan, Glynden, Glyndin, Glyndon, Glyndyn, Glynn, Glynndan, Glynnden, Glynndin, Glynndin, Glynndon, Glynndun, Glynndyn

Glenrowan (Gaelic/Celtic) from the rowan-tree valley.
Glennrowan, Glenrowen, Glenrowin, Glenrowyn, Glynnrowan, Glynnrowen, Glynnrowin, Glynnrowon, Glynnrowyn, Glynrowan,

Glynrowen, Glynrowin, Glynrowon, Glynrowyn

Glenton (Scottish/Old English) from the valley town.
Glennton, Glynnton, Glynton

Glenville (Scottish/Old English) from the village in the glen (valley).
Glennville, Glenvyl, Glenvyle, Glenvylle, Glynnville, Glynville

Glenworth (Scottish/Old English) from the homestead in the valley.
Glennworth, Glynnworth, Glynworth

Glyn (Welsh) small valley.
Glin, Glinn, Glynn

Goddard (Teutonic) firm in God.
Godard (Fren), Godewin, Godewyn (Dut), Gotthard (Dut), Gotthart (Ger)

Godfrey (Teutonic) divine peace.
Goddfree, Goddfrey, Godfree, Godfreed, Gotryd (Pol), Godofredo (Span), Goffredo (Ital), Goraidh (Scott), Gottfrid (Swed), Gottfried (Ger)

Godwin (Old English) God's friend.
Godwen, Godwinn, Godwyn, Godwynn

Goel (Hebrew) redeemer; to regain.

Gold (Old English) golden-haired, blond.
Goldi, Goldie, Goldy

Golding (English) little gold.
Goldan, Golden, Goldin, Goldyn

Goldwin (English) gold friend.
Goldwinn, Goldwinne, Goldwyn, Goldwyne, Goldwynn, Goldwynne

Goliath (Hebrew) giant.
Golliath, Golyath, Gully (Eng)

G

Gomda (Kiowa) wind.
Gomdah

Gomer (Hebrew) finishing.
(O/Eng) famous battle.

Gomez (Spanish) man.
Gomaz

Gommata (Sanskrit) strong-armed.
Gomata

Gondol (Norse) good.

Gonstan (Breton) from the hill
stone.

Gothier (French) war army.
Gonthyer

Gonza (Rutooro) love.
Gonzah

Gonzales (Spanish) wolf.
Goncalve, Gonsalve, Gonsalvo
(Ital), Gonzales (Fren), Gonzalo,
Gonzalos, Gonzalous

Goodman (Old English) good man.
Goodmen

Gool (Old English) from the
stream.

Gopal (Sanskrit) herd of cows.
Gopala

Gordon (Old English) from the
great hill.
Gordan, Gorden, Gordin, Gordun,
Gordyn

Gore (Old English) from the spear
field; from the triangular-shaped
field.

Gorm (Norse) war serpent.

Gorman (Irish) little one with the
blue eyes.
Gormen

Goro (Japanese) fifth-born child.

Gotardo (Italian) good; firm.

Gotzon (German/Greek) angel;
God's messenger.

Gough (Welsh) red-haired.
Gof, Goff

Govert (Dutch) heavenly peace.

Govinda (Sanskrit) keeper of the
cows.
Govynda

Gower (Old Welsh) purity.

Gowon (Tiv) rain maker.
Gowan, Gowen, Gowin, Gowyn

Gozol (Hebrew) soaring bird.
Gozal

Grady (Irish) noble; illustrious.
Gradee, Gradey, Gradi, Gradie,
Graidee, Graidey, Graidi, Graidie,
Graidy, Graydee, Graydey, Graydi,
Graydie, Graydy

Graeme/Graham (Old English)
from the grey home.
Graeham, Graehame, Graem,
Graham, Grahame, Grahme,
Grahem Graheme, Grahim,
Grahym, Graiam, Graiham,
Graihame, Grayham, Grayhame,
Grayhim, Grayhym, Greyham,
Greyhame, Greyhem, Greyheme,
Greyh

Grande (Portuguese) grand.
Grand

Granger (Old English) farmer.
Grainger, Graynger

Grant (French) grand.
Grand, Grandt, Grantham,
Granthem, Grantlea, Grantleah,
Grantlee, Grantley, Grantli,
Grantlie, Grantly

Grantland (English) from the grand
land.
Granlan, Granland, Grantlan

Grantley (Old English/French) from the grand meadow.
Grantlea, Grantleah, Grantlee, Grantleigh, Grantli, Grantlie, Grantly

Granville (French) from the grand village.
Granvil, Granvile, Granvyl, Granvyll, Granvylle

Gratian (Latin) thankful.
Gratiano, Gratien

Gray (Old English) grey colour.
Grae, Grai, Grey, Greye

Graydon (English) from the grey hill.
Graedan, Graeden, Graedin, Graedon, Graedyn, Graidan, Graiden, Graidin, Graidon, Graidyn, Graydan, Grayden, Greydin, Greydon, Greydyn

Grayson (English) the judge's son; the grey one's son.
Graeson, Graison, Greyson

Greeley (English) from the grey meadow.
Greelea, Greeleah, Greeleigh, Greeli, Greelie, Greely

Greenwood (English) from the green woods.
Gree, Greene, Greenewood, Greener, Greenerwood

Greg/Gregory (Greek) watchful.
Graig, Graigg, Greggori, Greggorie, Greggory (Lat), Gregoire (Fren), Gregor (Ger), Gregori (Ital/Port), Gregorie (Span/Ital), Gregorijie (Illy), Gregorio (Span), Gregorios (Ital/Port), Gregos (Dan), Greggson, Gregson, Gregus (Ger), Greig (Scott), Greigg (Scott), Greigoor (Scott), Greigor (Scott), Greigore (Scott), Grigori (Russ),

Grigorij (Russ), Grigory (Russ), Grigoris (Grk), Grzegorz (Pol)

Gresham (Old English) from the grassy homestead.

Gribbon (Irish/German) Robin's son; son of the robin bird keeper.
Gribon, Grybbon, Grybon

Griffin (Latin) hooked nose.
Griffen, Griffon, Griffyn, Gryffin,, Gryffyn

Griffith (Welsh) strong Lord.
Griffith, Gryffith, Gryphon

Grimshaw (English) from the dark woods.
Grymshaw

Grindal (Old English) from the green valley.
Gryndal

Grisha (Russian/Greek) watchful. A form of Gregory.
Grigoi, Grigor, Grigori (Bul), Grigorios, Grigorov, Grigory, Grysha

Griswold (German) Christ's power. (Fren) from the grey forest.
Griswald, Griswaldo, Griswoldo, Gryswald, Gryswaldo

Grosvenor (Old French) great chief hunter.

Grover (Old English) from the grove.

Guard (Old English) guardian; protector.
Gard, Garde

Guildford (Old English) from the yellow flower ford.
Guild, Guildford

Guire (Irish) beige colour.
MacGuire, Macguire, MacGuyre, Macguyre

Gulzar (Arabic) flowering.

Gunnar (German/Scandinavian)
bold.
Gun, Guna, Gunah, Gunner,
Gunter, Gunthar

Gunther (Teutonic) battle army.
Guenter, Guenther, Gunnar,
Gunner, Guntar, Gunter, Guntero,
Gunthar

Guntur (Indonesian) thunder.

Gur (Hebrew) lion cub.

Gurion (Hebrew) strength of a lion.
Guriel, Guryon

Gus (Scandinavian) staff (stick).

Gustav (Swedish) noble staff (stick)
bearer.
Gustaf, Gustave, Gustavius (Ger),
Gustavo (Ital)

Guthre (Irish) from the windy area.
Guthree, Guthrey, Guthri, Guthrie,
Guthry

Guy (French) guide from the forest.
(Eng) man.
Guie, Guion, Guyan

Gwern (Welsh) alder tree.

Gwesyn (Welsh) little friend.

Gwidon (Polish) life.
Gwydon

Gwyn (Welsh) fair-haired; blond.
Gwinn, Gwinne, Gwynn, Gwynne

Gwynfor (Welsh) fair lord.
Gwinfor

Gwynne (Welsh) white.
Gwin, Gwinn, Gwyn, Gwyne

Gyula (Hungarian) youthful.
Gyala, Gyuszi

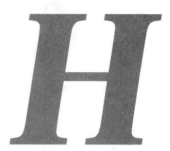

Haakan (Scandinavian) chosen son.
Hagan, Hagen, Hagin, Hagon,
Hagyn, Hakan, Haken, Hakin,
Hakon, Hakyn

Habib (Arabic) beloved.
Habyb

Hacket (German) little woodcutter.
Hackett, Hackit, Hackitt, Hackyt,
Hackytt

Hackman (German/French) cutter
of wood.
Hackmen

Haddad (Arabic) blacksmith.
Hadad

Haddon (Old English) from the
heather-covered hill.
Hadan, Haddan, Hadden, Haddin,
Haddyn, Haden, Hadin, Hadlee,
Hadleigh, Hadley, Hado, Hadon,
Hadun, Hadyn

Hadi (Arabic) guidance to the right.
Haddi, Had, Hadd

Hadley (Old English) from the
heather meadow.
Hadlea, Hadleah, Hadlee,
Hadleigh, Hadly

Harian (Latin) dark; mysterious;
from the Adriatic Sea. A
masculine form of Adriana.
Hadrien, Hadrion, Hadryan,
Hardyen, Hadryon, Hadryn

Hadriel (Hebrew) God is glory.
Hadriell, Hadryel, Hadryell

Hadwin (Old English) war friend.
Hadwen, Hadwinn, Hadwyn,
Hadwynn, Hadwynne, Hedwin,
Hedwyn

Hafiz (Arabic) remembering;
protection.
Hafyz

Hagan (Irish) ruler of the home.
Hagen, Hagin, Hagon, Hagyn

Hagar (Hebrew) forsaken.
Hager, Hagir, Hagor, Hagyr

Hagen (Irish/Gaelic) little; young.
Hagan, Hagin, Hagon, Hagun,
Hagyn

Hagley (Old English) from the
hedged meadow.
Haglea, Hagleah, Haglee, Hagleigh,
Hagli, Haglie, Hagly

Hahnee (Native American) one who
begs.

Hai (Vietnamese) sea.

Haidar (Arabic) lion.

Haig (Old English) dweller at the
hedged enclosure.
Hayg

Hailama (Hawaiian) famed brother.
Hairama, Hairamah, Hailamah,
Hilaman, Hilamah, Hirama

Haines (Old English) fence.
Hanes, Haynes

Haji (Swahili) born on the
pilgrimage to Mecca.

Hakan (Native American) fiery.

Hakeem (Arabic) wise ruler.
Kacim, Hackim

Hakim (Ethiopian) doctor.
Hackeem, Hakeem, Hakiem, Hakym

Hakon (Scandinavian) chosen;
praised. (O/Nrs) useful.
Haakon, Hakan, Hakin, Hako
(Nrs), Hakyn

Hal (Old English) dweller at the
hall. The short form of names
starting with 'Hal' e.g. Halford.

Hala (Greek/Latin) salty.
Halah

Halbert (Old English) brilliant one;
hero.
Halbirt, Halburt, Halbyrt

Halcyon (Latin/Greek) quiet.
Halcion

Halden (Scandinavian) half Danish.
Haldan, Haldane, Haldin, Haldon,
Haldyn

Hale (Old English) hero from the
hall.
Hael, Haele, Hail, Haley, Halford,
Hallie, Halsey, Halsy, Hayl, Hayle,
Hollis, Holly

Halen (Swedish) hall.
Hailan, Hailen, Hailin, Hailon,
Hailyn, Hale, Hallen, Hatlan,
Haylen

Haley (Scandinavian) hero.
(Old Eng) ingenious; from the
hay meadow.
Hailea, Haileah, Hailee, Haileigh,
Haily, Hale, Halea, Haleah,
Haleigh, Halle, Halley, Halli,
Hallie, Hally

Halford (Old English) from the ford
in the side valley.
Haleford

Hali (Greek) sea.
Halea, Haleah, Halee, Haleigh,
Haley, Halie, Haly

Halian (Zuni) young.
Halyan

H

Halifax (Old English) from the holy field.
Halyfax

Halil (Turkish) close friend.
Halyl

Halim (Arabic) gentle.
Haleem, Halym

Hall (German) dweller at the hall. (O/Eng) from the stone manor.
Hal

Hallam (Old Norse) from the rock. (O/Eng) from the sloping valley.
Halam

Hallan (English) hall dweller; dweller from the manor.
Halan, Halen, Halin, Hallen, Hallin, Hallon, Hallyn, Halon, Halyn

Halley (Old English) from the manor; hall in the meadow; from the holy meadow.
Halea, Haleah, Halee, Haleigh, Haley, Hallea, Halleah, Hallee, Halleigh, Hally, Haly

Halliwell (Old English) dweller near the holy stream.
Haliwel, Haliwell, Halliwel, Hallywel, Hallywell, Halywel, Halywell

Hallward (Old English) guardian of the hall.
Halward

Halola (Hawaiian) army power.
Halolah, Harola, Harolah

Halse (Old English) neck of land; from Hal's island.
Hallsea, Hallsey, Hallsy, Halsea, Halsy

Halstead (Old English) from the manor in the grounds.
Halsted

Halton (English) from the town on the hill.
Haltan, Halten, Haltin, Haltyn

Halvor (Norwegian) rock; guardian, protector.
Halvar, Halvard

Halyard (Scandinavian) rock defender.
Hallvar, Hallvard, Hallor, Halvar, Halvor

Ham (Old English) home; town. (Heb) dark-complexioned and warm one. The short form of names starting with 'Ham' e.g. Hamlet.

Hamal (Arabic) lamb. A star in the Aries constellation.
Hamel, Hamil, Hamol, Hamyl

Hamer (Old Norse) hammer.
Hama, Hamar, Hammar, Hammer

Hamford (Old English) from the rocky ford.

Hamid (Arabic) thanking God.
Haamid, Hamadi, Hamdrem, Hamed, Hameed, Hamidi, Hammad, Hammed, Hamyd, Hamydd, Humayd

Hamidi (Kenyan) one who is admired.
Hamidie, Hamidy

Hamill (English) from the proud mill.
Hamel, Hamell, Hamil, Hammil, Hamyl, Hamyll

Hamilton (Old English) from the proud town; from the crooked hill.
Hamel, Hamelton, Hamil, Hamill, Hamiltan, Hamilten, Hamiltun, Hamiltyn, Hamylton

Hamish (Scottish) remover.
Hamysh

Hamisi (Swahili) born on a Thursday.
Hamisie, Hamisy

Hamlet (Old French) little home.
Amleth, Amlothi, Haimes, Hamelin, Hames, Hamil, Hamilton, Hamlin, Hamlit, Hamlot, Hammond, Hamnet, Hamon, Hamond, Hampden, Hampton, Haymund

Hamlin (Old French/German) little home lover.
Hamlan, Hamlen, Hamlon, Hamlyn

Hammet (English/Scandinavian) village.
Hammett, Hamnet, Hamnett

Hammond (English) village.
Hamon, Hamond, Hammon, Hamund

Hamon (Teutonic) home.
Amon, Hamlet, Hamlin, Hamlyn, Hammond, Hamnet, Hamund, Hemelen, Hamony

Hampton (English) from the proud town.
Hamptan, Hampten, Hamptin, Hamptyn

Hamza (Arabic) powerful.
Hamzah

Hanale (Hawaiian/German) ruler of the house. A form of Henry.
Haneke

Hanan (Hebrew) graceful.
Hananel, Hanania, Hananiah, Johan, Johanan

Hanbal (Arabic) purity.
Hanbel, Hanbil, Hanbyl

Handel (German/English) God is gracious. A form of John.
Handal, Handil, Handol, Handyl

Handley (Russian) from the clearing in the forest.
Handlea, Handleah, Handlee, Handleigh, Handli, Handlie, Handly

Hanford (Old English) from the high ford.

Hani (Arabic) happy.
Hanee, Haney, Hanie, Hany

Hanif (Arabic) true believer.
Haneef, Hanef, Hanifa, Hanyfa

Hank (American/Teutonic) head person; chief.

Hanley (Old English) of the high meadow.
Hanlea, Hanleah, Hanlee, Hanleigh, Hanly, Henlea, Henleah, Henlee, Henleigh, Henley, Henly

Hannes (Finnish) God is gracious. A form of John.
Hanes

Hannibal (Phoenician) with the grace of God.
Anibal, Hanibal, Hannybal, Hanybal

Hanno (German/Hebrew) God is gracious. A form of John/Johann.
Hano

Hans (Scandinavian/Hebrew) God is gracious. The Scandinavian form of John.
Hannes, Hannus (Est), Hanschen, Hansel, Hansli (Swiss), Hnats, Hanz

Hansel (Scandinavian) God is gracious. A form of John/Johann.
Haensel, Hannsel, Hansal, Hansil, Hansol, Hansl, Hansyl

Hanson (Scandinavian) son of Hans; son of the gracious one.
Hansan, Hansen, Hansin, Hansun, Hansyn

Hanus (Czech) God is gracious. A form of John/Johann.

Hao (Chinese) good.

Haoa (Hawaiian/English) watcher; guardian. A form of Howard.

Haral (Scottish) army leader.
Arailt, Harall, Harell

Haram (Hebrew) mountaineer.

Harath (Arabic) provider.
Harith, Haryth

Harb (Arabic) warrior.

Harbin (Teutonic) glorious, little warrior.
Harban, Harben, Harbon, Harbyn

Harcourt (Old English) from the hawker's cottage. (O/Fren) fortified dwelling.
Harcort

Harden (Old English) from the valley of the hares.
Hardan, Harde, Hardie, Hardin, Harding, Hardon, Hardun, Hardy, Hardyn

Harding (Old English) son of the brave one.
Hardin, Hardyng

Hardwin (Old English/Teutonic) strong, loyal friend.
Hardwen, Hardwenn, Hardwinn, Hardwyn, Hardwynn

Hardy (Teutonic) bold; daring; hardy. (O/Fren) courageous.
Hardee, Harden, Hardey, Hardi, Hardie, Hardin, Harding

Harel (Hebrew) from God's mountain.
Haral, Harell, Hariel, Hariell, Harrel, Harrell, Haryel, Haryell

Harford (English) from the hare ford.
Hareford

Hargrove (English) from the hare grove.
Haregrove

Hari (Sanskrit) remover of sin. (Hind) tawny.
Hariel, Harin, Hary, Haryn

Harim (Hebrew) contracted.
Hareem, Harym

Harish (Hindi) lord.
Haresh, Harysh

Harith (Arabic) cultivator.
Haryth

Harkin (Irish) dark red colour; red-haired.
Harkan, Harken, Harkon, Harkyn

Harlan (Old English) from the hare's land; from the battle land.
Harland, Harle, Harlen, Harley, Harlin, Harlyn

Harlequin (Old English) brightly masked.
Harliwuin, Harlyquin

Harley (Old English) from the wooded hare meadow.
Harlan, Harlea, Harleah, Harlee, Harleigh, Harly

Harlow (Old English) from the rough hare's hill; battle hill.
Harlo

Harmens (Dutch) harmonious. The masculine form of Harmony.
Harmensz

Harmon (German) man of the army.
Harman, Harmen, Harmin,
Harmyn

Harold (Old Norse) powerful army
commander.
Arald, Araldo (Ital), Aralt (Ir),
Haldon, Harailt (Ir), Harald
(Swed/Dan), Haraldas (Lith),
Haraldo (Span/Port), Haralds,
Haralpos, Hareld, Harild, Haroldo
(Ital), Harral, Harrel, Harris, Harry,
Haryld, Haryldo, Herald, Hereld,
Herold (Dut), Herrick, Herris,
Herry, Heryld, Heryldo

Haroun (Arabic) highly praised.
Haaroun, Haarun, Harin, Haron,
Haroon, Harron, Harrun, Harun

Harper (Old English) player of harps.
Harpo

Harrington (English) from Harry's
town; from the army ruler's town.
Harringtown

Harris (Old English) Harry's son;
son of the army ruler.
Haris, Harrys, Harys, Heris, Herris,
Herrys, Herys

Harrison (Old Norse) Harry's son;
son of the army ruler.
Harison, Harryson, Haryson

Harrod (Hebrew) conquering hero.
Harod

Harry (English/Scandinavian) army
ruler. The short form of Harold.
Hari, Harie, Harri, Harrie, Hary

Harshad (Hindi) joy giver.

Hart (Old English) male deer; stag.
Hart, Harte, Hartley, Hartleigh,
Hartley, Hartwel, Hartwell,
Hartwig, Harwel, Harwell, Harwil,
Harwill, Heart, Heartlea, Heartleah,
Heartlee, Heartleigh, Heartlyey,
Heartli, Heartlie, Heartly, Hersch,

Herschel, Hersh, Hershel, Hertz,
Hertzl, Herzl, Heschel, Heshel,
Hirsch, Hirsh, Hyrt

Hartford (English) from the hare's
ford.

Hartley (Old English) from the
deer-wood clearing in the
meadow.
Hart, Harte, Hartlea, Hartleah,
Hartlee, Hartleigh, Hartli, Hartlie,
Hartly, Hartman

Hartman (German) strong; hard.
Hartmen

Hartwell (Old English) from the
deer stream.
Hartwel, Hartwil, Hartwill,
Hartwyl, Hartwyll

Hartwig (German) strong advisor.
Hartwyg

Hartwood (English) from the hare
woods; from the hard woods;
from the deer woods.

Harue (Japanese) born in the spring
time.
Haru

Harun (Arabic) praised highly.
Haroun

Harvey (Teutonic) army warrior.
(Celt) eager for battle.
Harve, Harvee, Harveson, Harvi,
Harvie, Harvy, Herve, Herevey,
Hervey, Hervi, Hervie, Hervy

Harwood (English) from the hare's
forest.
Hardwood, Hardtwood

Hasad (Turkish) harvesting.
Hassad

Hasant (Swahili) handsome.
Hasan, Hasen, Hasin, Hassan,
Hassani, Hassen, Hasson, Hassyn

H

Hashim (Arabic) destroyer of evil.
Haashim, Hasheem, Hashym

Hasib (Arabic) reckoner.
Hasyb

Hasim (Arabic) determined.
Hasam, Hasem, Hasom, Hasym

Hasin (Sanskrit) laughing.
Hasen, Hasin, Hassin, Hassyn,
Hasyn

Haskel (Hebrew) understanding.
Haskell

Haslett (Old English) from the
hazel-tree land.
Haslet, Hazel, Hazet, Hazett,
Hazlet, Hazlett

Hassan (Arabic) handsome.
Hasan

Hassel (English) from the witches'
corner. (Geographical) from
Hassall, England.
Hasel, Hasell, Hassell

Hastin (Hindi) elephant.
Hastan, Hasten, Hason, Hastyn

Hastings (Old English) son of the
stern one. (Ger) fast.
Hasting

Hatdar (Hindi) lion.
Haider, Hayder, Hyder

Hatiya (Native American) bear.
Hatiyah

Hau (Vietnamese) desired.

Havea (Polynesian) chief.

Havelock (Scandinavian) contest at
sea; battle.
Haveloc, Haveloch (Scott),
Havloche, Havlocke

Haven (English) refuge.
Hagan, Hagen, Hagin, Hagon,
Hagun, Hagyn, Havan, Havin,
Havon, Havun, Havyn, Hazan,
Hazen, Hazin, Hazon, Hazun,
Hazyn

Havgan (Celtic) white.
Havgen, Havgin, Havgon, Havgun,
Havgyn

Havika (Hawaiian/Hebrew) beloved.
A form of David.
Havyka

Hawley (English) from the hedged
meadow.
Hawlea, Hawleah, Hawlee,
Hawleigh, Hawli, Hawlie, Hawly

Hawthorne (English) the hawthorn
tree.
Hawthorn

Hayden (Old English) from the
valley with the hedges.
Hadan, Haden, Hadin, Hadon,
Hadun, Hadyn, Haidan, Haiden,
Haidin, Haidn, Hadon, Haidun,
Haidyn, Haydan, Haydin, Haydn,
Haydon, Haydun, Haydyn,
Heydan, Heyden, Heydin, Heydn,
Heydon, Heydun, Heydyn

Hayes (Old English/Irish) from the
place with hedges.
Hais, Haise, Haiz, Haize, Hays,
Hayz

Haytham (Arabic) proud.
Haitham

Hayward (Old English) from the
forest with hedges.
Haiward, Heiward, Heiwood,
Heyward, Heywood

Hearne (Scottish/English) horse
worker.
Ahearn, Ahearne, Ahern, Aherne,
Hearn, Herin, Hern, Herne

Heath (Old English) from the field
of heather. The short form of
names starting with 'Heath' e.g.
Heathcote.
Heaf, Heaff, Heathcliff, Heathcote,
Heathe

Heathcliffe (Old English) from the
field of heather.
Heafclif, Heafcliff, Heaffclif,
Heaffcliff, Heaffcliffe, Heaffclyffe,
Heathclif, Heathcliffe, Heathclyffe

Heathcote (Old English) from the
cliff cottage on the heather.
Heathcot

Heaton (English) from the high
town.
Heatan, Heaten, Heatin, Heatyn

Heber (Hebrew) associate.
Habar, Hebar

Hector (Greek) steadfast.
Ector, Ectore, Ettor, Ettore, Hectar,
Heckter, Hecktir, Hecktore, Hectori,
Hecktur, Hektar, Hekter, Hektir,
Hektor, Hektore, Hektori, Hektur

Heddwyn (Welsh) friend of peaceful
blessings.
Heddwen, Heddwin, Heddwyn,
Hedwen, Hedwin, Heddwin,
Hedwyn

Hedeon (Russian) tree cutter.
Hedion, Hedyon

Hedley (Old English) from the
meadow with hedges; sheep
meadow.
Heddlea, Heddleah, Heddlee,
Heddleigh, Heddley, Heddli,
Heddlie, Heddly, Hedlea, Hedleah,
Hedlee, Hedleigh, Hedli, Hedlie,
Hedly

Hedwig (Teutonic) fighter.
Heddwig, Heddwyg, Hedwyg

Heinrich (German) ruler of the
house. A form of Henry.
Heindric, Heindrick, Heiner,
Heinric, Heinrick, Heinrik,
Heynric, Heynrich, Heynrick,
Hinricm, Hinrich, Hinrick, Hynric,
Hynrich, Hynrick, Hynrik

Hekeka (Hawaiian) holding fast.
Hekekah, Heketa, Heketah

Helaku (Native American) sunny
day.

Helge (Russian) holy.
Helg

Helgi (Scandinavian) happy.

Heli (Greek) sun.
Helli

Helier (Latin) happy.

Helki (Moquelumnan) touch.

Helmer (German) famous.

Helmut (German) famous;
courageous. (Fren) warrior.
Hellmut, Helmuth

Heman (Hebrew) faithful.
Hemen

Hemene (Nez Perce) wolf.

Henderson (Scottish/English)
Henry's son; son of the ruler of
the house.
Hendri, Hendrie, Hendries,
Hendron, Henryson

Hendrick/Hendrix (Dutch/German)
ruler of the home. A form of
Henry.
Hendric, Hendricks, Hendrickson,
Hendrik, Hendriks, Hendrikus,
Hendrixx, Hendryc, Hendryck,
Hendrycks, Hendryk, Hendryks,
Hendryx, Hendryxx, Henning
(Ger), Hennings

Heneli (Hawaiian) ruler of the home. A form of Henry.
Henelie, Henely

Henley (English) from the high meadow.
Henlea, Henleah, Henlee, Henleigh, Henli, Henlie, Henly

Henning (German) ruler of the house. A form of Henry.
Hennings

Henoch (Yiddish) initiator.
Enoch

Henry (German) ruler of the house.
Arrigo, Eanruig (Scot), Enrico (Ital), Enrik, Enrikas, Enrique (Span), Enriquo, Enselius, Ensilis, Ensilo (Ger), Enskys (Balt), Enzio (Ital), Ezio, Guccio, Haimirich, Halkin, Hank, Hanraoi (Ir), Hedric, Hedrick, Hein, Heindrick, Heindrich, Heinriche, Heinrik, Hein (Ger), Heinje, Heinrich (Ger), Heinriche, Heinrick, Heintje (Dut), Heinz (Ger), Hendri, Hendrick (Dut), Hendrick, Hendrik (Dut), Heneli, Henke, Henning, Henny, Henri (Fren), Henric, Henricus, Henrik (Dan/Nor), Henrikus (Lith), Henryc, Henryck, Henryk

Herald/Heraldo (English) news bringer. (Span) army ruler.
Haroldo, Herald, Hiraldo, Hyroldo

Herb/Herbe/Herbert (German) brilliant warrior.
Ebert, Eberte, Eberto, Harbert, Herbe, Herbee, Hebert, Herbertas (Lith), Heberto (Span), Herberte, Herbertus, Herbi, Herbie, Herbirt, Herburt, Herby, Herbyrt, Hilbert, Hirbirt, Hirburt, Hirburt, Hoireabard (Ir), Hyrbert, Hyrbirt, Hyrburt, Hyrbyrt

Herbrand (Teutonic) army; sword.
Herbran, Herbrandt, Herbrant

Hercules (Greek) gift of glory; strength.
Ercole, Heracles, Hercule

Hereward (English) army.
Herward

Herman (Teutonic) noble warrior. (Lat) high ranking. (Heb) faithful.
Armand (Fren), Armando (Ital), Armandus, Armanno (Ital), Armant, Armin, Ermannis, Ermanno (Ital), Ermas, Erme, Ermin (Fren), Ermine (Fren), Ermolaj (Rus), Ermonas, Harman, Harmann, Harmen, Herma (Swiss), Hermando (Port), Hermann (Ger/Dan), Hermannus, Hermano (Span), Hermanus (Dut), Hermeli (Swiss), Hermi, Hermie, Hermin, Hermon, Hermy, Hermyn

Hermes (Greek) messenger.
Herm, Herme

Hern (Middle English) the heron bird.
Ahearn, Ahearne, Ahern, Aherne, Hearn, Hearne, Herin, Herne

Hernando (Spanish/German) adventurer; peace maker. (Goth) life adventure. The feminine form of Ferdinand.
Hernandes, Hernandez

Herod (Greek) protector.

Herrick (Teutonic) army ruler.
Herick, Herik, Herrik, Herryc, Herryck, Herryk

Hersh/Hershel (Hebrew) deer.
Hersch, Herschel, Hirsch, Hirschel, Hirshel, Hyrchel, Hyrshel

Hertz (Yiddish) trouble.
Herts

Herve (French/German) army
warrior. (Celt) eager for battle. A
form of Harvey.
Herv

Herzog (Teutonic) duke.

Hesperos (Greek) evening star.
Hespero

Hesutu (Moquelumnan) yellow
jacket's nest being picked up.

Hevel (Hebrew) breath.
Hevell

Hew (Welsh/German) intelligent.
(O/Ger) heart; mind. A form of
Hugh.
Hewe, Hiu (Haw), Hugh, Huw,
Huwe

Hewett (Teutonic) little Hugh;
intelligent. (O/Ger) heart; mind.
A form of Hugh.
Hewet, Hewit, Hewitt (Fren),
Hughet, Hughett, Hughit, Hughitt,
Hughyt, Hughytt

Hewney (Irish) green.
Hewnee, Hewni, Hewniw, Hewny

Hewson (Welsh/German) Hugh's
son; son of the intelligent one.
Hueson, Hughson

Heywood (Old English) from the
high woods.
Haiwood, Haywood, Heiwood

Hezekiah (Hebrew) God is my
strength.
Hezekia

Hiamovi (Cheyenne) high chief.
Hyamovi

Hiawatha (Iroqois) river maker.

Hibah (Arabic) gift.
Hiba, Hyba, Hybah

Hideaki (Japanese) clever.
Hydeaki

Hideo (Japanese) the best.

Hien (Vietnamese) sweet.

Hieu (Vietnamese) respectful.
Hyeu

Hiew (Vietnamese) religious.
Hyew

Hilal (Arabic) new moon.
Hylal

Hilary (Latin) cheerful.
Alair, Hilar, Hilare, Hilarius
(Ger/Dan/Dut/Swed), Hilaire
(Fren), Hilario (Span/Port), Hilery,
Hillary, Hillery, Hylari, Hylarie,
Hylary, Ilario (Ital)

Hilderic (Gothic) warrior. The
masculine form of
Hilda/Hilgegarde, battle
stronghold.
Hilderic, Hildriche (Ger), Hylderic,
Hylderych, Hylderyche

Hilel (Arabic) new moon.
Hylel

Hillard (German) tough warrior.
Hilard, Hylard, Hyllard

Hillel (Hebrew) highly praised;
renowned.
Hilel, Hylel, Hyllel

Hilliard (Gothic) warrior guardian
of war.
Hiliard, Hillard, Hilliar, Hillyer,
Hyliar, Hyliard, Hylliar

Hilmar (Swedish) famous; noble.
Hillmar, Hilmer, Hylmar, Hylmer

Hilmer (Old English) from the far,
remote hill.
Hylmer

Hilton (Old English) from the town on the hill.
Hillton, Hylton

Himesh (Hindi) king of the snow.
Hymesh

Hina (Tongan) spider.
Hinah

Hinto (Dakota) blue.
Hynto

Hinun (Native American) the storm's spirit.
Hynun

Hiram (Hebrew) most noble; God is high.
Ahiram, Hirom, Huram, Hyram, Hyrum

Hiroshi (Japanese) generous; person from Hiroshima.
Hyroshi

Hisoka (Japanese) shy.
Hysoka

Hiu (Hawaiian) intelligent. (O/Ger) heart; mind. A form of Hugh.
Hyu

Ho (Chinese) river; good.

Hoa (Vietnamese) peace loving.
Hoah

Hoang (Vietnamese) finish.

Hobart (Teutonic) bright mind or heart. A form of Hubert.
Hobard, Hoebard, Hoebart

Hobert (German) from Bert's hill; from the bright, shining, illustrious one's hill.
Hobirt, Hoburt, Hobyrt

Hobson (English) good; beautiful; Robert's son; son of the bright, famous one.
Hobsan, Hobsen, Hobsin, Hobsyn

Hoc (Vietnamese) studious.
Hock, Hok

Hod (Hebrew) splendour from God.
Hodiya

Hodaka (Japanese) mountain.
Hodakah

Hodgson (English) Roger's son; son of the renowned spearsman.

Hoffman (German) one with influence.
Hoffmen, Hofman, Hofmen

Hogan (Irish/Gaelic) young.
Hogen, Hogin, Hogun, Hogyn

Holata (Native American) alligator.
Holatah

Holbrook (Old English) from the brook near the hollow.
Holbrooke

Holcomb (Old English) from the deep valley.
Holcombe

Holden (Old English) from the hollow in the deep valley.
Holdan, Holdin, Holdon, Holdun, Holdyn

Holger (Teutonic) rich spear.

Holic (Czech) hair cutter; barber.
Holick, Holik, Holyc, Holyck, Holyk

Holland (English) from Holland.
Holan, Holand, Hollan

Holleb (Polish) dove.
Hollub, Holub

Hollis (Old English) from the holly-tree grove.
Holliss, Hollys, Hollyss

Holm (Old English) meadow; small island.
Holme, Holmes, Hume

Holman (Norse) from the hollow.
Hollman, Hollmen, Holmen

Holmes (Middle English) from the
river islands. (O/Nrs) from the
river flat.

Holt (Old English) from the forest.
Holtan, Holten, Holtin, Holton,
Holtyn

Homer (Greek) promise.
Holmer, Homa, Homar, Homere
(Fren), Homero, Homerus
(Ger/Dut), Omero (Ital)

Hondo (Shona) warrior.

Honester (Old English) stone; tool
sharpener.
Honesterr

Honesto (Filipino) honest.
Honest

Honi (Hebrew) gracious.
Honie, Hony

Honon (Moquelumnan) bear.

Honore (Latin) honourable.
Honor

Honovi (Native American) strength.

Honza (Czech) God is gracious. A
form of John.

Hop (Chinese) one who agrees.

Horace/Horatio (Latin) time keeper.
(Grk) promise.
Horacio (Span/Port), Horation,
Horatius (Ger), Horats (Dut),
Horaz, Horazio, Oratio, Orazio
(Ital)

Horimir (Bohemian) from the hill.
Horemer, Horemir, Horimer,
Horymer

Horst (Teutonic) thicket; nest;
leaping.
Hurst

Horton (Old English) from the grey
town. (Lat) garden.
Hartan, Horten, Hortin, Hortun,
Hortyn

Horus (Egyptian) God of the sky.
Horuss

Hosa (Native American) crow.
Hosah

Hosea (Hebrew) salvation; one who
is kept from harm.
Hoseia, Hoshal, Osia, Osias

Hotah (Lakota) white.
Hota

Hotaia (Polynesian) mine.
Hotaiah

Hoto (Native American) the
whistler.
Hototo

Houghton (Old English) from the
grey town on the steep bank.
Houghtan, Houghten, Houghtin,
Huetan, Hueten, Huetin, Hueton,
Hughtan, Hughten, Hughtin,
Hughton

Houston (Old English) from the
hill town; from Hugh's town;
from the intelligent one's town.
Houstan, Housten, Houstin,
Houstun, Houstyn

Howard (Old English) watcher;
guardian.
Howerd

Howe (Teutonic) distinguished.
Howey, Howi, Howie, Howy

Howell (Welsh) little; alert.
Hoel, Hoell, Hoelle, Howal,
Howall, Howel, Huel, Huell,
Hywel, Hywell

Howi (Moquelumnan) dove.
Howee, Howey, Howie, Howy

Howie (English) watcher; guardian. The short form of Howard.
Howee, Howey, Howi, Howy

Howin (Chinese) swallow who is loyal.
Howyn

Howland (Old English) from the hills.
Howlande

Hoyle (Old English) from the hollow.
Hoil, Hoile, Hoyl

Hoyt (Irish) mind; spirit.
Hoyts, Hoytz

Hsu (Chinese) promise; composed.

Hsuang (Chinese) yellow; supreme.

Hu (Chinese) tiger.

Hua (Chinese) flower.

Hubert (Teutonic) bright mind or heart.
Hobard, Hobart, Hobarte, Hoibeard (Ir), Huberto (Span), Hubertus (Ger), Hubirt, Huburt, Hubyrt, Hugibert (Ger), Hugo, Umberto (Ital)

Hudson (English) son of the hooded one.
Hudsan, Hudsen, Hudsin, Hudsyn

Huelo (Tongan) ray of light.

Huey (English) intelligent. (O/Ger) heart; mind. A form of Hugh.
Hughee, Hughey, Hughi, Hughie, Hughy

Hugh (Old English) intelligent. (O/Ger) heart; mind.
Aodh (Ir), Aoidh (Scot), Hew, Hewe, Hiu (Haw), Hosch, Hubbell, Hubert, Huberto, Hue, Huego, Hues, Huet, Huey, Hughe,

Hughes, Hugibert, Hugo (Ger/Span/Swed/Dut/Dan), Hugon, Hugues (Fren), Huig, Huw (Wel), Hughi, Hughie, Hughy, Hutchin, Huw (Wel), Ugo (Ital), Ugon, Ugues

Hugo (Latin/Old English) intelligent. (O/Ger) heart; mind.
Aodh (Ir), Aoidh (Scot), Huego, Hugho, Hugo (Ger/Swed/Span/Dut/Dan), Hugues (Fren), Ugo (Ital)

Hula (Osage) eagle.
Hulah

Hulbert (Teutonic) brilliant grace.
Holbard, Holbert, Holberte, Holbirt, Holburt, Holbyrt, Hulbard, Hulbert, Hulberte, Hulbirt, Hulburt, Hulbyrt, Ulberto (Ital)

Hulda (Scandinavian) covered.
Huldah

Humbert (Teutonic) bright giant.
Humberto (Span), Humbirt, Humburt, Humbyrt, Umberto (Ital)

Hume (Old Norse) from the river island. (Ger) one who loves the home.

Humphry (Teutonic) peace loving guardian; peaceful home.
Homfree, Homfrey, Homfroi, Homphree, Homphrey, Homphry, Humfree, Humfrey, Humfri, Humfrid (Swed), Humfrie, Humfried (Ger/Dut), Humphree, Humphrey, Hunfredo (Span), Onfre (Span), Onfredo, Onfree, Onfrey, Onfroi (Fren), Onofredo (Ital), Onufry

Hunt/Hunter (Old English) hunter.
Hunta, Huntar, Huntington, Huntly

Huntingdon (Old English) from the hunter's hill.
Huntington

Huntington (Old English) from the hunter's town.
Huntingdon

Huntly (Old English) from the hunter's meadow.
Huntlea, Huntleah, Huntlee, Huntleigh, Huntley, Huntli, Huntlie

Hurd (English) strong-minded.
Herd

Hurley (Old English) from the clearing in the woods; from the hare meadow. (Ir/Gae) sea tide.
Hurlea, Hurleah, Hurlee, Hurleigh, Hurli, Hurlie, Hurly

Hurst (Middle English) dweller in the forest.
Hearst, Hirst, Hyrst

Husam (Arabic) sword.

Husani (Swahili) handsome.

Hush (Hebrew) quick.
(O/Eng) quiet.
Husha, Hushi, Hushie, Hushy

Huslu (Native American) shaggy bear.

Hussein (Arabic) little handsome one.
Husain, Hussain, Husein

Hute (Native American) star.

Hutton (Old English) from the house on the overhanging ledge.
Hutan, Huten, Hutin, Huton, Huutan, Hutten, Huttin, Huttun, Hutun, Huttyn, Hutyn

Huxford (Old English) from Hugh's ford; from the intelligent one's ford.

Huxley (Old English) from Hugh's meadow; from the intelligent one's meadow.
Huxlea, Huxleah, Huxlee, Huxleigh, Huxli, Huxlie, Huxly

Huy (Vietnamese) glory.

Huyu (Japanese) writer.

Hy (Vietnamese) hope.
Hi, Hye

Hyacinthe (French) hyacinth; purple.

Hyatt (Old English) from the high gate.
Hiat, Hiatt, Hiatte, Hyat, Hyatte

Hyde (Old English) measure of land; acreage.
Hide

Hyder (English) tanner of hides.
Hyde

I chih (Chinese) intelligent; honourable.

Iago (Spanish/Hebrew) replacer. The Spanish form of James.
Santiago

Iakona (Hawaiian) healer.
Iakonah

Iakeka (Hawaiian) descendant.
Ialekah

Ian (Scottish/Hebrew) God is gracious. The Scottish form of John.
Ean, Ein, Eoin, Iain (Scot), Iin, Ion

Ibn (Arabic) son.

Ibrahim (Arabic/Hebrew) father of the multitudes. The Arabic form of Abraham.
Abraham, Ibraham

Ibsen (German) son of the archer.
Ibsan, Ibsin, Ibson, Ibsyn

Ichabod (Hebrew) glorious.

Ichiro (Japanese) first-born son.

Iden (Old English) pasture woods.
Idan, Idin, Idon, Idun, Idyn

Idi (Swahili) born during a festival.

Idris (Welsh) fiery Lord.
Idriss, Idrys, Idryss

Ieke (Hawaiian) wealthy.

Ielemia (Hawaiian) God is lifting up.
Ielemiah

Ifor (Welsh) archer.

Igal (Hebrew) God will avenge.
Igale

Igasho (Native American) one who travels.

Ignatius (Greek) fiery.
Eegnatie, Eneco (Lat), Ennicus, Ignaas (Scan), Ignace (Pol), Ignacey, Ignas (Scan), Ignascha, Ignasha, Ignatas, Ignatus, Ignatys, Ignaz (Ger), Ignazio (Ital/Span), Inigd

Igor (Russian/Old Norse) famous son; hero.
Egor

Ikaia (Hawaiian) God is my saviour.
Ikaiah

Ikale (Polynesian) eagle.

Ike (Hebrew) laughter; God smiles. The short form of Isaac.
Ikke

Iklal (Arabic) crown of believers.

Ilario (Italian/Greek) cheerful. The Italian masculine form of Hilary.
Ilaryo

Ilbert (Teutonic) distinguished warrior.
Ilbirt, Ilburt, Ilbyrt

Ilom (Nigerian) one with enemies.

Ilya (Russian) Jehovah is God.
Ilyah

Imad (Arabic) pillar.

Imam (Indonesian) leader of religion.

Imbert (Teutonic) poet.
Imbirt, Imburt, Imbyrt

Imran (Arabic) host.
Imren, Imrin, Imrym

Imri (Hebrew) tall.
Imric, Imrick, Imrie, Imry

Inar (English) individual.

Ince (Hungarian) innocent.

Incencio (Spanish) white.

Ing (Old Norse) famous.
Igamar (Nrs), Igor (Rus), Ingar,
Ingemar, Inger, Ingmar

Inger (Old Norse) son's army.
Ingar, Ingvar (Scan)

Inglebert (Teutonic) brilliant angel.
Englebert, Engleberte, Engelbert,
Engelberte, Engelbirt, Engelburt,
Engelburte, Engelbyrt, Ingleberte,
Ingelbert, Ingelberte, Ingelbirt,
Ingelburt, Ingelburte, Ingelbyrt

Inglis (Scottish) English.
Ingliss, Inglys, Inglyss

Ingmar (Old Norse) Ing's son; son
of the famous one.
Igamar (Nrs), Igor (Rus), Ingar,
Ingemar, Inger, Ingmar

Ingram (Old Norse) raven; angel.
Ingrem, Ingrim, Ingrym

Inir (Welsh) honourable.
Inyr

Inkata (Australian Aboriginal) elder.
Inkatah

Innes (Celtic) island.
Inis, Inness, Inis, Innis, Inniss,
Innys, Innyss

Innocent (Latin) innocent;
harmless.
Innocenz (Ger), Innocentz,
Innocenz, Innocenzio (Ital),
Innocenzyo, Inocent, Inocentz,
Inocenz, Inocenzio, Inocenzyo

Inteus (Native American) without
shame.

Intrepid (Latin) fearless.
Intrepyd

Iokia (Hawaiian) God will heal.
Iokiah, Iokya, Iokyah

Iokina (Hawaiian) God will help
develop.

Iokua (Hawaiian) God will help.

Iolo (Welsh) worthy Lord.

Iona (Hawaiian) dove.

Iongi (Polynesian) young.

Ipyana (Tanzanian) graceful.
Ipyanah

Ira (Australian Aboriginal) camp.
(Heb) watchful. (Arab) stallion.
Irah

Iram (English) shining.

Irmin (German) strong; mighty.
Irman, Irmen, Irmun, Irmyn

Irvin (Gaelic) from the green river.
Earvin, Earvine, Ervin, Ervine,
Ervyn, Ervyne, Erwin, Erwyn,
Irvine, Irving, Irvyn, Irvyne, Irwin,
Irwyn

Irving (English) boar friend; green
river; friend of the sea.
Earvin, Ervin, Ervine, Erving, Ervyn,
Ervyne, Ervyng, Erwin, Erwyn,
Irvin, Irvine, Irvyn, Irvyng, Irvyne,
Irwin, Irwyn

Isa (Sanskrit) lord.
Isah

Isaac (Hebrew) laughter; God smiles.
Isaack, Isaak (Rus), Isac, Isacco
(Ital), Isack, Izaac, Izaack, Izak,
Yitzhak

Isaiah (Hebrew) God is generous;
God is my helper.
Esai, Essaia, Essaiah, Ikaia, Isaias,
Isaya, Isayah, Yeshaya, Yeshayahu

Isambard (Greek/German) iron
giant.
Imbard, Imbart, Isambart

Isham (Old English) from the iron
estate.

Ishaq (Arabic) laughing.

Isi (Hebrew) God smiles. The short
form of names starting with 'Isi'
e.g. Isidore.
Isie, Issi, Issie, Issy, Izi, Izie, Izzi,
Izzie, Izzy, Izy

Isidore (Greek) gift of Isis.
(Eng) adored.
Eesidor, Esidor, Esidore, Ezador,
Ezadore, Ezidor, Ezidore, Isador,
Isadore, Isidor (Ger), Isidoro
(Span/Ital), Isidro (Span), Isodoro,
Izador, Izadore, Izidor, Izidore,
Izydor (Pol)

Iskemu (Native American) river.

Ismael (Hebrew) God will hear;
wanderer.
Ismal, Ismale

Israel (Hebrew) God's warrior.
Israele, Israelos, Yisrael, Ysrael

Issa (Swahili) one who has
protection.
Isa, Isah, Issah

Issur (Hebrew) from Israel.

Istu (Native American) sap from a
pine.

Italia (Latin) from Italy.

Itamar (Hebrew) palm-grove island.
Ittamar

Iterika (Australian Aboriginal)
green.
Iterikah

Ithel (Welsh) generous Lord.
Ithell

Itiel (Hebrew) God is with me.

Ivan (Hebrew) God is gracious. A
form of John.
Iva, Iven, Ivin, Ivon, Ivun, Ivyn,
Yvan, Yvann

Ivanhoe (Hebrew) God's gracious
tiller of the soil.
Ivanho, Ivanhow

Ivar (Danish/Scandinavian) archer
with a yew bow.
Iver, Iviy, Ivor, Yvon, Yvor (Rus),
Yves

Iven (Old French) little yew bow.
Ivan, Ivin, Ivon, Ivun, Ivyn

Ives (Old English) archer with a yew
bow.
Yves

Ivo (Old French) yew tree. (O/Ger)
archer.
Ivor, Yves, Yvon

Ivor (Scandinavian) God.

Ivory (African American) ivory;
white.
Ivoree, Ivorey, Ivori, Ivorie

Iye (Native American) smoke.
Iy

Izod (Celtic) fair-haired.
Izad, Ized, Izid, Izud, Izyd

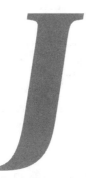

J

Ja (Korean) one who attracts.

Jaali (Swahili) powerful.
Jali

Jaan (Estonian/Greek) Christian.

Jaap (Dutch/Hebrew) replacer. The Dutch form of Jim.
Jape

Jabari (Swahili) fearless.
Jabaar, Jabare, Jabbar, Jabier, Jabary

Jabbar (Arabic) repairer.
Jaba, Jabar, Jabba

Jabez (Hebrew) born in sorrow.
Jabe, Jabes, Jabesh

Jabin (Hebrew) God has created.
Jabiri, Jabori, Jabyn

Jabir (Arabic) comforting.
Jabyr

Jabiru (Australian Aboriginal) stork.
Jabyru

Jacan (Hebrew) trouble.
Jacen, Jacin, Jacon, Jacyn

Jace (Australian/Greek) healer. The short form of Jason.
Jacee, Jacey, Jaci, Jacie, Jacy, Jaec, Jaece, Jaic, Jaice, Jaicee, Jaicey, Jaici, Jaicie, Jaicy, Jayce, Jaycee, Jaycey, Jayci, Jaycie, Jaycy

Jacinto (Spanish) hyancinth; purple. The masculine form of Jacinta.
Jacint, Jacynt, Jacynto

Jack (French) replacer. A form of James.
Jaac, Jaack, Jaak, Jac, Jacke, Jacki, Jackie, Jacky, Jacque, Jacques (Fren), Jak, Jakk

Jackson (Old English) Jack's son; son of the replacer.
Jackman, Jakman, Jakson

Jacob (Hebrew) replacer. A form of James.
Gemmes, Giocobbe, Jacobb, Jacobo (Ital/Span), Jacobos, Jacobs, Jacobson, Jacobus, Jacoby, Jacopo, Jaecob, Jaekob, Jaicob, Jaikob, Jakob, Jakobus (Grk), Jakov (Russ), Jakub (Indones), Jaume, Jaycob, Jaycobb, Jaykob, Jayme (O/Span), Jaykob, Jaykobb

Jacques (French/Hebrew) replacer. The French form of Jack.
Jacot, Jacquan, Jacquees, Jacquet, Jacquez, Jaques, Jarques, Jarquis, Jarquys

Jacy (Tupi-Guarani) moon.
Jaecee, Jaecey, Jaeci, Jaecie, Jaecy, Jaice, Jaicee, Jaicey, Jaici, Jaicie, Jaicy, Jayce, Jaycee, Jaycey, Jayci, Jaycie, Jaycy

Jade (Spanish) the jade stone.
Jaed, Jaid, Jaide, Jayd, Jayde

Jadon (Hebrew) God has heard.
Jadan, Jaden, Jadin, Jadyn

Jadrien (American/Latin) black jay bird. A combination of Jay/Adrian.
Jaedrian, Jaedrien, Jaidrian, Jaidrien, Jaydrian, Jaydrien

J

Jaegar (German) hunter.
Jaager, Jagur, Jaigar, Jaygar

Jaehwa (Korean) prosperous.

Jael (Hebrew) mountain goat; ascending.
Jail, Jayl

Jafar (Sanskrit) small stream.
Jafar, Jafari, Jaffar

Jagger (English) teamster; driver of horses.
Gaggar, Gaggor, Jaggar

Jago (Australian Aboriginal) complete. The Spanish/ Portuguese form of James, replacer.
Jaego, Jaigo, Jaygo

Jaguar (Spanish) jaguar.
Jagguar

Jahan (Hindi) world.

Jahdal (Hebrew) directed by God.
Jaidal

Jahdo (Hebrew) union.
Jaido

Jahi (Swahili) one who is dignified.

Jai (Hebrew) God has enlightened. The short form of Jairus.
Jae, Jay

Jaiden (Hebrew) God has heard.
Jaedan, Jaeden, Jaedin, Jaedon, Jaedyn, Jaidan, Jaidin, Jaidon, Jaidyn, Jaydan, Jayden, Jaydin, Jaydon, Jaydyn

Jaidev (Hindi) victory.
Jaedev, Jaydev

Jaimini (Hindi) victory.
Jaemini, Jaymini

Jairo (Spanish) God will enlighten.
Jair (Heb), Jairas, Jairo, Jairus, Jarius, Jayr, Jayro, Jayrus

Jaja (Ibo) honoured.
Jajah

Jajuan (African American/Hebrew) God is gracious. A form of John/Juan.
Jaejuan, Jaijuan, Jayjuan

Jake (Hebrew) replacer. A form of James.
Jaik, Jayck, Jayk

Jakeem (Arabic) uplifting.
Jakeam, Jakim, Jakym

Jakome (Basque) replacer. A form of James.
Jakom

Jal (Gypsy) wanderer.
Jall

Jala (Arabic) clarity.
Jalah

Jalaad (Arabic) glory.
Jalad

Jalal (Arabic) great; majestic.
Galal, Galeel, Jaleal, Jaleel, Jalel

Jalen (African American) calm.
Jalan, Jalin, Jalon, Jalyn

Jalil (Hindi) God-like.
Jahlee, Jahleel, Jahlil, Jalaal, Jalal

Jalon (Hebrew) one who dwells.
Jalan, Jalen, Jalin, Jalon, Jalyn

Jamaine (Arabic/French) from Germany.
Jamain, Jamayn, Jamayne

Jamal (Arabic) beautiful.
Jahmal, Jahmall, Jahmalle, Jajmel, Jahmil, Jahmile, Jahmill, Jahmille, Jamaal, Jamael, Jamahl, Jamail, Jamal, Jamala, Jamale, Jamall, Jarman, Jamar, Jamel, Jamil, Jammaal, Jamyl, Jamyle, Jarmal, Jaumal, Jemal, Jermal

J

Jamar (Arabic/AfricanAmerican) handsome.
Jam, Jamaar, Jamaari, Jamaarie, Jamahra, Jamahrae, Jamara, Jamari, Jamarr, Jamarvis, Jamaur, Jarmar, Jarmara, Jarmarr, Jarmarra, Jaumar, Jemaar, Jemar, Jimar, Jimara

Jamarcus (Latin) of Mars; warrior. A form of Marcus.
Jamarc, Jamarco, Jamark, Jemarcus, Jimarcus, Jymarcus

Jamario (Italian/French/American) sailor. A form of Mario, dedicated to the Virgin Mary.
Jamari, Jamarie, Jamariel, Jamarius, Jamaryo, Jemario, Jemarus

James (Hebrew) replacer.
Dago, Diego (Span), Gaymes, Giacobbe, Giacomo (Ital), Giacopo, Giocomo, Hamish, Iachimo, Iago, Jaak (Est), Jaako (Finn), Jack, Jackson, Jaemes, Jagli, Jago, Jahus (Dut), Jaime (Span), Jaimie, Jaimes, Jakab, Jakez, Jakobus (Grk), Jakov (Russ), Jalm (Bret), Jamelia, Jamesy, Jamille, Jamin, Jaques (Fren), Jasderika (Russ), Jascha (Russ), Jaschis, Jaserika, Jayme, Jaymee, Jaymes, Jeames (O/Eng), Jeka (Lith), Jekups (Lett), Jesiz, Kubinsch, Kubinschu, Seamus (Ir), Seumas, Shamus, Yago, Zebedee

Jameson (English/Hebrew) James' son; son of the replacer.
Jaemeson, Jaemison, Jaemyson, Jaimeson, Jaimison, Jaimyson, Jamerson, Jamesyn, Jamison, Jamyson, Jaymeson, Jaymison, Jaymyson

Jamie (Hebrew) replacer. A form of James.
Jaem, Jaemee, Jaemey, Jaemi, Jaemie, Jaemy, Jaim, Jaime, Jaimee, Jaimey, Jaimy, Jamey, Jami, Jamie, Jamey, Jammey, Jammy, Jamy, Jaym, Jayme, Jaymee, Jaymey, Jaymi, Jaymie, Jaymy, Jemi, Jemie, Jemm, Jemmi, Jemmie, Jemmy (Eng), Jemy, Jimbo, Jimi, Jimie, Jimm, Jimmbo, Jimme, Jimmee, Jimmey, Jimmi, Jimmie, Jimmy, Jimy, Jym, Jyme, Jymee, Jymey, Jymi, Jymie, Jymm, Jymme, Jymmee, Jymmey, Jymmi, Jymmie, Jymmy, Jymy

Jamil (Arabic) beautiful.
Jameal, Jameel, Jamile, Jamyl, Jamyle

Jamin (Hebrew) right hand.
Jaman, Jamen, Jamon, Jamyn

Jamison (English/Hebrew) James' son; son of the replacer.
Jaemeson, Jaemison, Jaemyson, Jaimeson, Jaimison, Jaimyson, Jamerson, Jameson, Jamesyn, Jamyson, Jaymeson, Jaymison, Jaymyson

Jamond (English) wise, mighty protector. A form of Raymond.
Jaemon, Jaemond, Jaemun, Jaemund, Jaimon, Jaimond, Jaimun, Jaimund, Jamon, Jamond, Jamun, Jamund, Jarmon, Jarmon, Jarmond, Jarmun, Jarmund, Jaymon, Jaymond, Jaymun, Jaymund

Jamsheed (Persian) from Persia.
Jamshead

Jan (Dutch/Slavic) God is gracious. A form of John.
Jaan, Jane, Jann, Janne (Finn), Jano, Jansen, Janson, Jenda, Yan

Janaka (Sanskrit) born of the ancestor.
Janakah

J

Jandah (Hebrew) rest.
Janda

Jando (Czech/Greek) defender of humankind. A form of Alexander.
Jandin, Jandino, Jandyn, Jandyno

Janek (Polish/Hebrew) God is gracious. A form of John.
Janik, Janika, Janka, Jankiel, Jankiela, Janko

Janesh (Hindi) the people's Lord.

Janis (Latvian/Hebrew) God is gracious. A form of John.
Ansis, Jancis, Janyc, Janyce, Janys, Zanis, Zanys

Janne (Finnish/Hebrew) God is gracious. A form of John.

Janos (Hungarian/Hebrew) God is gracious. A form of John.
Jancsi, Jani, Janie, Jankia, Jano, Jany, Janys

Jansen (Scandinavian) John's son; God is gracious.
Jansan, Jansin, Janson, Jansyn, Janssan, Janssen, Janssin, Jansson, Janten, Jantzen, Janzen, Jensan, Jensen, Jensin, Jenson, Jensyn

Janus (Latin) gateway; born in January.
Janario, Januarius, Janis, Janos, Janys

Jaquan (Comanche) fragrant. A form of Quana.
Jacquin, Jacquyn, Jaquana, Jaquanah, Jaquin, Jaquon, Jaquyn, Jaqwan

Jarah (Hebrew) sweet like honey.
Jara, Jarra, Jarrah, Jera, Jerah, Jerra, Jerrah

Jarara (Australian Aboriginal) rock with water flowing over it.
Jararah

Jardine (French) garden dweller.
Jardin, Jardyn, Jardyne, Gardin, Gardine, Gardyn, Gardyne

Jareb (Hebrew) maintaining.
Jarib, Jaryb

Jared (Hebrew) descendant of the inheritor. (Grk) rose.
Jara, Jarah, Jaret, Jarett, Jarod, Jarrad, Jarred, Jarret, Jarrett, Jarrod, Jarryd

Jarek (Slavic) born in January.
Janiuszck, Januarius, Januisz, Jarec, Jareck, Jaric, Jarick, Jarik, Jaryc, Jaryck, Jaryk

Jarell (Scandinavian/German) brave spear carrier. A form of Gerald.
Jaerel, Jaerell, Jaeril, Jaerill, Jaeryl, Jaeryll, Jairel, Jairell, Jareil, Jarel, Jarelle, Jarrell, Jarryl, Jarryll, Jayryl, Jayryll, Jerel, Jereli, Jerell, Jharel, Jharell

Jareth (Hebrew/Welsh) gentle descendant.
Jaref, Jareff, Jarif, Jariff, Jarith, Jarref, Jarreff, Jarreth, Jarrif, Jarriff, Jarrith, Jarryf, Jarryff, Jarryth, Jaryf, Jaryff, Jaryth, Jereth

Jarib (Hebrew) one who strives.
Jaryb

Jarl (Norse) noble.
Jarlea, Jarleah, Jarlee, Jarleigh, Jarley, Jarli, Jarlie, Jarly

Jarlath (Latin) in control.
Jarl, Jarlaf, Jarlen

Jarman (Teutonic) from Germany.
Jarmen, Jarmin, Jarmon, Jarmyn, Jerman, Jermen, Jermin, Jermon, Jermyn

Jaron (Hebrew) to cry or sing out.
Jaaron, Jaeron, Jairon, Jaran, Jaren, Jarin, Jarone, Jayron, Jayrone,

J

Jayronn, Je Ron, Je Ronn, J'ron,
Yartron

Jaroslav (Czech) spring glory.
Jarda, Jardah

Jarrah (Australian Aboriginal)
mahogany tree.
Jara, Jarah, Jarra

Jarratt (Teutonic) strong spear.
Jarat, Jaret, Jarit, Jarot, Jarrat, Jarret,
Jarrett, Jarrit, Jarritt, Jarrot, Jarrott,
Jaryt, Jarytt

Jarrell (English/German) brave
spear carrier. A form of Gerald.
Jaerel, Jaerell, Jaeril, Jaerill, Jaeryl,
Jaeryll, Jairel, Jairell, Jareil, Jarel,
Jarelle, Jarryl, Jarryll, Jayryl, Jayryll,
Jerel, Jereli, Jerell, Jharel, Jharell

Jarrett (English/Hebrew)
descendant.
Jairet, Jairett, Jaret, Jareth, Jarette,
Jarhet, Jarhett, Jarrat, Jarratt, Jarret,
Jarrette, Jarrot, Jarrote, Jarrott,
Jarrotte, Jerret, Jerrete, Jerrett. Jerrette

Jarvis (Teutonic) war leader.
Gary, Gervaise, Gervase, Gervice,
Jarus, Jaruss, Jary, Jarvice, Jarvise,
Jarvyc, Jarvyce, Jarvys, Jarvyse, Jerve,
Jervice, Jervis, Jervise

Jas (Polish/Hebrew) God is
gracious. A form of John. The
short form of names starting with
'Jas' e.g. Jason.
Jasi, Jasio, Jasy, Jasyo

Jasha (Russian/Hebrew) replacer.
Jascha

Jashawn (Irish/Hebrew) God is
gracious. A form of Shawn.
Jasean, Jashaun

Jason (Greek) healer.
Jaasan, Jaasen, Jaasin, Jaason,
Jaasun, Jaasyn, Jaesan, Jaesen,
Jaesin, Jaeson, Jaesun, Jaesyn,
Jahsan, Jahsen, Jahson, Jaisan,
Jaisen, Jaisin, Jaison, Jaisun, Jaisyn,
Jasan, Jasen, Jasin, Jasun, Jasyn,
Jaysan, Jaysen, Jaysin, Jayson,
Jaysun, Jaysyn

Jaspal (Punjabi) virtuous lifestyle.
Jaspel

Jasper (Persian) guardian of the
treasure. (Eng) gem stone.
Caspar, Casper, Gaspard,
Gaspardo, Gaspare, Gasper, Jaspar,
Jasper

Jassan (Native American) wolf.
Jassen, Jassin, Jasson, Jassyn

Jatinra (Hindi) sage plant.
Jatinrah

Javan (Hebrew) clay.
Jaavon, Jahvaughan, Jahvine,
Jahvon, JaVaughn, Javen, Javin,
Javine, Javion, Javoanta, Javon,
Javona, Javonah, Javone, Javoney,
Javoni, Javonie, Javonn, Javyn,
Jayvin, Jayvine, Jayvon, Jevan

Javaris (English/German) skilled
with a spear.
Javaor, Javar, Javares, Javario,
Javarios, Javarius, Javaro, Javaron,
Javarous, Javarre, Javarrious,
Javarro, Javarros, Javarte, Javarus,
Javays, Javoris, Javouris, Javourys

Javas (Sanskrit) quick.
Jav, Java

Javier (Arabic) bright.
Jabier, Javyer, Xavier, Xavyr

Javon (African American) son of
Joseph; God will increase; God has
added a child. A form of Joseph.
Javan, Javen, Javin, Javyn

Jawaun (Spanish) God is gracious. A form of John/Juan.
Jajaun, Jawaa, Jawan, Jawann, Jawn, Jawon, Jawuan, Jejuan, Jujuan, Juwan

Jawdat (Arabic) good.
Gawdat

Jawhar (Arabic) jewel.
Jawha

Jay (Old French) the blue jaybird.
Jae, Jai, Jaie, Jayd, Jayde

Jayant (Hindi) victory.
Jaeant, Jaiant

Jaydon (Hebrew) God has heard.
Jaedan, Jaeden, Jaedin, Jaedon, Jaedyn, Jaidan, Jaiden, Jaidin, Jaidon, Jaidyn, Jaydan, Jayden, Jaydin, Jaydyn

Jaydrien (Latin/French) dark-blue jaybird.
Jader, Jadrien, Jadryen, Jaidrian, Jaidrien, Jaidrion, Jaidryon, Jaydrian, Jaydrion, Jaydryan

Jaylee (English) from the jaybird meadow.
Jaelea, Jaeleah, Jaelee, Jaeleigh, Jaeley, Jaeli, Jaelie, Jaely, Jailea, Jaileah, Jailee, Jaileigh, Jailey, Jaili, Jailie, Jaily, Jaylea, Jayleah, Jayleigh, Jayley, Jayli, Jaylie, Jayly

Jayson (Greek) healer. (O/Eng) son of the jaybird.
Jaycent, Jaysen, Jaysin, Jayssen, Jaysson, Jayssyn

Jazon (Polish) healer.
Jazan, Jazen, Jazin, Jazyn

Jazz (English/American) lover of jazz music.
Jaz, Jaze, Jazze, Jazzlea, Jazzlee, Jazzman, Jazzmen, Jazzmin, Jazzmon, Jazzmyn, Jazztin, Jazzton

Jean (French/Hebrew) God is gracious. A form of John.
Gean, Geen, Gene, Jeannot, Jeanot, Jeanty, Jeen, Jene

Jebediah (Hebrew) friend; beloved of the Lord.
Jebadia, Jebadiah, Jebidia, Jebidiah, Jebidya, Jebydia, Jebydiah, Jebydya, Jebydyah, Jedidia, Jedediah, Jededia, Jedediah, Jedidi,

Jed (Hebrew) beloved of the Lord. The short form of Jedaiah, God knows.
Jedd

Jedaiah (Hebrew) God knows.
Jedah, Jedaya, Jedayah, Yehiel

Jedi (American) warrior.

Jedrek (Polish) strength.
Jedrec, Jedreck, Jedric, Jedrick, Jedrik, Jedrus, Jedryc, Jedryck, Jedryk

Jedynak (Polish) one son.
Jedinak

Jeff (French) divine peace. The short form of Jeffery.
Gef, Geff, Geof, Geoff, Jef, Jefer, Jeffer, Jeffers, Jeph

Jefferson (Old English) son of Jeffrey, son of divine peace.
Gefferson

Jeffery/Jeffrey (French) divine peace.
Gefaree, Gefarey, Gefari, Gefarie, Gefary, Geffaree, Geffarey, Geffari, Geffarie, Geffary, Geferi, Gerferie, Gefery, Gefferee, Gefferey, Gefferi, Gefferie, Geffery, Geffree, Geffrey, Geffri, Geffrie, Geffry, Geoffrey, Geoffri, Geoffrie, Geoffry, Geofrey, Geofri, Geofrie, Geofry, Godfrei, Godfrey, Goffredo, Gottfried,

J

Jefaree, Jefarey, Jefari, Jefarie, Jefary, Jeffaree, Jeffarey, Jeffari, Jeffarie, Jeffary, Jeferee, Jeferi, Jeferie, Jeffer, Jefferee, Jefferey, Jefferee, Jefferey, Jefferi, Jefferie, Jeffrey, Jeffri, Jeffrie, Jeffry

Jefford (English) from the divinely peaceful ford.
Jeford

Jehan (French/Hebrew) God is gracious. A form of John.
Jehann

Jehiel (Hebrew) God lives.

Jehu (Hebrew) the Lord is He.

Jehudi (Hebrew) of Judah, God's leader.

Jela (Swahili) father is in jail during the birth.
Jelah, Jella, Jellah

Jelani (Swahili) mighty.
Jelanee, Jelaney, Jelanie, Jelany

Jem (English) jewel.

Jemond (French) worldly.
Jemon, Jemonde, Jemone, Jemun, Jemund

Jen (Chinese) able.

Jenkin (Flemish) little John; God is gracious.
Jenkins, Jenkyn, Jenkyns, Jenning, Jennings

Jeno (Hungarian/Greek) noble; well born. A form of Eugene.
Jenci, Jencie, Jency, Jenoe, Jensi, Jensy

Jens (Scandinavian) God is gracious. The Dutch form of John.
Jenz

Jensi (Hungarian) noble; well born.
Jensee, Jensey, Jensie, Jensy

Jeovanni (Italian/Hebrew) God is gracious. A form of John.
Giovani, Jeovani, Jeovanie, Jeovanny, Jeovany, Jiovani, Jiovanie, Jiovanni, Jiovannie, Jiovanny, Jiovany, Jyovani, Jyovanie, Jyovany

Jerald (English/German) brave spear carrier. A form of Gerald.
Jeraldo, Jerold, Jeroldo, Jerral, Jerrald, Jerraldo, Jerrold, Jerroldo, Jerryld, Jeryld

Jerara (Australian Aboriginal) waterfall.
Jerarah

Jeremiah (Hebrew) chosen by God.
Diarmuit, Geremiah, Geremias, Jereme, Jeremee, Jeremey, Jeremi, Jeremia, Jeremias, Jeremie, Jeremy, Jeremya, Jeremyah, Jeremyas, Jeriamias (Austri), Jermias

Jeremy (Hebrew) praised highly by God.
Gerami, Geramie, Geramy, Geremi, Geremie, Geremy, Geromi, Geromie, Geromy, Jeramee, Jeramey, Jerami, Jeramia, Jeramiah, Jeramias, Jeramie, Jeramy, Jereme, Jeremee, Jeremey, Jeremi, Jeremia, Jeremiah, Jeremias, Jeremie, Jerom, Jerome, Jeromee, Jeromey, Jeromi, Jeromia, Jeromiah, Jeromias, Jeromie, Jeromy, Jeromya, Jeromyah, Jeromyas, Yirmeeyahu

Jeriah (Hebrew) God has seen.
Jeria, Jerya, Jeryah

Jericho (Arabic) moon city.
Jeric, Jerick, Jericko, Jerico, Jerik, Jeriko, Jerric, Jerrico, Jerrick, Jerricko, Jerriko, Jerryco, Jerrycko, Jerryko

Jeriel (Hebrew) vision of God.
Jeryel

J

Jermaine (German) from Germany.
Germain, Germiane, Jermain,
Jermayn, Jermayne

Jermal (Arabic) handsome.
Jermaal, Jermael, Jermail, Jermal,
Jermall, Jermaul, Jermel, Jermell

Jeroboan (Hebrew) enlarger.

Jerolin (Basque/Latin) holy.
Jerolyn

Jerome (Greek) sacred name; of God.
Geremia (Ital), Gerome,
Geronimo, Heironom,
Heironymus, Hiernonimo, Jarom,
Jarome, Jarrom, Jarrome, Jeremias
(Span/Ger/Dut), Jeriamiasz,
Jeroan, Jeromene, Jeromina,
Jeronim (Russ), Jeronimo,
Jeronimus (Lith), Jeromino (Span),
Jeromo, Jeronim, Jerram, Jerrold,
Jerrome

Jeron (English/Latin) holy.
Jerone, Jeronimo, Jerron, J'ron

Jerrawa (Australian Aboriginal)
goanna (large lizard).
Jerawa

Jerrell (English) strong; open-
minded.
Jerel, Jeril, Jerrel, Jerril, Jerryl, Jeryl

Jerrick (German) brave spear carrier
who is the ruler of the people.
Jeric, Jerick, Jerik, Jerric, Jerrik,
Jerryc, Jerryc, Jerryck, Jerryk

Jerry (German) sacred name; of
God. The short form of names
starting with 'Jer' e.g. Jerome.
Geree, Gerey, Geri, Gerie, Gerree,
Gerrey, Gerri, Gerrie, Gerry, Gery,
Jeree, Jeri, Jerie, Jerree, Jerri, Jerrie,
Jery

Jervis (German) skilful with a spear.
Jarvis, Jarvys, Jervys

Jerzy (Polish) earth worker.
Jersey, Jerzi, Jerzy

Jess (Hebrew) wealthy. The short
form of Jesse.

Jesse (Hebrew) wealthy.
Jescee, Jescey, Jesee, Jesi, Jesie, Jess,
Jessee, Jessey, Jessi, Jessie, Jessy,
Jezze, Jezzee, Jezzey, Jezzi, Jezzie,
Jezzy

Jesus (Hebrew) God will help.
Jezus

Jethro (Hebrew) abundant.
Jetro, Jetrow, Jettro

Jett (English) black.
Jet, Jetson, Jette (Scand), Jetter,
Jetty

Jevan (Welsh) young warrior. A
form of Evan, well born.
Jevaun, Jeven, Jevin, Jevohn, Jevon,
Jevonn, Jevonne, Jevyn, Jevynn

Ji (Chinese) order.

Jiao-Long (Chinese) dragon.

Jibade (Yoruba) born near royalty.
Jibad, Jybad, Jybade

Jie (Chinese) wonderful.

Jilt (Dutch) money.
Jylt

Jim/Jimmy (Hebrew) replacer. A
form of James.
Jem, Jemee, Jemey, Jemi, Jemie,
Jemm, Jemmee, Jemmey, Jemmi,
Jemmie, Jemmy, Jemy, Jimee,
Jimey, Jimi, Jimie, Jimm, Jimmee,
Jimmey, Jimmi, Jimmie, Jimmy,
Jimy, Jymee, Jymey, Jymi, Jymie,
Jymm, Jymmee, Jymmey, Jymmi,
Jymmie, Jymmy, Jymy

Jimell (Arabic) handsome.
Jimel, Jimelle, Jimmil, Jimmill,
Jimmyl, Jimmyll, Jymel, Jymell,

J

Jymil, Jymill, Jymmel, Jymmell, Jymmil, Jymmill, Jymmyl, Jymmyll, Jymyl, Jymyll

Jimeoin (Irish/Hebrew/Australian) replacer who is born to nobility. A combination of Jim/Owen. Jimeoine, Jimowen, Jimowyn, Jymoin, Jymoine, Jymowen, Jymowyn

Jimiyu (Abaluhya) born during the dry season.

Jimoh (Swahili) born on a Friday. Jimo, Jymo, Jymoh

Jin (Chinese) gold. Jinn, Jyn, Jynn

Jinan (Arabic) garden. Jinen, Jinon, Jinyn

Jindra (Czech/Scandinavian) army ruler. Jindrah

Jing-Quo (Chinese) the country's ruler.

Jirair (Armenian) strong; hard-working. Jyrair

Jiri (Czech) farmer. A form of George. Jirka

Jiro (Japanese) second-born son.

Jivin (Hindi) giver of life. Jivan, Jivanta, Jiven, Jivon, Jivyn, Jyvan, Jyven, Jyvin, Jyvon, Jyvyn

Joab (Hebrew) God is my father. Joaby

Joachim (Hebrew) God will establish. Joacheim, Joakim, Joaquim, Joaquin, Jokin, Jov

Joah (Hebrew) his brother is God. Joa

Joao (Portuguese) God is gracious. A form of John.

Joaquim (Portuguese/Hebrew) God will establish. Jehoichin, Joaquin, Joaquyn, Joaquynn, Jocquin, Jocquinn, Jocquyn, Jocquynn, Juaquin, Juaquyn

Job (Hebrew) distressed; afflicted. Jobe, Jobee, Jobert, Jobey, Jobi, Jobie, Joby

Joben (Japanese) clean. Joban, Jobin, Jobon, Jobyn

Jock (Hebrew/American) replacer. A form of Jack. Jocko, Joco, Jocobi, Jocobie, Jocoby, Jocolbee, Jocolbey, Jocolbi, Jocolbie, Jocolby

Jodan (Hebrew) God is my judge. Joden, Jodin, Jodon, Jodyn

Jody (Hebrew) God will increase. A form of Joseph. Jodee, Jodey, Jodi, Jodie, Joedee, Joedey, Joedi, Joedie, Joedy

Joe (Hebrew) God will increase. A short form of Joseph. Jo, Joey, Jow

Joel (Hebrew) God is willing. Joell, Joelle, Joely, Jole, Yoel

Joergen (Scandinavian) farmer. A form of George. Jorgen

Johann (German) God is gracious. A form of John Joahan, Johan (Dan), Johanan, Johane, Johanna, johannas, Johannes, Johansen, Johanson, Johanthan, Johatan, Johathan, Johathon, Johaun, Johon, Johonson, Yohan, Yohann, Yohannon

Johar (Hindi) jewel.

John (Hebrew) God is gracious.
Eoin, Evan, Gian, Giankos,
Giannakos, Gianni, Giannini,
Gianninno, Gianozzi, Giovanni
(Ital), Gon, Hanan, Hanka,
Hankos, Hans, Hanns, Hannus,
Hansel, Hansli, Hanson, Iain, Ian,
Ievan, IfanIoannes, Ion, Ivan,
Ivanjuscha, Ivanku, Ivor, Iwan,
Jackie, Jackson, Jacky, Jan, Janos,
Jean (Fren), Jehan (Bel), Jen,
Jenicek (Boh), Jenkin (Wel),
Jenkins, Jens, Jevon (Wel), Joao
(Braz), Joan, Joanico, Joaninho,
Joannoulos, Jock, Jocko, Joh,
Johan, Johann (Ger), Johannes
(Dut), Johanon, Johnson, Jon,
Jovica (Illy), Juan (Span), Juha,
Juhani, Jukka, Jvan, Jveica, Nannos,
Nozzo, Sean, Seon, Shane,
Shaughn, Shaun, Shawn, Yahya,
Zane

Johnny (Hebrew/English) God is
gracious. A form of John.
Johnee, Johney, Johni, Johnie,
Johnier, Johnni, Johnnie, Johnsi,
Johnsie, Johnny, Johnsy, Johny,
Jonee, Joney, Joni, Jonie, Jonnee,
Jonney, Jonni, Jonnie, Jonny, Jony

Johnson (Hebrew) John's son; son
of the one whose God is gracious.
Jonson

Joji (Japanese) farmer. A form of
George.

Jojo (Fanti) born on a Monday.
Joejoe, Johjoe

Jokim (Hebrew) God sets up.
Jokeam, Jokeem, Jokym

Jolon (Native American) from the
valley of dead oaks.
Jolyon

Jomei (Japanese) spreading light.
Jomey

Jonah (Hebrew) dove.
Jona, Yona, Yonah

Jonas (Hebrew) accomplisher. The
Lithuanian form of John, God is
gracious.
Jonelis, Jonukas, Jonus, Jonutis,
Jonys, Joonas

Jonathon (Hebrew) gift of God.
Janathon, Jhonathan, Johathe,
Johnatan, Johnathan, Johnathaon,
Johnathen, Johnathon, Johnatten,
Johniathin, Johnothan, Jonaton,
Jonatan, Jonatane, Jonate, Jonatha,
Jonathen, Jonathon, Jonattan,
Jonethen, Jonnatha, Jonnathan,
Jonnattan, Jonothan, Jonothon

Jones (Welsh) John's son; son of the
one whose God is gracious.
Joenes, Joennes, Jonesy

Jonigan (African American/Hebrew)
gift from God.

Jontae (Hebrew) God is gracious. A
form of John.
Johntae, Jontai, Jontay, Jontea,
Jonteau, Jontez

Jonte (African American/Hebrew)
gift from God.

Joop (Dutch/Hebrew) God will
increase; God has added a child.
A form of Joseph.
Jopi, Jopie, Jopy

Joost (Dutch) just.

Jora (Hebrew) child born at the
time of the autumn/fall rains.
Jorah, Yora, Yorah

Joram (Hebrew) God is highly
praised.

J

Jordan (Hebrew) flowing down; descending.
Giordano (Ital), Jared, Jered, Jorden, Jordin, Jordon, Jordyn, Jourdain (Fren)

Jordy (Hebrew) flowing down; descending. The short form of Jordan.
Jordi, Jordie, Jory

Jorell (American) one who saves.
Jorel, Jorelle, Jorrel, Jorrell, Jorrelle

Jorg (German/Greek) farmer. A form of George.
Jeorg, Jois (Dut), Jorrin (Span), Juergen, Jungen, Jurgen

Jorin (Sanskrit/Hebrew) child of freedom.
Joryn

Joscelin (Teutonic) small Goth (East German people from Scandinavia who invaded the Roman Empire).
Joscelyn

Jose (Spanish/Hebrew) God will increase; God has added a child. A form of Joseph.
Hosae, Hose, Josean, Josecito, Josee, Joseito, Joselito, Josey

Joseph (Hebrew) God will increase; God has added a child.
Chepito, Gioseffa, Giuseppe (Ital), Iosep (Ir), Joergen, Jose (Span), Josef (Ger/Port/Czech/Scan), Joseff, Josephus, Joses, Josip (Illy), Joska (Slav), Jossif (Russ), Jozef (Pol), Jozeff, Juozapas (Lith), Jusepe, Jusuf, Pepito, Seosaidh (Scott), Septh, Seth

Josha (Hindi) satisfied.
Joshah

Joshi (Swahili) to gallop.
Joshee, Joshey, Joshie, Joshy

Josh/Joshua (Hebrew) God is my salvation.
Johsua, Johusa, Josh, Josha, Joshau, Joshaua, Joshauh, Joshawa, Joshawah, Joshe, Joshee, Joshi, Joshia, Joshu, Joshuaa, Joshuah, Joshuea, Joshula, Joshus, Joshusa, Joshuwa, Joshwa, Joshy, Josua, Josue (Heb), Jousha, Jozshua, Jozsua, Jozua, Jushua, Yasser, Yusha

Josiah (Hebrew) God will heal and protect.
Josia, Josias, Josya, Josyah, Yasser

Joss (Chinese) fate.
Jos

Jotham (Hebrew) God is perfect.
Jothem, Jothim, Jothom, Jothym

Joubert (Old English) bright; shining.
Joubirt, Jouburt, Joubyrt

Jovan (Latin) love; majestic. The Slavic form of John, God is gracious.
Jovaan, Jovaann, Jovani, Jovanic, Jovanie, Jovann, Jovanni, Jovannic, Jovannie, Jovannis, Jovanny, Jovany, Jovenal, Jovenel, Jovi, Jovian, Jovin, Jovito, Jovoan, Jovon, Jovonn, Jovonne, Yovan

Jovi (Latin) happy.
Jovee, Jovey, Jovie, Jovy

Juan (Spanish) God is gracious. A form of John.
Juanch, Juanchito, Juanito, Juann, Juaun

Jubah (African) ant hill.
Juba

Jubal (Hebrew) source of joy.

Judah (Hebrew) God leads.
Jud, Juda, Judas, Judd, Judda, Juddah, Jude

Judas (Hebrew) praised.
Judas, Juddas

Judd (Hebrew) praised. A form of
Judah, God leads.
Jud

Jude (Latin) right with the law.
Jood, Joode

Judson (English) Judd's son; son of
the praised.
Juddson

Juhana (Finnish/Hebrew) God is
gracious. A form of John.
Johana, Johanah, Johanna,
Johannah, Juhanah, Juhanna,
Juhannah

Juku (Estonian/English) rich,
powerful, hard ruler. A form of
Richard.
Jukka

Jules (French/Greek/Latin) youthful.
Jewels, Joles, Jule

Julian (Latin) belonging to the
youth. The masculine form of
Julia.
Giuliano, Giulio, Gulian, Gulien,
Guiliano, Gulio, Jellon, Jewelian,
Jewelien, Jolian, Jolin, Jollan,
Jollanus, Jolyon, Juliano (Port),
Julien (Fren), Julijonas, Julio,
Julion (Wel), Juliois, Julyan,
Julyen, Julyin, Julyon

Julio (Hispanic/Latin/Greek)
youthful.
Juleo, Julyo

Julius (Greek) youth with a shabby
beard.
Gulias, Gulious, Juilios (Span),
Julas, Juliao, Julias, Jules (Fren),
Julious, Juliyo, Julot, Julyo

Jumaane (Swahili) born on a
Tuesday.
Jumane

Jumah (Swahili) born on a Friday.
Juma

Jumbo (African) elephant. (O/Eng)
large.
Jamba, Jambo, Jumba

Jumoke (Nigerian) beloved of
everyone.
Jumok

Jun (Chinese) truth. (Jap) pure.

June (Chinese) true. (Jap)
obedience. (Eng) born in the
month of June.
Joon

Jungay (Australian Aboriginal) west
wind.
Jungae, Jungai

Junior (Latin) young.
Junious, Junius, Junyor

Junipero (Spanish) the juniper
berry.

Junius (Latin) youthful; born in
June.
Gunius, Junyus

Jupp (German/Hebrew) God will
increase; God has added a child.
A form of Joseph.
Jup

Jur (Czech/Greek) farmer. A form of
George.
Juraz, Juree, Jurek, Juri (Lat), Jurie,
Jurik, Jury

Jurgen (German) farmer. A form of
George.

Juro (Japanese) best wishes for a
long life.

Jurrien (Dutch) God will uplift.
Jore, Joree, Jurian, Jurion, Juryan,
Juryen, Juryin, Juryon

Justice (Old French) judge; justice.
Giusto (Ital), Juste (Fren), Justis,

Justise, Justo (Span), Justus (Ger), Justyce, Justys, Justyse

Justin (Old French) righteous; just.
Giustino (Ital), Giusto, Jestan, Jesten Jestin, Justinas (Lith), Justinian, Justino (Ital/Span), Justo (Port), Justus, Justyn (Pol), Justyno, Yestin, Yestyn

Juventino (Latin) youthful.
Juvenal, Juventin, Juventine, Juventyn, Juventyne, Juventyno, Juvon, Juvone

Juwan (American/Hebrew) God is gracious. A form of John.
Juwann, Juwaun, Juwon, Juwuan

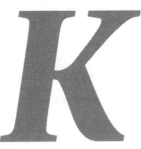

Kabiito (Rutooro) born when foreigners visited.
Kabito, Kabyto

Kabil (Turkish/Hebrew) spear gatherer.
Kabyl

Kabir (Arabic) great; history.
Kabyr, Kadbar, Khabir

Kabonesa (Rutooro) baby of a difficult birth.
Kabonesah

Kabr (Hindi) grass.

Kacancu (Rukonjo) first-born child.

Kacey (Irish) brave.
Kace, Kacee, Kacy, Kaecee, Kaecey, Kaeci, Kaecie, Kaecy, Kaesee, Kaesy, Kaesi, Kaesie, Kaesy, Kaicee, Kaicey, Kaici, Kaicie, Kaicy, Kase, Kasee, Kasey, Kasi, Kasie, Kasy, KC, K.C.

Kadar (Arabic) powerful.
Kader, Kadir, Kador, Kadyr

Kade (Scottish) from the wetlands.
Cade, Cadee, Caed, Caid, Caide, Cayd, Cayde, Kadee, Kaed, Kaid, Kaide, Kayd, Kayde, Kaydee

Kadeem (Arabic) servant.
Kadim, Kadym, Khadeem

Kadin (Arabic) friend.
Kadan, Kaden, Kadon, Kadyn

Kadir (Arabic) spring.
Kadeer, Kadyr

Kadish (Aramaic) holy; sacred.
Kadysh

Kadmiel (Hebrew) God first.
Kadmiell

Kado (Japanese) gateway.

Kaelan (Gaelic) powerful warrior.
Kaelen, Kaelin, Kaelon, Kaelyn, Kailan, Kailen, Kailin, Kailyn, Kalan, Kalen, Kalin, Kalon, Kalyn, Kaylan, Kaylen, Kaylin, Kaylon

Kaemoon (Japanese) joyful.
Kaimon, Kaymon

Kafele (Ngoni) worth dying for.

Kafir (Arabic) unbeliever.
Kafyr

Kaga (Native American) writer.
Kagah

Kahale (Hawaiian) home.
Kahail, Kahayl

Kahana (Hawaiian) priest.
Kahanah, Kahanna, Kahannah

Kahil (Turkish) young; naive.
Kahleel, Kahleil, Kahlill, Kahyl,
Kalel, Kalil, Kalyl

Kaho (Tongan) reed. (Poly) arrow.

Kaholo (Hawaiian) runner.

Kahua (Hawaiian) sea.
Kahauah

Kai (Native American) willow tree.
(Jap) to forgive. (Wel) keeper of
keys. (Haw) sea.
Cai

Kaihau (Polynesian) chief.

Kaikara (Runyoro) a god.
Kaikarah

Kailao (Tongan) war dance.
Kaelo, Kaylo

Kailen (Irish) mighty warrior.
Kaelan, Kaelen, Kaelin, Kaellan,
Kaellen, Kaellin, Kaellon, Kaellyn,
Kaelon, Kaelyn, Kailan, Kallan,
Kallen, Kallin, Kallon, Kallyn,
Kaylan, Kaylin, Kayllan, Kayllen,
Kayllin, Kayllon, Kayllyn, Kaylon,
Kaylyn

Kaili (Hawaiian) a god.
Kaelea, Kaeleah, Kaelee, Kaeleigh,
Kaeley, Kaeli, Kaelie, Kaely, Kailea,
Kaileah, Kailee, Kaileigh, Kailey,
Kailie, Kaily, Kaylea, Kayleah,
Kaylee, Kaylei, Kayleigh, Kayli,
Kaylie, Kayly

Kain (Hawaiian) spear thrower.
Cain, Caine, Cayn, Cayne, Kain,
Kayn, Kayne

Kaine (Welsh) beautiful.
(Ir) tribute. (Haw) eastern sky.
(Jap) golden.
Caen, Cain, Caine, Cane, Cayn,
Cayne, Kaen, Kahan, Kain, Kainan,
Kaine, Kainen, Kane, Kaney, Kayn,
Kayne

Kainga (Tongan) relative.
Kaynga

Kaipo (Hawaiian) sweet heart.
Kaypo

Kaiser (Bulgarian) hairy.
Kayser

Kaivai (Tongan) mariner; sea
worker.
Kaivay, Kayvai, Kayvay

Kaivao (Tongan) wild.
Kayvao

Kaj (Danish) earth.
Kai

Kaka (Tongan) climb.
Kakah

Kakaea (Tongan) tall.
Kakaeah

Kakaio (Hawaiian) God will
remember.

Kakana (Hawaiian) power.
Kakanah

Kakar (Hindi) grass.

Kakau (Polynesian) swim.

Kala (Hawaiian) sun. (Hin) black;
time.
Kalah

Kalama (Hawaiian) torch.
Kalam, Kalamah

Kalameli (Tongan) caramel.
Kalamelie, Kalamely

Kalani (Hawaiian) heaven; chief.
Kalan, Kalanee, Kalaney, Kalanie,
Kalany

Kalat (Arabic) castle.
Kalatt

Kalauka (Hawaiian/Latin) weak. A
form of Claude.

K

Kalawina (Hawaiian) bald.

Kale (Arabic) naive.
Kael, Kaelea, Kaeleah, Kaelee, Kaeleigh, Kaeli, Kaelie, Kaely, Kalea, Kaleah, Kalee, Kaleigh, Kaleu, Kaley, Kali, Kalie, Kalin, Kayl, Kayle, Kaylea, Kayleah, Kaylee, Kayleigh, Kayley, Kayli, Kaylie, Kayly

Kalea (Hawaiian) happy.
Kaleah, Kalee, Kalei, Kaleigh, Kaley, Kali, Kalie, Kaly

Kaleb (Hebrew) dog. (Arab) brave.
Kaelab, Kaeleb, Kailab, Kalab, Kalb, Kale, Kalev, Kalib, Kalyb, Kaylab, Kayleb, Kilab, Kylab

Kalechi (Nigerian) praise to God.

Kalen (Arabic) naive.
Kaelan, Kaelen, Kaelin, Kaelon, Kaelyn, Kailan, Kailen, Kailin, Kailon, Kailyn, Kalan, Kalin, Kalon, Kalyn, Kaylan, Kaylen, Kaylin, Kaylon, Kaylyn, Len, Leni, Lenie, Leny

Kaleo (Hawaiian) voice.
Caleo

Kalepa (Hawaiian) faith.
Kalepah

Kalevi (Finnish) hero.
Kalevee, Kalevey, Kalevie, Kalevy

Kalhana (Hindi) poet.
Kalhanah

Kalid (Arabic) eternal; everlasting.
Kalyd

Kalikau (Polynesian) athlete.

Kalil (Arabic) good friend.
Kahaleel, Kahlil, Kalyl

Kalinga (Hindi) bird.
Kalingah

Kalino (Hawaiian) brilliant.

Kaliq (Arabic) creative.
Kalique, Kaliqu, Kalique, Khaliq, Khaliqu, Khalique

Kalkin (Hindi) tenth-born child.
Kalkyn

Kalle (English/Scandinavian) strong; courageous. (Ger) farmer.
Kale

Kallen (Irish) mighty warrior.
Kalan, Kalen, Kalin, Kallan, Kallin, Kallon, Kallun, Kallyn, Kalon, Kalun, Kalyn

Kalmin (Scandinavian) man.
Kalman, Kalmen, Kalmon, Kalmyn

Kaloosh (Armenian) blessed event.

Kamaha (Hawaiian) asleep.
Kamahah

Kamaka (Hawaiian) face.
Kamakah

Kamakani (Hawaiian) wind.
Kamakanee, Kamakaney, Kamakanie, Kamakany

Kamal (Hindi) lotus. (Arab) perfection.
Kamaal, Kameel, Kamel, Kamil, Kamyl

Kamau (Kikuyu) quiet warrior.

Kambara (Australian Aboriginal) crocodile.
Kambarah

Kamekona (Hawaiian) strength.

Kami (Hindi) loving.
Kamee, Kamey, Kamie, Kamy

Kamilo (Tongan/French) ceremonial attendant. (Lat) freedom.
Camillo, Camilo, Kamillo, Kamyllo, Kamylo

Kamoku (Hawaiian) island.

Kamuela (Hawaiian/Hebrew) his name is God; asked for. A form of Samuel.
Kamuelah, Kamuele

Kamuzu (Ngoni) medicine.

Kana (Japanese) powerful.
Kanah

Kanai (Hawaiian) winner.

Kanale (Hawaiian) from the stony meadow. A form of Stanley.
Kanal

Kanaloa (Hawaiian) a god.

Kane (Irish/Gaelic) tribute. (Wel) beautiful. (Jap) golden. (Haw) eastern sky.
Caen, Cain, Caine, Cane, Cayn, Cayne, Kaen, Kahan, Kain, Kainan, Kaine, Kainen, Kaney, Kayn, Kayne

Kang (Chinese) healthy.

Kanga (Australian Aboriginal/Australian) kangaroo.

Kangan (Australian Aboriginal) to cut.

Kangi (Lakota Sioux) raven.
Kanga, Kange, Kangee, Kangie, Kangy

Kaniel (Hebrew) stalk.
Kaniell, Kannyel, Kanyel

Kanji (Japanese) tin.

Kanku (Australian Aboriginal) boy.

Kanoa (Polynesian) freedom.
Kanoah

Kantu (Hindi) happy.

Kanu (Swahili) wild cat.

Kanya (Australian Aboriginal) rock.
Kania, Kaniah, Kanyah

Kaori (Japanese) strength.
Kaoru

Kapali (Hawaiian) cliff.
Kapalee, Kapalie, Kapaly

Kapeni (Malawian) knife.
Kapenee, Kapenie, Kapeny

Kapila (Hindi) ancient prophet.
Kapil, Kapill, Kapilla, Kapyla, Kapylla

Kapo (Tongan) self taught.

Kapono (Hawaiian) righteous.
Kapena

Karam (Arabic) charitable.
Kareem, Karim, Karym

Kardal (Arabic) mustard seed.
Kardel

Kare (Norwegian) enormous.
Karee

Kareem (Arabic) noble.
Karee, Karem, Kareme, Karim, Karreem, Karriem, Karrym

Karey (Welsh) from the rocky island. (Grk) purity.
Carey, Karee, Kari, Karree, Karrey, Karri, Karrie, Karry, Kary

Karif (Arabic) born in autumn/fall.
Kariff

Karim (Arabic) noble; generous.
Karee, Karem, Kareme, Karreem, Karriem, Karrym, Karym

Karl (English) strong; courageous. (Ger) farmer.
Carl, Carle, Kaarl, Kaarle, Kaarlo, Kale, Kalle, Kalman, Karcsi, Karel, Karlen, Karlitis, Karlo, Karlos, Karlow, Karlton, Karius, Karol, Kjell

Karlif (Arabic) born in autumn/fall.
Kareef, Karlyf

Karlisa (Runyankore) herder.
Karlisah, Karlysa, Karlysah

K

Karmai (Australian Aboriginal) spear.
Karma, Karmae, Karmay

Karnak (Hindi) heart.

Karney (Irish) winner.
Karnee, Karni, Karnie, Karny

Karnik (Hindi) control.
Karnika

Karr (Scandinavian) marsh.

Karsten (Greek) anointment.
Karstan, Karstein, Karstin, Karston, Karstyn

Karu (Hindi) cousin.
Karun

Kaseem (Arabic) divided.
Kasceem, Kaseym, Kasim, Kazeem

Kaseko (Zimbabwean/Rhodesian) one who teases or ridicules.

Kasem (Thai) happy.
Kaseme

Kasen (Basque) helmet; head protection.
Kasan, Kasin, Kason, Kasyn

Kasey (Irish) brave.
Kace, Kacee, Kacy, Kaecee, Kaecey, Kaeci, Kaecie, Kaecy, Kaesee, Kaesy, Kaesi, Kaesie, Kaesy, Kaicee, Kaicey, Kaici, Kaicie, Kaicy, Kase, Kasee, Kasey, Kasi, Kasie, Kasy, KC, K.C.

Kasi (Hindi) bright.
Kasee, Kasey, Kasie, Kasy

Kasib (Arabic) fertile.
Kasyb

Kasim (Arabic) divided.
Kasym

Kasimir (Slavic) commander of peace.
Kasimyr, Kasymir, Kasymyr

Kasiya (Ngoni) separate.
Kasiyah

Kasper (Persian) guardian of the treasure. A form of Casper.
Caspar, Casper, Caspir, Caspor, Caspyr, Kaspar, Kaspir, Kaspor, Kaspyr

Kass (German) black bird.
Kaese, Kasch, Kase

Kassidy (Irish) clever; curly-haired.
Cassidy, Kassadee, Kassadey, Kassadi, Kassadie, Kassady, Kassedee, Kassedi, Kassedie, Kassedy, Kassidee, Kassidey, Kassidi, Kassidie, Kassydee, Kassydey, Kassydi, Kassydie, Kassydy

Kateb (Arabic) writer.

Kato (Runyankore) second born of twins.

Katoa (Polynesian) completed.
Katoah

Katode (Yoruba) bringer of joy.
Kaiode

Katriel (Hebrew) God is my crown. (Arab) peace.
Katryel

Katungi (Runyankore) wealthy.
Katungie, Katungy

Kaufman (German) merchant; trader.
Kaufmann

Kaukau (Tongan) surfer.

Kaul (Arabic) trusted.

Kaulana (Hawaiian) famous.
Kaulanah

Kaulo (Hawaiian) borrower.

Kauri (Polynesian) forest tree.
Kauree, Kaurie, Kaury

Kava (Tongan) beard.
Kavah

Kavan (Irish) handsome.
Cavan, Caven, Cavin, Cavon,
Cavun, Cavyn, Kavanagh, Kaven,
Kavenaugh, Kavin, Kavon, Kavun,
Kavyn

Kavanagh (Irish) Kevin's follower;
follower of the handsome one.
Cavanagh, Kavenagh

Kaveh (Persian) ancient hero.
Kava, Kavah

Kavi (Hindi) poet.
Kavee, Kavey, Kavie, Kavy

Kavindra (Hindi) god of poets.
Kavindrah

Kawika (Hawaiian/Hebrew)
beloved. A form of David.
Kawyka

Kay (Greek) purity.
Kai (Wel), Kayde, Kayden, Kayle,
Kaylen, Kaylid, Kayne, Kaynen

Kayam (Hebrew) stable.

Kayin (Nigerian) celebrated.
(Yoruba) long hoped-for child.
Kaiyan, Kaiyen, Kaiyin, Kaiyon,
Kayan, Kayen, Kayon

Kayinga (Runyankore) great warrior.
Kaionga

Kayle (Hebrew) faith.
Kaile

Kazuo (Japanese) peace.

Ke (Irish) handsome one from
birth; gentle.
Keavan, Keaven, Keavin, Keavon,
Keavun, Keavyn, Keevan, Keeven,
Keevin, Keevon, Keevun, Keevyn,
Keivan, Keiven, Keivin, Keivon,
Keivyn, Kevan, Keven, Kevin,
Kevinn, Kevion, Kevis, Kevlon,

Kevon, Kevron, Kevun, Kevyn,
Keyvan, Keyven, Keyvin, Keyvon,
Keyvyn

Keahi (Hawaiian) flames.

Keal (Old Norse) ridge.
Keal, Keale, Keel, Keele

Kealoha (Hawaiian) fragrance;
perfume.
Ke'ala, Keala, Kealoha, Kealohah,
Keela, Keelah

Keane (Old English) keen; sharp.
Kean, Keanan, Keanen, Keen,
Keene, Kienan, Kienen, Keyan,
Keyen, Keyin, Keyon

Keanu (Hawaiian) sea breeze.
Keani, Keanie, Keany

Kearn (Irish) dark-haired.
Kearne, Kern, Kerne, Kerrn, Kerrne

Keaton (English) from the town
where hawks fly.
Keatan, Keaten, Keatin, Keatun,
Keatyn, Keetan, Keeten, Keetin,
Keeton, Keetun, Keetyn, Keitan,
Keiten, Keitin, Keiton, Keitun,
Keityn, Keytan, Keyten, Keytin,
Keyton, Keytun, Keytyn

Keaziah (African American/Hebrew)
cassia tree.
Keazia

Keb (Egyptian) earth.
Kebb

Kedar (Hebrew) dark-haired. (Arab)
powerful. (Hind) mountain lord.
Kadar, Keder

Keddy (English) of the red earth. A
form of Adam.
Keddi, Keddie

Kedem (Hebrew) ancient.
Kedeam, Kedeem, Kedim, Kedym

Kedrick (English) gift; splendour.
(O/Eng) war chief. A form of
Cedric.
Keddric, Keddrick, Keddrik,
Keddryc, Keddryck, Keddryk,
Kedric, Kedrik, Kedryc, Kedryck,
Kedryk

Keeaka (Hawaiian/Hebrew)
replacer. A form of Jack.
Keakah

Keefe (Irish) enjoyment.
Keef, Keeff, Keif, Keifer, Keiff,
Keiffer, Keith, Keithe, Keyf, Keyff,
Keyffe, Keyth

Keegan (Irish/Gaelic) small; fiery.
Kaegan, Keagan, Keagen, Keagin,
Keagon, Keegan, Keegen, Keegin,
Keegon, Kegan, Kegen, Keghan,
Keghen, Kegun, Kegyn, Keigan,
Keigen, Keigin, Keigon, Keigun,
Keigyn, Keygan, Keygen, Keygin,
Keygon, Keygyn

Keelan (Irish/Gaelic) slender;
islander.
Kealan, Kealen, Kealin, Kealon,
Kealyn, Keelen, Keelin, Keelin,
Keelon, Keelun, Keelyn, Keilan,
Keilen, Keilin, Keilon, Keilyn,
Keylan, Keylen, Keylin, Keylon,
Keylyn

Keeley (English/Irish/Gaelic)
handsome meadow.
Kelea, Keleah, Kealee, Kealeigh,
Kealen, Keali, Kealie, Kealy, Keelea,
Keeleah, Keelee, Keeleigh, Keelen,
Keeli, Keelie, Keely, Keilea, Keileah,
Keilee, Keileigh, Keiley, Keili, Keilie,
Keily, Keylea, Keyleah, Keylee,
Keyleigh, Keyley, Keyli, Keylie,
Keyly

Keelin (Chinese) little dragon.
(Eng) from the handsome pool.
Kee-Lyn

Keenan (Irish/Gaelic) little ancient
one.
Cianan, Keanan, Keanen, Keannan,
Keannen, Keenon, Kenan, Keynan,
Keynen, Keynin, Keynon, Kienan,
Kienen, Kienon, Keynan, Keynen,
Keynin, Keynon, Keynyn

Keene (German) bold; sharp.
Kean, Keane, Keen, Keenan, Kein,
Keine, Keyn, Keyne

Kees (Dutch/Greek) the cornel tree.
(Lat) horn-coloured.
Keas, Kease, Keese, Keesee, Keis,
Keys, Keyse

Kefir (Hebrew) lion cub.

Kefu (Polynesian) blond-haired.

Kehind (Yoruba) second-born twin.
Kehynd

Keiffer (German) cooper; barrel
maker.
Keefer, Keifer, Kiefer, Kieffer, Keyfer,
Keyffer

Keiji (Japanese) cautious ruler.
Keyjy

Keir (Gaelic) small, dark hair/
complexioned. A short form of
Kieran.
Kerr, Keyr

Keitaro (Japanese) blessed.
Keata, Keataro, Keita, Keyta, Keytaro

Keith (Gaelic) forest.
Keaf, Keafe, Keaff, Keaffe, Keif,
Keife, Keifer, Keiffer, Keiff, Keiffe,
Keyf, Keyfe, Keyff, Keyffe

Keka (Hawaiian) appointed.
Kekha

Kekapa (Hawaiian) rebel.
Kekapah

Kekoa (Hawaiian) bold; courageous.
Kekoah

Kelala (Hawaiian) spear leader.
Kelalah

Kelaya (Hebrew) grain that is dried.

Kelby (German) from the farm near the spring.
Kelbee, Kelbey, Kelbi, Kelbie, Kellbee, Kellbey, Kellbi, Kellbie, Kellby

Kele (Hopi) sparrow hawk.
Kelle

Kelemen (Hungarian) gentle; kind.
Kelleman, Kellemen, Kellieman, kelliemen, Kelliman, Kellimen, Kellman, Kellmen, Kellyman, Kellymen, Kelmen, Kelyman, Kelymen

Kelept (Polynesian) faithful.
Kelep

Kelevi (Finnish) hero.
Kelevee, Kelevey, Kelevie, Kelevy

Kelham (Old Norse) ridge.
Kellham

Keli (Hawaiian) chief.
Kealea, Kealeah, Kealee, Kealeigh, Keali, Kealie, Kealie, Kealy, Keelea, Keeleah, Keelee, Keeleigh, Keeli, Keelie, Keely, Kelea, Keleah, Kelee, Keleigh, Keley, Kelie, Kely, Keilea, Keileah, Keilee, Keileigh, Keiley, Keili, Keilie, Keily, Keylea, Keyleah, Keylee, Keyleigh, Keyli, Keylie, Keyly

Keli'i (Hawaiian) chief.

Kelile (Ethiopian) protected.
Kelyle

Kell (Old Norse) dweller from the spring.
Kel, Kelda, Keldah, Kellda, Kelldah

Kellagh (Irish) war.

Kellen (Irish) mighty warrior.
Kaelan, Kaelen, Kaelin, Kaelon, Kaelyn, Kailan, Kailan, Kalan, Kalen, Kalin, Kallan, Kallen, Kaylen, Keelan, Keilan, Keillan, Kelden, Kellan, Kelle, Kellin, Kelynn

Keller (Irish/Gaelic) little companion warrior.
Keler

Kelly (Irish/Gaelic) warrior; dweller from the meadow near the woods.
Kealea, Kealeah, Kealee, Kealeigh, Keali, Kealie, Kealie, Keallea, Kealleah, Keallee, Kealleigh, Kealley, Kealli, Keallie, Keally, Kealy, Keelea, Keeleah, Keelee, Keeleigh, Keeli, Keelie, Keelea, Keeleah, Keelee, Keeleigh, Keylley, Keelli, Keellie, Keelly, Keely, Kelea, Keleah, Kelee, Keleigh, Keley, Kelie, Kellee, Kelley, Kelli, Kellie, Kely, Keilea, Keileah, Keilee, Keileigh, Keiley, Keili, Keilie, Keillea, Keilleah, Keillee, Keilleigh, Kelley, Kelli, Kellie, Keily, Keylea, Keyleah, Keylee, Keyleigh, Keyli, Keylie, Keyllea, Keylleah, Keyllee, Keylleigh, Keylley, Keylli, Keyllie, Keylly, Keyly

Kelmen (Basque) merciful.
Kellman, Kellmen, Kelman

Kelsey (Old Norse) dweller at the island of ships.
Kelcey, Kelci, Kelcie, Kellci, Kellcie, Kellcy, Kelli, Kellie, Kelly, Kellog, Kellow, Kelo, Kelson, Keltan, Kelten, Keltin, Kelton

Kelton (English) from the port; from the keel maker's town.
Keldan, Kelden, Keldin, Keldon, Kelson, Keltan, Kelten, Keltin, Keltonn, Keltyn

K

Kelvin (Irish/Gaelic) from the narrow river.
Calvan, Calven, Calvin, Calvon, Celvan, Celven, Celvin, Celvon, Kalvan, Kalven, Kalvon, Kalvyn, Kelvan, Kelven, Kelvon, Kelvyn

Kelwin (Old English) friend from the ridge.
Kelwen, Kelwinn, Kelwyn, Kelwynn, Kelwynne

Kemal (Turkish) highest honour.
Kemel

Kemen (Basque) strength.
Keaman, Keamen, Keeman, Keemen, Keiman, Keimen, Keman, Keyman, Keymen

Kemp (Middle English) warrior.
Kempe

Kempton (English) from the warrior's town.
Kemptan, Kempten, Kemptin, Kemptyn

Kemuel (Hebrew) helper of God.

Ken (Japanese) relation; clear; bright water. The short form of names starting with 'Ken' e.g. Kenneth.
Kena, Kenn, Kenno, Keno

Kenan (Hebrew) attainment.
Kenen, Kenin, Kenon, Kenyn

Kenaz (Hebrew) bright.

Kendal (Celtic) chief leader of the valley.
Kendale, Kendali, Kendall, Kendan, Kendel, Kendell, Kendral, Kendrall, Kendrel, Kendrell, Kendryl, Kendryll

Kendrew (Scottish) strong; brave; courageous. A form of Andrew.
Kandrew

Kendrick (Irish) son of Ken; son of the relative; clear, bright water.
Kendric, Kendrick, Kendricks, Kendrik, Kendrix, Kendryc, Kendryck, Kendryk, Kenric, Kenrick, Kenrik, Keondric, Keondrick, Keondrik, Keondryc, Keondryck, Keondryk

Keneke (Hawaiian) handsome.

Kenelm (Old English) defender of the relations.

Kenete (Hawaiian) handsome.
Kenet

Kenji (Japanese) second-born son.
Kenjee, Kenjie, Kenjy

Kenley (English) from the royal meadow; from the meadow of the relatives.
Kenlea, Kenleah, Kenlee, Kenleigh, Kenli, Kenlie, Kennlea, Kennleah, Kennlee, Kennleigh, Kennley, Kennli, Kennlie, Kennly, Kenly

Kenn (Old Welsh) relation; bright, clear water. The short form of names starting with 'Kenn' e.g. Kenneth.
Ken

Kennan (Scottish) little Ken; the little relative; little bright, clear water.
Kenan, Kenen, Kenin, Kennen, Kennin, Kennon, Kennyn, Kenon, Kenyn

Kennard (Old English) strength.
Kenard, Kenerd, Kenner, Kennerd

Kennedy (Old English) royal ruler. (Ir) helmeted chief.
Kenman, Kennadie, Kennady, Kennard, Kennedey, Kennedi, Kennedie, Kent, Kenton, Kenyon

Kenneth (Irish/Gaelic) handsome.
(Eng) royal oath.
Canice, Cennydd, Cenydd, Kene,
Kenly, Kenley, Kennan, Kennen,
Kennin, Kennon, Kennyn,
Kennyth, Kent, Kenton, Kenward,
Kenworth, Kenyth

Kenrick (English) bold, royal ruler.
Kennric, Kennrick, Kennrik,
Kennryc, Kennryck, Kennryk,
Kenric, Kenricks, Kenrik, Kenriks,
Kenryc, Kenryck, Kenrycks, Kenryk,
Kenryks

Kent (Celtic) lord. (O/Wel) white;
bright.
Kentan, Kenten, Kentin, Kenton,
Kentyn

Kentaro (Japanese) big boy.

Kentigern (Gaelic) lord.
Kentygern

Kenton (Old English) from the
royal town.
Kentan, Kenten, Kentin, Kentoon,
Kentyn

Kentrell (English) from the king's
estate.
Kentrel

Kenward (Old English) brave
warrior.

Kenway (Old English) from the
brave warrior's estate.
Kenwai

Kenwood (Old English) from the
warrior's forest.

Kenya (Africa) jewel.
(Geographical) country in Africa.
Kenia, Keniah, Kenja, Kenyat,
Kenyata, Kenyatt, Kenyatta

Kenyon (Irish) blond-haired.
Kenyan, Kenyen, Kenyin

Kenzie (Scottish) wise leader.
Kensi, Kensie, Kensy, Kenzi, Kenzie,
Kenzy

Keo (Hawaiian) God will increase.

Keoia (Hawaiian) life.
Keola, Keola

Keoki (Hawaiian/Greek) farmer. A
form of George.

Keon (Irish) young warrior. A form
of Ewan/Evan, well born.
Keaon, Keeon, Keion, Keionne,
Keondre, Keone, Keontae,
Keontrye, Keony, Keyon, Kian,
Kion, Kyon

Keoni (Hawaiian) God is gracious.
A form of John.
Keonee, Keonie, Keony

Kerel (African) youth.
Kerell

Kerem (Turkish) noble; kind.

Kerey (Gypsy) homeward bound.
Keree, Keri, Kerie, Kery

Kerman (Basque) from Germany.
Kermen, Kerrman, Kerrmen

Kermit (Irish) freedom.
Kermitt, Kermyt, Kermytt

Kern (Old Irish) infantry unit.
Kearn, Kearne, Kearney, Kearny,
Keirn, Keirne, Kernan, Kernen,
Kernin, Kernon, Kerran, Kerren,
Kerrin, Kerron, Kerryn, Keryn,
Keyrn, Keyrne

Kerr (Scandinavian) from the
marsh.

Kerrick (English) the king's rule.
Keric, Kerick, Kerik, Kerric, Kerrik,
Kerryc, Kerryck, Kerryk, Keryc,
Keryck, Keryk

K

Kerry (Celtic) dark-haired.
Keary, Keri, Kerie, Kerray, Kerree, Kerrey, Kerri, Kerrie, Kery

Kers (Hindi) plant.

Kersen (Indonesian) cherry.
Kersan, Kersin, Kerson, Kersyn

Kerstan (Dutch) Christian. A form of Christian/Kirstan.
Kersten, Kerstin, Kerston, Kerstyn

Kerwin (Irish) dark-haired friend.
Kerwan, Kerwane, Kerwain, Kerwaine, Kerwon, Kerwyn, Kerwynn, Kerwynne

Kes (English) falcon.

Kesava (Sanskrit) long-haired.
Kesavah

Keshawn (Hebrew) God is gracious. A form of Sean/Shawn.
Kesean, Keshaun, Keshaune, Keshon

Keshon (African American/Hebrew/Gaelic) God is gracious. A form of Sean.
Kesaun, Kesean, Keshughn, Keshawn

Kesin (Hindi) long-haired beggar.
Kesyn

Kesse (Native American/Fanti) chubby baby.
Kessey, Kessi, Kessie, Kessy, Kezi, Kezie, Kezy, Kezzi, Kezzie, Kezzy

Kester (Old English) from the Roman army camp.

Kestrel (English) falcon.
Kestrell

Kettil (Scandinavian) kettle.
Kettel, Kettle, Kettyl

Keung (Chinese) the universe.

Kevin (Irish/Gaelic) handsome.
Kevan, Keven, Kevern, Keverne, Kevin, Kevinah, Kevine, Kevirn, Kevirne, Kevon, Kevyn, Kevyrn, Kevyrne

Kewini (Hawaiian) the birth is beautiful.

Key (Irish) son of the fiery one. (Eng) son of the key holder.
Kea, Kei, Key, Keye, Keynan, Keynon

Khalif (Arabic) king.
Khalyf

Khalil (Arabic) friend.
Kahil, Kahill, Kaleel, Kalid, Kalil, Khalee, Khali, Khalial, Khaliyl, Khalyd

Khaliq (Arabic) creative.
Kaliq, Khaliqu, Khalique, Khalyq, Khalyqu, Khalyque

Khamisi (Swahili) born on a Thursday.
Khamisy, Khamysi, Khamysy

Khan (Turkish) prince.
Cahn, Chan, Chanh, Kahn, Khanh

Khang (Vietnamese) strength.

Kharald (Russian/German) mighty spearman.

Khoury (Arabic) priest; holy.
Khori, Khorie, Khory, Khouri, Khouri

Khristos (Greek) Christ bearer. A form of Christopher.
Christo, Christofer, Christoffer, Christopher, Christos, Christous, Cristo, Cristos, Cristous, Crysto, Crystos, Crystous, Khristo, Khristofer, Khristoffer, Khristoph, Khristopher, Khrysto, Khrystos, Khrystous, Kristous, Krysto, Krystos, Krystous

Kibo (Uset) worldly; wisdom.
Kybo

Kibuuka (Luganda) brave warrior.
Kybuuka

Kidd (English) child; young goat.
Kid, Kida, Kidah, Kidda, Kiddad,
Kiddo, Kido, Kyd, Kyda, Kydah

Kiele (Hawaiian) the gardenia
flower.
Kyele

Kieran (Irish) small with dark hair
or complexion.
Ciaran, Ciaren, Ceiran, Ceiren,
Ceirin, Ceiron, Keeran, Keeren,
Keerin, Keeron, Kielan, Keiran,
Keiren, Keirin, Keeiron, Kiernan,
Kyran, Kyren, Kyrin, Kyron, Kyryn

Kiet (Thai) honourable.
Kyet

Kifeda (Luo) only boy amongst
many girls.
Kyfeda

Kiho (Dutooro) child born on a
foggy day.
Kyho

Kijika (Native American) one who
walks quietly.
Kijyka, Kyjika, Kyjyka

Kika (Hawaiian/Welsh) forest. A
form of Keith.
Kikah, Kyka, Kykah

Kiki (Spanish/German) ruler of the
house. A form of Henry.

Kilab (Arabic) dog.
Kylab

Kiley (English) from the narrow
land.
Kilea, Kileah, Kilee, Kilei, Kileigh,
Kiley, Kili, Kilie, Kily

Killian (Gaelic) small but warlike.
Kilian, Kiliane, Kilien, Killian,
Killienn, Kilmer, Kylian, Kylien,
Kyllian, Kyllien

Kilohana (Hawaiian) supreme.
Kilohanah

Kim (English) warrior chief.
Kimbal, Kimbel, Kimbele, Kimbell,
Kym, Kymbal, Kymbel, Kimbele,
Kimbell, Kymbal, Kymbel,
Kymbele, Kymbell, Kymbelle

Kimba (Australian Aboriginal) bush
fire; wild fire.
Kimbah, Kymba, Kymbah

Kimbal (Greek) vessel that is
hollow. (Eng) warrior chief.
Kimball, Kimbel, Kimbele,
Kimbell, Kymbal, Kymbel,
Kymbele, Kymbell

Kimberley (Old English) royal
meadow.
Kimbalea, Kimbaleah, Kimbalee,
Kimbaleigh, Kimbaley, Kimbali,
Kimbalie, Kimbaly, Kimberlea,
Kimberleah, Kimberlee,
Kimberleigh, Kimberli, Kimberlie,
Kimberly, Kymbalea, Kymbaleah,
Kymbalee, Kymbaleigh, Kymbaley,
Kymbali, Kymbalie, Kymberlea,
Kymberleah, Kymberlee,
Kymberleigh, Kymberley, Kymberli,
Kymberlie, Kymberly

Kimeona (Hawaiian) he heard.
Kimeonah

Kimo (Hawaiian/Hebrew) replacer.
A form of James.

Kimokeo (Hawaiian/Greek)
honouring God. A form of
Timothy.

Kin (Japanese) golden.
(Eng) relative.
Kyn

K

Kincaid (Celtic/Scottish) battle chief.
Kincaide, Kincayd, Kincayde, Kyncaid, Kyncayd, Kyncayde

Kinchen (Old Norse) relative.
Kynchen

Kindin (Basque) fifth-born child.
Kindyn, Kyndin, Kyndyn

King (Old English) king; ruler.
Kyng

Kingman (English) the king's man.
Kingmen

Kingsley (Old English) from the king's meadow.
King, Kings, Kingslea, Kingsleah, Kingslee, Kingsleigh, Kingsli, Kingslie, Kingsly, Kinslea, Kinsleah, Kinslee, Kinsleigh, Kinsley, Kinsli, Kinslie, Kinsly, Kyng, Kyngs, Kyngslea, Kyngsleah, Kyngslee, Kyngsley, Kyngsli, Kyngslie, Kyngsly

Kingston (English) from the king's town.
Kinston, Kyngston, Kynston

Kingswell (Old English) one who lives at the king's stream.
Kingswel, Kyngswel, Kyngswell

Kinnard (Irish) from the king's high hill.
Kinard, Kynard, Kynnard

Kinsey (English) victorious king.
Kinsee, Kinsi, Kinsie, Kynsee, Kynsey, Kynsi, Kynsie, Kynsy

Kinta (Native American) beaver.
Kintah, Kynta, Kyntah

Kinton (Hindi) crowned.
(Eng) from the king's town.
Kynton

Kioshi (Japanese) quiet.

Kip (Old English) dweller at the pointed hill; sleep.
Kipp, Kippa, Kippar, Kipper, Kippi, Kippie, Kippy, Kyp, Kypp

Kiral (Turkish) king.
Kyral

Kiran (Sanskrit) light beam.
Kiren, Kirin, Kiron, Kirun, Kiryn, Kyran, Kyren, Kyrin, Kyron, Kyrun, Kyryn

Kirby (Old Norse) from the church by the village. (O/Eng) from the cottage by the water.
Kerbbee, Kerbbey, Kerbbi, Kerbbie, Kerbby, Kerbee, Kerbi, Kerbie, Kirbee, Kirbey, Kirbi, Kirbie, Kyrbbee, Kyrbbey, Kyrbbi, Kyrbbie, Kyrbby, Kyrbee, Kyrbey, Kyrbi, Kyrbie, Kyrby Ker, Kerb, Kerbb, Kerbbi, Kerbbie, Kerbby, Kerbi, Kerbie, Kerby, Kir, Kirb, Kirbb, Kyr, Kyrb, Kyrbb, Kyrbbi, Kyrbbie, Kyrbby, Kyrbi, Kyrbie, Kyrby

Kiri (Cambodian) mountain.
Kiry, Kyri, Kyry

Kiril (Slavic/Greek) lordly ruler. A form of Cyril.
Ciril, Cyril, Kirill, Kiryl, Kiryll, Kyril, Kyrill, Kyrillos, Kyryl, Kyryll

Kiritan (Hindi) crown wearer.
Kiriten, Kiritin, Kiriton, Kirityn

Kirk (Old Norse/Scandinavian) dweller in the church.
Kerc, Kerck, Kerk, Kirc, Kirck, Kirklan, Kirkland, Kirtly, Kurc, Kurck, Kurk, Kyrc, Kyrck, Kyrk

Kirkland (English) from the church land.
Kerklan, Kerkland, Kirklan, Kurklan, Kurkland, Kyrklan, Kyrkland

K

Kirkley (English) from the church meadow.
Kerklea, Kerkleah, Kerklee, Kerkleigh, Kerkli, Kerklie, Kerkly, Kirklea, Kirkleah, Kirklee, Kirkleigh, Kirkley, Kirkli, Kirklie, Kirkly, Kurklea, Kurkleah, Kurklee, Kurkleigh, Kurkley, Kurkli, Kurklie, Kurkly, Kyrklea, Kyrkleah, Kyrklee, Kyrkleigh, Kyrkley, Kyrkli, Kyrklie, Kyrkly

Kirkwell (English) from the church stream.
Kerkwel, Kerkwell, Kirkwel, Kurkwel, Kurkwell, Kyrkwel, Kyrkwell

Kirkwood (Old Norse) from the church forest.
Kerkwood, Kurkwood, Kyrkwood

Kirstur (Gypsy) rider.
Kystur

Kirton (English) from the town with a church.
Kerston, Kurston, Kyrston

Kistna (Hindi) sacred; holy.
Kisstna, Kysstna, Kystna

Kito (Swahili) precious jewel.
Kitto, Kyto, Kytto

Kitroon (Hebrew) crown.
Kytron

Kitwana (Swahili) promised to live.
Kitwanah

Kiva (Hebrew) replacer. A form of James.
Akiva, Kivah, Kyva, Kyvah

Kiyiyah (Nez Perce) howling wolf.

Kiyoshi (Japanese) peace.

Kizil (Turkish) red.
Kizyl, Kyzil, Kyzyl

Kizza (Fanti) born after twins.
Kiza, Kizah, Kizzi, Kizzie, Kizzy, Kyza, Kyzah, Kyzza, Kyzzah, Kyzzi, Kyzzie, Kyzzy

Klah (Navajo) one who is left-handed.

Klaus (German) victory of the people. A form of Nicholas.
Claus, Klaas, Klaes, Klas, Klause

Kleef (Dutch) cliff.

Kleng (Norwegian) claw.
Klen

Kline (German) small.
Cline, Clyne, Klyne

Klinger (Hebrew) collector of discarded objects.
Clinger

Knight (Old English) warrior; knight.
Knightee, Knightleigh, Knightly, Knyght

Knoton (Native American) wind.

Knowles (English) from the grassy sloping hill.

Knox (Irish/Gaelic) from the hill.
Knol, knoll, Knoxx

Knud (Danish) kind.

Knute (Old Danish) relative.
Cnut, Cnute, Knud, Knut

Ko (Chinese) change.

Koby (Polish) replacer. A form of Jacob.
Cobee, Cobey, Cobi, Cobie, Coby, Kobee, Kobey, Kobi, Kobie

Kodwo (Ghanian) born on a Monday.

Kody (English) cushion.
Codee, Codey, Codi, Codie, Cody, Kodee, Kodey, Kodi, Kodie

K

Kofi (Twi) born on a Friday.

Kohana (Native American) fast.
Kohanah

Koi (Hawaiian/English) water.

Kojo (Akan) born on a Monday.

Koka (Hawaiian) from Scotland.
Kokah

Kokayi (Shona) to bring together.

Kole (Tongan) plea.

Kolet (Australian Aboriginal) dove.
Kolett

Koloa (Tongan) wealth.
Koloah

Kolya (Australian Aboriginal) winter.
Kolein, Kolyen, Kolia

Kolyah (Russian/Greek) victory of the people. A form of Nikolai/Nicholas.
Kolia, Koliah, Kolya

Komaki (Tongan) bay.
Komakie, Komaky

Kona (Hawaiian/Scottish) little ruler. A form of Don.
Konah

Konane (Hawaiian) bright moonlight.
Konan

Kondo (Swahili) war.
Kond

Kong (Chinese) sky that is glorious.

Kono (Moquelumnan) squirrel who eats pine nuts.

Kontar (Akan) only child.
Konta

Kootchal (Australian Aboriginal) dew.

Kopano (Botswana) union.

Koppel (Hebrew) little Jacob; the little replacer.
Kopel

Korah (Hebrew) bold.
Kora

Korb (German) basket.

Korong (Australian Aboriginal) canoe.
Koron

Kort (Scandinavian) wisdom.

Kory (Irish) from the hollow; head protection; helmet used for battle.
Coree, Corey, Cori, Corie, Cory, Koree, Korey, Kori, Korie

Kosey (Swahili) lion.
Kossee, Kossey

Kosumi (Moquelumnan) spear fisher.

Kovit (Thai) expert.
Kovyt

Kpodo (Ghanian) first-born twin.

Krishna (Hindi) delightful.
Kistna, Kistnah, Krisha, Krishnah, Kryshna, Kryshnah

Krun (African) mountain.

Kruz (Spanish/Portugese) cross.
Cruz

Kuei (Chinese) spirit.

Kueili (Tongan) quail.
Kueilie, Kueily

Kueng (Chinese) universe.

Kui (Tongan) grandparent; fish.

Kuka (Tongan) crab.
Kukah

Kukane (Hawaiian) masculine.
Kukain, Kukaine

Kulapo (Tongan) fish.

Kuli (Tongan) dog.

Kuma (Tongan) mouse.
Kumah

Kumala (Tongan) sweet potato;
yam.

Kumar (Sanskrit) prince.

Kumi (Tongan) quest.

Kun (Chinese) universe.

Kunle (Yoruba) honourable home.

Kuo (Chinese) person.

Kuper (Yiddish) copper; red-haired.
Copper, Cuper, Kopper, Kupor,
Kupper

Kuracca (Australian Aboriginal)
white cockatoo (parrot).
Kuraccah

Kurao (Japanese) mountain.

Kurt (Latin/German/French)
courteous; from the enclosure.
Curt, Kort

Kuruk (Pawnee) bear.

Kuusi (Tongan) goose.

Kwach (Ngoni) morning time.
Kwacha, Kwachah

Kwakou (Ghanian) born on a
Wednesday.
Kwako, Kwaku

Kwam (Native American) God is
gracious. A form of John.

Kwasi (Akan/Ghanian) born on a
Sunday. (Swa) wealthy.
Kwas, Kwesi

Kwintyn (Polish) fifth-born child.

Ky (Irish/Gaelic) from the strait.
The short form of Kyle.
Ki

Kyan (African American/Irish) little
king. A form of Ryan.
Kian

Kyle (Irish/Gaelic) from the strait.
Kiel, Kilan, Kile, Kilen, Kiley,
Kylan, Kyel, Kyele, Kylan, Kylar,
Kylen, Kyler (Eng), Kylon

Kyloe (Old English) from the
meadow of cows.
Kilo, Kiloe, Kilow, Kilowe, Kylo,
Kylow, Kylowe

Kynan (Welsh) chief.
Kinan

Kyne (Old English) royal.
Kine

Kyros (Greek) master.
Kiro, Kiros

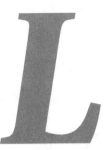

Laban (Hebrew) white.
Laben, Labin, Labon, Labyn

Labib (Arabic) intelligent; sensible.
Labid, Labyb, Labyd

Lachlan (Scottish/Celtic) from the
land of the lakes.
Lach, Lache, Lachee, Lachey, Lachi,
Lachie, Lachlann, Lachlun,
Lachlunn, Lachunn, Lachy,
Lakelan, Lakeland, Loch, Loche,
Lochee, Lochey, Lochi, Lochie,
Lochlan, Lochlen, Lochlin,
Lochlon, Lochlyn, Lochy

Lacy (Latin) from the Roman
manor.
Lacey

Ladd (Middle English) page; young
attendant.

Ladislaus (Slavic) glory.
Lachman (Ger), Laczko (Hung),
Ladislao, Ladislas (Pol), Ladislav,
Ladyslas, Ladyslaus, Lako, Laszolo,
Wladislav, Wladislaw

Ladislav (Czech/German) army
ruler. (Eng) from the woods.
Ladislaus, Ladyslav, Ladyslaus

Lado (Fanti) second-born son.

Lael (Hebrew) belonging to the
Lord.

Laffit (Old French) faithful.
Lafayette, Lafitte

Lafrance (Italian/German) freedom.
Lafrance

Laibrook (English) from the path
by the stream.
Laebrook, Laybrook

Laidley (English) from the path by
the watery meadow.
Laedlea, Laedleah, Laedlee,
Laedleigh, Laedley, Laedli, Laedlie,
Laedly, Laidlea, Laidleah, Laidlee,
Laidleigh, Laidli, Laidlie, Laidly,
Laydlea, Laydleah, Laydlee,
Laydleigh, Laydli, Laydlie, Laydly

Laione (Tongan) lion.
Laion

Laird (Scottish) land owner; lord of
the manor.
Layrd

Lais (Arabic) lion.
Lays

Lajos (Hungarian) holy; famous.
Lajcsi, Laji, Lajie, Lali

Lake (Latin) from the pond.
Laek, Laik, Layk

Lakepi (Tongan) rugby player
(footballer).

Laki (Samoan) lucky.

Lamani (Tongan) lemon.
Lamanee, Lamaney, Lamanie,
Lamany

Lamar (Teutonic) famous through
the land. (Fren) from the sea.
LaMarr, Lamarr, Lemar, Lemarr,
Limar, Limarr, Lymar, Lymarr

Lambert (Teutonic) bright rich
land; owner of many estates.
Lamberts (Ital), Lamberto (Ital),
Lambirt, Lambirto, Lamburt,
Lamburto, Lambyrt, Lambyrto,
Landbert (Ger), Landberto,

Lambert cont.
Landbirt, Landbirto, Landburt,
Landburto, Landbyrt, Landbyrto,
Landebert, Landeberto, Landebirt,
Landebirto, Landeburt,
Landeburto, Landebyrt, Landebyrto

Lamech (Hebrew) powerful
strength.
Lamec

Lami (Tongan) to conceal.
Lamee, Lamey, Lamie, Lamy

Lamond (French) the world.
Lammond, Lamondre, Lamund,
Lemond, Lemund

Lamont (Scandinavian) lawyer.
(O/Fren) mountain.
Lammond, Lamond, LaMont,
Lamont, Lamonte, Lemmont,
LeMont, Lemont, Lemonte

Lamorna (French/Gaelic) beloved.
Lamornah

Lance/Lancelot (Latin/Old French)
the knight's spear attendant.
Lancelott, Lancelotte, Lancey,
Lancilot, Lancilott, Lancilotte,
Lancilotto (Ital), Lancing, Lancylot,
Lancylott, Lancylotte, Lanse,
Lansing, Launce, Launcelot,
Launcelott, Launcelotte

Landan (Teutonic) from the open
land.
Landen, Lander, Landers, Landin,
Landis, Landman, Landon, Landor,
Landors, Landry, Landun, Landyn,
Langtry, Lunds, Lunt

Lander (English) owner of the
grassy plain.
Landar, Landers, Landor, Launder,
Launders

Lando (Portuguese/Spanish/
German) famous through the
land.
Landow

Landon (Old English) owner of the
grassy land; dweller on the hill.
Landan, Landen, Lander, Landers,
Landin, Landis, Landman, Landor,
Landors, Landry, Landun, Landyn,
Langtry, Lunds, Lunt

Landric (Teutonic) land ruler.
Landrick, Landrik, Landryc,
Landryck, Landryk

Landry (French/English) ruler of the
land.
Landre, Landrew, Landri, Landrie,
Landrue

Lane (Middle English) narrow road.
(Aust/Abor) good.
Laine, Laney, Lani, Lanie, Layn,
Layne, Layni, Laynie, Layny

Lang (Scottish/Scandinavian) long;
tall. (Aust/Abor) tree.
Laing, Langdon, Langer, Langford,
Langhorne, Langlee, Langleigh,
Langley, Langsdon, Langston,
Langstone, Langtry, Longfellow

Langdon (Old English) from the
long hill.
Langdan, Langden, Langdin,
Langdun, Langdyn, Langlea,
Langleah, Langlee, Langleigh,
Langley, Langli, Langlie, Langly,
Langsdon, Langston

Langford (English) dweller by the
long river crossing.
Laingford

Langi (Tongan) heaven.
Langee, Langey, Langie, Langy

L

Langley (Old English) of the long meadow.
Lainglea, Laingleah, Lainglee, Laingleigh, Laingley, Laingli, Lainglie, Laingly, Lang, Langlea, Langleah, Langlee, Langleigh, Langli, Langlie, Langly

Langston (Old English) from the long, narrow town; farm that belongs to the tall one.
Laingston, Langsdon, Langsdown

Langundo (Native American) peaceful.
Langund

Langworth (English) from the long enclosure.
Laingworth

Lani (Hawaiian) sky; heaven.
Lanee, Laney, Lanie, Lany

Lann (Celtic) sword.
Lan

Lanny (American/Latin) crown of laurel leaves; victory. A form of Laurence.
Lannee, Lanni, Lannie, Lany

Lanu (Moquelumnan) running around a pole.

Lanz (Italian/French) knight. A form of Lance, the knight's spear attendant.
Lanzo, Lonzo

Lanzo (German) land servant.
Lancelot, Lancilott, Lancilotto (Ital), Landa, Landza, Launce, Launcelot, Launcelott

Lao (Spanish/Latin) glorious stand. (Ton) law.

Lap (Vietnamese) independent.

Laquintin (Latin/American) fifth-born child.
Laquentin, Laquenton, Laquintas, Laquintise, Laquintiss, Laquinton, Laquyn, Laquynt, Laquyntan, Laquynten, Laquyntin, Laquynton, Laqyuntun, Laquyntyn

Laramie (French) one who cries tears of love.
Laramee, Laramey, Larami, Laramy

Laris (Latin) happy.
Larris, Larrys, Larys

Larkin (Irish) rough; fierce.
Larkan, Larken, Larklin, Larklyn, Larkyn

Larnell (Latin) beloved victory. A combination of Larry/Daryl.
Larnel

Larron (Old French) thief.
Laran, Laraun, Laren, Larin, Laron, Laronn, Larun, Laryn, Latheron, Lathron

Larry (Latin) crown of laurel leaves; victory. A short form of Laurence.
Lari, Larie, Larri, Larrie, Larry, Lary

Lars/Larson (Swedish) Lars' son; son of the one crowned with laurel; victorious one. The Norse form of Laurence.
Laris, Larris, Larse, Larsen, Larson, Larsson, Larz, Larzon, Lasse, Laurans, Laurits, Lavrans, Lorens

Larvall (Italian) to wash.
Larvell

Lasalle (French) hall.
Lasal, Lasale, Lasall

Lascelles (Old French) cell.
Lascel, Lascele, Lascell, Lascelle

Lash (Gypsy/German) famous
warrior. A form of Louis.
Lasher, Lashi, Lasho

Lashawn (Irish/American) God is
gracious. A form of Shawn.
Lasean, Lashajaun, Lashaun,
Lashon, Lashonne

Lasse (Finnish/Greek) victory of the
people. A form of Nicholas.
Lase

Laszlo (Hungarian) famous ruler.
Laci, Lacko, Lasio, Laslo, Lazlo

Lateef (Arabic) gentle; subtle.
Latif, Latyf, Letif, Letyf

Latham (Scandinavian) from the
barn at the homestead.
Laith, Lathe, Lather, Lathrop,
Latimer, Latymer

Lathan (Hebrew/American) gift of
God. A form of Nathan.
Lathanial, Lathaniel, Lathen,
Lathin, Laythyn, Leathan

Lathom/Lathrop (Old Norse) from
the home with the barn.
Lath, Lathe, Lathrope, Latholme

Latimer (Old French) language
teacher; interpreter.
Latimor, Latymer

Latravis (American/French) keeper
at the crossroads; tax or toll
collector. A form of Travis.
Latavious, Latavers, Latavious,
Latravers, Latraviaus, Latravious,
Latravys

Laudalino (Portuguese) praised.
Laudalin, Laudalyn, Laudalyno

Laughlin (Irish) servant.
Lauchlin, Laughlyn, Leachlain,
Leachlainn

Laurie/Laurence/Lawrence (Latin)
crown of laurel leaves; victory.
Labhras (Ir), Labhruinn, Larrance,
Lars (Swed), Larson, Larz, Laurans,
Lauree, Lauren, Laurencio (Span),
Laurens (Dut), Laurent (Fren),
Laurenz (Ger/Dan), Laurey, Lauri,
Lauriston, Lauritj, Lauris (Swed),
Lauritz (Dan), Lauro (Fili), Laurri,
Laurrie, Laurry, Laurus (Est), Laury,
Laurynas (Lith), Lavrenty (Russ),
Lavreuty (Russ), Lawrance, Lawree,
Lawrence, Lawrey, Lawri, Lawrie,
Lawry, Lawson, Loren, Lorenco
(Span), Lorencs, Lorenis (Hung),
Lorens, Lorenz (Ger), Lorenzo
(Ital/Span), Lori, Lorie, Lorit,
Loritz, Lorri, Lorrie, Lorry, Lorus,
Lory, Lourenco (Port), Lowrance,
Lowree, Lowrence, Lowrey, Lowri,
Lowrie, Lowry, Raulus, Vavrinec

Laval (Old English) lord.
Lave, Lavrans

Lavalle (French) from the valley.
Lavail, Laval, Lavall, Lavalei,
Lavalley

Lavan/Lavaughan (Hebrew) white.
Lavaughan, Laven, Lavin, Lavon,
Lavyn, Levan, Leven, Levin, Levon,
Levyn

Lave (Italian) lava. (Eng) lord.
Laev, Laeve, Laiv, Laive, Layv, Layve

Lavern (Latin) spring time.
Laverne, LaVern, LaVerne, Lavyrn,
Lavyrne, Lavrans, Luvern, Luverne

Lavi (Hebrew) lion.
Lavee, Lavey, Lavie, Lavy

Lavon (American/Hebrew) white.
Lavan, Lavaughan, Laven, Lavin,
Lavon, Lavyn, Levan, Leven, Levin,
Levon, Levyn

L

Lavrenti (Russian/Latin) crown of laurel leaves; victory. A form of Laurence.
Larent, Larenti, Lavrentij, Lavrusha, Lavrik, Lavro

Lawford (Old English) from the low ford on the hill.

Lawler (Gaelic) mumbler of words; softly spoken.
Law, Ler, Leri, Lerie, Lery

Lawley (Old English) from the low meadow on the hill.
Lawlea, Lawleah, Lawlee, lawleigh, Lawley, Lawli, Lawlie, Lawly

Lawson (Old English) Lawrence's son; son of the victorious one crowned in laurel leaves.

Lawton (Old English) from the town on the hill; refinement.
Laughton

Lazaro (Italian/Greek) resurrection.
Lazarillo, Lazarilo, Lazarito, Lazzaro

Lazarus (Hebrew) God will help.
Eleazar, Lazar (Russ), Lazarasz, Lazare (Fren), Lazaro (Ital/Span), Lazarsz (Pol), Lazer, Lazlo, Lazzaro (Ital), Lazzo (Illy), Lesser

Lazhar (Arabic) best appearance.

Leaf (English) leaf from a tree.
Leath, Leef, Leeth, Leif, Leighth, Leyf, Leyth

Leal (English) loyal, faithful friend.

Leander (Greek) like a lion.
Ander, Leandre (Fren), Leandro (Ital/Span), Leanther

Leben (Yiddish) life.

Lech (Polish) forest spirit.

Ledyard (German) guardian of the nation.

Lee/Leigh (English) from the meadow.
Lea, Leah, Lei, Ley

Leeland (Old English) shelter.
Layland, Layton, Lealan, Lealand, Leelan, Leighlan, Leighland, Leighton, Lelan, Leland, Letant, Leylan, Leyland

Leggett (Old French) ambassador.
Lagat, Lagate, Leggitt, Liggett, Lyggett

Legrand (Old French) the great one.
Legran, Legrant

Lei (Chinese) thunder. (Haw) king. (Ton) ivory.
Leigh, Ley, Leygh

Leib (Yiddish) lion roaring.
Leibel

Leif (Scandinavian) beloved. (Scot/Gae) broad river.
Laif, Leyf, Leif, Leiff, Leith (Scot/Gae), Lief

Leighton (Old English) from the meadow town.
Laeton, Laiton, Layton, Leaton, Leeton, Leiton, Leyton

Lek (Thai) small.

Lekeke (Hawaiian) ruler who is powerful.
Likeke

Leks (Estonian) defender of humankind. A form of Alexander.
Leksik, Lekso

Lel (Hindi) beloved.

Leland (Old English) from the meadow.
Layland, Layton, Lealan, Lealand, Leelan, Leighlan, Leighland,

Leland cont.
Leighton, Lelan, Letant, Leylan,
Leyland

Lele/Lalo (Latin) lullaby.

Lemar (French) ocean.
Lamar, Lemario, Lemarr, Limar,
Limarr, Lymar, Lymarr

Lemuel (Hebrew) devoted to God.

Len/Lenny (Old English) house with
tenants. The short form of names
beginning with 'Len' e.g. Lennor.
Len, Lenee, Leney, Leni, Lenie,
Lenn, Lennee, Lenney, Lenni,
Lennie, Leny

Lencho (Spanish/Latin) crown of
laurel leaves; victory. A form of
Lawrence.
Lenci, Lencie, Lenzy

Lenis (Latin) gentle; soft.
Lenys

Lenno (Native American) man.
Leno

Lennon (Gaelic) little cap; cloak.
Lenna, Lannan, Lennen, Lennin,
Lennyn

Lennor (Gypsy) spring/summer
time.
Lenor

Lennox (Gaelic) grove of elm trees.
Lenox

Lensar (Gypsy) from his parents.
Lansa, Lensah, Lenza, Lenzah,
Lenzar

Leo (Latin) lion.
Lav, Leaho, Leao, Leeo, Leigho,
Leio, Leodis, Leon (Fren),
Leondaus, Leone, Leonid (Russ),
Leonidas, Leonis, Lev (Russ), Lio,
Lion, Lyo, Lyon

Leofric (Old English) beloved ruler.
Leofrick, Leofrik, Leofryc, Leofryck,
Leofryk

Leofwin (Old English) beloved
friend.
Leofwen, Leofwyn

Leon (French) lion-like.
Leahon, Leaon, Leighon, Leion,
Leonas, Leonce, Leoncio, Leondris,
Leone, Leonek, Leonetti, Leoni,
Leonid, Leonidas, Leonirez,
Leonidas, Leonirez, Leonizio,
Leonon, Leons, Leontes, Leontios,
Leontrae, Levin (Russ), Leyon,
Lion, Lionel, Lionelle, Lionello,
Lyon, Lyonal, Lyonel

Leonard (Teutonic) bold; strong
like a lion.
Leanard, Leanardas (Lith),
Leanardus (Lat), Leanhard,
Lennard, Leonardo (Ital/Span),
Leonerd, Leongard (Russ),
Leonhard (Ger), Leonid (Russ),
Leonidas (Grk), Leonide,
Lienhardt, Lionard, Lionardo,
Lonnard, Lonnardo, Lyonard

Leonel (French) lion cub; bold;
strong like a lion. A form of
Leonard.
Leaonal, Leaonall, Leaonel,
Leaonell, Leional, Leionall,
Leionel, Leionell, Lional, Lionall,
Lionel, Lionell, Lyonal, Lyonall,
Lyonel, Lyonell

Leopold (German) brave people.
Leopoldo, Leorad, Lipot, Lopolda,
Luepold, Luitpold

Leor (Hebrew) light of mine.
Leory, Lior

Lepati (Tongan) leopard.

Leron (Old French) circle.
Lerond, Leron, Lerin, Lerrin, Leryn

L

Leroy (Old French) king.
Learoi, Learoy, Lee-Roy, Leeroy,
Leighroi, Leighroy, Leiroi, Leiroy,
Leroi, Lerol, Leyroi, Leyroy

Les (Scottish/Gaelic) from the grey
fortress; garden court by the pool
meadow. The short form of names
starting with 'Les' e.g. Leslie.
Less

Lesharo (Pawnee) chief.

Leshawn (Irish/American) God is
gracious. A form of Shawn.
Lesean, Leshajaun, Leshaun,
Leshon, Leshonne

Leshem (Hebrew) precious stone.

Leslie (Scottish/Gaelic) from the
grey meadow; garden court by the
stream meadow.
Leslea, Lesleah, Leslee, Leslei,
Lesleigh,Lesley, Lesli, Lesly, Lezlea,
Lezleah, Lezlei, Lezleigh, Lezley,
Lezli, Lezlie, Lezly

Lester (Latin) from the chosen
camp. (O/Eng) shining lamp.
Leichester

Lev (Hebrew) he heard. The short
form of names starting with 'Lev'
e.g. Levant.
Leb, Leva, Levah, Levka, Levko,
Levushka

Levander (Hebrew) rising from the
sea.

Levant (Latin) rising.
Lavant, Lavante, Lebert, Levandar,
Levante, Lavender, Lavendor, Lever,
Leveret, Leverett, Leverette

Leveni (Tongan) raven.
Levenee, Leveney, Levenie, Leveny

Leverett (Old French) young rabbit.
Leveret, Leverit, Leveritt, Leveryt,
Leverytt

Levi (Hebrew) united in harmony;
promise.
Lavi, Lavy, Leavitt, Leevi, Lever,
Levic, Levy, Lewi

Levin (Old English) dearest friend.
Leevon, Levon, Levone, Levonn,
Levonne, Levyn, Levynn, Lew,
Lewan, Lewen, Lewon, Lewyn,
Louan, louen, Louin, Louon,
Louyn, Lyvon. Lyvonn, Lyvonne

Lewis (German) renowned battle.
The short form of Llewelyn, lion
like friend; lightning.
Lewys, Louis, Louys

Lex (Greek) word.
Laxton, Lexan, Lexen, Lexton

Leyati (Moquelumnan) abalone
shell-shaped.
Leyatie, Leyaty

Li (Chinese) strength.

Liam (Teutonic) helmet of
resolution. (Irish) wilful.
A short form of William.
Lyam

Lian (Irish) protector.
Liam, Lyam, Lyan

Liang (Chinese) excellent.
Lyang

Lias (English) rock.
Lyas

Liberio (Portuguese) freedom.
Liberaratore, Libero (Ital), Liberty,
Lyberio, Lyberyo

Liddon (Old English) shelter.
Lidon, Lyddon, Lydon

Lieb (German) love.
Lyeb

Ligongo (Yao) who is he?
Lygongo

Liko (Hawaiian) bud of a flower.
(Chin) protected.
Like, Lyko

Limu (Tongan) seaweed.
Lymu

Lin (Burmese) bright.
Linh, Linn, Linni, Linnie, Linny,
Lyn, Lynn

Linc (English) from the place near
the pool. The short form of
Lincoln.
Link, Lynk

Lincoin (Old English) from the
place near the pool.
Lincon, Lincoyn, Lyncoin, Lyncoyn

Lind (Old English) dweller by the
linden tree.
Lynd

Lindall/Lindel (English) from the
linden or lime trees.
Linlind, Lindal, Lindberg,
Lindbergh, Lindel, Lindell, Lindsay,
Linsey, Lyndal, Lyndall, Lyndel,
Lyndell, Lyndsay, Lyndsey

Lindberg (German) hill with linden
trees.
Lindbergh, Lindburg, Lynberg,
Lynbergh, Lynburg

Lindbert (Teutonic) from the
linden-tree hill.
Linbert, Linbirt, Linburt, Linbyrt,
Lindberg, Lindbirt, Lindburg,
Lindburt, Lynbert, Lynbirt,
Lynburt, Lynbyrt, Lyndbert,
Lyndbirt, Lyndburt, Lyndbyrt

Linden (Old English) from the
linden- or lime-tree valley.
Lindan, Lindin, Lindon, Lindyn,
Lyndan, Lynden, Lyndin, Lyndon,
Lyndyn

Lindley (Old English) from the
meadow with linden or lime
trees.
Lindlea, Lindleah, Lindlee,
Lindleigh, Lindli, Lindlie, Lindly,
Lyndlea, Lyndleah, Lyndlee,
Lyndleigh, Lyndley, Lyndli, Lyndlie,
Lyndly

Lindsay (Old English) from the
linden-tree island.
Lindsee, Lindsey, Linsey, Lyndsay,
Lyndsee, Lyndsey

Linford (Old English) from the
linden-tree river crossing.
Lynford

Linfrid (German) gentle peace.
Linfryd, Lynfrid, Lynfryd

Lingrel (Old English) river bank;
rising hill.
Lyngrel

Link (Old English) from the river
bank.
Linc, Linck, Lync, Lynck, Lynk

Linley (Old English) from the flax
field (a blue flowering plant).
Linlea, Linleah, Linlee, Linleigh,
Linli, Linlie, Linly, Lynlea, Lynleah,
Lynlee, Lynleigh, Lynley, Lynli,
Lynlie, Lynly

Linton (Old English) from the flax
town (a blue flowering plant).
Lynton

Linu (Hindi) lily.
Lynu

Linus (Greek) flax (a blue flowering
plant); yellow-coloured/haired.
Linas, Linis, Liniss, Linous, Lynis,
Lyniss, Lynus

Lio (Hawaiian/French) lion cub.
Lyo

Lionel (Old French) young lion; cub.
Lionello (Ital/Span), Lyonell, Lyonelle, Lyonello

Lipman (Teutonic) lover of human kind.
Lieber, Lypman

Liron (Hebrew) my song.
Lyron

Lise (Moquelumnan) salmon poking its head out of the water.
Lyse

Lisimba (Yao) lion.
Lasimba, Lasimbah, Lisimbah, Lysimba, Lysymba, Simba, Simbah, Symba, Symbah

Lisle (Old French) from the island town.
Lysle

Lister (English) cloth dyer.
Lyster

Litton (Old English) from the farm on the little hillside town.
Lyle, Lytel, Lytten, Lytton

Lius (Polish) light.
Lyus

Livingston (English) from the lively stone town.
Livingston, Livinston, Livinstone

Liwanu (Moquelumnan) growling bear.
Lywanu

Llewelyn (Welsh) lion-like friend; lightning.
Leoline, Lewelan, Lewelen, Lewis, Llewellyn, Llywellyn

Lleyton (Old English) from the meadow town.
Leaton, Leahton, Leeton, Leighton, Leyton

Lloyd (Welsh) grey-haired.
Floyd, Loyd

Loa (Tongan) storm clouds.
Loah

Lobo (Spanish) wolf; fierce.

Loch/Lochie (Irish/Scottish) from the land of the lakes. The short form of Lachlan.
Lachi, Lachie, Lachy, Lochey, Lochi, Lochy

Locke (Old English) from the forest or enclosure.
Loc, Lock, Lockwood

Lockwood (Old English) from the enclosed forest.
Locwood, Lokwood

Loe (Hawaiian/French) king. A form of Roy.

Lofa (Tongan) storm bird.
Lofah

Logan (Irish/Gaelic) from the hollow.
Logen, Login, Logon, Logyn

Lok (Chinese) happy.

Lokela (Hawaiian/German) renowned spear user. A form of Roger.
Lokelah

Lokni (Moquelumnan) rain coming in through the roof.

Loman (Celtic) enlightened. (Ir) brave. (Slav) sensitive.
Lomen

Lombard (Teutonic) long beard.
Lombarda, Lombardi, Lombardo (Ital)

Lon (Irish/Gaelic) strong; fierce. The short form of Alonzo/Lawrence.
Loni, Lonie, Lonni, Lonnie, Lonny, Lony

Lonan (Zuni) cloud.
Lonen, Lonin, Lonon, Lonyn

Lonato (Native American) flint
stone.

London (Middle English)
(Geographical) the capital of
Britain; fortress of the moon.
Longdon

Long (Chinese) dragon. (Viet) hair.

Longo (Tongan) quiet.

Lono (Hawaiian) god of farming;
peace.

Lootah (Lakota) red.
Loota

Lorcan (Celtic) little fierce one.
Lorcen, Lorcin, Lorcon, Lorcyn

Lord (English) noble one with a
title.

Lorenzo (Italian/Spanish/Latin)
crown of laurel leaves; victory. A
form of Lawrence.
Larinza, Laurenzo, Laurinzo,
Laurynzo, Leranzo, Lerenzo,
Lerinzo, Leronzo, Lerynzo, Lorant,
Lorantso, Lorantzo, Lorenc,
Lorence, Lorenco, Lorencz,
Lorenczo, Lorens, Lorenso, Lorent,
Lorentz, Lorentzo, Lorenz,
Lorenza, Lorenzo, Loretto, Lorinc,
Loricao, Lorinzo, Loritz, Lorrenzo,
Lorrynzo, Lorynzo

Loretto (Italian/Latin) crown of
laurel leaves; victory. A form of
Lawrence.
Loreto

Lorimer (Old French) saddler; spur;
bit maker.
Lorimer, Lorrimer, Lorrymer,
Lorymer

Loring (Teutonic) son of the
famous warrior.
Lorrin, Lorring, Lorryin, Lorrying,
Loryng

Loris (Dutch) clown.
Lorys

Loritz (Danish/Latin) crown of
laurel leaves; victory. A form of
Lawrence.
Lauritz, Laurytz, Lorytz

Lorne (Latin) crown of laurel leaves;
victory. A form of Lawrence.
Lorn, Lornie, Lorny

Lorry (English/Latin) crown of
laurel leaves; victory. (Eng) truck.
A form of Lawrence.
Lauri, Laurie, Laury, Lorri, Lorrie,
Lory

Lot (Hebrew) hidden.
Lotan

Lothar (Teutonic) warlike.
Lotair, Lotaire, Lottario, Lothair,
Lothaire, Lothario

Lotu (Tongan) to pray.

Lou (German) famous warrior. The
short form of names starting with
'Lou' e.g. Louis.
Lew

Loudon (German) from the low
valley.
Lewdan, Lewden, Lewdin, Lewdon,
Lewdyn, Loudan, Louden, Loudin,
Loudyn, Lowdan, Lowden, Lowdin,
Lowdon, Lowdyn

Louis (Teutonic) famous warrior.
Aloys, Aloysius, Clodoveo, Clovis,
Elois, Lajos (Hung), Lasho,
Lewellen, Lewes, Lewis, Lewys,
Ljudevit, Llewelyn, Llwellyn, Lodde
(Nrs), Lodewyck (Dut), Lodoe,
Lood (Dut), Lodovico (Ital),

Lodowick (Scott), Loeis, Lowes, Ludeg, Ludevit, Ludovicus, Ludvick, Ludvick, Lugaidh (Ir), Ludvig (Swed), Ludvik (Swed), Ludwik, Lui, Luigi (Ital), Luis (Span), Luiz, Luthais (Scott)

Lourdes (French) (Geographical) from Lourdes in France.
Lordes, Lords

Louvain (English) vain.
Louvayn

Lovell/Lowel (French/English) young wolf; fierce.
Lovel, Lovelle, Low, Lowe, Lowel, Lowell (O/Fren), Lowelle

Loyal (French/English) faithful.
Loial, Loy, Lyal, Lyall, Lyel, Lyell

Luber (German) beloved.

Lubomir (Polish) peace lover.
Lubomyr

Luc/Lucas (German/Irish/Danish/Dutch) bringer of light. A masculine form of Lucy.
Luca (Ital), Lucah, Lucassie, Lucca (Ital), Luciano (Ital), Lucio (Ital), Luckas, Lucus, Lucys, Lukas, Lukus, Lukys

Lucian (Latin) bringer of light. A masculine form of Lucy.
Lucan, Lucianus, Luciano, Lucien, Lucio (Ital/Span), Lucyan, Lucyen, Luzian, Luzien (Fren), Luzio, Luzius

Lucius (Latin) bringer of light. A masculine form of Lucy.
Luca (Ital), Lucais, Lucas (Ger), Lucca, Luce, Lucian (Lat), Luciano (Ital), Lucia, Luciah, Lucias, Lucien (Fren), Lucio, Lucyas, Lucyus, Lukas, Lukash, Luke, Lukey

Lucky (Middle English) fortunate; fate.
Lucki, Luckie, Luki, Lukie, Luky

Lucretius (Latin) gain.
Lucretyus

Ludlow (English) from the hill of the prince.

Ludwig (German) famous warrior.
Ludovic, Ludovico, Ludvig, Ludvik, Ludwik, Ludwyg, Lui (Haw/Ger), Luigi (Ital/Ger), Luigino, Lutz

Luke (Latin) bringer of light. A masculine form of Lucy.
Luc, Luca (Ital), Lucano, Lucca, Lucais (Scott), Lucas (Ger/Dut/Dan/Irish), Lucio (Span), Luka, Lukas (Swed), Lukaz, Lukela (Haw), Luken, Luki (Bas), Lukyn

Lukman (Arabic) prophet.
Luqman

Lulani (Hawaiian) highest point in heaven.
Lulanee, Lulaney, Lulanie, Lulany

Lumo (Ewe) born face down.

Lundy (Scottish) from the grove at the island.
Lundee, Lundey, Lundi, Lundie

Lunn (Irish) warlike.
Lon, Lonn, Lonni, Lonnie, Lonny, Lony, Lunni, Lunnie, Lunny, Luny

Lunt (Swedish) from the grove.
Lont

Lupus (Latin) wolf; fierce.

Lusila (Hindi) leader.
Lusyla

Lusio (Zuni) light.
Lusyo

Lutalo (Luganda) warrior.

Lutfi (Arabic) kind friend.

Luther (Old French) renowned warrior.
Lotario (Ital), Lothaire (Fren), Lothar, Lothaiire, Lothario, Lother, Lothur, Lutero (Span)

Luyu (Moquelumnan) head shaker.

Lyall (Scottish) loyal.
Loyal, Loyel, Lyel, Lyell

Lyceus (Greek) light.
Lycius

Lyle (Old French) from the island.
Lisle, Lyal, Lyall, Lyel, Lyell

Lyman (Old English) from the meadow valley.
Leaman, Leamen, Leeman, Leemen, Leiman, Leimen, Leyman, Liman, Limen, Limin, Limon, Limyn, Lymen, Lymin, Lymon, Lymyn

Lynch (Irish) mariner.
Linch

Lyndal (English) from the valley of the linden trees.
Lindal, Lindall, Lindel, Lyndale, Lyndall, Lyndel, Lyndell

Lyndon (English) from the linden-tree hill.
Lindan, Linden, Lindin, Lindon, Lindyn, Lyndan, Lynden, Lyndin, Lyndyn

Lynn (Celtic) from the stream with the waterfall.
Lin, Linn, Linlee, Linleigh, Linley, Linly, Linwood, Lyn, Lynford, Lynton, Lynwood

Lyron (Hebrew/French) round circle.
Liron

Lysander (Greek) freedom maker.
Lisander

Lytton (Old English) place on the loud torrent; town by the loud stream.
Liton, Litton, Lyton

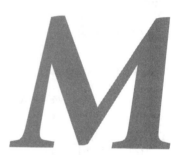

Maake (Polynesian) warrior.

Maau (Tongan) poet.

Mabry (Latin) worthy of love. A short form of Amabel, lovable. The masculine form of Mabel.
Mabri, Mabrie

Mac (Scottish/Gaelic) son.
Mack, Mak

Macabee (Hebrew) hammer.
Maccabee, Mackabee, Makabee

Macadam (Old English/Scottish) son of Adam; son of the earth.
Mackadam, Makadam

Macalla (Australian Aboriginal) full moon.
Macala, Macalah, Macallah

Macallister (Irish) Allister's son; son of the avenger.
Macalaster, MacAlistair, Macalister, Mackalistair, Mackalister, Makalistair, Makalister, McAlister, McAllister

Macardle (Irish) bravery's son.

Macario (Spanish) blessed; happy.
Macaryo

Macarthur (Irish) Arthur's son; son
of the noble strength. (Scot/Wel)
son of the bear.
MacArthur, Mackarthur, Makarthur,
McArthur

Macauley (Scottish) son of
righteousness.
Macaulea, Macauleah, Macaulee,
Macaulei, Macauleigh, Macauley,
Macauli, Macaulie, Macauly,
Mackaulea, Mackauleah,
Mackaulee, Mackaulei,
Mackauleigh, Mackauley, Mackauli,
Mackaulie, Mackauly, McCaulea,
McCauleah, McCaulee, McCaulei,
McCauleigh, McCauley, McCauli,
McCaulie, McCauly

MacBeth (Scottish) Elizabeth's son;
son who is holy, sacred to God.
Mackbeth, Makbeth

MacBride (Scottish/English) Bride's
son; son of the bridle maker.
Macbryd, Macbryde, Mackbride,
Mackbryde, Makbride, Makbryde,
McBride, McBryde

MacCoy (Irish) Coy's son; son of
the shy, sweet and modest one.
MacCoi, MacCoy, Mackoi, Mackoy,
Makcoi, Makcoy, Mccoy, McCoi,
McCoy

Maccrea (Irish) Grace's son; son of
the graceful, blessed one.
MacCrae, MacCrai, MacCray,
Macrae, MacCrea, Mackrea,
Makcrea, Mccrea, McCrea

MacDonald (Gaelic) Donald's son;
son of the world ruler.
MackDonald, Mackdonald,
MakDonald, Makdonald,
McDonald

MacDougal (Scottish) Dougall's
son; son of the dark one.
MacDougall, Macdougal,
MackDougal, MackDougall,
Mackdougall, MakDougal,
MakDougal, MakDougall,
Makdougall

Mace (Old French) club; aromatic
spice.
Macey, Macon, Macy (O/Fren)

MacFarlane (Old English) Farlane's
son; son of the dweller at the far
lane. (Scot/Gae) son of Parlan;
son of the farmer.
Mackfarlan, Mackfarlane,
Mackpharlan, Mackfarlane,
Macpharlane, Makfarlan,
Makfarlane, Makpharlan,
Makpharlane, Mcfarlan, Mcfarlane,
Mcpharlan, Mcpharlane

McGeorge (Scottish) George's son;
son of the farmer.
MacGeorge, Mackgeorge,
MakGeorge, Makgeorge

Macharios (Greek) blessed.
Macarius, Macharyos, Makarios,
Makcarius

Mack (Scottish) son. The short form
of names starting with 'Mack' e.g.
Mackenzie.
Mac, Mak

McKay (Scottish) Kay's son; son of
purity.
Macai, Macay, Mackai, Mackaye,
Makkai, Makkay, Makkaye

MacKenzie (Irish) Kenzie's son; son
of the wise, handsome leader.
Mackenzee, Mackenzey, Mackenzi,
Mackenzy, Makenzee, Makenzey,
Makenzi, Makenzie, Makenzy,
McKenzee, McKenzey, McKenzi,
McKenzie, McKenzy

MacKinley (Irish) Kinley's son; son of the skilful leader. (O/Eng) son of the relative from the meadow.
Mackinlea, Mackinleah, Mackinlee, Mackinlei, Mackinleigh, Mackinli, Mackinlie, Mackinly, Mackynlea, Mackynleah, Mackynlee, Mackynlei, Mackynleigh, Mackynli, Mackynlie, Mackynly, Makinlea, Makinleah, Makinlee, Makinlei, Makinleigh, Makinley, Makinli, Makinlie, Makinly, Makynlea, Makyleah, Makynlee, Makynlei, Makynleigh, Makynli, Makynlie, Makynly

Maclean (Gaelic) Leander's son; son of the lion-like one.
MacKlean, Macklean, MaKlean, Maklean, McClean

MacMahon (Irish) Mahon's son; son of the one who is strong like a bear.
Mackmanon, MacMahon, Makmahnon, McMahon

MacMurray (Irish) Murray's son; son of the sailor.
Mackmuray, Mackmurray, Macmuray, Macmurry, Makmuray, Makmurray, Mcmurray, Mcmurry

MacNair (Scottish/Gaelic) Nair's son; son of the heir.
Macknair, Macknayr, McNair, McNayr, Maknair, Maknayr

Maco (Hebrew) God is with us. A form of Emmanuel.
Macko, Mako

Macon (Old English) creating; to perform.
Macan, Macen, Macin, Macun, Macyn

Macy (Old French) from the estate owned by Matthew; gift of God.
Mace, Macey, Maci, Macie, Macy

Maddock (Welsh) fortunate; generous.
Maddoc, Maddoch, Maddok, Maddox, Madoc, Madoch, Madock, Madox

Madeep (Punjabi) mind that is full of light.
Mandee, Mandieep

Madison (Old English) son of the powerful warrior.
Maddison, Maddyson, Madyson

Madoc (Welsh) fortunate; lucky.
Maddoc, Maddoch, Maddock, Maddok, Maddox, Madoch, Madock, Madok, Madox

Madon (Celtic) charitable.
Maddan, Madden, Maddin, Maddon, Maddyn, Madan, Maden, Madin, Madyn

Madu (Ibo) people.

Mafu (Tongan) heart.

Magar (Armenian) attendant of the groom.
Magarious

Magee (Irish) Hugh's son; son of the intelligent one. (O/Ger) heart; mind.
MacGee, MacGhee, McGee

Magnar (Norwegian) warrior.
Magah, Magne

Magnus (Latin) great.
Manus (Ir), Magnuss, Manasses (Ir)

Magomu (Luganda) the youngest twin.

Maguire (Irish) Gurie's son; son of the beige one.
MacGuire, McGuire, McGwire

Magus (Latin) wizard of knowledge.

Mahir (Hebrew) expert; hard-working.
Mair

Mahkah (Lakota) earth.
Maka, Makah

Maholi (Tongan) powerful.
Maoli

Mahon (Irish) strong like a bear.
Mahoney

Mahpee (Lakota/Sioux) sky.

Maidoc (Welsh) fortunate.
Maedoc, Maedock, Maidock, Maidok, Maydoc, Maydock, Maydok

Mailen (Latin) mesh; chain.
Maylen

Maimon (Arabic) lucky.
Maymon

Maitland (Old French) from the meadow pastureland.
Maitlan, Maytlan, Maytland

Majid (Arabic) glorious.
Majyd

Major (Latin) great.
Majar, Majer, Mayar, Mayer, Mayor

Maka (Tongan) rock.
Makah

Makaio (Hawaiian/Hebrew) gift of God. A form of Matthew.
Makayo

Makalani (Mwera) writer.
Makalanee, Makalaney, Makalanie, Makalanie, Makalany

Makani (Hawaiian) wind.
Makanie, Makany

Makara (Sanskrit) crocodile.
Makarah

Makarios (Greek) blessed with happiness.
Makari, Makarie, Makary (Pol), Makaryos

Makin (Arabic) strength.
Makyn

Makis (Greek/Hebrew) likeness to God. A short form of Michael.
Makys

Maksim (Russian/Latin) greatest.
Mac, Mack, Macka, Mak, Makimus (Pol), Maks, Maksim, Maksimka, Maksym (Pol), Maksymilian (Pol), Maxim, Maximilian

Makya (Hopi) eagle hunter.
Makia, Makiah, Makyah

Malcom (Irish/Scottish/Gaelic) follower of Saint Columba.
Malcolm, Maolcolm

Malach (Hebrew) angel; messenger of God.
Malac, Malachi, Malachie, Malachy

Malawi (Native American) flames.

Maldon (Old English) meeting place in the wood hollow.
Maldan, Malden, Maldin, Maldun, Maldyn

Maleko (Hawaiian/Latin) warrior of Mars. A form of Mark.

Malik (Arabic) king.
Malic, Malick, Malyc, Malyck, Malyk

Malin (Old English) little warrior.
Malen, Malin, Mallen, Mallin, Mallon, Mallyn, Malon, Malyn

Malise (Gaelic) servant of Jesus.
Malice, Malyca, Malyse

Malleson (Hebrew) Mary's son; son of the wished-for one; star of the sea; bitter.
Maleson

Mallory (Teutonic) fated; army counsellor.
Mallorey, Mallori, Mallorie, Malorey, Malori, Malorie, Malory

Malo (Tongan) thank you.

Malohi (Tongan) strength.

Malone (Irish) St John's servant.
Malon

Maloney (Irish) devoted to worship on Sundays.
Malonee, Maloni, Malonie, Malony

Maloo (Australian Aboriginal) thunder.
Malo

Malory (Old French) wild duck.
Mallori, Mallorie, Mallori, Mallorie, Mallory

Malu (Tongan) shadow.

Malvern (Welsh) from the bare hill.
Malverne, Malvirn, Malvirne, Malvyrn, Malvyrne

Malvin (Irish/Gaelic) chief.
Malvan, Malven, Malvon, Malvyn, Melvan, Melven, Melvin, Melvon, Melvyn

Mamafa (Tongan) serious.
Mamafah

Mamani (Tongan) the Earth.
Mamanie, Mamany

Mamo (Hawaiian) yellow; the saffron flower; yellow bird.

Mana (Maori) prestigious; successful. (Tong) miracle; charm. (Arab) rock.
Manah (Arab)

Manawa (Maori) heart.
Manawah

Manchu (Chinese) purity.

Manco (Peruvian) supreme leader; an Incan king.

Mandala (Yao) flower.
Manda, Mandah, Mandel, Mandela, Mandelah

Mandek (Polish/German) warrior.

Mandel (German) almond.
Mandell

Mander (Gypsy) myself.
Mandar, Mandir, Mandor, Mandyr

Mandu (Australian Aboriginal) sun.

Manford (Old English) from the man's river crossing.
Manforde, Menford, Menforde

Manfred (Old English) man of peace.
Manfredo, Manfrid, Manfried, Manfryd, Manifred, Manifrid, Manifryd, Manyfred, Manyfrid, Manyfryd

Manger (Old English) trough for animals; where Jesus slept after being born.
Mangar, Mangor

Mango (Spanish/Hebrew) God's gift; a sweet tropical fruit.

Manheim (Teutonic) servant.

Manipi (Native American) walking wonder.

Manley (Old English) from the masculine one's meadow.
Manlea, Manleah, Manlee, Manleigh, Manli, Manlie, Manly

Mann (German) masculine. (O/Eng) hero.
Man

Mannaw (Australian Aboriginal) honey.
Manaw

Manning (Old English) Mann's son; son of the masculine one.
Maning

Mannix (Irish) monk.
Mainchin, Mannox, Mannyx, Manox, Manyx

Mano (Hawaiian) shark.
Manno, Manolo

Manolis (Greek) God is with us.
Mano, Manolys

Manrico (Italian/Old English) masculine ruler.
Manricko, Manriko, Manrycko, Manryco, Manryko

Mansa (Swahili) king.
Mansah

Mansel (English) the clergy's house.
Mansell

Mansfield (Old English) from the masculine one's field.
Mansfyeld

Manton (Old English) from the masculine one's town.
Mantan, Manten, Mantin, Mantyn

Manu (Hawaiian/Tongan) bird. (Hind) maker of laws. (Af/Ghan) second born son.

Manuel (Spanish/Hebrew) God is with us. French/Spanish form of Emmanuel.
Emanuel, Emmanuel, Manuell

Manville (Old French) from the great village.
Manvile, Manvyl, Manvyle, Manvyll, Manvylle

Manzo (Japanese) third-born son.

Mapira (Yao) grass; animal fodder.
Mapirah

Maralinga (Australian Aboriginal) thunder.
Maralynga

Marama (Polynesian) moon.
Maramah

Marar (Watamare) dust; mud.

Marbilling (Australian Aboriginal) wind.
Marbiling

Marcel/Marcellus (Latin) warrior; war-like one; of Mars.
Marc, Marceau, Marcel, Macele, Marceles, Marcelin, Marcelino, Marcelis, Marcell, Marcelle, Marcellin, Marcellino, Marcelle,Marcello (Ital), Marcellous, Marcelluas, Marcellus (Fren), Marcely, Marciano (Ital), Marcilka (Hung), Marcsseau, Marzel, Marzell, Marzellos, Marzellous, Marzellus.

March (English) boundary dweller.

Marcus (Latin) of Mars; warrior.
Marcuss, Marian, Mario (Ital), Marion, Markis, Markise, Markos, Markous, Markus, Markys

Marden (Old English) from the warrior's valley.
Mardan, Mardin, Mardon, Mardun, Mardyn

Marek (Czech) warrior.

Maren (Basque) sea.
Maran, Marin, Maron, Maryn

Marian (Polish/Latin) warrior. A form of Mark.
Mariano (Ital), Maryan, Maryano

Marid (Arabic) rebel.
Maryd

Marin/Marinus (Latin) belonging to the sea; mariner. (Fren) sailor.
Marina, Marien, Marinos, Marion, Mariono, Marriner, Marryner, Maryn, Maryna, Maryner, Marynos, Marynus

Mario (Latin) dedicated to the Virgin Mary. The Italian form of Mark, warrior; war-like one; of Mars.
Mareo, Maryo

Marion (Old French) Mary's son; wished for; star of the sea; bitter. The masculine form of Mary.
Mariano (Span), Maryon

Mark (Latin) warrior; warlike one; of Mars.
Marc (Fren), Marceau, Marcel, Marcele, Marcelino, Marcell, Marcelle, Marcellino, Marcello, Marcelluas, Marcellus, Marcelo, Marck, Marco (Ital), Marcos (Span/Port), Marcous, Marcus, Marczi (Hung), Marek (Pol/Boh), Mario (Ital), Marious, Marius, Marke (Eng), Marki, Markie, Markk, Markku (Fin), Marko, Markos (Grk), Markous, Markus (Ger/Hung), Marq, Marqu, Marque, Marx (Ger)

Markham (English) fenced homestead.
Markam, Markem

Marlan/Marland (Old English) from the warrior's land.
Mahlan, Mahland, Mahlen, Mahlend, Mahlin, Marlind, Mahlon, Mahlyn, Marland, Marlen, Marlend, Marlin, Marlind, Marlon, Marlond, Marlyn, Marlynd

Marley (English) from the warrior's meadow.
Marlea, Marleah, Marlee, Marleigh, Marli, Marlie, Marly

Marlon (Old French) little falcon; hawk.
Marlan, Marland, Marlen, Marlin, Marlyn

Marlow (Old English) from the hill near the lake.
Marlo, Marlowe

Marmaduke (Irish) servant of Madoc; lucky. (O/Eng) noble; mighty.
Marmaduc, Marmaduk, Melmidoc

Marmion (Old French) tiny. (Ir) sea bright.
Marmien, Marmyon

Marnin (Hebrew) singer who brings joy.
Marnyn

Maro (Japanese) myself.
Marow

Marr (Spanish) divine. (Arab) forbidden.
March

Marron (Australian Aboriginal) leaf.
Maran, Maren, Marin, Maron, Marran, Marren, Marrin, Marryn, Maryn

Mars (Latin) war warrior; the God of war.

Marsden (Old English) from the warrior's valley.
Marsdan, Marsdin, Marsdon, Mardyn

Marsena (Persian) worthy.
Marsenah

Marsh (Old English) from the marsh area.

Marshall (Old French) horse groomer. (Amer) law keeper.
Marshal, Marshel, Marshell

Marston (Old English) from the town by the lake or marsh; from the warrior's town.
Marstan, Marsten, Marstin, Marstyn

M

Mart (Turkish) born in the month of March.

Martell (English) one who hammers.
Martal, Martall, Martel

Martin/Marty (Latin) warrior; warlike one; of Mars.
Maartan, Maarten (Dut), Maartin, Maarton, Maartyn, Martan, Martain, Martainho (Port), Martainn (Scott), Marte, Martee, Marten, Martey, Marti, Martie, Martii (Fin), Martijn (Dut), Martili (Swis), Martine, Martino (Ital/Span), Martinos, Martinous, Martinus (Indo), Martnet, Marton, Marty, Martyn, Martynas (Lith), Martyne, Martynis, Martynos, Martynous, Martynus, Martynys, Mertan, Merten, Mertin, Merton, Mertyn

Marv (English) sea lover. The short form of names starting with 'Marv', e.g. Marvin.
Marvein, Marven, Marvyn, Marvyne, Marwin, Marwyn, Marwynn, Marwynne, Mervin, Mervine, Mervyn, Mervyne

Marvell (Latin) wondrous.
Marvel, Marvele, Marvelle

Marvin (Old English) famous friend.
Marvan, Marven, Marvon, Marwen, Marwin, Marwon, Marwyn, Mervan, Merven, Mervin, Mervon, Mervyn, Marvyne, Merwin, Merwyn, Murvan, Murven, Murvin, Murvine, Murvon, Murvyn, Murvyne, Murwin, Murwyn

Marwan (Arabic) history.
Marwen, Marwin, Marwon, Marwyn

Marwood (Old English) from the forest near the marsh; from the warrior's forest.

Masaccio (Italian) twin.
Masaki

Masahiro (Japanese) broad-minded.
Masahyro

Masamba (Yao) one who leaves.
Masambah

Masao (Japanese) righteous.
Masato

Mascot (French) talisman; magical powers.
Mascott

Mashama (Shona) surprise.
Mashamah

Mashema (Native American) elk antlers.
Mashemah

Masio (African American) twin. A form of Thomas.

Maska (Native American) powerful.
Maskah

Maskil (Hebrew) educated.
Maskyl

Maslin (Old French) little Thomas; son of the twin.
Maslan, Maslen, Maslon, Maslyn

Mason (Old French) stone mason.
Maisan, Maisen, Maisin, Maison, Maisun, Maisyn, Masan, Masen, Masin, Masun, Masyn

Massey (English) twin.
Massi, Massie, Masy

Massimo (Italian) great.
Massimiliano, Massymo

Massing (Old English) place of warriors.
Massey, Massin

M

Masud (Swahili) lucky.
Masood, Masoud, Mhasood

Mata (Tongan) blade.
Matah

Matai/Mataniah (Basque/Bulgarian/ Hebrew) gift of God. A form of Matthew.
Matania, Matanya, Matanyah

Mateen (Afghani) polite.
Matin, Matyn

Mather (Old English) army power.
Mathers

Mato (Native American) brave warrior.
Matto

Matong (Australian Aboriginal) strength.
Maton

Matope (Rhodesian) the last-born child.
Matop

Matson (English/Hebrew) Matt's son; son of the gift of God.
Mattson

Matt/Matthew (Hebrew) gift of God.
Macias (Span), Macie (Pol), Macisk (Slav), Mado, Mafew, Maffew, Mafthew, Mat, Mata, Matausas (Lith), Mate (Hung), Matej (Boh), Mateo (Span/Ital), Mateoz (Slav), Mateusz (Pol), Matfei (Rus), Mathes (Bav), Mathew, Mathia, Mathias (Swed/Swiss/Fren), Mathies, Matius (Indo), Mathieu, Matta, Matte, Mattea (Ital), Matteo, Mattey, Matthes (Ger), Matthias (Lat), Matthieu (Fren), Matthiew, Matti, Mattie, Mattis, Mattius, Matty, Matui (NZMaori), Maty, Matya (Serb), Matyas (Hung), Thies (Swed)

Matu (Native American) brave warrior.
Mattu

Mauli (Tongan) Maori, native New Zealander. (Lat/Haw) dark-haired; from the moor. A form of Maurice.

Mauri (Greek) twilight. The Finnish form of Maurice, dark-haired; from the moor.

Maurice (Latin) dark-haired; from the moor.
Maolmuire (Scot), Mauri (Fin), Mauricio (Span), Mauritius, Maurits (Dut/Neth), Mauritz (Ger), Maurizio, Mauryc, Mauryce, Maurys, Mauryse, Meuric, Meurisse, Moreno, Moris, Morris, Moritz, Morrys, Morys, Morytz

Maverick (American/English) independent; wild.
Maveric, Maverik, Maveryc, Maveryck, Maveryk, Mavric, Mavrick, Mavrik, Mavryc, Mavryck, Mavryk

Mawake (Maori) breeze from the southern sea.

Max (Latin) extreme. The short form of names starting with 'Max' e.g. Maxwell.
Maxx

Maxfield (English) from Mack's field; from the son's field; from the extreme one's field.
Macfield, Mackfield, Mackfyld, Makfield, Makfyld

Maximilian/Maximus (Latin) extreme; maximum.
Maksimilian, Maksimillian (Slav), Maksymilian (Pol), Massimiliano (Ital), Missimo, Maxam, Maxamilian, Maxem, Maxim, Maximilianos, Maximilianus,

Maximilien (Fren), Maximino, Maximo, Maximos, Maxymilian, Maxymos, Maxymus

Maxwell (Old English/Latin) from the extreme stream.
Maxwel

Mayer (Hebrew) light. (O/Ger) dairy worker.
Maier, Mayar, Mayir, Mayor

Mayes (English) from the field.
Maies, Mays

Mayfield (Old English) from the warrior's field.
Maefield, Maifield

Mayhew (Old French) gift of God. A form of Matthew.
Maehew, Maihew

Maynard (Teutonic) brave; powerful; strength.
Mainard, Maynard, Menard

Mayo (Irish) from the yew-tree plain. (Eng) relation.
Maio

Mayon (Hindi) a god.
Maion

Mazi (Ibo) sir.

Mazin (Arabic) proper.
Mazan, Mazen, Mazinn, Mazon, Mazyn

Meade (Old English) from the meadow.
Mead, Meed

Medgar (German/English) successful with a spear.
Edgar, Edger, Medger

Medric (Old English) from the flourishing meadow.
Mead, Meade, Medard, Medford, Medrick, Medrik, Medryc, Medryck, Medryk

Medwin (Teutonic) powerful, strong, worthy friend.
Medwyn

Meged (Hebrew) sweetness; perfection.

Meinhard (German) beloved.
Meynhard

Meinrad (German) counsel of strength.
Meinhard, Meinhardt, Meinke, Meino, Mendar, Meynrad

Meir (Hebrew) shining.
Meiri, Meyr, Meyri

Meka (Hawaiian) eyes.
Mekah

Mel (English/Irish) friend; mill chief. The short form for names starting with 'Mel' e.g. **Melvin.**
Mell

Melbourne (Old English) from the mill stream.
Melborn, Melborne, Melburn, Melburne, Melden, Meldon, Milbourne, Milburn, Milburne

Meldon (Old English) from the mill hill.
Meldan, Melden, Meldin, Meldyn

Meldrick (Old English) from the powerful mill.
Meldric, Meldrik, Meldryc, Meldryck, Meldryk

Melea (Greek) abundance.
Meleah, Melee, Meleigh, Meley, Meli, Melie, Mely

Melino (Tongan) peace.
Melin, Melinos, Melyn, Melyno, Melynos

Melrose (Old English) rose from the mill; from the bare moor.
Melros

Melvern (Native American) great
chief.
Melverne, Melvirn, Melvirne,
Melvyrn, Melvyrne

Melville (Old French) from the
village near the mill.
Malvil, Malvill, Malville, Melvil,
Melvill

Melvin (Irish/Gaelic) Mel's friend
from the mill. (O/Eng) sword
friend.
Melvan, Melven, Melvern,
Melverne, Melvine, Melvirn,
Melvirne, Melvyn, Melvyrn,
Melvyrne

Mendel (Semitic/Hebrew) wisdom.
Mendal, Mendil, Mendyl

Menewa (Creek) great warrior.
Menewah

Mensah (Ewe) third-born son.
Mensa

Mercer (Latin) shopkeeper;
merchant. (Fren) textile dealer.
Merce

Mercury (Roman) messenger of the
gods.
Mercurino (Ital), Mercuryno

Meredith (Welsh) from the sea.
Meredeth, Meredyth, Merideth,
Merydeth, Merydith, Merydyth

Mereki (Australian Aboriginal)
peacemaker.

Merivale (Old English/Old French)
pleasant valley.
Merival, Meryval, Meryvale

Merle (French) blackbird.
Merl, Murl, Murle

Merlin (Welsh) from the sea fort.
(M/Eng) hawk.
Marlin, Marlyn, Merlo, Merlyn

Merrick (English) ruler of the sea.
Meril, Merle, Merric, Merrik, Merrill,
Merrington, Merryc, Merryck,
Merryk, Merton, Meryl, Myril, Myrl

Merrill (French) famous.
(Eng) water.
Merle, Merrel, Merrell, Merril,
Meryl, Meryll

Merritt (Old English) little famous
one. (Lat) deserving.
Merit, Meritt, Merrit, Merryt

Merton (English) town by the sea.
Mertan, Merten, Mertin, Mertyn

Merv (Irish/English) famous friend.
The short form of Mervin.
Merve

Mervin (Old French) famous friend.
Mervan, Merven, Mervon, Mervyn

Meyer (German) head servant;
farmer. (Heb) bringer of light.
Mayeer, Mayer, Mayor, Meir, Meier,
Myer

Mhina (Swahili) delightful.
Mhinah

Micah (Hebrew) likeness to God. A
form of Michael.
Mica, Myca, Mycah

Michael/Mick/Mike (Hebrew)
likeness to God.
Meikal, Meikel, Meikil, Meikyl,
Mekal, Mekel, Mekele, Mekil,
Mekyl, Mic, Mica, Micah (Heb),
Michal, Michale, Michail, Michan
(Ital), Michel,Micheil, Michel,
Michele, Mick, Micki, Mickie,
Micky, Miekal, Miekel, Miekil,
Miekil, Miekyl, Miguel (Span),
Mihael, Mik, Mika, Mikael, Mikail
(Rus), Mike, Mikel, Mikhail (Rus),
Miki, Mikie, Mikkel, Miklos, Mikol,
Miky, Mischa (Slav), Misshael

M

(Heb), Myc, Mychal, Myck,
Myckael, Myckaele, Myckaell,
Mycki, Myckie, Mycky, Mykael,
Mykaele, Mykaell, Mykaelle, Myke,
Mykey, Myki, Mykie, Mykil, Mykill,
Mykyl, Mykyle, Mykyll, Mykyle

Michio (Japanese) with the strength
of three thousand.

Micke (Australian Aboriginal) tree
struck by lightning.
Mick, Mickee, Mickey, Micki,
Mickie, Micky, Myc, Mycke,
Myckee, Myckey, Mycki, Myckie,
Mycky, Myk, Myke, Mykee, Mykey,
Myki, Mykie, Myky

Midgard (Old Norse) from the
middle garden.
Midgarth, Midrag, Mithgarthr,
Mydgard

Midgee (Australian Aboriginal)
acacia tree.
Midge, Mydge, Mydgee

Miguel (Portuguese/Spanish/
Hebrew) likeness to God. A form
of Michael.
Migeal, Migeel, Migel, Miguelly,
Migui, Myguel, Myguele, Myguell,
Myguelle

Mika (Ponca) raccoon. The Russian
form of Michael, likeness to God.
Miika, Mikah, Myka, Mykah

Mikasi (Omaha) coyote.
Mykasi

Miki (Japanese) tree.
Mikio

Miksa (Hungarian/Latin) extreme;
maximum. A form of Max.
Miks, Myksa

Milan (Slavic) beloved.
Milen, Millan, Millen, Mylan,
Mylen, Mylon, Mylyn

Milborough (English) from the
middle borough town.
Milbrough, Mylborough,
Mylbrough

Milburn (Old English) from the
mill stream.
Milborn, Milborne, Milbourn,
Milbourne, Milburne, Millborn,
Millborne, Millbourn, Millbourne,
Millburn, Millburne

Milek (Polish/Greek) victory of the
people. A form of Nick.
Mylek

Miles (Latin) warrior.
(O/Ger) merciful.
Maolmuire (Ir), Mile, Milesius,
Milon, Myle, Myles, Mylo

Milford (English) from the mill by
the ford.
Millford, Mylford, Myllford

Mililani (Hawaiian) heavenly caress.
Mililanee, Mililaney, Mililanie,
Mililany

Millard (Latin/Old English) caretaker of the mill.
Millar, Miller, Mylard, Myllard

Miller (English) grain grinder.
Mellar, Meller, Mellor, Milar, Miler,
Millar, Millard, Millen, Millon,
Milor, Mylar, Myler, Myllar, Myller,
Myller, Mylor

Millin (Australian Aboriginal)
charm.
Millyn, Myllin, Myllyn

Millington (Old English) from the
mill town.
Milington

Mills (English) from the mill.
Mils, Mylls, Myls

Millyn (Aramaic) words. (O/Eng) from the mill pool.
Millin, Myllin, Myllyn

Milner (Middle English) miller.
Milnar, Mylner

Milo (Teutonic) merciful. (Lat) miller.
Mylo

Milos (Greek/Slavic) pleasant.
Milo, Mylo, Mylos

Miloslav (Slavic) crowned with glory.
Myloslav

Milton (Old English) from the mill town.
Millard, Miller, Mills, Millton, Myllton, Mylton, Nillton, Nilton, Nyllton, Nylton

Milward (Old English) mill keeper.
Mylward

Min (Burmese) king.
Mina, Minah, Myn, Myna, Mynah

Miner (English) worker in the mine.
Myner

Minet (Old French) delightful.
Minett, Mynet, Mynett

Mingan (Native American) grey wolf.
Myngan

Minh (Vietnamese) light.
Mynh

Minkah (Akan) fair-haired.
Minka, Mynka, Mynkah

Minster (Old English) from the monastery church.
Mynster

Miron (Polish) peace.
Myron

Miroslav (Czech) peace; glory.
Myroslav

Mishiki (Egyptian) apricot; from the east.
Myshiki

Mister (English) mister.
Mista, Mistah, Mistar, Mistur, Mysta, Mystah, Mystar, Mystur

Misu (Native American) rippling water.
Mysu

Mitch/Mitchell (Old English) big.
Mitchel, Mytch, Mytchel, Mytchell

Mitford (Middle English) from the big river crossing.
Mytford

Modeste (French) modest. The masculine form of Modesty.
Modesti, Modestie, Modesto (Ital), Modesty

Modred (Teutonic) brave, courageous counsel. (Lat) to consume.
Mordred, Modris, Mordred, Mordryd

Moe (Hebrew) saved; taken from the water. (Egypt) child. The short form of Moses.
Mo, Mow

Mogens (Dutch) powerful.
Mogen

Mogul (Persian) from Mongolia.

Mohammed (Arabic) prophet.
Mohammad, Muhammed, Mohomet (Turk)

Mohan (Hindi) delightful.
Mohana

Mohe (Native American) elk.

Moiag (Native American) loud-crying baby.

M

Moki (Australian Aboriginal) cloudy.
Mokee, Mokey, Moki, Mokie, Moky

Molan (Irish) servant of the storm.

Mona (Moquelumnan) gathering the jimson weed seed.
Monah

Monahan (Irish) monk.
Monaghan, Monoghan

Monford (Old English) from the monk's river crossing.
Montford, Mountford

Mongo (Yoruba) famous.

Monita (Italian/Greek) alone.
Minitah

Monroe (Irish) from the red swamp.
Monro, Monrow, Munro, Munroe, Munrow

Montague (Old French) from the pointed mountain.

Montana (Spanish) mountain.
Montanah

Montago (Japanese) big boy.

Monte (Latin) mountain. The short form of names starting with 'Monte' e.g. Montega.
Montee, Montey, Monti, Montie, Monty

Montega (Native American) new arrow.
Montegah

Montez (Spanish) dweller at the mountain.
Monteiz, Monteze, Montise, Montiz, Montize, Montyz, Montyze

Montgomery (Old French) from the wealthy one's mountain.
Mountgomery

Monti (Australian Aboriginal) stork.
Monte (Lat), Montee, Montey, Montie, Monty

Montre (French) show.
Montrai, Montray, Montres, Montrez

Montreal (French) royal mountain.
Montrail, Montrale, Montrall, Montrel, Montrell

Montsho (Tswana) black.

Monty (English) from the rich one's mountain. The short form of names starting with 'Mont' e.g. Montgomery.
Monte (Lat), Montee, Montey, Monti, Montie

Moorak (Australian Aboriginal) mountain.

Moore (Old French) dark complexioned. (O/Eng) from the wetlands or moor.
Moar, Moare, Moor, More, Morre

Mootska (Hopi) yucca plant.

Morandoo (Australian Aboriginal) sea.
Moran, Morando

Mordred (Latin) pain.
Modred

Morel (French) mushroom.
Morell

Moreland (English) from the marshland.
Moarlan, Moraland, Morelan, Moreno (Span), Morino, Moorelan, Mooreland, Moorlan, Moorland, Morlan, Morland, Moryno

Morey (English/Greek) dark one from the moor. The short form of Morris.
Moree, Mori, Morie, Morree, Morrey, Morri, Morrie, Morry, Mory

M

Morgan (Celtic) sea bright; of the sea. (O/Wel) white sea dweller.
Morgen, Morgin, Morgon, Morgun, Morgyn

Morio (Japanese) woods.
Moryo

Morland (Old English) from the marsh meadow.
Moarlan, Moraland, Morelan, Moreland, Moorelan, Mooreland, Moorlan, Moorland, Morlan, Morland

Morley (Old English) from the meadow near the marsh.
Morlea, Morleah, Morlee, Morleigh, Morli, Morlie, Morly

Morrell (Old French) dark-coloured.
Morel, Morell, Morrel

Morris (Latin/Old English) dark one from the moor.
Moris, Morison, Morrys, Morys

Morrison/Morse (Old English) son of Morris; son of the dark one from the moor.

Mort (Middle English) stump. The short form of names starting with 'Mort' e.g. Mortimer.

Morten (Norwegian/Latin) warrior; warlike one; of Mars. A form of Martin.
Mortan, Mortin, Morton, Mortyn

Mortimer (Old French) still waters. (Ir) sea director.
Mortymer

Morton (Old English) from the town near the marsh.
Mortan, Morten, Mortin, Mortun, Mortyn

Morven (Scottish/Gaelic) sea mariner. (Celt) sea raven.
Morvan

Moses (Hebrew) saved; taken from the water. (Egypt) child.
Maiziesius, Moise (Fren/Ital), Moises (Span), Mose, Moyse, Mozes (Dut), Musa (Arab) Mos, Moz

Mosi (Swahili) first-born child.
Mosee, Mosey, Mosie, Mosy

Moss (Irish) from the area with moss.
Mos

Moswen (African) light in colour.
Moswin, Moswyn

Motega (Native American) new arrow.
Motegah

Moulton (Old English) mule stable town.

Mozart (Italian) breathless.
Mozar

Mpasa (Ngoni) mat.
Mpasah

Mposi (Nyakusa) blacksmith.

Muata (Moquelumnan) sixth-born child; nesting yellow jackets (bird).
Mutah

Mubdi (Arabic) beginner.

Muid (Arabic) restorer.
Muyd

Muir (Scottish/Gaelic/Old English) from the marsh.
Muire, Muyr, Muyre

Muirhead (Scottish/Gaelic) from the top of the marsh.
Muyrhead

Mukasa (Luganda) the chief administrator of God.
Mukasah

Mukul (Sanskrit) blossom; soul.
Mukull

M

Mulga (Australian Aboriginal) acacia tree.
Mulgah

Mullion (Australian Aboriginal) eagle.
Mullyon

Mulogo (Musoga) wizard.

Muluk (Indonesian) praised.

Mulwala (Australian Aboriginal) rain.
Mulwalah

Mundan (Rhodesian) garden.
Mundana

Mundo (Spanish/English) prosperous protector.

Mundy (Irish) from Reamonn in Ireland.
Mund, Munde, Mundee, Mundey, Mundi, Mundie, Mundo (Span)

Mungo (Celtic) lovable.

Munir (Arabic) brilliant.
Munyr

Munny (Cambodian) wisdom.
Munee, Muney, Muni, Munie, Munnee, Munney, Munni, Munnie, Muny

Munte (Australian Aboriginal) thunder.
Mundara, Munt

Muraco (Native American) white moon.
Muracco

Murat (Turkish) wish that came true.

Murdock (Scottish/Gaelic) wealthy sea mariner.
Murdoc, Murdock, Murdox, Mutagh (Ir)

Murphy (Celtic) from the sea.
Murffey, Murffi, Murffie, Murffy, Murphee, Murphey, Murphi, Murphie

Murray (Scottish/Gaelic) sailor from the settlement.
Murae, Murai, Muray, Murrae, Murrai, Murree, Murrey, Murri, Murrie, Murry

Murrobo (Australian Aboriginal) thunder.
Murobo

Murtagh (Irish/Scottish) wealthy sailor.
Murdoc, Murdock, Murdok, Murtaugh

Mustafa (Arabic) royal; chosen.
Mostafa, Mostafah, Mostaffa, Mostaffah, Moustafa, Mustafah, Mustapha

Myall (Australian Aboriginal) drooping acacia.
Mial, Miall, Myal

Myer (Hebrew) light. (Eng) from the swamp.
Mier, Mieres, Mires, Myers

Mykal (American/Hebrew) likeness to God. The short form of Michael.
Mikaal, Mikal, Mikall, Mikael, Mykaal, Mykall, Mykel, Mykell, Mykil, Mykill, Mykyl, Mykyll

Myles (Latin) warrior.
Miles

Myron (Greek) fragrance.
Miron

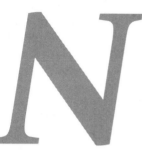

Naal (Irish) birth.
Nal

Naaman (Hebrew) pleasant.
Naman

Naarai (Hebrew) youthful.
Narai

Nabiha (Arabic) intelligent.
Nabihah

Nabil (Arabic) noble prince.
Nabill, Nabyl, Nabyll, Nadiv, Nagid

Naboth (Hebrew) high; prominent; prophecy.

Nacoma (Comanche) wanderer.
Nacomah

Nada (Arabic) generous; noble.
Nadah, Nadav (Heb), Nadiv

Nadim (Arabic) friend.
Nadym

Nadir (Arabic/Afghani) rare; dear.
Nadar, Nader, Nadyr

Nadisu (Hindi) river of beauty.
Nadysu

Naeem (Arabic) kind.
Naim, Naiym, Nieem

Nagid (Hebrew) one who leads.
Nagyd

Naham (Hebrew) sighing.

Nahele (Hawaiian) forest.

Nahma (Native American) the sturgeon fish.
Nahmah

Nahor (Hebrew) light.

Nahum (Hebrew) consoling.
Nehemiah, Nemiah, Nahym

Naija (Ugandan) next to be born.
Naijah

Nailah (Arabic) successful.
Naila, Nayla, Naylah

Naim (Arabic) happy.
Naym

Nain (Australian Aboriginal) lookout.
Nayn

Nair (Old English) heir.
Nayr

Nairn (Celtic) can't swim. (Scott) dweller at the alder-tree river.
Nairne, Nayrn, Nayrne

Naite (Tongan) knight.
Nait, Nayt, Nayte

Naji (Arabic) safety.
Najee, Najey, Najie, Najy

Najib (Arabic) born into nobility.
Najeeb, Najyb, Nejib, Nejeeb, Nejib, Nejyb

Najji (Ugandan) second-born child.
Naji

Nakai (Navajo) from Mexico.

Nakos (Arapaho) wisdom; sage herb.

Naljor (Tibetan) holy.

Nalong (Australian Aboriginal) the river's source.
Nalon

N

Nalren (Dene) melting.

Nam (Vietnamese) to scrape off.

Namaka (Hawaiian) eyes.
Namakah

Namid (Chippewa) star dancer.
Namyd

Namir (Arabic) swift like a leopard.
Namer, Namyr

Namur (Australian Aboriginal) tea tree.

Nandin (Hindi) God of destruction.
Nandyn

Nando (Teutonic) adventurer; peacemaker. A form of Ferdinand.
Nandor

Nangila (Abaluhya) born while parents were travelling.
Nangilah, Nangyla, Nangylah

Nansen (Swedish/English) graceful; Nancy's son. The masculine form of Nancy.
Nansan, Nansen, Nansin, Nanson, Nansyn

Nantai (Navajo) chief.
Nantay

Nantan (Apache) spokesperson.
Nanten, Nantin, Nanton, Nantyn

Naoko (Japanese) honest; straight.

Napa (Greek) taken by a wolf.
Napah

Napier (Spanish) from the new city.
Napyer, Neper, Nepier, Nepyer

Napoleon (Italian) from Naples. (Grk) lion from the forest dell.
Napoleone

Narain (Hindi) protector; guardian.
Narayan

Narcissus (Greek) daffodil; self-love.
Narciso (Span), Narcisse, Narcisso (Ital), Narcyso, Narcyss, Narcysse, Narcyssus, Narkis, Narkissos

Nard (Persian) player of chess.

Nardo (German) strength.
Nard (Per)

Nardoo (Australian Aboriginal) clover.

Narn (Australian Aboriginal) sea.

Narrie (Australian Aboriginal) bushfire.
Narree, Narrey, Narri, Narry

Narve (Dutch) healthy strength.
Narv

Nash (American) from Nashville.
Nashville

Nashoba (Choctaw) wolf.
Nashobah

Nasim (Persian) breeze.
Naseem, Nasym

Nasser (Arabic) victorious.
Naseer, Nasir, Nassor, Nassyr

Nat (English/Hebrew) gift of God. The short form of Nathan/Nathanial.
Natt

Natal (Latin) birth. The Spanish form of Noel, born at Christmas time.
Natale, Natalino, Natalio, Nataly

Natane (Polynesian) gift.
Natain, Nataine, Natan, Natayn, Natayne

Nate (Hebrew) little gift. A short form of Nathan/Nathaniel.
Nait, Naite, Nayt, Nayt

Nathan (Hebrew) gift. The short form of Nathaniel.
Naethan, Naethen, Naethin, Naethon, Naethun, Naethyn, Naithan, Naithen, Naithin, Naithon, Naithun, Naithyn, Natham, Nathann, Nathean, Nathen, Nathian, Nathin, Nathon, Nathun, Nathyn, Natthan, Naythan, Naythern, Naython, Naythun, Naythyn

Nathaniel (Hebrew) gift of God.
Nafanael (Rus), Nafanail, Nafanyl, Nafanyle, Naethanael, Naethanial, Naithanael, Naithanyael, Naithanyal, Naithanyel, Natalianou (Samo), Nataneal (Span), Nataniel (Span), Natanielas, Natanielias (Lith), Nataniello, Nathan, Nathanael, Nathaneal, Nathaneil, Nathanel, Nathaneol, Nathanial (Heb), Nathanie (Heb), Nathanielle, Nathanuel, Nathanyal, Nathanyel, Nathel, Nathel, Nathinel, Natthanial, Natthaniel, Natthanielle, Natthaniuel, Natthanyal, Natthanyel, Nayfanial, Naythaneal, Naythanial, Naythaniel, Nethanial, Nethaniel, Nethanielle, Nethanuel, Nithanial, Nithaniel, Nithanyal, Nithanyel, Nothanial, Nothaniel, Nothanielle, Nothanyal, Nothanyel

Nattai (Australian Aboriginal) water.
Nattay

Navarro (Spanish) from the plains.
Navara, Navarah, Navaro, Navarra, Navarrah

Naveed (Hindi) bringer of good thoughts.
Naved

Navin (Hindi) new one.
Navyn

Nawat (Native American) left-handed.

Nawkaw (Winnebago) wood.

Nayati (Native American) wrestler.
Nayaty

Nayland (English) dweller from the island.
Nailan, Nailand, Naylan

Naylor (Old English) nail maker.
Nailor

Nazareth (Hebrew) from Nazareth in Israel.
Nazair, Nazaire, Nazaret, Nazari, Nazarie, Nazario, Nazaryo

Nazih (Arabic) purity.
Nazim, Nazir, Nazyh

Ndale (Ngoni/Malawian) trickster.
Ndal

Neal (Irish) champion.
Neale, Neall, Nealle, Nealon, Nealy, Nealye, Neel, Neele, Neell, Neelle, Neil, Neile, Neill, Neille (Scand), Nel, Nels (Scand), Nial, Niale, Niall (Scott), Nialle, Niel, Niele, Niell, Nielle, Niels (Dan/Scand/Nrs), Niilo (Finn), Nil (Russ), Nile, Niles, Nill, Nille, Nils (Scand), Nilo (Finn), Njal, Nyal, Nyale, Nyall, Nyalle, Nyeal, Nyeale, Nyeall, Nyealle, Nyl, Nyle (Ir), Nyles, Nyll, Nylle, Nylles

Nebraska (Sioux) flat water.
Nebraskah

Neco (Egyptian) unseeing.
Neko

Ned (English) wealthy ruling guardian. The short form of Edward.
Nedd, Neddym, Nedric, Nedrickm,

N

Nedric, Nedrick, Nedrik, Nedryc,
Nedryck, Nedryk

Nedaviah (Hebrew) the Lord's
charity.
Nedavia, Nedavya, Nedavyah

Neel (Hindi) blue.

Neenan (Australian Aboriginal)
grasshopper.

Neerim (Australian Aboriginal)
long.
Neerym

Negasi (Ethiopian) to become
royalty.

Negev (Hebrew) from the south.

Nehemiah (Hebrew) with the
compassion of God.
Nahemia, Nahemiah, Nechemya,
Nehemia, Nethemias, Nehmia,
Nehmiah, Nemo, Neyamia,
Neyamiah, Neyamya, Neyamyah

Nehru (Hindi) canal.

Neil (Irish/Gaelic) champion.
Neal (Ir), Neale, Neall, Nealle,
Nealon, Nealy, Nealye, Neel, Neele,
Neell, Neelle, Neile, Neill, Neille
(Scand), Nel, Nels (Scand), Nial,
Niale, Niall (Scott), Nialle, Niel,
Niele, Niell, Nielle, Niels
(Dan/Scand/Nrs), Niilo (Finn), Nil
(Russ), Nile, Niles, Nill, Nille, Nils
(Scand), Nilo (Finn), Njal, Nyal,
Nyale, Nyall, Nyalle, Nyeal, Nyeale,
Nyeall, Nyealle, Nyl, Nyle (Ir),
Nyles, Nyll, Nylle, Nylles

Neka (Native American) wild goose.
Nekah

Nektarios (Greek) sweet nectar.
Nektario, Niktario, Nyktario

Nelek (Polish/Latin) horn colour;
horn blower; cornell tree. A form
of Cornelius.
Nelius (Lat), Nelik

Nelo (Spanish/Hebrew) God is my
judge.
Nello

Nels/Nelson (Scandinavian/English)
Neil's son; son of the champion.
Neal, Neals, Nealsan, Nealsen,
Nealso, Nealson, Nealsun,
Nealsyn, Neel, Neelsan, Neelsen,
Neesin, Neeson, Neelsun, Neelsyn,
Neils, Neilsan, Neilsen, Neilsin,
Neilson, Neilsun, Neilsyn, Nel,
Nels, Nelsen, Nelsin, Nelsun,
Nelsyn, Neyl, Neylsan, Neylsen,
Neylsin, Neylson, Neylsun,
Neylsyn, Nile, Niles, Nils, Nilsan,
Nilsen, Nilsin, Nilson, Nilsun,
Nilsyn, Niul, Nyle, Nyles, Nylsan,
Nylsen, Nylsin, Nylson, Nylsun,
Nylsyn

Nemesio (Spanish) just one.
Nemesyo

Nemo (Greek) from the valley.
Nimo, Nymo

Nemuel (Hebrew) the spreading sea
of God.
Nemuele, Nemuell, Nemuelle

Nen (Egyptian) ancient water.

Neper (Spanish) new town.

Nepo (Australian Aboriginal) friend.

Neptune (Latin) ruler of the sea.
Neptuna, Neptunah

Nerang (Australian Aboriginal)
little.
Neran

Nereus (Greek) by the water.

Nero (Latin) black. (Span) stern.
Neron, Nerone, Nerron, Nerrone,
Niro, Nyro

Nerville (French/Irish) from the sea
village.
Nervil, Nervile, Nervill, Nervyl,
Nervyle, Nervyll, Nervylle

Nesbit (English) river bend which is
nose-shaped.
Naisbit, Naisbitt, Naisbyt, Naisbytt,
Nesbitt, Nesbyt, Nesbytt, Nisbet,
Nisbett, Nysbet, Nysbett, Nysbit,
Nysbitt, Nysbyt, Nysbytt

Nester (Greek) wise traveller.
Nestar, Nestor, Nestyr

Netaniah (Hebrew) gift of God.
Netania, Netanya, Netanyah

Neto (Spanish) earnest.

Nevada (Spanish) covered in snow.
Nevadah, Nevadia, Nevadiah,
Navadya, Nevadyah

Nevan (Irish) holy.
Neven, Nevin, Nevon, Nevun,
Nevyn

Neville (Old French) from the new
village.
Neval, Nevall, Nevall, Nevel,
Nevele, Nevell, Nevelle, Nevil,
Nevile, Nevill, Nevyl, Nevyle,
Nevyll, Nevylle

Nevin (Irish/Gaelic) little saint.
(O/Eng) nephew.
Nefan, Nefen, Nefin, Nevan,
Neven, Nevins, Nevon, Nevyn,
Nivan, Niven (Eng), Nivon, Nivyn,
Nyvan, Nyven, Nyvin, Nyvon,
Nyvyn

Newbold (Old English) from the
new building.

Newell (Old English) from the new
spring.
Newel

Newland (Old English) from the
reclaimed land.
Newlan

Newlin (Old English) from the new
pool.
Newlyn

Newman (English) new man.
Neuman, Neumann (Ger),
Newmann, Newmen

Newton (Old English) from the new
town.
Naunton, Newborough,
Newburrie, Newburry, Newtown

Ngai (Vietnamese) herb.

Nghi (Vietnamese) suspicion.

Nghia (Vietnamese) forever.

Ngozi (Ibo) blessed one.

Ngu (Vietnamese) sleeping.

Ngunda (Malawian) dove.

Nhean (Cambodian) self-
knowledge; ego.

Niagara (Native American) thunder
water.
Niagra, Niagrah

Niaz (Hindi) present.

Nibal (Arabic) arrow.
Nybal

Nibaw (Native American) one who
stands tall.
Nybaw

Nicabar (Gypsy) cunning.
Nycabar

N

Nicho (Spanish/Greek) follower of Dionysos, the God of wine; celebration. A form of Denis.
Nycho

Nicholas/Nicolai/Nicky (Greek) victory of the people.
Claes, Claus, Clobes, Colas, Klaas (Dut), Flaasje (Dut), Klas, Klassis, Klaus, Kolinka, Neacail (Scot), Nic, Nicc, Niccolo (Ital), Nicholaj, Nicholo (Ital), Nichals, Nick, Nicke (Bav), Nicki, Nickie, Nicky, Nicol (Scot), Nickola, Nicodeme (Fren), Nicodemer, Nicodemus, Nicol, Nicola (Ital), Nicolai (Slav/Russ/Nor), Nicolaio (Port), Nicolas (Fren), Nicolau, Nickolaus, Nicole, Nicolo (Ital), Nicomedus (Grk), Niikodem (Pol), Nik, Nikel (Bav), Niki (Hung), Nikie, Nikita (Rus), Nikkelis, Nikki (Finn), Niklaas (Dut), Niklaus (Dan/Ger), Nikola (Slav), Nikolai (Slav), Nikolaon (Esp), Nikolas, Nikolaus (Ger), Niku, Niky, Nolascha, Nyc, Nycholas, Nyck, Nycki, Nyckie, Nyckolas, Nycomdeus (Grk), Nykolas, Nycky, Nyk, Nyki, Nykie, Nyky

Nicholson (English/Greek) Nicholas' son; son of the victorious people.
Nickelson, Nickoles, Nickoleson, Nycholson, Nyckolson, Nykolson

Nien (Vietnamese) year.
Nyen

Nigan (Native American) aged.
Nigen, Nigin, Nigyn, Nygan, Nygen, Nygin, Nygon, Nygyn

Nigel (Latin) black; dark-haired. (Gae) champion.
Niegal, Niegel, Nigal, Nigiel, Nigil, Niglie, Nijel, Nygal, Nygel

Nika (Yoruba) ferocious.
Nica, Nicah, Nicka, Nickah, Nikah, Nyca, Nycah, Nycka, Nyckah, Nyka, Nykah

Nike (Greek) victorious.
Nikee, Nikey, Niki, Nikie, Niky, Nyke, Nykee, Nykey, Nyki, Nykie, Nyky

Nikita (Russian/Greek) victory of the people. A form of Nicholas.
Nakita, Nakitah, Nakitas, Nikula, Nikulah, Nykita, Nykitah, Nykyta, Nykytah

Nikiti (Native American) smooth; round like the abalone shell.
Nikity, Nikyti, Nikyty, Nykiti, Nykity, Nykyty

Nila (Hindi) blue.
Nilah, Nyla, Nylah

Niles (English) Neil's son; son of the champion.
Niel, Niels, Nile, Nilese, Nilesh, Nyle, Nyles

Nimrod (Hebrew) fiery rod; brave; great hunter.
Nymrod

Nino (Spanish) young child.
Neno, Nyno

Nir (Hebrew) ploughed field.
Niral, Niria, Nirel, Nyr, Nyra, Nyral, Nyrel, Nyria, Nyrial

Niran (Thai) eternal.
Niren, Nirin, Niron, Niryn, Nyran, Nyren, Nyrin, Nyron, Nyryn

Nirvan (Hindi) happy.
Nyrvan

Nishan (Armenian) sign; cross.
Nyshan

Nissan (Hebrew) emblem.
Nisan, Nissim, Nyssan

Nissim (Hebrew) miracle.
Nisan, Nissym, Nyssim, Nyssym

Nitis (Native American) good friend.
Netis, Nytis, Nytys

Nitya (Sanskrit) constant.
Nityah, Nytya, Nytyah

Niu (Tongan) coconut.
Niutei (Poly), Nyu

Niv (Arabic) speech.
Nyv

Nixon (Old English) Nicholas' son;
son of the victorious people.
Nixan, Nixen, Nixin, Nixson,
Nixun, Nixyn, Nyxan, Nyxen,
Nyxin, Nyxon, Nyxyn

Nizam (Arabic) leader.
Nyzam

Njau (Kenyan) youthful bull.

Nkunda (Runyankore) loves those
who dislike him.
Nkundah

N'namdi (Ibo) his father's name
will live on.

Noadiah (Hebrew) to meet with
God.
Noadia, Nodya, Nodyah

Noah (Hebrew) long rest.
Noach (Dut), Noak (Swed), Noe
(Czech/Fren/Span), Nohah

Noam (Hebrew) pleasant.

Noble (Latin) noble; respected.
Nobel

Nocona (Comanche) one who
wanders.
Noconah

Nodin (Native American) wind.
Knoton, Nodyn, Noton

Noe (Hebrew/Spanish) peace.

Noel (French) born at Christmas
time. The masculine form of
Noelle.
Natal (Span), Natale (Ital), Noele,
Noell, Noelle, Nowel, Nowele,
Nowell, Nowelle

Noga (Hebrew) star; famous.
Nogah

Nohea (Hawaiian) handsome.

Nolan (Irish/Gaelic) descended
from nobility; famous.
Nolen, Nolin, Nolon, Nolyn

Nompie (Australian Aboriginal)
wedge-tailed eagle.
Nompi

Noor (Hebrew) light.

Norbert (Scandinavian) brilliant
hero.
Norberto, Norburt, Norburto,
Norbyrt, Norbyrto, Northbert,
Northberto, Northburt,
Northburto, Northbyrt, Northbyto

Noriss (Old French) northerner.
Norice, Noris, Norreys, Norrys

Norman (Old French) man from the
north; Norse man.
Normand, Normen, Normin,
Normon, Normyn

North (Old English) from the north.

Northcliff (Old English) from the
north cliff.
Northclif, Northcliffe, Northclith,
Northclithe, Northclyf, Northclife,
Northcliff, Northcliffe

Northrop (Old English) from the
north farm.
Northrup

Norton (Old English) from the
northern town.
Northton, Northtown

N

Norville (Old English) from the northern village.
Norvale, Norvil, Norvile, Norvill

Norvin (Old English) friend from the north.
Norvyn, Norwin, Norwyn

Norward (Old English) guardian of the north.
Norwald, Norword

Norwell (Old English) from the north stream.
Northwel, Northwell, Norwel

Norwood (Old English) from the northern forest.
Northwood

Notaku (Moquelumnan) growling bear.

Nouri (Persian) the prince of light.

Nova (Latin) new.
Novah

Nowles (English) from the grassy slope.
Knowl, Knowle, Knowles, Nowl, Nowle

Noy (Hebrew) beautiful; bountiful.
Noi

Nsoah (African) seventh-born child.
Nsoa

Nudge (Old English/Australian) gentle push.
Nudg

Nudgee (Australian Aboriginal) green frog.
Nudge

Nugent (English) shoving.
Nugant

Nui (Maori) great.

Numa (Arabic) pleasant.
Numah

Numair (Arabic) panther.
Numayr

Numid (Native American) star dancer.
Numyd

Nuncio (Italian) messenger; bearer of news.
Nuntius, Nunzio

Nunnally (Old English) from the valley of the nuns.
Nunnaly, Nunally

Nuri (Hebrew) fire.
Neri, Neria, Nery, Noori, Nuriel, Nuris, Nurism, Nury

Nuria (Hebrew) fire of the Lord.
Nuriah, Nurya, Nuryah

Nuriel (Hebrew/Arabic) the Lord's fire.
Nuria, Nuriah, Nuriya, Nuryel

Nuru (Swahili) born in the day-time light.

Nusair (Arabic) bird of prey.
Nusayr

Nwake (Nigerian) born on the market day.

Nye (Old English) islander.
Nyle

Nyo (Burmese) from the city.
Nio

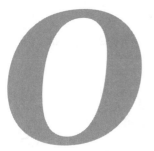

Oakes (Old English) dweller by the oak trees.
Oak, Oake, Oaklea, Oakleah, Oaklee, Oakleigh, Oakley, Oakli, Oaklie, Oakly, Oaks, Oaky

Oakley (Old English) from the field of oak trees.
Oak, Oaklea, Oakleah, Oaklee, Oakleigh, Oakli, Oaklie, Oakly

Oalo (Spanish/Latin) small.

Oba (Yoruba) king.
Obah

Obadele (Yoruba) king arriving at the wooded hollow.
Obadel

Obadiah (Hebrew) servant of God.
Obadia, Obadias, Obadya, Obadyah, Obadyas, Obediah, Obedias, Obedya, Obedyah, Obedyas

Obasi (Nigerian) honours God.

Obed (Hebrew) working.
Obad

Oberon (French) obedient; the king of the fairies.
Oberan, Oberen, Oberin, Oberun, Oberyn

Obert (Teutonic) wealthy; bright leader.
Obirt, Oburt, Obyrt

Obie (English) servant of God. The short form of Obadiah.
Obee, Obey, Obi, Oby

Ocan (Luo) hard times.

Oceanus (Greek) God of the sea; ocean dweller.
Ocean, Oceana, Oceanah, Oceane, Oceanis, Oceanos, Oceanous, Oceanys

O'Connor (Irish/Celtic) high will; desire.
O'Conor

Octavio/Octavius (Latin) eighth-born child.
Octave, Octavee, Octavey, Octavian (Fren), Octavien, Octavio (Lat), Octavious, Octavo, Octavous, Octavus (Lith), Octavyo, Octavyos, Octavyous, Octavyus, Oktawiusz (Pol), Ottavio, Ottavios, Ottavious, Ottavius

Odakota (Native American) friendly.
Dakota, Dakotah, Odakotah

Odam (Middle English) son-in-law.

Odd (Norwegian) point.
(Eng) strange.
Oddvar, Oddver

Ode (Benin) born on the road while travelling.
Odee, Odey, Odi, Odie, Ody

Oded (Hebrew) encouraging.

Odell (Scandinavian) wealthy; little.
(O/Eng) one who lives in the valley.
Odel, Odele, Odelle

Odhran (Irish) green.

Odin (Scandinavian) ruler.
Odyn

Odinan (African) fifteenth-born child.

Odion (Benin) first born of twins.
Odyon

Odissan (African) thirteenth-born son.

Odo (Old English) wealthy. A form of Otto.
Aodh, Audo, Odoh

Odom (Ghanian) oak tree.

Odon (Hungarian) wealthy protector.

Odran (Irish) pale green colour.
Odhran, Odran, Odren, Odrin, Odron, Odryn

Odulf (German) noble wolf.
Odolf, Odolfe, Odolph, Odolphe

Odwin (German) wealthy, noble friend.
Odwinn, Odwyn, Odwynn

Odysseus (Greek) wrath.
Odyseus

Ofer (Hebrew) young deer; fawn.
Opher

Ogbay (Ethiopian) don't take him away.
Ogbae, Ogbai

Ogbonna (Ibo) the image of his father.
Ogbonnah

Ogden (Old English) from the valley with the oak trees.
Ogdan, Ogdin, Ogdon, Ogdyn

Oghe (Irish) horse worker.

Ogier (Teutonic) wealthy warrior.
Oger, Ogyer

Ogilvie (Welsh) high. (Gae) from the high hill or peak.
Ogil, Ogyl, Ogylvie

Ogima (Chippewa) chief.
Ogimah, Ogyma, Ogymah

Oglesby (Old English) awe-inspiring one
Oglesbi, Oglesbie

Ogun (Nigerian) god of war.
Ogunkey, Ogunkeye, Ogunsanwo, Ogunsheye

Ohanko (Native American) restless.

Ohannes (Turkish/Hebrew) God is gracious. A form of John.
Ohan, Ohane, Ohanes, Ohann, Ohanne

Ohanzee (Lakota) shadow which is comforting.
Ohanze

Ohin (African) chief.
Ohan, Ohyn

Ohio (Native American) beautiful river.
Ohyo

Ohitekah (Lakota) brave.
Ohiteka

Ohiyesa (Sioux) victory.

Oisin (Irish) small deer.
Oisyn, Oysin, Oysyn

Oistin (Irish/Latin) little but majestic. A form of Austin.
Oistan, Oisten, Oistyn

Ojo (Yoruba) baby of a difficult birth.

Okapi (Swahili) animal with horns, a reddish-brown coat and horizontal white stripes on its legs.
Okapie, Okapy

Oke (Hawaiian/Scandinavian) divine spearer. (Tong) oak tree. A form of Oscar.
Okee, Okey, Oki, Okie, Oky

Okeke (Ibo) born on market day.

Okemos (Native American) little chief.

Oketa (Tongan) orchid.
Oketah

Oko (Yoruba) god of war.

Okoon (African) born during the night.

Okoth (Nigerian) born during a storm.

Okpara (Ibo) first-born son.
Okparah

Okuth (Luo) born during a rain shower.

Ola (Hebrew) eternity.
Olah, Olla, Ollah

Olaf (Old Norse) ancestral heritage.
Olaph, Olop (Est)

Olamina (Yoruba) my wealth.
Olaminah, Olamyna, Olamynah

Olando (Italian) from the famous land.
Olan, Oland

Oleg (Latvian/Russian) holy.
Olezka

Oleksandr (Russian/Greek) defender of humankind. A form of Alexander.
Olek, Oles (Pol), Olesandr, Olesko

Olin (English) holly.
Olen, Olney, Olyn

Olindo (Italian) (Geographical) from Olinthos in Italy.
Olin, Olind, Olyn, Olynd, Olyndo

Oliver (Old French/Latin) olive tree. (Scand) affectionate; kind.
Hiliver, Holivar, Holivaer, Oliva, Olivah, Olivar, Olier (Fren), Olivarius, Oliveras (Lith), Olivero (Ital), Oliveros (Span), Olivier

(Fren), Olivieras, Oliverio (Span), Oliviero (Span), Oliwa (Haw), Olliva, Ollivah, Ollivar, Olliver, Ollyva, Ollyvah, Ollyvar, Ollyver, Ollyvir, Ollyvyr, Olvan, Olven, Olvin, Olyva, Olyvah, Olyvar

Ollie (English) olive tree. (Scand) affectionate; kind. A short form of names starting with 'Ol' e.g. Oliver.
Olea, Oleah, Olee, Oleigh, Oley, Oli, Olie, Ollea, Olleah, Ollee, Olleigh, Olley, Olli, Olly, Oly

Olney (Old English) from the old island.

Olujimi (Yoruba) God gave me this.
Olujimy

Olishola (Yoruba) God has blessed.
Olusholah

Olympas (Greek) of Olympus; heavenly.

Omar (Arabic) first-born son. Follower of the prophet, speaker.
Omer, Omir, Omri, Omyr, Umar, Umer

Omari (African/Swahili/Arabic) highest follower of the prophet; speaker. A form of Omar.
Omar, Omaree, Omarey, Omarie, Omary

Omolara (Benin) child born during the night.
Omolarah

On (Chinese) peace. (Bur) coconut.

Ona (Latin/Irish/Gaelic) unity. (Lith) graceful. (Grk) donkey.

Onacona (Cherokee) white owl.
Onaconah

Onan (Turkish) prosperous.
Nan, Nani, Nanie, Nany, Onen, Onin, Onon, Onyn

O

Onani (African) to look quickly.
Onanee, Onanie, Onany

Onaona (Hawaiian) fragrance which is pleasant.
Onaonah

O'Neil (Irish) Neil's son; son of the champion.
O'Neal, O'Neale, O'Neel, O'Neele, O'Neile, O'Nel, O'Nel, O'Niel, O'Neile, O'Nil, O'Nile, O'Nyel, O'Nyele, O'Nyl, O'Nyle

Ongo (Tongan) spirited.

Onike (Tongan) onyx, semi-precious stone.

Onilwyn (Welsh) ash-grove friend.
Onilwin

Onkar (Hindi) purity.

Onslow (Old English) from the zealous one's hill.

Onhur (Turkish) honourable.

Ophir (Hebrew) faith.
Ophyr

Opio (Ateso) first born of twin boys.
Opyo

Oran (Irish) green.
Oren, Orin, Oron, Orran, Orren, Orrin, Orron, Orryn, Oryn

Oratio (Latin) time keeper. (Grk) promise. A form of Horatio.
Horatio, Oratyo, Orazio, Orazyo

Orban (Hungarian) urban. (Lat) circle; globe.
Orben, Orbin, Orbon, Orbyn

Ord (Old English) spear.
Orde

Orde (Latin) peaceful; logical.
Ordel, Ordele, Ordell, Ordelle

Ordell (Latin) beginning.
Orde, Ordel, Ordele, Ordelle

Ordway (Old English) spear path.
Ordwai

Oreb (Hebrew) raven; black.

Orel (Russian) eagle. (Lat) listener. (O/Eng) from the hill of ore.
Oran, Oreel, Orele, Orell, Orelle, Orenthal, Oriel, Oriele, Orielle, Orin, Orran, Orrel, Orrele, Orrell, Orrelle, Orren, Orrin, Orryn, Oryn

Oren (Hebrew) pine tree. (Gae) pale-complexioned.
Oran, Orin, Oron, Oryn

Orestes (Greek) mountaineer.
Orest, Orest

Orev (Hebrew) raven.

Orford (Old English) from the upper river crossing.

Ori (Hebrew) light.
Oree, Orey, Orie, Ory

Orien (Latin) visitor from the east.
Orian, Orin, Orion, Oris, Oran, Oren, Orin, Oron, Orono, Orran, Orren, Orrin, Orryon, Orryn, Oryn

Orin (Celtic) white.
Oran, Oren, Oron, Orran, Orren, Orrin, Orron, Orryn, Oryn

Orion (Greek) son of fire; son of light.
Orian, Orien, Oryan, Oryen, Oryin, Oryon

Orlan (English) from the pointed land.
Orland, Orlando

Orlando (German) famous.
Lando, Oland, Olando, Orlan, Orland, Orlanda, Orlande, Orlandous, Orlandus, Orlon, Orlond, Orlondo, Orlondon

O

Orman (Teutonic) mariner.
(O/Eng) spearman.
Ormen

Ormond (Old English) from the
bear mountain.
Ormon, Ormondo

Oro (Spanish) golden.

Oroiti (Polynesian) slow-footed.

Oron (Hebrew) light.
Oran, Oren, Orin, Orun, Oryn

Orono (Latin) from Oren.
Oron

Orpheus (Greek) ear.
Orfeus

Orrick (English) dweller at the old
oak tree.
Oric, Orick, Orik, Orric, Orrik,
Orryc, Orryck, Orryk, Oryc, Oryck,
Oryk

Orrin (English) river.
Orin, Orryn, Oryn

Orris (Latin) time keeper. (Grk)
promise. A form of Horatio.
Oris, Orris, Orriss, Orrys, Orryss

Orry (Latin) from the Orient.
Oarri, Oarrie, Orrey, Orri, Orrie,
Ory

Orsino (Italian/Latin) bear. A form
of Orson.
Orsine, Orsyne, Orsyno

Orson (Latin) bear.
Orsin, Orsino, Orsoch, Orsyn,
Ursen, Ursin, Urson

Orton (Old English) from the
riverside town.
Ortan, Orten, Ortin, Ortyn

Ortzi (Basque) sky.
Ortzy

Orunjan (Yoruba) born under the
midday sun.

Orville (Old French) from the
golden city.
Orvil, Orvile, Orvill, Orvyl, Orvyle,
Orvyll, Orvylle

Orvin (English) friend with a spear.
Orvan, Orven, Orvon, Orvyn,
Orwin, Orwyn

Osahar (Benin) God will hear.

Osaze (Benin) God likes.
Osaz

Osbert (Old English) clever; bright;
divine. (O/Nrs) bright god.
Osbirt, Osborne, Osbyrt, Osric

Osborn (Old English) divine
warrior. (O/Nrs) divine bear.
Osborne, Osbourn, Osbourne,
Ozborn, Ozborne, Ozbourn,
Ozbourne, Osburn, Osburne

Oscar (Old English/Scandinavian)
divine spear.
Oke, Osgar (Gae), Oscer, Oskaras
(Lith), Oskar, Osker

Osei (Fanti) noble.
Osee, Osey, Osi, Osie, Osy

Osgood (Old English) divinely
good; creator.

O'Shea (Irish) Shea's son; son of
the majestic one.
Osean, Oshae, Oshai, Oshane,
Oshaun, Oshawn, O'Shay, O'Shaye

Osiris (Egyptian) mythological god
of rebirth, resurrection, fertility
and the after-life.
Osirys, Osyris, Osyrys

Osman (Turkish) ruler.
(Eng) servant of God.
Osmanek, Osmen, Osmin,
Osmon, Osmyn, Otthmor, Ottmar,
Ottmor

O

Osmand (Old English) protected by God.
Esman, Esmand, Osman, Osmond, Osmondo, Osmund, Osmundo, Oswin, Oswyn

Osmar (Old English) divinely glorious.
Osmer, Osmir, Osmor, Osmyr

Osmond (Old English) divine protector.
Osmonde, Osmondo, Osmont, Osmonte, Osmund, Osmunde, Osmundo, Osmunt, Osmunte

Osred (Old English) divine advisor.

Osric (Old English) divine ruler.
Osric, Osrick, Osrig, Osrik, Osryc, Osryck, Osryg, Osryk

Ossian (Irish) fawn.
Ossyan, Osyan

Osten (Latin) held in high regard.
Ostan, Ostin, Ostun, Ostyn

Oswald (Old English) divinely ruled by God; God of the forest.
Osvald, Osvaldo, Osvalds, Oswal, Oswaldo, Oswall, Oswel, Osweld, Osweldo, Oswell

Oswin (Old English) divine friend.
Oswyn

Ota (Czech) prosperous.
Otah, Otik

Otadan (Native American) many.

Otaktay (Lakota) many strikes.
Otaktai

Otayba (Australian Aboriginal) bird.
Otaybah

Otem (Luo) born away from home.

Othello (German/Spanish) wealthy.
Otello (Ital)

Othman (German) wealthy.
Othmen

Othniel (Hebrew) lion of God.
Othnyel

Otis (Old English) son of Otto; son of the wealthy, prosperous one. (Grk) keen of hearing.
Oates, Otes, Ottis, Ottys, Otys

Otskai (Nez Perce) going.
Otskae, Otskaie, Otskay

Ottah (Nigerian) baby who is thin.
Ota, Otah, Otta

Ottar (Norwegian) point warrior; maker of arrows.
Otar

Ottmar (Turkish) ruler.
Otman, Otomar, Otomars, Otmen, Ottmer, Ottmen, Ottoma, Ottomar

Otto (Teutonic) wealthy.
Oddo, Odo, Osman, Osmand, Othello (Ital), Othman, Othmar, Oto, Otoe, Otow, Otteran, Ottone (Ital), Ottorina, Ottmar, Ottmer

Ottokar (German) happy warrior.
Otokar

Otu (Native American) sea shells being collected into a basket.
Ottu

Otway (Teutonic) lucky in battle.
Otwai

Ouray (Native American) arrow.
Ourae, Ourai

Overton (Middle English) from the high town.
Overtan, Overten, Overtin, Overtyn

Ovid (Latin) life.
Ovyd

Oviedo (Spanish) applause.
Ovyedo

P

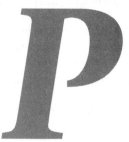

Owen (Welsh) well born. A form of Evan.
Evan, Even, Evin, Evon, Ewen, Owan, Owain, Owaine, Owan, Owayn, Owayne, Owin, Owine, Owon, Owone, Owyn, Owyne, Ywain, Ywaine, Ywayn, Ywayne

Owney (Irish) elder.
Onee, Oney, Oni, Onie, Ony, Ownee, Owni, Ownie, Owny

Oxford (Old English) from the oxen river crossing.
Oxforde

Oxley (Old English) from the meadow of the oxen.
Oxlea, Oxleah, Oxlee, Oxleigh, Oxli, Oxlie, Oxly

Oxton (Old English) from the ox town.
Oxtan, Oxten, Oxtin, Oxtyn

Oya (Moquelumnan) talking of the snake.
Oyah

Oystein (Norwegian) rock of joy.
Ostein, Osten, Ostin, Oston, Ostyn

Oz (Hebrew) strength.
Ozz

Ozias (Hebrew) strength of the Lord.
Ozia, Oziah, Ozya, Ozyah, Ozyas

Ozni (Hebrew) ear.
Ozny

Ozuru (Japanese) stork.
Ozuro, Ozuroo

Ozzie (Old English) divinely ruled by God; God of the forest. The short form of names starting with 'Os' or 'Oz' e.g. Oswald.
Osi, Osie, Oss, Ossi, Ossie, Ossy, Osy, Ozi, Ozie, Ozy, Ozz, Ozzi, Ozzy

Paavo (Finnish/Latin) small. A form of Paul.
Paav

Pablo (Latin/Spanish) small. The Spanish form of Paul.

Pace (English/French) born at Easter time.
Paice, Payce

Pachomai (Australian Aboriginal) grey.
Pachomay

Pacifico (Filipino) peaceful.
Pacifica, Pacific, Pacifyc, Pacyfyc

Paco (Native American) bold eagle. (Ital) to pack.
Packo, Pako

Paddy (Irish) noble. The Irish form of Patrick.
Paddee, Paddey, Paddi, Paddie, Padi, Padie, Padriac, Pady

Padget/Page/Paget (English) attendant; young child. The masculine form of Paige.
Padge, Padgett, Paeg, Paege, Page, Paget (Fren), Pagett, Paig, Paige, Paiget, Paigett, Payg, Payge, Payget, Paygett

Padilpa (Australian Aboriginal) parrot.
Padilpah

Padre (Spanish) priest.

P

Padulla (Australian Aboriginal) stone.
Padula, Padulah, Padullah

Pagan (Latin) country dweller.
Paegan, Paegen, Paegin, Paegon, Paegyn, Paganel, Pagen, Pagin, Pagon, Pagun, Paigan, Paige, Paigen, Paigin, Paigon, Paigyn, Pain, Paine, Payn, Payne, Paynel

Pagiel (Hebrew) worships God.
Paegel, Paegell, Pagiell, Paigel, Paigell, Paygel, Paygell

Paine (Old French) country person.
Pane, Pain, Painey, Payn, Payne

Painter (English) artist who works with paint.
Paintar, Paintor, Payntar, Paynter, Payntor

Paki (African) witness.

Pakile (Hawaiian) royal.
Pakil, Pakill, Pakyl, Pakyll

Pal (Swedish/Latin/Hungarian) small. A form of Paul.
Pali, Palika

Palaina (Hawaiian/Irish) strong honour.
Palainah

Palaki (Polynesian) black.
Palakee, Palakey, Palakie, Palaky

Palani (Hawaiian/English/Latin) freedom. (O/Eng) honest. A form of Frank.
Palanee, Palaney, Palanie, Palany

Palash (Hindi) flowery tree.

Palauni (Polynesian) brown.
Palaunie, Palauny

Palben (Basque) blond-haired.

Palladin/Pallaton (Native American) warrior.
Pallaton, Palladyn, Palleten

Pallano (Australian Aboriginal) new moon.
Palano

Palmer (Old English) palm bearer; pilgrim.
Palm, Palma, Palmah

Palmiro (Latin) born on Palm Sunday.
Palmira, Palmirow, Palmyro

Palti (Hebrew) God frees.

Panas (Russian) immortal.

Pancho (Spanish/English) freedom. (O/Eng) honest. A form of Frank.
Panchito

Pancras (Greek) powerful strength.

Pandu (Sanskrit) pale.
Pandue

Pangari (Australian Aboriginal) soul.
Pangary

Panos (Greek) stone. A form of Peter.
Pano

Paolo (Italian/Latin) small. A form of Paul.

Papa (Polynesian) earth.
Pappa

Papacy (Latin) from the Pope's office.

Papahi (Tongan) mischievous; smart.
Papahy

Papiano (Hawaiian/Latin) prosperous bean grower. A form of Fabian.
Papian

Pare (English) peeler.

Paris (French) (Geographical) the capital of France.
Parys

Park/Parker (Middle English)
guardian of the park.
Parc, Parke, Parker, Parkman

Parkin/Parnell (English) little Peter;
little stone.
Parkyn, Perkin, Perkyn, Parnel,
Parnele, Parnell, Parnelle

Parlan (Scottish) farmer.
Parlen, Parlin, Parlon, Parlyn

Parr (English) from the barn.

Parri (Australian Aboriginal)
stream.
Pari, Parrie, Parry, Pary

Parrish (English) district of the
church.
Parish, Parrisch, Parrysh, Parysh

Parry (Welsh) Harry's son; son of
the army ruler. (Eng) warding off
an attack.
Paree, Parey, Pari, Parie, Parree,
Parrey, Parri, Parrie, Pary

Parson (English) parish priest.

Pas (Latin) dance.

Pascal/Pasch (Italian) born at
Easter time.
Pascale, Pascall, Pascalle, Pasch,
Paschal, Pascoe, Pascual (Span),
Pashel, Pascoli, Pasquale (Ital)

Pasha (Russian/Latin) small. A form
of Paul.
Pashah, Pashenka, Pashka

Pastor (English) drawing.

Pastor (Latin) spiritual leader.
Pastar, Paster, Pastir, Pastyr

Pat (Latin) little noble one. The
short form of names beginning
with 'Pat' e.g. Patrick.
Patt

Patamon (Native American) angry.
Pataman, Patamen, Patamin,
Patamyn

Pati (Sanskrit) master.
Patie, Patt, Patti, Pattie, Patty, Paty

Patonga (Australian Aboriginal)
small wallaby (a member of the
kangaroo family).
Patongah

Patrick (Latin) noble.
Patric, Patryc, Patryck

Patrobas (Greek) life of his father.
Pad, Padd, Paddi, Paddie, Padi,
Padie, Paddy, Pady, Pat, Pati, Patie,
Patt, Patti, Pattie, Patty, Paty, Ric,
Rici, Ricie, Rick, Ricki, Rickie,
Ricky, Rik, Riki, Rikie, Riky, Ryc,
Ryck, Rycki, Ryckie, Rycky, Ryc,
Ryck, Rycki, Ryckie, Rycky, Ryk,
Ryki, Rykie, Ryky

Patterson (Irish) Pat's son; son of
the noble one.
Paterson, Patteson

Pattin (Gypsy) leaf.
Patin, Pattyn, Patyn

Patton (Old English) from the
warrior's town.
Patan, Paten, Patin, Paton, Pattan,
Patten, Pattin, Pattun, Pattyn,
Patyn

Patwin (Native American) man.
(O/Eng) noble friend.
Patwyn

Paul (Latin) small.
Paal, Paavo (Fin), Pablo (Span),
Padra, Padlo (Ital), Paley, Pal, Pall,
Paolo (Ital), Paova (Poly), Pauley,
Pauli, Paulie, Paulin (Grk),
Paulinas, Paulino (Span), Paulinus
(Lith), Paulis, Paull, Paulle, Paulo
(Ital/Port), Paulot (Fren), Paultje
(Dut), Paval, Pavel (Rus/Boh/Pol),

P

Pavelek (Slav), Pavelik, Pavlenka (Rus), Pavil, Pavils (Lett), Pavli (Est), Pavlik (Boh), Pavlo, Pavlos (Grk), Pavluschka (Rus), Pavol, Pawl (O/Eng), Pawley, Paz, Pewlen, Pol, Poul (Dan), Pouvylas, Pouw (Dut), Pouwl, Pouvylas

Pave (English) paver.
Paver

Pavit (Hindi) purity.
Pavitt, Pavyt, Pavytt

Pawel (Polish) small. A form of Peter.
Pawelek, Pawell, Pawl

Pax/Paxton (Latin) from the town of peace.
Paxtan, Paxten, Paxtin, Paxtun, Paxtyn, Paxx

Payat (Native American) he is coming.
Payatt

Payne (Latin) from the country.
Pain, Paine, Payn

Paytah (Lakota) fire.
Pita, Paitah, Payta

Paz (Spanish/Latin) peace.
Pax

Peatea (Tongan) polar bear.

Peadar (Irish) stone. A form of Peter.
Peader, Peadir, Peador, Peadyr

Pearson (Scottish) Peter's son; son of the stone.
Pearsson, Pehrson, Peterson, Pierson, Piersson, Pyerson

Pedahel (Hebrew) God will redeem.
Pedahil, Pedahyl

Peder (Scandinavian/Latin) stone. A form of Peter.
Peadar, Peader, Pedey, Pedro

(Span), Peers (Eng), Peet (Est), Peeter (Est), Peir (Fren), Peirce (Eng), Pekeio (Haw), Pete (Eng), Petr (Bul), Petras (Laith), Petros (Grk), Petru (Rom), Petter (Nor)

Peel (Old French) from the castle on the Scottish border. (Celt) stronghold.
Peal, Peil, Peyl

Peka (Hawaiian) stone. A form of Peter.
Pekelo

Pekeri (Australian Aboriginal) dream.

Pelagius (Greek) of the sea.
Pelagyus

Peleke (Hawaiian) wise helper.

Pelham (Old English) from the stream village. (Celt) pelt; hide.
Pelhem, Pelhim, Pelhon, Pelhym

Peli (Latin/Basque) happy.
Pelie, Pely

Pelias (Greek) leader.
Pelyas

Pell (English) paper.
Pel

Pello (Greek/Basque) stone.

Pelton (English) from the town by the pool.
Peltan, Pelten, Peltin, Peltyn

Pembroke (Celtic/Welsh) from the headland; from the hill stream.
Pembrock, Pembrok

Pendle (Old English) hill.
Pendal, Pendel, Penndal, Penndel, Penndle

Penley (English) from the enclosed meadow.
Penlea, Penleah, Penlee, Penleigh, Panli, Panlie, Panly

Penmina (Hawaiian/Hebrew) favourite son. A form of Benjamin.
Penminah, Penmyna, Penmynah

Penn (Old English) from the enclosure. (O/Ger) commander. (Lat) quill; pen.
Pen

Penrith (Old Welsh) from the chief river crossing.
Penryth

Penrod (Teutonic) renowned commander.
Pennrod

Peopeo (Nez Perce) bird.

Pepe (Spanish/Hebrew) God will increase; God has added a child. The Spanish form of Joseph.
Pepa (Czech), Pepee, Pepey, Pepi, Pepie, Peppe (Ital), Peppee, Peppey, Peppi, Peppie, Peppy, Pepy

Pepin (German) preserver.
Pepan, Pepen, Penon, Pepyn

Per (Swedish/Latin) stone. A form of Peter.

Perach (Hebrew) flower.
Pera, Perah

Perben (Greek/Danish) stone.
Perban, Perbin, Perbon, Perbyn

Percival/Percy (Old French) perceptive.
Parsefal, Parsifal, Pededur, Percee, Percey, Perceval, Perci, Percie, Percivale, Percy, Percyval

Peregrine (Latin) foreigner.
Pelaijo (Ital), Pelgrim (Dut), Pellegrino, Peregrin (Fren), Peregrino, Peregryn, Perergrin, Perergryn,, Pilgrim

Peretz (Hebrew) to leap.
Perez

Perez (Hebrew) to break through.
Perezz

Pericies (Greek) just leader.
Perycies

Perkin (English) little Peter; little stone.
Perka, Perkah, Perkins, Perkyn, Perkyns

Perry (Old English/Greek) stone. A form of Peter. The short form of Peregrine, foreigner.
Peree, Perey, Peri, Perie, Perree, Perrey, Perri, Perrie, Pery

Persis (Greek) from Persia.
Persys

Perth (Scottish) from the thorn-bush thicket.
Pirth, Pyrth

Pervis (Latin) passage.
Pervys

Pesach (Hebrew) one who is spared.
Pesac, Pessach

Pesekava (Polynesian) song.

Pete/Peter (English/Latin) stone.
Feoris, Panos, Parnal, Parnel, Parrie, Parry, Peadair (Scot), Pearce (Eng), Peat, Peate, Peater, Pedar (Nor/Dan), Peder, Pedo (Est), Pedr (Wel), Pedrinho (Port), Pedro (Span/Port), Peet, Peete, Peeter, Peer, Peira, Peirce (Eng), Peit, Peite, Peiter, Pejo (Illy), Pekka (Fin), Per (Swed), Perez, Perkin, Perkins, Perrie (Eng), Pernal, Pernael, Pero, Perrin (Fren), Perromik (Bret), Perry (Eng), Petai (Illy), Petar, Pete, Peteras, Peterus, Petr (Rus), Petri, Petrol (Corn), Petros (Grk), Petru (Rum), Petrus (Ger), Petruscha, Petruschka, Pewlin (Wel), Peyt,

P

Peyte, Peyter, Piera (Fren), Pieter, Piter, Pyet, Pyete, Pyeter

Pethuel (Hebrew) with an open mind towards God.

Petiri (Shona) here.
Petri, Petyri, Petyry

Peton (Old English) from the warrior's town.
Peatoan, Peaten, Peatin, Peaton, Peatun, Peatyn, Petan, Peten, Petin, Petun, Petyn

Peverell (French) piper.
Peverall, Peverel, Peveril, Peveryl,

Pewlin (Welsh) small.
Pewlan, Pewlen, Pewlon, Pewlyn

Peyton (English) from the warrior's estate; from the toll keeper's town.
Paeton, Paiton, Payton, Peiton

Pezi (Sioux) grass.

Pharaoh (Latin/Egyptian) ruler.
Faro, Faroh, Pharo, Pharoh

Phelan (Irish/Celtic) wolf.
Felan, Feland, Pheland

Phelps (English) Philip's son; son of the one who loves horses.
Felp, Felps, Phelp

Phil/Philip (Hebrew) Philip's son; son of the one who loves horses; spokesperson.
Feeleep, Felep, Felip, Felipe, Felide, Filandras, Filep, Filip, Filippinho, Filippo, Filypas, Fulip, Fulup, Lip (Ital), LipstsPhil, Phelippe, Phelp, Phelps (Eng), Philipp, Philippe (Fren), Philippos (Grk), Phillip (Scot), Phillipe (Fren), Phillippe (Fren), Pip, Piripi (NZMaori), Phyleap, Phyleep, Phylip, Phylleap, Phylleep, Phyllip,

Phyllyp, Phylyp, Pip, Piripi (NZMaori)

Philander (Greek) lover of humankind. A combination of Phil/Alexander.
Filander, Fylander, Phylander

Philart (Greek) one who loves virtue.
Filart, Filarte, Fylart, Fylarte, Philaret, Philarte, Phylart, Phylarte

Philemon (Greek) kiss.
Philamin, Philamina, Philamine, Philamyn, Philamyna, Philmon, Philmyn, Philmyna, Philmyne, Phylmin, Phylmina, Phylmine, Phylmon, Phylmyn

Philibert (Teutonic) bright.
Filbert, Filberte, Filbirt, Filbirte, Filburt, Filburte, Filibert, Filiberte, Filibirt, Filibirte, Filiburt, Filiburte, Fylbert, Fylberte, Fylbirt, Fylbirte, Fylburt, Fylburte, Fylibert, Fyliberte, Fylibirt, Fylibirte, Fyliburt, Fyliburte, Philberte, Philbirt, Philberte, Philburt, Philburte, Philibert, Philiberte, Philibirt, Philibirte, Philiburt, Philiburte, Phillbert, Phillberte, Phillbirt, Phillbirte, Phillburt, Phillburte, Phillibert, Philliberte, Phillibirt, Phillibirte, Philliburt, Philliburte, Phylbert, Phylberte, Phylbirt, Phylbirte, Phylburt, Phylburte, Phylibert, Phyliberte, Phylibirt, Phylibirte, Phyliburt, Phyliburte, Phyllbert, Phyllberte, Phyllbirt, Phyllbirte, Phyllburt, Phyllburte, Phyllibert, Phylliberte, Phyllibirt, Phyllbirte, Phylliburt, Phylliburte

Philiman (Greek) lover of humankind.
Phileman, Philleman, Philliman, Phyliman, Phylliman

Philo (Greek) long friend.
Filo, Fylo, Phylo

Phineas (Egyptian) dark-skinned.
(Heb) prophecy; mouth of brass.
Fineas, Fyneas, Phyneas

Phirun (Cambodian) rain.

Phoebus (Greek) shining; pure;
bright. The masculine form of
Phoebe.
Phoebas, Phoebius

Phoenix (Greek) purple; immortal.

Piao (Chinese) handsome.

Pickford (English) from the river
crossing near the pick.

Picton (Old English) from the town
near the pointy hill.
Pictan, Picten, Picktown, Pickun,
Picktyn, Piktan, Pikten, Piktin,
Pikton, Piktown, Piktun, Piktyn,
Pyckton, Pycton, Pyctin, Pyctyn,
Pyktin, Pykton, Pyktyn

Pie (French/Latin) dutiful. The
French form of Pius, devout.
Pye

Pier (English) from the pier.

Pierce (English) sharp.

Piercy (English) from the pier
hedge.

Pikoka (Tongan) peacock.
Pikokah, Pykoka, Pykokah

Pila (Hawaiian) wilful. A form of
Bill.
Pilah

Pilar (Latin/Spanish) pillar;
column.
Pillar, Pylar, Pyllar

Pili (Swahili) second-born child.
Pyli, Pyly

Pillan (Native American) supreme
essence.
Pilan, Pylan, Pyllan

Pilpo (Hawaiian/Greek) one who
loves horses.

Pin (Vietnamese) faithful.
Pyn

Pinchas (Egyptian) dark-haired.
(Heb) oracle.
Phineas, Pincas, Pinchos, Pincus,
Pinkas, Pinkus, Pynchas

Pindari (Australian Aboriginal)
from the high ground.
Pyndari, Pyndary

Pino (Italian) God adds.

Pinon (Native American) star
constellation.

Pinpi (Australian Aboriginal)
parrot.
Pynpi, Pynpy

Pinto (Native American) horse with
white patches.

Pio (Latin) purity.
Pyo

Pip (English) seed.

Pippin (German) father.
Pippyn

Piram (Hebrew) fast.
Pyram

Piran (Irish) prayer.
Peran, Pieran, Pieren, Pieryn, Pyran

Pirrin (Australian Aboriginal) cave.
Pirryn, Pyrrin, Pyrryn

Pirro (Greek/Spanish) one with the
flaming red hair.
Piro, Pyro, Pyrro

P

Pitney (English) from the island of the strong-willed.
Pitnee, Pitni, Pitnie, Pitny, Pytnee, Pytney, Pytni, Pytnie, Pytny

Pitt (Old English) from the hollow or pit.
Pit

Pius (Latin) devout.
Pie (Fren), Pinz (Bret), Pye, Pyus

Pizi (Sioux) middle son.

Placid/Placidius (English/Latin) peaceful. The short form of Placidus.
Placidio (Ital), Placido (Span), Placyd (Pol), Placydius

Plato (Greek) broad; flat-shouldered.
Platan, Platen, Platin, Platon, Platun, Platyn

Platt (French) flat land.
Platte

Pledge (English) promise.

Pocano (Pueblo) the spirits are coming.

Poesy (Latin) poetry.

Polar (Latin) from the polar region.

Pollard (Norse) short-haired.
Polard, Polerd, Pollerd

Pollock (Old English) small. (Grk) crowned.
Polick, Pollick, Polloch, Pollok, Polock, Polok

Pollux (Greek) crowned.
Polux

Polo (Tibetan) brave wanderer.
Pollo

Polona (Australian Aboriginal) hawk.
Polonah

Pomeroy (French) from the apple orchard.
Pomaroy, Pomaroi, Pmeroi

Ponce (Spanish) fifth-born child.

Pontus (Greek) sea god.

Pony (Scottish) small horse.
Ponee, Poney, Poni, Ponie

Porfirio (Greek) dressed in purple; purple stone.
Porfiryo, Porfryio, Porfryo

Porter (Latin) gate keeper; to carry.

Pshita (Sanskrit) cherished.
Poshitah

Posin (Chinese) old grandfather elephant.

Posoa (Polynesian) friendly; flirt.
Posoah

Potiki (Maori) youngest child.
Potily

Poutini (Polynesian) green stone.
Poutiny, Poutyny

Pov (Gypsy) earth.

Powa (Native American) wealthy.
Powah

Powell (Celtic) son of Howell; little alert one.
Powal, Powall, Powel, Powil, Powill, Powyl, Powyll

Powhatan (Algonquin) where the powwow is being held.

Prabhat (Hindi) dawn light.

Pradeep (Hindi) light.

Pradosh (Hindi) night light.

Pramad (Hindi) joy.

Praman (Polynesian) wisdom.
Pramanah

Pramod (Hindi) happy.

Prantin (Australian Aboriginal) wonder.
Prantyn

Prasad (Hindi) brilliant.

Pratap (Hindi) great.

Pravat (Thai) history.

Pravin (Hindi) capable.
Pravyn

Praxedes (Greek) active.
Praxiteles

Prem (Hindi) love.

Premysl (Czech) first born.

Prentice (Middle English) apprentice.
Prentis, Prentise, Prentiss, Prentyc, Prentyce, Prentys, Prentyse

Prescott (Old English) from the priest's cottage.
Prescot

President (English) leader of a nation.

Presley (English) from the meadow of the priest.
Preslea, Presleah, Preslee, Presleigh, Presli, Preslie, Presly

Preston (English) from the priest's town.
Prestan, Presten, Prestin, Prestyn

Prewitt (French) little brave.
Preuet, Prewet, Prewett, Prewit, Prewyt, Prewytt, Pruit, Pruitt, Pruyt, Pruytt

Price (Welsh) son of the ardent one.
Pryce

Primo (Italian) first-born child. The masculine form of Prima.
Primus, Prymo

Prince (Latin) chief; first in rank.
Prins, Prinse, Prynce, Pryns, Prynse

Priscus (Latin) ancient.
Pryscus

Proctor (Latin) leader.
Proctar, Procter

Prokop (Czech) progressive.

Prometheus (Greek) forethought.

Prosper (English) wealthy.

Pryor (Latin) the head of the monastery.
Prior

Puluke (Hawaiian/English) dweller at the dense shrubs. A form of Bruce.
Puluc, Puluc

Puluno (Hawaiian) brown.

Pumeet (Sanskrit) purity.

Punawai (Hawaiian) water.

Prudy (Hindi) recluse; hidden.

Puriri (Maori) New Zealand sheoak tree.

Purusha (Sanskrit) man.
Purushah

Purvis (English/French) provider.
Purvise, Purviss, Purvys, Purvyss

Pushkara (Sanskrit) blue lotus.
Pushkarah

Putnam (Old English) dweller by the pond. (Lat) tree pruner.
Putnem, Putnum

Pwyll (Welsh) prudent.
Pwill

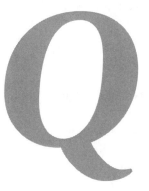

Qabic (Arabic) able.
Quabic, Quabick, Quabik, Quabyc, Quabyck, Quabyk

Qabil (Arabic) able.
Qabill, Qabyl, Qabyll

Qadim (Arabic) ancient.
Qadym

Qadir (Arabic) powerful.
Qadeer, Quadeer, Quadir

Qamar (Arabic) moon.

Qasim (Arabic) divider.
Qasym

Qayyim (Arabic) rightful; generous.
Qayim

Qimat (Hindi) valuable.
Qymat

Qing-Nan (Chinese) young generation.

Quaashie (Ewe) born on Sunday.
Quaashi, Quashi, Quashie

Quabiz (Arabic) restrainer.
Quabyz

Quadree (African American) fourth-born child.
Quadrees

Quahhar (Arabic) dominant.

Quain (French) clever.
Quayn

Quamby (Australian Aboriginal) shelter.
Quambi

Quan (Comanche) fragrant.
Quanah

Quab (Vietnamese) allowed.
Quan-van

Quana (Native American) fragrant.
Quanah

Quant (Greek) quantity.
Quanta, Quantae, Quantah, Quantai, Quantay, Quante, Quantea, Quantey, Quantez

Quay (English) from the wharf.
Quey

Qudamah (Arabic) courageous.
Qudam, Qudama

Quddus (Arabic) holy.
Qudus

Qued (Kiowa) decorated robe.

Quenby (Scandinavian) from the woman's estate.
Quenbi, Quenbie

Quennel (Old French) dweller by the little oak.
Quenal, Quenall, Quenel, Quenell, Quennal, Quennall, Quennell

Quentin (Latin) fifth-born child.
Kvintinuas, Quantin, Queintin, Queinten, Quienton, Quent, Quenten, Quenton, Quentyn, Quintan, Quinten, Quintin, Quinton, Quintus, Quyntan, Quynten, Quyntin, Quynton, Quyntyn, Qwentan, Qwenten, Qwentin, Qwenton, Qwentyn, Qwyntan, Qwynten, Qwyntin, Qwynton, Qwyntyn

R

Quenton (English) from the queen's town.
Quentan, Quenten, Quentin, Quentyn

Quigley (Old English) from the queen's meadow.
Quiglea, Quigleah, Quiglee, Quigleigh, Quigli, Quiglie, Quigly

Quill (English) feather.
Quil, Quyl, Quyll

Quillan/Quillian (Irish) cub.
Quilan, Quilen, Quilin, Quille, Quillin, Quillon, Quillyn, Quilon, Quilyn

Quiller (Old English) writer.
Quiler

Quillon (Latin) sword.
Quilon, Quyllon, Quylon

Quimby (Norse) dweller by the queen's estate.
Quembee, Quembey, Quemby, Quenbee, Quenbey, Quenby, Quinbee, Quinby, Quymbee, Quymbey, Quymbi, Quymbie, Quymby, Quynbee, Quynbey, Quynbi, Quynbie, Quynby

Quincy (Old French/Latin) from the fifth son's estate; fifth-born child.
Quincee, Quincey, Quinn, Quinnsey, Quinnsy, Quyncee, Quyncey, Quynn, Quynnsey, Quynnsy, Qunnsy, Quynsy

Quinlan (Irish) strong; well-formed; athletic.
Quindlen, Quinlen, Quinlin, Quinn, Quinnlan, Quynlan, Quynlen, Quynlin, Quynlon, Quynlyn

Quinn (Irish/Gaelic) wisdom.
Quin, Quyn, Quynn

Quinto (Spanish) home ruler.

Quiqui (Spanish/German) ruler of the house. A form of Henry.
Quinto, Quiquin, Quyqu y

Quirin (English) magic spell.
Quiryn

Quiver (English) arrow holder.
Quyver

Quon (Chinese) bright.

Qusay (Arabic) distant.
Qusai

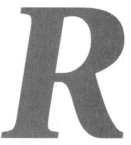

Raamah (Hebrew) thunder.
Raama, Rama, Ramah

Raanan (Hebrew) fresh.
Ranan

Rabbi (Hebrew) master.
Rabby, Rabi

Rabi (Arabic) breeze.
Rabee, Rabey, Rabie, Raby

Raby (Scottish) brightly famous.
Rabee, Rabey, Rabi, Rabie

Race (English) competitive; one who races.
Racee, Racel, Racer

Rachamin (Hebrew) compassionate.
Racham, Rachaman, Rachamin, Rachamyn, Rachim, Rachman,

R

Rachmiel, Rachmyel, Rachum,
Raham, Rahamim, Rahamym

Rad (Old English) counsellor.
Radd, Radel, Radell

Radbert (Old English) brilliant
counsellor.
Radbirt, Radburt, Radbyrt, Raddbert,
Raddbirt, Raddburt, Raddbyrt

Radburn (Old English) from the
red, reedy brook.
Radbern, Radborn, Radborne,
Radburne, Radbyrn, Radbyrne

Radcliffe (Old English) from the red
cliff.
Radclif, Radcliff, Radclith,
Radclithe, Radclyth, Redclif,
Redcliff, Redcliffe, Redclyth

Radek (Czech) famed ruler.
Radec, Radeque

Radimir (Czech) the joy of fame.
Radymir

Radley (Old English) from the red
meadow.
Radlea, Radleah, Radlee, Radleigh,
Redlee, Redleigh, Redley, Redli,
Redlie, Redly

Radman (Slavic) happy.
Raddman, Reddman, Redman

Radnore (Old English) from the red
shore.
Radnore, Rednor, Rednore

Radolf (Old English) swift wolf
counsellor.
Radolph

Radomil (Czech) one who loves
peace.
Radomyl

Radoslav (Polish) gloriously happy.
Radik, Rado, Radoslav, Radzmir,
Radzmyr

Radwan (Arabic) delightful.
Radwen, Radwin, Radwon, Radwyn

Rafa (Hebrew) to cure.
Rafah

Rafael/Rapheal (Spanish/Hebrew)
God has healed.
Rafaele (Ital), Rafaell, Rafaelle
(Fren), Rafaello, Rafaelo, Rafal
(Pol), Rafel, Rafeal, Rafee, Rafelle,
Rafello, Rafer (Heb), Raffael,
Raffael (Ital), Raffaelius (Lith),
Raffaell, Raffaello (Ital), Raffer
(Heb)

Rafat (Arabic) one who is merciful.

Rafferty (Irish/Gaelic) rich; son of
prosperity.
Rafertee, Rafertey, Raferti, Rafertie,
Raferty

Rafi (Arabic) highly praised.
Rafee, Rafey, Raffee, Raffey, Raffi,
Raffie, Raffin, Raffy, Raffyn, Rafie,
Rafin, Rafy, Rafyn

Rafiq (Arabic) friend.
Rafeeq, Rafic, Rafique, Rafyq,
Rafyqu, Rafyque

Rafu (Japanese) net.

Raghib (Arabic) desired.
Raghyb, Raquib, Raquyb

Raghid (Arabic) happy.

Raghnall (Irish) wise; powerful.
Raghnal, Ragnal, Ragnall

Ragnar (Norwegian/Swedish)
mighty army.
Ragner, Ragnir, Ragnor, Ragnyr,
Rainer, Raynar, Rayner, Raynor,
Rainier

Ragnvald (Scandinavian) judgment
that is powerful.

Rago (Hausa) ram.

R

Raguso (Italian) from the city of Ragusa in Sicily.

Raheem/Rahim (Punjabi) God is compassionate. (Arab) merciful.
Raeman, Raemen, Raemin, Raemon, Raemyn, Raheem, Raheim, Rahiim, Rahmatt, Rahmen, Rahmet, Rahmin, Rahmon, Rahmyn, Raiman, Raimen, Raimin, Raimon, Raimyn, Raman, Ramen, Ramin, Ramon, Ramyn, Rayman, Raymen, Raymin, Raymon, Raymyn

Rahul (Arabic) one who travels.

Raid (Arabic) leader.
Rayd

Raiden (Japanese) god of thunder.
Rayder

Rain (English) precipitation; rain.
Raen, Raene, Raine, Rayn, Rayne

Raine (English) lord; wisdom.
Raen, Raene, Raines, Rain, Rains, Rayn, Rayne

Rainer (Old German) warrior of judgment; counsellor.
Rain (Eng), Raina, Raine, Raineier, Rainey (Ger)Ranier (Fren), Ranieri (Ital), Ranierie, Raynar, Rayner, Raynier, Raynor, Reignier (Fren), Reinar, Reiner, Reynar, Reyner, Reynir, Reynor

Rainhart (German) judgment that is great.
Raynhart

Raini (Native American) creator god.
Rainee, Rainie, Rainy, Raynee, Rayney, Rayni, Raynie, Rayny

Raja (Australian Aboriginal) the stars. (Hindi) king.
Rajah, Raji

Rajabu (Swahili) born in the seventh month of the Islamic calendar.

Rajak (Hindi) pure.

Rajiv (Hindi) stripe.

Rakin (Arabic) respectable.
Rakeen, Rakyn

Raktim (Hindi) bright red.
Raktym

Raleigh (Old English) from the clearing in the red roe-deer (small graceful deer) meadow.
Raelea, Raeleah, Raelee, Raeleigh, Raeley, Railea, Raileah, Railee, Raileigh, Railey, Rawlea, Rawleah, Rawlee, Rawleigh, Rawley, Raylea, Rayleah, Raylee, Rayleigh, Rayley

Ralph (Old Norse) wolf counsellor.
Radulf, Raffe, Rafe, Ralf, Raoul (Fren), Raul (Rom), Roelof (Dut), Rolf, Rolph, Rou (Fren)

Ralston (Old English) dweller at Ralph's town; dweller at the wolf counsellor's town.
Ralfston, Ralfstone, Ralfton, Ralftone, Ralphstone, Ralphton, Ralphtone, Ralstone, Ralstyn

Ram (English) male sheep.

Rambert (Old German) mighty brilliant.
Rambirt, Ramburt, Rambyrt

Ramelan (Indonesian) prophecy.
Rameland

Rameses (Egyptian) sun.

Ramiah (Hebrew) praise the Lord.
Ramia, Ramya, Ramyah

Ramiro (Portuguese/Spanish) supreme judge.
Rameriz, Ramirez, Ramos, Ramyro

R

Ramon (Spanish/English) mighty and wise protector.
Ramone, Ramones, Remon, Remone, Remones, Romon, Romone, Romones

Ramsay (Old English) from the ram or raven island; the wild garlic island.
Ramsee, Ramsey, Ramsi, Ramsie, Ramsy

Ramsden (Old English) from the ram's valley.
Ramsdan, Ramsdin, Ramsdon, Ramsdyn

Ranan (Hebrew) fresh; luxuriant.
Ranen, Ranin, Ranon, Ranun, Ranyn

Rance (African) borrowed. (Fren) marble.
Rancel, Rancell, Ransel, Ransell

Rand (English) warrior.
Rando

Randall/Randolph/Randy (Old English) shield; wolf.
Randal, Randall, Randee, Randel, Randell, Randey, Randi, Randie, Randolf, Randolfe, Randolphe, Randolpus, Randulf, Randulfe, Randulph, Randulphe

Ranen (Hebrew) happy singer.
Ranan, Ranin, Ranon, Ranun, Ranyn

Ranger (Old French) protector of the forest.
Rainger, Range, Raynger, Reinger, Reynger

Rangi (Maori) sky.
Rangee, Rangey, Rangie, Rangy

Rangle (American/English) cowboy.
Rangla, Ranglah, Ranglar, Rangler, Wrangla, Wranglah, Wranglar, Wrangler

Rangsey (Cambodian) seven colours.
Rangslea, Rangsleah, Rangslee, Rangleigh, Rangsli, Rangslie, Rangsly

Rani (Hebrew) my song of happiness.
Ranee, Ranen, Raney, Ranie, Ranit, Ranon, Rany, Ranyt

Ranier (English) great army.
Ranyer

Ranjit (Hindi) delightful.

Rankin (Old English) little shield; little protector.
Rankyn

Ranon (Hebrew) happy.
Ranan, Ranen, Ranin, Ranyn

Ransford (Old English) from the raven's river crossing.
Ransforde, Rensford, Rensforde

Ransley (Old English) from the raven's meadow.
Ranslea, Ransleah, Ranslee, Ransleigh, Ransli, Ranslie, Ransly, Renslee, Rensleigh, Rensley, Rensli, Renslie, Rensly

Ransom (Old English) son of the shield; son of the warrior.
Randsom, Randsome, Ransome

Ranwul (Australian Aboriginal) ancient.
Ranwil, Ranwyl

Raoul/Raul (French/German) famous wolf. A form of Rudolph. (O/Nors) wolf counsel.
Raol, Raulas (Lith), Reuel

Raphah (Hebrew) high; tall.
Rapha

Rapier (French) sharp as a blade.
Rapyer

Raquib (Arabic) protecting guardian.
Raquyb

Ras (Arabic) cape.
Raz

Rashad (Arabic) wise counsellor.
Raashad, Rachad, Rachard, Rachaud, Raeshad, Raishard, Rashaad, Rashaud, Rashid, Rashod, Rayshaad, Rayshod, Rhasaad, Rhasad

Rashaun (African American/Irish) God is gracious. A form of Shaun.
Rasean, Rashaughn, Rashawn, Rashon

Rashid (Arabic) giver of directions.
Rasheed, Rasheid, Rasheyd, Rashida, Rashidah, Rashied, Rashieda, Rashyd, Raushaid

Rashida (Swahili) righteous.
Rasheed, Rasheeda, Rasheid, Rasheyd, Rashidah, Rashied, Rashieda, Rashyda, Raushaida

Rashidi (Swahili) sound advice.

Rasmus (Greek) loved.

Ratan (Hindi) gem.

Rauf (Arabic) kind-hearted.

Rav/Ravi (Hindi) sun.
Ravee, Ravijot, Ravy

Raven (Old English) the raven bird; black-haired.
Ravan, Ravin, Ravon, Ravone, Ravonne, Ravyn, Ravynn

Ravia (Hebrew) fourth-born child.
Raviah, Raviya, Raviyah

Ravid (Hebrew) rain or dew; adorned with jewellery.
Raviv, Ravyd, Ravyv

Rawdon (Old English) from the rough hill.
Rawdan, Rawden, Rawdin, Rawdyn

Rawleigh (English) from the meadow of the deer.
Rawlea, Rawleah, Rawlee, Rawley, Rawli, Rawlie, Rawly

Rawlins/Rawson (Old English) son of the little wolf counsellor.
Rawlin, Rawling, Rawlings, Rawlyn, Rawlyng, Rawlyngs, Rawsan, Rawen, Rawsin, Rawsyn

Ray (Old French) king. The short form of names starting with 'Ray' e.g. Raymond.
Rae, Rai, Raie, Raye, Rey

Rayburn (Old English) from the roe-deer (small graceful deer) stream.
Raebourn, Raebourne, Raeburn, Raeburne, Raibourn, Raibourne, Raiburn, Raiburne, Raybourn, Baybourne, Rayburne, Reibourn, Reinourne, Reiburn, Reiburne, Reybourn, Reybourne, Reyburn, Reyburne

Raydon (Old English) from the rye hill.
Raedan, Raeden, Raedin, Raedon, Raedyn, Raidan, Raiden, Raidin, Raidon, Raidyn, Reidan, Reiden, Reidin, Reidon, Reidyn, Reydan, Reyden, Reydin, Reydon, Reydyn

Rayfield (English) from the stream in the field.
Raefield, Raifield, Reifield, Reyfield

Rayford (Old English) from the stream ford (shallow river crossing).
Raeford, Raeforde, Raiford, Raiforde, Reiford, Reiforde, Reyford, Reyforde

Rayhan (Arabic) favoured by God.
Raehan, Raihan

Raymond (Old English) mighty,
wise protector.
Raimo (Finn), Rainmond (Fren),
Raimondo (Ital), Raimous,
Raimund (Ger), Raimundas (Lith),
Raimundus, Raimundo (Span/Ital),
Ramon (Span), Raymund,
Raymundo, Reaman, Reamonn
(Ir), Reamyn, Redmon, Redmond,
Reidman, Reidmond, Reimond,
Reimund (Dut/Ger), Reymon,
Reymond, Reymondo, Reymun,
Reymund, Reymundo

Raynor (Scandinavian) mighty
army.
Ragnar, Rainar, Rainer, Rainier
(Ger), Rainor, Ranier, Ranieri,
Raynar, Rayner, Raynier, Raynieri,
Regnier

Rayshod (Arabic/American) wise
counsellor.
Raeshod, Raishod

Raz/Razi (Hebrew) secret.
Razee, Razey, Razie, Raziel, Raziq,
Razy

Raza (Hindi) contented.
Razah

Razzaq (Arabic) provider.
Razaq

Reade/Red/Reed (Old English/
Australian) red-haired.
Read, Redd, Reid, Reide, Reyd,
Reyde

Reading (Old English) Reade's son;
son of the red-haired one.
Redding, Reedeing, Reiding

Reagan (Irish) little king.
Raegan, Raegin, Raegon, Raegyn,
Raigan Raigen, Raigin, Raigon,
Raigyn, Raygan, Raygen, Raygin,
Raygon, Raygyn, Reegan, Reegen,
Reegin, Reegon, Reegyn, Regan,
Regen, Regin, Regon, Regyn,

Reigan, Reigen, Reigin, Reigon,
Reigyn, Reygan, Reygen, Reygin,
Reygon, Reygyn

Reba (Hebrew) fourth-born child.
Rebah

Rebel (English/American)
rebellious.
Rebell, Rebil, Rebill, Rebyl, Rebyll

Rechab (Hebrew) rider of horses.

Reda (Arabic) satisfied.
Redah, Rida, Ridah

Redford (Old English) from the red
shallow river crossing.
Radford

Redley (Old English) dweller at the
red meadow.
Radlea, Radleah, Radlee, Radleigh,
Radley, Radli, Radlie, Radly, Redlea,
Redleah, Redlee, Redleigh, Redley,
Redli, Redlie, Redly

Redman (Old English) red-haired
man.
Radman, Radmann, Redmann

Redmund (Old (German))
protecting counsellor. The Irish
form of Raymond, mighty, wise
protector.
Radmon, Radmond, Radmondo,
Radmun, Radmund, Radmundo,
Redmon, Redmond, Redmondo,
Redmun, Redmundo

Redpath (English) from the red
path.
Raddpath, Radpath, Reddpath

Redwald (Old English) mighty
counsellor.
Radwald, Radweld, Radwold,
Redwold

Reece (Welsh) enthusiastic; ardent.
Reace, Rease, Rees, Reese, Reice,
Reyce, Reyse, Rhys, Rhyse

Reeve (Middle English) steward.
Reav, Reave, Reeves, Reive, Reyve,
Rhyve

Reg (English) advisor of the king.
The short form of names starting
with 'Reg' e.g. Reginald.
Regg, Reggi, Reggie, Reggy, Regi,
Regie, Regy

Regan (Irish/Gaelic) little king.
Raegan, Raegin, Raegon, Raegyn,
Raigan Raigen, Raigin, Raigon,
Raigyn, Raygan, Raygen, Raygin,
Raygon, Raygyn, Reegan, Reegen,
Reegin, Reegon, Reegyn, Regen,
Regin, Regon, Regyn, Reigan,
Reigen, Reigin, Reigon, Reigyn,
Reygan, Reygen, Reygin, Reygon,
Reygyn

Regin (Scandinavian) judge.
Regan, Regen, Regon, Regyn

Reginald (Old English) powerful;
mighty.
Raghnall (Ir), Rajnold (Pol),
Raonmill, Raynold, Reginauld,
Reginaldas, Reginaldus (Lith),
Regnaud (Fren), Rein (Est), Reinald
(Ger), Reinaldo (Span), Reinhold
(Swed/Dan), Reinis (Lett), Reinold
(Dut), Reinoldos (Span), Reinwald
(Ger), Renato (Span), Renault
(Fren), Rene (Fren), Reynald,
Reynold, Rinaldo (Ital), Ryginald,
Ryginaldo

Regis (Latin) regal.
Regiss, Regys, Regyss

Rehema (Swahili) second-born
child.
Rehemah

Rei (Japanese) law.
Rey

Reidar (Norwegian) warrior of the
nest.
Reydar

Reinhart (German/French) wise;
bold; courageous.
Rainert, Rainhard, Rainhardt,
Rainhart, Reinart, Reinhard,
Reinhardt, Renke, Reynart,
Reynhard, Reynhardt

Reju (Finnish/English) rich,
powerful, hard ruler. A form of
Richard.

Remi/Remington (French/English)
from the raven's town.
Remee, Remey, Remie, Remmee,
Remmey, Remmi, Remmie,
Remmy, Remy

Remigius/Remus (Latin) fast.
Remas, Remigyus, Remos,
Remygius, Remygyus

Renald/Renalds/Renaldo (Spanish/
English) advisor of the king. A
form of Reynold, powerful;
mighty.
Rainald, Rainaldo, Raynold,
Raynaldo, Reinald, Reinaldo,
Reynoldo, Rinald, Rinaldo, Rynald,
Rynaldo

Renato (Italian) reborn.
Renatis, Renatus (Lat), Renatys

Renaud (French) powerful.

Rendor (Hungarian) police officer.
Rendar, Render, Rendir, Rendtr

Rene (French) reborn.
Renee

Renfred (English) strong peace.
Ranfred, Ranfrid, Ranfryd, Rinfred,
Rinfryd, Ronfred, Ronfryd, Rynfred,
Rynfryd

Renfrew (Old English) from the still
river.
Ranfrew

Renjiro (Japanese) virtuous.
Renjyro

R

Renny (Irish) small strength. The short form of names starting in 'Ren' e.g. Renato, reborn.
Renee, Reney, Reni, Renie, Rennee, Renney, Renni, Reny

Reno (English) fame. (Amer) one who gambles.
Renos, Renot, Rino, Rinos, Ryno

Renshaw (Old English) from the raven's forest.
Ranshaw, Ranshore, Renshore

Renton (Old English) from the roe-deer (small graceful deer) town.
Rentown

Renzo (Latin) crown of laurel leaves; victory. The short form of Lorenzo.

Reuben (Hebrew) son.
Reaven, Reuven (Heb), Rouvin, Ruban, Ruben (Span), Rubin, Rubon, Rubun, Rubyn

Reuel (Hebrew) friend of God.
Ruel

Rex (Latin) king.
Rei (Span), Rexx, Rey (Span), Roi (Fren)

Rexford (Old English) dweller at the king's ford.
Rexforde

Rexton (English) from the king's town.

Reyhan (Arabic) favoured by God.
Reihan, Reiham, Reyham

Reynard (Old French) fox. (Ger) mighty.
Raenard, Rainard, Raynard, Reinhard (Ger), Reiyard, Renard (Fren), Renaud (Fren)

Reynold (Old English) powerful; mighty.
Raenold, Rainold, Raynold, Reinold, Renard, Renardo, Renato, Renaud, Reynolds

Rez (Hungarian) red-haired; copper.

Rezin (Hebrew) delightful.
Rezan, Rezen, Rezi, Rezie, Rezon, Rezy, Rezyn

Rhesa (Greek) chief.
Rhesah

Rhett (Old English) mighty; red. (Wel) ardent; enthusiastic.
Rhet

Rhidian (Welsh) dweller by the river crossing.
Rhydian

Rhodes (Greek) from where the roses grow; from Rhodes.
Rhoads, Rhodas, Rodas

Rhodri (Welsh) wheel ruler.

Rhun (Welsh) grand.
Rhu

Rhydwyn (Welsh/Old English) friend from the white river crossing.
Rhiwin, Rhiwyn

Rhys (Old Welsh) ardent; enthusiastic.
Reace, Rease, Reece, Reese, Reice, Reise, Reyce, Reyse, Rhyse

Rice (English) rich; noble.
Reace, Reece, Reice, Reyce, Ryce

Rich/Richie/Richard/Ricardo (Old German) rich, powerful, hard ruler.
Racardo, Recardo, Ric, Ricard, Ricardo (Ital/Port), Riccard, Riccardo, Ricco, Ricehard, Rich, Richee, Richey, Richi, Richie, Richards, Richardo, Richardus (Lith), Richart, Riik (Neth), Riikard, Rijkard (Dut), Riocard,

R

Rich/Richie/Richard/Ricardo cont.
Ritchard, Ritchardt, Ritchee, Ritchey, Ritchi, Ritchie, Ritchird, Ritchy, Ritchyrd, Rych, Rychard, Rychardo, Rychardt, Rychee, Rychey, Rychi, Rychie, Rychird, Rychy, Rychyrd

Richman (English) wealthy man.
Richmen, Rychman, Rychmen

Richmond (Old French/Old English) from the powerful, hard mountain. (O/Ger) powerful protector.
Richman, Richmand, Richmando, Richmon, Richmondo, Richmondt, Richmound, Richmun, Richmund, Richmunde, Richmundo, Rychman, Rychmand, Rychmon, Rychmond, Rychmondo, Rychmont, Rychmun, Rychmund, Rychmundo, Rychmunt

Rick/Rickard (German) rich, powerful, hard ruler. A form of Richard.
Rashard (Af/Amer), Ric, Ricard, Ricardo (Ital/Port), Rickard (Swed), Rickardo, Rik, Rikard, Rikardo, Riki (Est), Riqui (Span), Ryc, Ryck, Ryckard, Ryckardo, Rykard, Rykardo

Ricker (English) powerful army.
Ricka, Rickah, Rickar, Rikar, Ryckar, Rykar

Rickward (English) great guardian.
Ricward, Ryckward, Rycward

Rico (Spanish) ruler of the home. The Spanish form of Henry.
Ricco, Rycco, Ryco

Rida (Arabic) favoured.
Raza, Ridah, Ryda, Rydar, Ryder

Riddock (Old English) from the smooth field.
Riddoc, Riddok, Ridoc, Ridock, Ridok, Rydoc, Rydock, Rydok

Rider (Old English) horse rider.
Ridar, Ridley, Rydar, Rydder, Ryder, Ryderson

Ridge (Old English) from the ridge.
Rydge

Ridgeway (Old English) from the road at the ridge.
Rydgeway

Ridgley (Old English) dweller by the ridged meadow.
Ridglea, Ridgleah, Ridglee, Ridgleigh, Ridgli, Ridglie, Ridgly, Rydglea, Rydgleah, Rydglee, Rydgleigh, Rydgli, Rydglie, Rydgly

Ridley (Old English) from the red meadow.
Ridlea, Ridleah, Ridlee, Ridleigh, Ridly, Rydlee, Rydleigh, Rydli, Rydlie, Rydly

Riel (Spanish/Hebrew) the strength of God. The short form of Gabriel.
Reill, Reille, Riell, Rielle, Ryel, Ryelle

Rigby (Old Norse) from the farm on the ridge; the ruler's valley.
Rigbee, Rigbey, Rigbi, Rigbie, Rygbee, Rygbey, Rygbi, Rygbie, Rygby

Rigel (Arabic) foot.
Rygel

Rigg (Old English) from the ridge.
Rig, Riggs, Rigo, Ryg, Rygg, Ryggs, Rygs

Riley (Irish/Gaelic) valiant; war-like.
Reilea, Reileah, Reilee, Reileigh, Reili, Reilie, Reillea, Reilleah, Reillee,

R

Reilleigh, Reilli, Reillie, Reilly, Reily, Rylea, Ryleah, Rylee, Ryleigh, Ryley, Ryli, Rylie, Ryly

Rimon (Hebrew) pomegranate, a shrub with red fruit.
Rymon

Rimu (Polynesian) tree.
Rymu

Ring (English) gold band.
Ryng

Ringo (Old English) bell ringer. (Jap) apple.
Ryngo

Rio (Spanish) river.
Ryo

Riordan (Irish/Gaelic) royal poet.
Ryordan

Rip (Dutch) full grown; ripe. The short form of Ripley.
Ripp, Ryp, Rypp

Ripley (Old English) from the shouter's meadow; from the strip of wood in the clearing.
Riplea, Ripleah, Riplee, Ripleigh, Ripli, Riplie, Riply, Ripplee, Rippleigh, Rippley, Rippli, Ripplie, Ripply, Ryplea, Rypleah, Ryplee, Rypleigh, Rypley, Ripli, Ryplie, Rypplea, Ryppleah, Rypplee, Ryppleigh, Ryppley, Ryppli, Rypplie, Rypply, Ryply

Rishi (Hindi) sage.
Ryshi

Risley (Old English) from the brushwood meadow.
Rislea, Riselah, Rislee, Risleigh, Risley, Risli, Rislie, Risly, Ryslea, Rysleah, Ryslee, Rysleigh, Rysley, Rysli, Ryslie, Rysly

Risto (Finnish/Hebrew) Christ bearer. A form of Christopher.
Christo, Rysto

Riston (Old English) from the brushwood town.
Ryston, Wriston, Wryston

Ritter (German) knight.
Rittar, Ryttar, Rytter

Rivai (Hebrew) conflict.
Ryvai

River (Latin) dweller at the river bank.
Riv, Riva, Rivah, Rivar, Rive (Fren), Rivers, Riverton, Rivington, Ryv, Ryva, Ryvah, Ryver

Riverina (Australian/English) from the river region.
Rivereena, Rivereenah, Riverinah, Riveryna, Riverynah, Ryvereena, Ryvereenah, Ryverina, Ryverinah, Riveryna, Ryverynah

Roadie (English/Australian) road worker.
Rhoadee, Rhodey, Rhodi, Rhodie, Rhody, Roadee, Roadey, Roadi, Roady

Roald (Old German) famous ruler.

Roan (English) dweller near the rowan tree.
Roen, Rowan, Rowen, Rowin, Rowon, Rowyn

Roana (Spanish) red/brown colour.
Roanah

Roar (Norwegian) warrior.

Roarke (Irish/Gaelic) famous ruler.
Rork, Rorke, Rourk, Rourke, Ruark

Rob/Robby/Robert/Roberto (English) famous; brilliant.
Riobard (Ir), Rob (Eng/Austra), Robars, Robart, Robb, Robbee,

R

Rob/Robby/Robert/Roberto cont.
Robbey, Robbi, Robbie, Robby,
Robee, Robertas (Lith), Robertino
(Ital), Roberto (Span/Ital/Port),
Roberts, Robey, Robi, Robie, Robin,
Robinson, Robirt, Robirte, Roby,
Robyn, Robyrt, Robyrt, Rupert,
Ruperto, Ruprecht (Ger)

Robertson (English) son of the
famous brilliant one.
Robirtson, Roburtson, Robyrtson

Robin (English) the robin bird. A
form of Robert.
Roban, Robban, Robben, Robbin,
Robbins, Robbon, Robbyn, Roben,
Robon, Robyn

Robinson (English) Robin's son;
son of the robin bird.
Robynson

Rocco (Italian) stone.
Rocca, Rocki, Rockie, Rocko, Rocky,
Rokko, Roko, Roqu, Roque

Roch (Old German) tranquility.
Rocco, Roche

Rochester (Old English) from the
stone camp.

Rock (Old English) from the stone.
Roc, Rockee, Rockey, Rocki, Rockie,
Rocky, Rok

Rockford (English) from the stony
river crossing.

Rockland (English) from the stony
land.
Rocklan

Rockledge (English) from the stony
ledge.
Ledg, Ledge, Roc, Rock, Rocki,
Rockie, Rocky

Rockley (English) from the stony
meadow.
Rocklea, Rockleah, Rocklee,
Rockleigh, Rockli, Rocklie, Rockly

Rockwell (Old English) from the
stone by the stream.
Rockwel, Rocwel, Rocwell, Rokwel,
Rokwell

Rocky (English) from the stone.
Rockee, Rockey, Rocki, Rockie,
Rokee, Rokey, Roki, Rokie, Roky

Rod (Old German) famous ruler.
The short form of names starting
with 'Rod' e.g. Roderick.
Rodd

Rodas (Greek/Spanish) where roses
grow.

Rodden (Old English) from the roe-
deer (small graceful deer) valley;
from the reed valley.
Rodan, Roden, Rodin, Rodon,
Rodyn, Roedan, Roeddan,
Roedden, Roeddin, Roeddon,
Roeddyn, Roeden, Roedin, Roedon,
Roedyn

Roderick/Rodrik (Old German)
famous ruler.
Hrorek, Rennell, Rhodri, Rhoderic,
Rhoderick, Rhoderik, Rhoderyc,
Rhoderyck, Rhoderyk, Rodaric,
Rodarick, Rodarik, Roderic,
Roderich (Ger), Roderigo, Rodric,
Rodrick, Rodrik, Roderikis (Lith),
Roderikus, Roderyc, Roderyck,
Roderyk, Rodrigo (Span/Ital),
Rodringo, Rodrigue (Fren),
Rodrique (Fren), Rodryc, Rodryck,
Rodryk, Ruaidhri (Ir), Ruric (Rus),
Rurik (Slav), Ruy (Span)

Rodmann (Old English) one who
rides with the knight; from the
clearing.
Rodman

R

Rodney (Old English) from the
famous one's clearing on the
island.
Roddnee, Roddney, Roddni,
Roddnie, Roddny, Rodnee, Rodni,
Rodnie, Rodny

Rodwell (Old English) dweller at
the cross near the stream.
Roddwel, Roddwell, Rodwel

Roe (Middle English) the roe-deer
(small graceful deer).
Row, Rowe

Rogan (Irish/Gaelic) red-haired.
Rogen, Rogin, Rogon, Rogun,
Rogyn

Rogelio (Spanish) famous warrior.
Rogelyo

Roger (Old German) renowned
spear user.
Hrodjier, Raadgjer (Nrs), Rekkerts
(Lith), Rodga, Rodgah, Rodgar,
Rodger, Rodgir, Rodgyr, Rogerio
(Span), Rogerius, Rogero (Ital),
Rogers, Rogier (Pol/Dut), Rogerio
(Span), Rogir, Rogyer, Rottgers
(Ger), Rozer (Rus), Rudiger (Ger),
Ruggiero (Ital), Rutger (Dut),
Rutgert, Ruttger, Rydygier

Rohan (Hindi) sandalwood.
Roan, Roane, Roen, Roene, Rowan

Rohin (Hindi) path leading upward.
Rohyn

Rohit (Hindi) big, beautiful fish.
Rohyt

Roja (Spanish) red.
Rojai, Rojay

Roka (Japanese) wave.
Rokah

Roland (Old German) from the
famous land.
Orland, Orlando (Ital), Roeland,
Rolandas (Lith), Rolando
(Ital/Span/Port), Roldan (Span),
Rodhlann (Ir), Roeland (Dut),
Rolland, Rollando, Rollin, Rollins,
Rowland (O/Eng), Ruland (Ger),
Rudlaud (Ger)

Rolf (Old German) famous wolf.
The short form of Rudolph.
Rolfe, Rolo (Nrs), Rolph, Rolphe

Rolon (Spanish) famous wolf.
Rollon

Rolt (Old German) famous power.

Romain/Roman (French/Latin)
from Rome.
Roma, Romane, Romas (Port),
Romain, Romano (Ital), Romayn,
Romayne, Romin, Romyn,
Rumanus

Romany (Gypsy) wanderer; gypsy.
Romanee, Romaney, Romani,
Romanie

Romeo (Italian) from Rome.
Romio, Romyo

Romney (Welsh) curving river.
Romaos, Romero, Romni, Romnie,
Romny

Romy (Italian/Latin) from Rome.
The short form of Roman.
Romee, Romey, Romi, Romie

Ron/Ronnie/Ronlad (Old Norse)
powerful. The short form of
names starting with 'Ron' e.g.
Ronald.
Raghnall (Ir), Ranald, Ranaldo,
Renaldo (Span), Ronaldo
(Span/Port), Ronee, Roney, Roni,
Ronie, Ronn, Ronnee, Ronney,
Ronni, Ronnie, Ronny, Rony,
Rynald, Rynaldo

Ronan (Celtic) little seal; promise.
Rona

Rondel (French) short poem.
Rondal, Rondale, Rondall,
Rondeal, Rondell

Rondre (African American)
powerful; strong; brave;
courageous. A combination of
Ronald/Andre.

Ronel (Hebrew) the joy of God's
song.
Ronal, Ronil, Ronnel, Ronnell,
Ronol, Ronyl

Roni (Hebrew) my song of joy.
Rani, Ranie, Roneet, Ronit, Ronyt

Ronson (Old English) son of the
mighty, powerful one.
Bronan, Bronsan, Bronsen,
Bronsin, Bronson, Ronan, Ronsen,
Ronsin, Ronsun, Ronsyn

Roone (Old English) mysterious,
magic sign. (O/Eng) counsel.
Roon, Rune

Rooney (Irish/Gaelic) red-haired.
Roonee, Rooni, Roonie, Roony,
Rowan, Rowen, Rowney

Roosevelt (Old Dutch) from the
rose field.

Roper (Old English) maker of rope.

Rory (Irish/Gaelic) the red king.
Roree, Rorey, Rori, Rorie, Ruaidhri
(Ir), Rurik (Slav)

Rosario (Portuguese) rosary.
Rosaryo

Roscoe (Scandinavian) from the
deer forest; red. (Scot/Gae)
headland. (O/Ger) famous.
Rosco, Roscow

Roshaun (African American/Irish)
red-haired one whose God is
gracious. A combination of
Ross/Shaun.

Roshe (Hebrew) chief.
Rak (Rus), Rosh

Rosito (Filipino) rose.
Rosyto

Roslin (Old French) from the cape;
headland meadow. (O/Eng) from
the rose pool. The masculine
form of Rosalin.
Roslyn, Rozlin, Rozlyn

Rosmer (Danish) seahorse.
Rozmer

Ross (Old French) red-haired.
(Scot/Gae) headland. (O/Ger)
famous. (Scot/Gae) from the
peninsula.
Ros, Rosse

Roswald (Old English) from the
field of roses. (Dan) horsepower.
Roswold

Roswel (English) from the roses by
the well.
Rosswel, Rosswell, Roswel

Roth (Old German) red-haired.
Rousse (Fren)

Rothwell (English) from the rose
well.
Rothwel

Roto (Maori) lake.

Rouke (Irish) might.
Roark, Roarke, Rork, Rorke

Rover (Middle English) one who
wanders; traveller.
Rova, Rovar, Rovir, Rovor

Row (Irish) red-haired.

Rowan (Old Norse) mountain ash
tree. (Celt) little red-haired one.
Rhoan, Rhoann, Roean, Roehan,
Rohan, Rohen, Rohin, Rohyn,
Rowen, Rowin, Rowon, Rowyn

Rowell (English) from the spring of the roe-deer (small and graceful deer).
Roewel, Roewell, Rowel

Rowland (English) from the rough land.
Roelan, Roeland, Rohlan, Rohland, Rowlan

Rowley (Old English) from the rough wood clearing.
Rowlea, Rowleah, Rowlee, Rowleigh, Rowli, Rowlie, Rowly

Rowson (Irish) Row's son; son of the red-haired one.
Rawson

Roxbury (Old English) from the castle fortress.
Roxburg, Roxburge, Roxburghe

Roy (Old French) king; royal. (Celt) red-haired. The short form of names starting with 'Roy' e.g. Royden.
Roi

Royal (Old French) royal.
Roial, Royale

Royce (Old English) prince.
Roice, Roise, Royse

Royd (English) from the clearing in the forest.
Roid, Royde

Royden (Old English) from the rye hill.
Roidan, Roiden, Roidin, Roidon, Roidyn, Royden, Roydin, Roydun, Roydyn

Royston (Old English) from the town by a stone cross.
Roiston, Roystown

Rozario (Latin) rosary.
Rozaryo

Rozen (Hebrew) leader.

Ruadhan (Irish) little one with red hair.

Rudd (Old English) red/brown-complexioned.
Ruddey, Ruddi, Ruddie, Ruddy

Rudo (African) love.

Rudolph (Old German) famous wolf.
Hrolf, Hrudolf, Raoul, Ridolfo, Rodolf, Rudolf (Ger/Swed/Hung/Pol), Rodol (Span/Ital), Rodolphe (Fren), Rohlops (Let), Rudi (Swis), Rudolf, Rudolfas (Lith), Rudolfe, Rudolfo (Span), Ruedolf

Rudy (Old English) red/brown-complexioned.
Rudee, Rudey, Rudi, Rudie, Rudy

Rudyard (Old English) from the red enclosure.

Ruff (French) red-haired.
Ruf (Pol), Ruffin, Ruffyn, Rufin, Rufyn

Ruford (Old English) from the red ford (shallow river crossing).

Rufus (Latin) red-haired.
Grifone, Ruefus, Ruffo (Ital)

Rugby (Australian) football player. (Eng) from the rock fortress.
Rugbee, Rugbey, Rugbi, Rugbie

Rule (Latin) ruler.
Reul, Reule, Ruel, Ruell, Ruelle

Rumford (English) from the wide ford.

Runako (Shona) handsome.

Rune (German/Swedish) secret.

Rungie (Australian Aboriginal) swan.
Rungi, Rungy

R

Rupert (Italian/English) famous; brilliant.
Roudbert (Fren), Ruberto, Ruepert, Ruperth (Ger), Ruperto (Ital/Span), Rupirt, Ruprat (Slav), Rupprecht (Ger), Rupyrt

Rurik (Scandinavian) famous king.
Rurek, Ruryk

Rush (French) red-haired. (O/Eng) from the rushes.

Rushford (English) from the rushes near the river crossing.
Rushforde

Rusk (Spanish) twisted beard.

Ruskin (Old French) red-haired relation.
Ruskyn

Russ/Russell (Old French) red-haired; fox.
Rusal, Rusel, Rusell, Ruskel, Ruskell, Russal, Russall, Russel, Russil, Russill, Russyl, Russyll

Rusty (Old English/Old French) red-haired.
Rust, Ruste, Rustee, Rustey, Rusti, Rustie

Rutherford (Old English) from the castle river crossing.
Ruverford

Rutland (Old Norse) from the stump.
Rutlan

Rutledge (Old English) from the red ledge.

Rutley (Old English) from the stumpy, red meadow.
Rutlea, Rutleah, Rutlee, Rutleigh, Rutli, Rutlie, Rutly

Ruud (Scandinavian) famous wolf.
Rud

Ruy (Spanish/German) famous ruler. A form of Roderick.
Rui

Ryan (Irish)/(Gaelic) little king.
Rian, Rien, Rion, Riun, Riyn, Rhian, Rhien, Rhion, Rhiun, Rhiyn, Ryann, Ryen, Ryin, Ryon, Ryun

Rycroft (Old English) from the rye field.
Ricroft

Ryder (English) rider of horses.
Rider, Rydder

Ryderson (Old English) Ryder's son; son of the horse rider.
Riderson

Rye (Polish) powerful ruler. (Eng) grain grass.
Ri, Rie, Ry

Rylan (English) dweller near the rye land.
Rilan, Riland, Ryland

Ryle (Old English) from the rye hill.
Riel, Riell, Rielle, Ryel, Ryele, Ryell, Ryelle

Ryman (Old English) seller of rye.
Riman

Rymer (Polish) saddle maker.
Rimer

Ryne (Irish) little king. A form of Ryan.
Rine

Ryton (Old English) from the rye town.
Riton

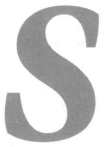

Saad (Arabic) lucky.
Sad, Sadd

Saarik (Hindi) bird.
Sarik

Saber (French) sword.
Saba, Sabah, Sabar, Sabir, Sabor,
Sabyr

Sabin (Latin) from Sabines (an
ancient Italian tribe).
Sabian, Sabyn

Sabir (Arabic) patient.
Sabar, Saber, Sabir, Sabor, Sabyr

Sabiti (Rutooro) born on a Sunday.
Sabit, Sabith, Sabyti

Sabola (Ngoni) pepper.
Sabol, Sabolah

Sabra (Hebrew) thorny cactus.
Sabrah

Saburo (Japanese) third-born child.
Saburow

Sacha (Greek) defender of
humankind. The short form of
Alexander.
Sasha

Saddam (Arabic) hard hitting.
Sadam

Sadiki (Swahili) faithful.
Saadiq, Sadiq, Sadiqua, Sadique,
Sadyki, Sadyky

Sadler (Old English) saddle maker.
Saddler

Sadoc (Hebrew) sacred.
Sadock, Sadok

Sadowy (Polish) gardener.
Sadowi, Sadowie, Sadowy

Saeed (Swahili) happy.
Saed

Safa (Arabic) purity.
Safah

Safford (English) from the willow-
tree ford.
Saford

Safwat (Arabic) selected.

Sagar (Teutonic) victorious people.
Sager, Sayar, Sayer

Sage (French) wisdom.
Saig, Saige, Sayg, Sayge

Sahaj (Hindi) natural.

Sahale (Native American) falcon
bird. (Hind) above.
Sahal, Sahan, Sahen, Sahin, Sahon,
Sahyn

Sahil (Hindi) one who leads.
Sahyl

Sahir (Arabic/Hindi) friend.
Sahyr

Sahn (Vietnamese) comparing.

Said (Arabic) happy; master.
Saeed, Saied, Sajid, Sajjid, Sayeed,
Sayid, Sayyid (Arab), Seyed

Saint (Latin) holy.
Sanche, Sanchez, Sancho, Santo,
Saynt

Sajag (Hindi) watchful.

Sajan (Hindi) loved.

Saka (Swahili) hunter.
Sakah

Sakaria (Scandinavian) God remembers.
Sakaree, Sakarey, Sakari, Sakarie, Sakary, Sakerl (Dan), Sakschej (Russ)

Sakhir (Arabic) rock.
Sakyr

Sakima (Native American) king.
Sakimah, Sakyma, Sakymah

Sal (Italian) saved. The short form of Salvatore.
Sall

Saladin (Arabic) goodness of faith.
Saladine, Saladyn, Saladyne

Salah (Arabic) virtue.

Salamao (Portuguese) little person of peace.
Salomo (Ger), Salomaun (Boh), Salomon (Fren/Hung)

Saleh (Indonesian) devout; religious.
Sale

Salene (Swahili) good.
Salin, Saline, Salyn, Salyne

Salid (Arabic) lucky.
Salyd

Salih (Arabic) just.

Salim (Arabic) peace; safety.
Salam, Salem, Salim, Salom, Salym, Salyn

Salisbury (Old English) from the fort by the willow pool.
Salisberi, Salisberie, Salisberri, Salisberrie, Salisberry, Salisbery, Salisburi, Salisburie, Salisburri, Salisburrie, Salisburry, Salysberry, Salysbery, Salysburry, Salysbury

Sallu (Swahili) safety.

Salmon (Hebrew) covering.
Salman, Salem, Salmin, Salmun, Salmyn

Salton (Old English) from the manor hall town; from the willow tree town.
Saltan, Salten, Saltin, Saltyn

Salu (Hebrew) basket.

Salvadore (Italian) saved.
Salvador (Span), Salvator, Salvatore (Ital), Sauveur (Fren)

Salvestro (Italian) found in the forest.
Sylvester

Sam (Hebrew) his name is God; asked for. The short form of names starting with 'Sam' e.g. Samuel.
Samm, Samolio (Russ)

Samani (Polynesian) salmon.
Samanie, Samany

Sambhu (Sanskrit) house of happiness.

Samgar (Persian) gracious.

Sami (Hebrew) highly praised.
Samee, Samey, Samie, Samy

Samir (Arabic) entertaining.
Samyr

Samisoni (Polynesian) sun.
Samisonie, Samisony

Samman (Arabic) food supplier.
Saman, Samen, Samin, Sammen, Sammin, Sammon, Sammun, Sammyn, Samon, Samun, Samyn

Samoset (Algonquin) walks a lot.

Samson (Hebrew) sun-like.
Sampsan, Sampsen, Sampsi, Sampson, Sampsun, Sampsyn, Sansao, Sansim (Fren), Sansom, Sansome, Sansum, Shem, Shimson, Shymson

Samuel (Hebrew) his name is God; asked for.
Samel, Samouel, Samuele, Samuell, Samuelle, Shemuel

Samuru (Japanese) sun.

Sanat (Hindi) ancient.

Sanborn (English) from the sandy stream.
Sanborne, Sanbourn, Sanbourne, Sanburn, Sanburne, Sandborn, Sandborne, Sandbourn, Sandbourne

Sancho (Spanish) saint.
Sanchaz, Sanchez, Sauncho

Sandeep (Punjabi) enlightened.

Sanders (Greek) Alexander's son; son of the defender of humankind. (O/Eng) from the beach.
Sanda, Sandas, Sander, Sanderson, Saunder, Saunders, Saunderson

Sanditon (English) from the beach town.
Sandyton

Sandler (Hebrew) shoe maker.

Sandor (Hungarian/Slavic/Greek) defender of humankind. A form of Alexander.
Sandar, Sander, Sandir, Sandur, Sandyr

Sandy (Greek) Alexander's son; son of the defender of humankind. (O/Eng) from the beach.
Sande, Sandee, Sandey, Sandi, Sandie

Sanford (English) from the beach sand bar.
Sanforde, Sansford

Sani (Hindi) saturn.
Sanee, Saney, Sania, Sanie, Sany

Sanjay (Sanskrit) one with a conscience.
Sanjai, Sanjaye, Sanjy, Sanjye

Sanjiv (Hindi) long-lived.
Sanjeev, Sanjyv

Sankara (Sanskrit) lucky; fortunate.
Sankarah

Santana (Spanish) saint.
Santanah, Santanio, Santanyo

Santerl (Bavarian) gold-coloured flower.
Santrel, Santrele, Santrell, Santrelle

Santiago (Spanish) Saint James.
Santia, Santiah, Santyago, Santya, Santyah

Santo (Spanish/Italian) Saint.
Santos

Santon (Old English) from the beach town.
Santan, Santen, Santin, Santun, Santyn

Santonia (Spanish) from San Antonio in Texas.
Santoniah, Sanantonio, Santonya, Santonyah, Santonya

Santosh (Hindi) satisfaction.
Santosha

Santoso (Indonesian) good peace.
Santosow

Sanyu (Luganda) happy.

Sanzio (Italian) Christian.
Anzio, Anzyo, Sanzyo

Saqr (Arabic) falcon.

Sarad (Hindi) born in the autumn/fall time.
Saradd

Sargent (English) military officer.
Sargant, Sarge, Sarjant, Sergeant, Sergent, Serjeant

Sargon (Persian) prince of the sun.
Sargan, Sargen, Sargin, Sargyn

Sariyah (Arabic) clouds at night time.
Sariya

Sarngin (Hindi) archer who gives protection.
Sarngyn

Sarojin (Hindi) lotus-like.
Sarojun, Sarojyn

Sasson (Hebrew) happy.
Sass

Sastra (Sanskrit) book of rules.
Sastrah

Satordi (French) saturn.
Satordia, Satordie, Satordy, Saturno (Span)

Saturn (Latin) saturn, the planet.
Saturne

Saul (Hebrew) borrowed; soul.
Saulius, Sawyl, Talut

Saula (Polynesian) ask.
Saul, Saulah

Sauts (Cheyenne) bat.

Savage (Irish/English) untamed.
Savag, Savaig, Savaige, Savyg, Savyge

Saverij (Illyrian) bright; brilliant.
Savero (Ital), Xavier, Zavier, Zavyer

Saville (French) from the village of the willow trees.
Savil, Savile, Savill, Savyl, Savyla, Savyll, Savylle

Saw (Burmese) early.

Sawney (Scottish) protector.
Sawnee,, Sawni, Sawniw, Sawny

Sawyer (English) one who works with a saw.
Sawer, Sawier, Soier

Sawyl (Welsh) child who was asked for.
Saul, Sawl

Saxby (Old Norse) from the farm with the short sword.
Saxbee, Saxbey, Saxbi, Saxbie

Saxon (English) a Saxon.
Saxan, Saxe, Saxen, Saxin, Saxus, Saxyn

Saxton (Old English) from the Saxon's town; from the town of the warrior's town.
Saxtan, Saxten, Saxtin, Saxtyn

Sayed (Arabic) prince.
Saied

Sayers (Welsh) carpenter.
Sayer, Sayre, Sayres

Scafer (German) shepherd.
Schaefer, Shaffar, Shaffer

Scanlon (Irish) little scandalous one.
Scanlan, Scanlen, Scanlin, Scanlyn

Sceva (Greek) covering.
Scevah

Schmidt (German) blacksmith.
Schmid, Schmit, Schmitt, Schmyt, Schmytt

Schmul (German) asked of God.
Schmull

Schneider (German) tailor of clothes.
Schnieder, Snider, Snyder, Snydley

Scholes (Old Norse) hut.
Schole

Schon (German) handsome.
Schonn, Shon

Schuman (German) shoe maker.
Schu, Schumann, Schumen, Schumenn, Shoe, Shoeman, Shoemann, Shoemen, Shoemenn,

S

Shoo, Shooman, Shoomann,
Shoomen, Shoomenn, Shue,
Shueman, Shuemann, Shuemen,
Shuemenn, Shu, Shuman,
Shumann, Shumen, Shumenn,
Shumyn, Shumynn, Shyman,
Shymann

Schuyler (Dutch) shield.
Schuylar, Schylar, Schyler, Schylor,
Skilar, Skiler, Skuylar, Skuyler,
Skylar, Skyler, Skylor

Scipio/Scipion (Latin) staff; stick.
Scipion (Fren), Scipione (Ital),
Scipyo, Scypion, Scypyo

Scoey (Old French) from the
Scottish one's village. The short
form of Scoville.
Scoee, Scoi, Scoie, Scowi, Scowie,
Scowy, Scoy

Scooby (English) from Scott's
nearby estate; from the Scottish
one's estate.
Scobee, Scobey, Scobi, Scobie,
Scoby, Scoobee, Scoobey, Scoobi,
Scoobie

Scorpio (Latin) scorpion.
Scorpeo, Scorpyo

Scott (Old English) from Scotland.
Scot, Skot, Skott

Scoville (Old French) from the
Scottish one's village.
Scovil, Scovile, Scovill, Scovyl,
Scovyle, Scovyll, Scovylle

Scribe (Latin) writer.
Scribner, Scrivener, Scryb, Scrybe

Scully (Irish) town crier.
Scullea, Sculleah, Scullee,
Sculleigh, Sculley, Sculli, Scullie

Seabert (English) from the shining
sea.
Seabirt, Seaburt, Seabyrt, Seebert,
Seebirt, Seeburt, Seebyrt, Seibert,

Seibirt, Seiburt, Seibyrt, Seybert,
Seybirt, Seyburt, Seybyrt

Seabrook (English) from the stream
by the sea.
Seabrooke, Seebrook, Seebrooke,
Seibrook, Seibrooke, Seybrook,
Seybrooke

Seafra (Irish) God's peace.
Seafrah

Seamus/Shamus (Irish) God is
gracious. A form of Sean/Shane.
James, Seamus (Scott), Shamis,
Shaimis, Shaimus, Shaymis,
Shaymus

Sean/Shaun/Shawn (Irish) God is
gracious. A form of John/Shane/
Shawn.
Schaun, Schaune, Schawn, Schawne,
Seaghan, Seanan, Seane, Seanen,
Seann, Seannan, Seannen, Seannon,
Seain, Seaine, Seatn, Seayne, Shane,
Shaughn, Shaun, Shaune, Shawn,
Shawne, Shon, Shorn, Shorne, Sion,
Syaun, Syawn, Syon, Syown

Seanan (Irish) old wisdom.
Senan, Sinan, Sinon, Sinyn

Searle (German) armed.
Searl, Searlas (Ir/Fren), Serl, Serle,
Serlo (Nrs)

Seaton (English) from the town
near the sea.

Seaward (English) victory peace.
Seeward, Seiward, Seyward

Seba (Greek) majestic.
Sebah

Sebastian (Latin) honoured above
all others.
Bastian, Bastien, Eigels, Sebastao
(Port), Sebaste (Fren), Sebastiano
(Ital), Sebastiao, Sebastien (Fren),
Sebastion, Sebastyn (Hung),
Sebestyen, Sepasetiano

S

Secundus (Latin) second-born child.
Secondas, Secondus, Secondys

Sed (Egyptian) saviour.
Sedd

Sedgley (Old English) from the meadow of the sword.
Sedglea, Sedgleah, Sedglee, Sedgleigh, Sedgli, Sedglie, Sedgly

Sedgwick (Old English) dweller from the place of the sword grass.
Sedgwic, Sedgwik, Sedgwyc, Sedgwyck, Sedgwyk

Seeley (Old English) blessed and happy one's meadow.
Sealea, Sealeah, Sealee, Sealeigh, Sealey, Seali, Sealie, Sealy, Seelea, Seeleah, Sealeigh, Seeli, Seelie, Seelie, Seely, Seilea, Seileah, Seilee, Seileigh, Seiley, Seili, Seilie, Seily, Seylea, Seyleah, Seylee, Seyley, Seyleigh, Seyley, Seyli, Seylie, Seyly

Seemeon (Russian) listening. A form of Simon.
Seameon, Seimein (Grk), Seymeon, Seymein, Seymon, Simeon, Simon

Sef (Egyptian) yesterday.
Seff

Sefton (Old Norse/Old English) from the place in the rushes.
Seftan, Seften, Seftin, Seftun, Seftyn

Sefu (Swahili) sword.

Segel (English) treasure.
Seagal

Seger (English) warrior of the sea.
Seagar, Seager, Seegar, Seeger, Segar

Segub (Hebrew) highly praised.

Segun (Yoruba) conquering.
Segan, Segen, Segin, Segon, Segyn

Segundo (Spanish) second-born child.

Seif (Arabic) religion's sword.
Seyf

Sein (Basque) innocent.
Seyn

Sekaye (Shona) laughing.
Sekai, Sekay

Selby (English) from the farmstead.
Selbee, Selbey, Selbi, Selbie

Selden (English) rare; strange one from the willow valley. (O/Eng) from the house on the hill.
Seldan, Seldin, Seldon, Seldyn

Seldon (Old English) from the house on the hill.
Seldan, Selden, Seldin, Seldun, Seldyn

Seled (Hebrew) to spring up.
Seledd

Selemaea (Polynesian) God will hear.

Selig (German) blessed.
Seligg, Selyg, Selygg

Selvaggio (Italian) wild.
Selvagio

Selway (Old English) rich way.
Selwai

Selwin (English) blessed friend.
Selwinn, Selwyn, Selwynn, Selwynne

Semanda (Luganda) cow.
Semandah

Semer (Ethiopian) farmer. A form of George.

Semi (Polynesian) character.
Semee, Semey, Semie, Semy

S

Sempala (Luganda) born during prosperous times.
Sempalah

Sen (Japanese) wood fairy.
Senh

Senior (Old English) lord of the manor.
Senyor

Sennett (French) old wisdom.
Senan (Ir), Senen, Senet, Senett, Senin, Senit, Senitt, Sennan, Sennen, Sennet, Sennin, Sennit, Sennyn, Sennyt, Senyn, Senyt

Senon (Spanish) live.
Senan, Senen, Senin, Senyn

Senwe (African) dry like a stalk of grain.

Seoirse (Irish) farmer. A form of George.

Sepp/Seppi (Hebrew/German/ Italian) God will increase; God has added a child. A form of Joseph.
Sep, Sepee, Sepey, Sepi, Sepie, Seppee, Seppey, Seppie, Seppy, Sepy

Septimus (Latin) seventh-born child.
Septimous

Serafino (Spanish/Italian) seraph, highest order of the angels.
Seraphino

Serapis (Egyptian) god of fertility.
Serapys

Sereno (Latin) peaceful.
Sereen, Serene, Serino, Seryno

Serge (French) moving forward.
Seargeoh, Serg, Serge, Sergei (Russ), Sergi, Serginio, Sergio (Ital), Sergios (Grk), Sergius, Sergiusz, Serguel, Serjio, Sirgio, Sirgios

Sersa (Illyrian) worthy of reverence; venerable king.
Sersah

Servaas (Scandinavian) save.

Setangya (Kiowa) sitting bear.

Seth (Hebrew) one who is appointed.

Setimba (Luganda) dweller by the river.
Setimbah

Setimkia (Kiowa) attacking bear.

Seton (English) from the place by the sea.
Seatan, Seaten, Seatin, Seaton, Seatun, Seatyn, Setan, Seten, Setin, Setun, Setyn

Severin/Seven/Severn (Latin) seventh-born child.
Seve, Severan, Sererian, Sereriano, Serero, Severen, Severyn, Sevien, Sevirn, Sevyrn, Sevrin, Sevryn

Sevilen (Turkish) loved.
Sevilan, Sevilin, Sevilon, Selilyn

Seward (English) guardian of the sea.
Seawrd, Seeward, Seiward, Seyward

Sewati (Moquelumnan) bear with curved claws.
Sewatee, Sewatey

Sewell (English) from the sea wall.
Seawal, Seawald, Seawall, Seawel, Seawell, Seewal, Seewald, Seewall, Seewel, Seewell, Seiwal, Seiwall, Seiwel, Seiwell, Sewal, Sewall, Sewel, Seywal, Seywall, Seywel, Seywell

Sexton (English) church official.
Sextan, Sexten, Sextin, Sextyn

S

Sextus (Latin) sixth-born child.
Sextis, Sextys

Seymour (French) from the moors
by the sea.
Seamoor, Seamoore, Seamor,
Seamore, Seamour, Seamoure,
Seemoor, Seemoore, Seemor,
Seemore, Seemour, Seemoure,
Seimoor, Seimoore, Seimor,
Seimore, Seimour, Seymoor,
Seymore, Seymour, Seymoure

Shachor (Hebrew) black.

Shad (Punjabi) happy, lucky one.
Shadd

Shade/Shadey/Shadoe/Shadow
(Old English) shadow cover;
dweller from the shady doe
enclosure.
Shaed, Shaede, Shaid, Shaide,
Shayd, Shayde

Shadrach (Babylonian) God-like.
Shadrac, Shadrach, Shadrack,
Shadrack, Shadrick, Shederick,
Shedrach, Shedrick, Shedrik,
Shedryc, Shedryck, Shedryk

Shadwell (Old English) from the
shad-fish stream.
Shadwal, Shadwall, Shadwel,
Shedwal, Shedwall, Shedwel,
Shedwell

Shafer (Arabic) beautiful; good.

Shah (Persian) king.

Shahid (Arabic) witness.
Shahyd

Shai/Shay (Hebrew) gift. (Ir) from
the fairy palace.
Shae, Shaye

Shaiming (Chinese) sunshine; life.
Shaimin, Shayming

Shaka (Zulu) founder of the Zulu
empire.
Shakah

Shakir (Arabic) thankful.
Shakeer, Shakur, Shakyr

Shalom (Hebrew) peace.
Shalmae, Shalmay, Shalum,
Shlomo, Sholem, Sholom

Shaman (Sanskrit/Native American)
holy one; medicine man.
Shaiman, Shaimen, Shamen,
Shayman, Shaymen

Shamin (Hebrew) perfume.
Shamym

Shanahan (Irish) wisdom.
Seanahan, Shaunahan, Shawnahan

Shandy (English) boisterous; loud;
part beer/part lemonade drink.
Shandea, Shande, Shandey, Shandi,
Shandie

Shane (Irish) God is gracious.
Chaen, Chaene, Chain, Chaine,
Chane, Chayn, Chayne, Cheyn,
Cheyne (Scott), Shaen, Shaene,
Shain, Shaine, Shayn, Shayne

Shani (Hebrew) red.
Shanee, Shaney, Shanie, Shany

Shank (Irish) God is good.

Shanley (Irish) old hero from the
meadow.
Shanlea, Shanleah, Shanlee,
Shanleigh, Shanli, Shanlie, Shanly

Shannon (Irish) hero who is wise;
small.
Shanan, Shanen, Shanin, Shanon,
Shannan, Shannen, Shannin,
Shannyn, Shanyn

Shantae (French) singer. A form of
Chante.
Shant, Shantai, Shantay, Shantel,

S

Shantell, Shantelle, Shanti, Shantie, Shanton, Shanty

Shapoor (Russian) prince.
Shapoora

Shappa (Native American) (Sioux) red thunder.
Shapa

Shaq/Shaquille (Arabic) handsome. The short form of Shaquille.
Scaq, Shaquil, Shaquile, Shaquill, Shaquyl, Shaquyle, Shaquyll, Shaquylle

Sharad (Pakistani) autumn/fall.
Sharid, Sharyd

Sharezer (Persian) prince of fire.

Sharif (Arabic) honest; noble.
Shareef, Sharef, Shareff, Shariff, Shariyf, Sharyf, Sharyff

Sharone (African American/ Hebrew) from the plains. The masculine form of Sharon.
Sharan, Sharen, Sharin, Sha Ron, Sha Rone, Sharon, Sharran, Sharren, Sharrin, Sharryn, Sharyn

Shastra (Sanskrit) giver of instructions.
Shastrah

Shattuck (Middle Eastern) little shad-fish.
Shatuck

Shavar (Hebrew) comet.
Shavara, Shavarah, Shaver, Shavir, Shavyr

Shaw (Old English) dweller at the grove.
Shawe, Shor, Shore

Shawnel (African American/Irish) God's gracious champion. A combination of Shawn/Nell.
Seanel, Shaughnel, Shaunel

Shawnta (Irish/American) God is gracious. A form of Shawn.
Seanta, Seantah, Shaunta, Shauntah, Shawntah

Shayla (Hindi) throne.
Shalyah

Shea (Irish) majestic.
Sheah

Sheach (Scottish/Irish) courteous.

Sheary (Irish) peaceful.
Shearee, Shearey, Sheari, Shearie

Shechem (Hebrew) incline.

Sheehan (Irish) little peace.
Sheehen

Sheffield (English) from the crooked field.
Sheffyeld, Shefield, Shefyeld

Shelby (Old English) from the estate by the ledge.
Shelbea, Shelbee, Shelbi, Shelbie

Sheldon (Old English) from the ledge.
Sheldan, Shelden, Sheldin, Sheldun, Sheldyn

Shelesh (Hebrew) third-born child.

Shelley (English) from the island of shells.
Shellea, Shelleah, Shellee, Shelleigh, Shelli, Shellie, Shelly

Shelpey (Old English) from the sheep meadow.
Shelpea, Shelpeah, Shelpee, Shelpeigh, Shelpi, Shelpie, Shelpy

Shelton (Old English) from the shelly beachside town.
Sheltan, Shelten, Sheltin, Sheltyn

Shem (Hebrew) reputation.

Shen (Egyptian) sacred amulet, worn to protect against evil. (Chin) meditation; spirit.

Sheng (Chinese) victory.

Shep (Old English) sheep.

Shepherd (English) sheep herder.
Shep, Shephard, Sheperd, Shepp, Sheppard, Shepperd

Shepley (Old English) from the sheep meadow.
Sheplea, Shepleah, Sheplee, Shepleigh, Shepli, Sheplie, Sheply

Sherborne (Old English) from the clear stream.
Sherborn, Sherbourn, Sherbourne

Sheridan (Irish) wild. (O/Eng) from the shire valley.
Sheriden, Sherisin, Sheridon, Sheridyn, Sherydan, Sheryden, Sherydin, Sherydon, Sherydyn

Sheriff (English) law keeper.
Sherif, Sherrif, Sherriff, Sherryf, Sherryff, Sheryf, Sheryff

Sherill (English) from the shire on the hill.
Sheril, Sheryl, Sheryll

Sherlock (Old English) one with the fair, short hair.
Sherloc, Sherloch, Sherloche, Sherlocke, Sherlok

Sherman (Old English) shearer.
Shermann, Shermen, Shirman, Shirmann, Shyrman, Shyrmann

Sherrod (English) land clearer.
Sherod

Sherwin (English) splendid friend.
Sherwinn, Sherwyn, Sherwynn, Sherwynne

Sherwood (English) from the bright woods.
Sharwood

Shihab (Arabic) fire.
Shyhab

Shilin (Chinese) intellectual.
Shilyn, Shylin, Shylyn

Shima (Japanese) island.
Shimah, Shyma, Shymah

Shimon (Hebrew) amazing.
Shimona, Shimonah, Shymon, Shymona, Shymonah

Shimshon (Hebrew) sun.

Shin (Korean) trusted.
Shyn

Shing (Chinese) victory.
Shingae, Shingo, Shyng

Shipley (Old English) dweller at the sheep meadow.
Shiplea, Shipleah, Shiplee, Shipleigh, Shipli, Shiplie, Shiply, Shyplea, Shypleah, Shyplee, Shypleigh, Shypley, Shypli, Shyplie, Shyply

Shipton (Old English) dweller at the sheep town.
Shiptan, Shipten, Shiptin, Shiptun, Shiptyn, Shyptan, Shypten, Shyptin, Shypton, Shyptyn

Shiro (Japanese) fourth-born child.
Shirow, Shyro, Shyrow

Shiva (Hindi) life; death.
Shivah, Shyva, Shyvah

Sholto (Irish/Gaelic) the teal duck. (Celt) sower of seeds.

Shomer (Hebrew) guardian.
Shomar, Shomir, Shomor, Shomyr

Shon (American/Hebrew) God is gracious. A form of Sean/John.
Shondae, Shoondai, Shondale, Shonday, Shondel, Shonntay

Shoni (Hebrew) changing.
Shonee, Shoney, Shonie, Shony

Shonkah (Osage) black dog.

Shovai (Hebrew) gem.
Shovay

Shri (Sanskrit) worthy of reverence.

Shunnar (Arabic) pheasant.
Shunar

Siaki (Polynesian) God is gracious.

Siaosi (Polynesian) farmer.
Sior

Siarl (Welsh) man.
Syarl

Sibran (Breton) from Cyprus.
Sybran

Sid (Phoenician) from St Denis. (Eng) wide. (Phoe) enchanter. A form of Sidney.
Sidd, Syd, Sydd

Siddartha (Sanskrit) accomplishment.
Sida, Siddhartha, Sidh, Sidharth, Sidhartha, Sidhdhardth, Sidhdhartha, Sydartha, Syddhartha

Siddell (Old English) from the wide valley. (O/Fren) from St Denis' valley.
Siddel, Sidel, Sidell, Sydel, Sydell

Sidney/Sydney (Old French) from St Denis. (Eng) wide. (Phoe) enchanter.
Sidnee, Sidni, Sidnie, Sidny, Sydnee, Syndey, Syndi, Sydnie, Sydny

Sidonius (Greek) fine cloth of linen.
Sidonis, Sydonis, Sydonius

Sidwell (English) from the wide stream.
Siddwal, Siddwall, Siddwel, Siddwell, Sidwal, Sidwall, Sidwel, Syddwal, Syddwall, Syddwel, Syddwell, Sydwal, Sydwall, Sydwel, Sydwell

Sierra (Irish) black. (Span) saw-like toothed. (Span/Arab) mountain.
Siera, Sierah, Sierrah, Syera, Syerah, Syerra, Syerrah

Siffredo (Italian) victorious peace.
Sifredo, Syffredo

Sigbjorn (Scandinavian) guardian bear of victory.

Sigfried (Teutonic) victorious peace.
Siffre (Fren), Sigefredo, Sigfrid (Ger), Sigfroi, Sigvard (Nor), Sygfred, Sygfreid, Sygfreyd, Sygfrid, Sygfryd, Ziegfried, Zigfrid, Zygfred, Zygfreid, Zygfid, Zygfried, Zygfryd

Sigmund (Teutonic) victorious protector.
Saegmon (Nrs), Saegmond (Nrs), Saegmun, Saegmund, Sigismond (Fren), Sigismondo (Ital), Sigismund (Ger), Sigismundo (Span), Sigismunus (Dut), Sigmundo (Ger), Sygmon, Sygmond, Sygmondo, Sygmun, Sygmund, Sygmundo, Sygismon, Sygismond, Sygimondo, Sygismun, Sygismund, Sygismundo, Sygysmon, Sygysmond, Sygysmondo, Sygysmun, Sygysmund, Sygysmundo, Zigimond, Zigimund, Zigmon, Zygismon, Zygismond, Zygismondo, Zygismun, Zygismund, Zygismundo,

Sigmund cont.
Zygysmon, Zygysmond,
Zygysmondo, Zygysmun,
Zygysmund, Zygysmundo

Sigurd (Old Norse) victorious
guardian.
Sygurd

Sigwald (Old Norse) victorious
ruler.
Sigwaldo, Sygwald, Sygwaldo

Sikueli (Tongan) squirrel.
Sykueli

Sikwaii (Cherokee) sparrow.

Silburn (Old English) child who is
blessed.
Silborn, Silborne, Silbourn,
Silbourne, Silburne, Sylborn,
Sylborne, Sylbourn, Sylbourne,
Sylburn, Sylburne

Silvan/Silvanus (Latin) forest
dweller.
Silas, Silvain (Fren), Silvano
(Ital/Span), Silvio (Ital/Span),
Sylas, Sylvanus (Eng), Sylvio-
Ital/Span)

Silvester (Latin) from the forest.
Sailbheastar (Ir), Silvestre
(Fren/Span), Silvestro (Ital),
Sylvester

Sima (Hebrew) treasure.
Simah, Syma, Symah

Simba (Swahili) lion.
Simbah, Symba, Symah

Simeon (German/French) monkey.
A form of Simon, listening.
Symeon, Symian, Symyan

Simmias (Greek) listening. A form
of Simon.
Simias, Symmias, Symmyas,
Symyas

Simms (Hebrew) Simon's son; son
of the listening one.
Sims, Symms, Syms

Simo (Finnish/Australian) obedient.
The short form of Simon,
listening.
Symo

Simon (Hebrew) listening.
Seemeon, Semein, Simanao,
Simanas, Simej (Illy), Simeon
(Fren), Simone (Ital/Fren), Simons,
Simonson, Siomon, Siomonn (Ir),
Sim (Scott), Ssemar (Russ),
Symon, Symond, Symonn,
Symonns, Szimon, Szymon (Pol),
Zimon, Zymon

Simpson (Hebrew/Old English)
Simon's son; son of the one who
listens.
Simpsan, Simpsen, Simpsin,
Simpsyn, Sympsan, Sympsen,
Sympsin, Sympson, Sympsyn

Sinbad (German) sparkling prince.
Sinbaldo, Sinbad, Sinibaldo,
Synbad, Synbald

Sinclaire (French) from St Clair's
town. (Lat) clear sign.
Sinclair, Sinclar, Sinclare, Synclair,
Synclaire, Synclar, Synckare,
Synclayr

Singer (Old English) singer.
Synger

Sinjon (English) saint.
Sinjun, Sjohn, Synjon

Sinou (Tongan) snow.
Synou

Sintram (Teutonic) sparkling raven.
Syntram

Sion (Hebrew) highly praised.
Syon

Sione (Tongan) God is gracious.
Sionee, Sioney, Sioni, Sionike,
Soane, Sone

Sipatu (Moquelumnan) pulling out.
Sypatu

Sipho (Zulu) present.
Sypho

Siraj (Arabic) light.
Syraj

Siroslav (Teutonic) famous glory.
Siroslav, Syroslav

Sisi (Fanti) born on a Sunday.
Sysi, Sysy

Sisto (Italian) sixth-born child.
Systo

Sitoake (Tongan) stork.
Sytoake

Sitriv (Norse) secure conqueror.
Sitrick, Sitrik, Sytric, Sytrick, Sytrik,
Sytryc, Sytryck, Sytryk

Sivan (Hebrew) born during the
ninth month of the Jewish year.
Syvan

Siward (English) victorious peace.
Syward

Siwili (Native American) fox's long
tail.
Siwilie, Siwily, Siwyli, Siwylie,
Siwyly, Sywili, Sywilie, Sywyly

Sixtus (Latin) sixth-born child.
Sixte, Syxte, Syxtus

Skeet (Middle English) swift
moving.
Skeat, Skeets, Skeeter

Skelly (Irish) teller of stories.
Skelea, Skeleah, Skelee, Skeleigh,
Skeley, Skeli, Skelie, Skell, Skellea,
Skelleah, Skellee, Skelleigh, Skelley,
Skelli, Skellie, Skely

Skender (Slavic) defender of
humankind. A form of Alexander.
Skendr (Slav)

Skene (Gaelic) bush.
Sken

Skerry (Norwegian) stone island.
Skery

Skip/Skipper (Old Norse) ship
owner.
Skip, Skipi, Skipie, Skipp, Skippi,
Skippie, Skippy, Skipy, Skyp, Skypi,
Skypie, Skypp, Skyppi, Skyppie,
Skyppy, Skypy

Skipton (Old English) from the
ship town.
Skippton, Skyppton, Skypton

Skule (Norse) shield.
Skul, Skull

Slade/Sladen (English) from the
valley.
Sladan, Sladein, Sladon, Sladyn,
Slaid, Slaidan, Slaiden, Slaidin,
Slaidon, Slaidyn, Slayd, Slaydan,
Slayden, Slaydin, Slaydon,
Slaydybn

Slane (Czech) salty.
Slain, Slaine, Slayn, Slayne

Slater (English) slater of roofs.
Slaiter, Slayter

Slava (Russian/Latin) glorious
stand.
Slavah, Slavik, Slavoshka

Slavin (Irish) mountain man.
Slavan, Slaven, Slavon, Slavyn

Slavomil (Slavic) friend who is
glorious.
Slavomilo, Slavomyl, Slavomylo

Slawek (Polish) gloriously happy. A
form of Radoslaw.

Sleeman (Old English) clever.
Sleaman

Slevin (Irish) mountain climber.
Slavan, Slaven, Slavin, Slavon,
Slavyn, Slevan, Sleven, Slevon,
Slevyn

Sloane (Irish) warrior.
Sloan

Smedley (Old English) from the
meadow.
Smedlea, Smedleah, Smedlee,
Smedleigh, Smedli, Smedlie,
Smedly

Smith (Old English) blacksmith.
Smithe, Smithey, Smithi, Smithie,
Smithy, Smitth, Smyth

Snow/Snowden (Old English) from
the snowy valley.
Snowdan, Snowdin, Snowdon,
Smowdyn

So (Vietnamese) first-born child.

Socrates (Greek) wisdom.
Socratis, Sokrates, Sokratis

Sofian (Arabic) devoted.
Sofyan

Sohan (Hindi) charming.

Sohrad (Persian) hero who is
ancient.
Sorad

Soja (Yoruba) warrior.
Sojah

Sol (Latin) sun.
Soll

Solomon (Hebrew) peace.
Salaman, Salamen, Salamon,
Salaun, Salman, Salmyn, Saloman,
Salomo, Salomon (Fren),
Salomone (Ital), Selim, Shelomoh,
Shlomo, Sholom, Solaman,

Solamh (Ir), Soloman, Solomo
(Ger/Dut), Solomyn, Sulaiman,
Zalman, Zalmen, Zalmin, Zalmon,
Zalmyn

Solon (Greek) wisdom; grave.
Solan, Solen, Solin, Solyn

Solve (Danish) warrior who is
healthy.

Somerled (Scottish) sailor.

Somerset (Old English) summer
place.
Sommerset, Sumerset, Summerset

Somerton (English) from the
summer town.

Somerville (Teutonic) from the
summer village.
Somervil, Somervill, Somervyl,
Somervyll, Somervylle, Sumervil,
Sumervill, Sumerville, Sumervyl,
Sumervyll, Sumervylle, Summervil,
Summervill, Summerville,
Summervyl, Summervyll,
Summervylle

Son (Native American) star.
(Viet) mountain. (Eng) son.

Songan (Native American) strength.
Song

Sonny (Old English) son.
Sonee, Soney, Soni, Sonie, Sonnee,
Sonney, Sonni, Sonny, Sony, Suni,
Sunie, Sunni, Sunnie, Sunny, Suny

Sono (Akan) elephant.

Sophocles (Greek) the glory of
wisdom.

Sophus (Greek) wisdom. The
masculine form of Sophia.
Sophis, Sophys

Soren (Danish) thunder; war.
Sorenson

Sorley (Old Norse) Viking; summer wanderer.
Sorlea, Sorleah, Sorlee, Sorleigh, Sorli, Sorlie, Sorly

Sorrell (Old French) reddish/brown-haired.
Sorel, Sorell, Soril, Sorill, Sorrel, Sorril, Sorrill, Soryl, Soryll

Sosaia (Polynesian) God will help.
Sosaiah

Soterios (Greek) saviour.

Southwell (Old English) from the south stream.
Southwal, Southwall, Southwel

Sovann (Cambodian) gold.
Sovan

Sowande (Yoruba) a wise healer found me.
Sowand

Spain (Latin) (Geographical) the country.
Spayn

Spalding (English) from the divided field.
Spaulding

Spangler (French) glittering. (Ger) tinsmith.

Spark (English) flash of light.
Sparkee, Sparkey, Sparki, Sparkie

Sparrow (Middle English) little sparrow bird.
Sparro

Spear (English) one who carries a spear.
Speer, Speir, Speyr

Speed (English) fast success.
Speedee, Speedey, Speedi, Speedie

Spencer (English) dispenser of provisions.
Spence, Spense, Spenser

Sperling (Middle English) little sparrow bird.
Sperlin

Spicer (Old French) spice seller.
Spycer

Spier (Old French) watcher.
Spyer

Spike (Latin) grain ear. (O/Eng) spike-haired.
Spyke

Spiro (Latin) breath of God.
Spiridion, Spiridone (Ital), Spyridion, Spyridone, Spyro

Spode (Old English) from the spear-shaped field.

Spooner (Old English) maker of spoons or roofing shingles.

Spoor (English) maker of spurs.
Spoors, Spur, Spurs

Spreckley (Old English) twigs.
Sprecklea, Spreckleah, Sprecklee, Spreckleigh, Spreckli, Sprecklie, Spreckly

Spring (English) from the spring; spring time.
Spryng

Springsteen (Old English) from the stone river.
Springstein, Springsteyn, Spryngsteen, Spryngstein, Spryngsteyn

Squire (English) attendant to a knight.
Squyre

Stable (Old French) reliable.
Stabel

Stacey (Latin) prosperous.
Stace, Stacee, Staci, Stacie, Stacy

Stack (Old Norse) stacker of hay.

Stafford (Old English) from the ford near the landing place.
Staford

Stamford (Old English) from the stone ford.
Stemford

Stamos (Greek) crown.

Stan (Old English) stone. The short form of names starting with 'Stan' e.g. Stanley.
Stann

Stanbury (Old English) from the stone fortress.
Stanberi, Stanberie, Stanberri, Stanberrie, Stanberry, Stanbery, Stanburi, Stanburie, Stanburri, Stanburrie, Stanburry

Stancil (Old English) beam or bar.
Stancile, Stancyl, Stancyle

Stancliff (Old English) from the stone cliff.
Stanclif, Stancyf, Stanclyff

Standish (Old English) from the stony enclosure.
Standysh

Standwood (Old English) from the stone woods.
Stanwood

Stanfield (Old English) from the stone field.
Stanfyeld

Stanford (Old English) from the stone ford.
Stanforde

Stanhope (Old English) from the stone hollow.
Stenhope

Stanislaus (Slavic) glorious stand.
Aineislis (Ir), Stanislao, Stanislas (Fren), Stanislav (Ger), Stanislavas (Lith), Stanislavs (Lett), Stanislaw (Pol), Stanislus, Stanko (Illy), Stanyslaus

Stanley (Old English) from the stony meadow.
Stanlea, Stanleah, Stanlee, Stanleigh, Stanli, Stanlie, Stanly

Stanmore (Old English) from the stony moor.
Stanmoar, Stanmoare, Stanmoor, Stanmoore, Stanmor

Stannard (Old English) hard like stone.
Stanard

Stanton (Old English) from the stone town.
Staunton

Stanway (Old English) dweller at the stone-paved road.
Stanwai, Stenwai, Stenway

Stanwick (Old English) dweller at the stone village.
Stanwic, Stanwik, Stanwyc, Stanwyck, Stanwyk

Stanwood (Old English) dweller at the stone forest.
Stenwood

Starbuck (Old English) stone road; from the deer star meadow.
Starrbuck

Stark (German) strength.
Starke

Starling (Old English) the starling bird.
Starlin, Starlyn, Starlyng

Starr (Old English) star.
Star

Stavros (Greek) crowned. A form of Stephen.
Stavro

Steadman (English) farmstead occupant; steady; reliable.
Stedman

Steele (Old English) one who works with steel.
Steal, Steale, Steel

Steenie (Scottish) crowned. A form of Stephen.
Steen, Steene, Steenee, Steeni, Steeny, Stein, Steine, Steinee, Steiney, Steini, Steinie, Steiny, Steyn, Steynee, Steyney, Steyni, Steynie, Steyny

Stefan (Polish/Russian/Swedish/Swiss) crowned. A form of Stephen.
Stefano, Stefen, Steffan, Steffano, Steffen, Steffin, Stefin, Stenka (Russ), Stephan, Stephano, Stephanos (Grk), Stephen, Steven

Stein (German) stone.
Stean, Steen, Steine, Steiner, Stene, Steyn, Steyne

Steinar (Norwegian) stone warrior.
Stean, Steane, Steanar, Steaner, Steenar, Steene, Steener, Stein, Steine, Steiner, Steyn, Steyne, Steynar, Steyner

Stephen/Steven (Greek) crowned.
Estaban, Estevan (Span), Etienne (Fren), Steaphan (Scott), Steav, Steave, Steaven, Stefan (Ger/Dan/Russ/Pol/Swed/Swiss), Stefano (Ital), Stefin, Stefinn, Stefyn, Stefynn, Stephan, Stephin, Stephyn, Stenka (Russ), Stenkia, Stephanus (Swed), Stephanos, Stephanus, Stepika, Stepka, Stepko, Stevan, Steve, Steven (Austr/Eng), Stevin, Stevon, Stevyn, Tiennot

Stephenson (English) Stephen's son; son of the crowned one.
Stravropoulos (Grk), Stevenson

Stephon (Greek) turner.
Strephonn

Sterling (English) silver penny.
Sterlin, Stirlin, Stirling, Styrlin, Styrling, Styrlyn, Styrlyng

Stern (German) star. (O/Eng) stern.
Sterne, Sturn, Sturne

Stewart (English) steward of the manor.
Stuart

Stig (Old Norse/Swedish) rising mount.

Stillman (English) still; quiet.
Stilman, Styllman, Stylman

Sting (English) grain spike.
Styng

Stinson (English) Stone's son; son of the stone one.
Stynson

Stockley (Old English) from the meadow with the stock.
Stocklea, Stockleah, Stocklee, Stockleigh, Stockli, Stocklie, Stockly

Stockman (English) remover of tree stumps.
Stockmen

Stockwell (English) from the well by the tree stump.
Stockwal, Stockwall, Stockwel

Stoddard (Old English) keeper of horses.
Stodard

Stoke (Old English) village.
Stok

Stoker (English) tender of the fire.
Stoke, Stokes

Stone (English) stone.
Stonee, Stoney, Stoni, Stonie, Stony

S

Storm (Old English) tempest.
Storme, Stormee, Stormey, Stormi,
Stormie, Stormy

Storr (Old Norse) great.

Stover (English) tender of the stove.
Stov, Stove

Stowe (Old English) from the place.
Stow

Strahan (Irish/Gaelic) poet;
wisdom.

Stratford (Old English) from the
street near the river ford; from
the straight river ford.
Strattford

Stratton (Scottish) from the river
valley town.
Straton

Stringfellow (Old English/Old
Norse) strong fellow.
Stryngfello

Strobe (Greek) twist.

Strom (German) river.

Strong (Old English) powerful.
Stonge

Stroud (Old English) from the
thicket.

Struthers (Irish/Gaelic) from the
stream.

Stuart (Old English) steward.
Stewart

Sturt (Old English) hill.

Styge (Norse) rising.
Stygge

Styles (Old English) dweller by the
stock enclosure.
Stiles

Subhi (Arabic) early morning.
Subhee, Subhie

Sudi (Swahili) lucky.
Suud

Sued (Arabic) chief.

Suffield (Old English) from the
south field.
Sufield

Sugen (English) valley of the sows.
Sugdan, Sugdin, Sugdon, Sugdyn

Suhail (Arabic) gentle.
Sohail, Sohayl, Souhail, Sujal

Suhuba (Swahili) friendly.
Suhubah

Sujay (Hindi) success; victory.
Sujae, Sujai

Sukru (Turkish) thankful.
Sukroo

Sullivan (Irish/Gaelic) one with the
black eyes.
Sullyvan

Sully (Old English) from the
meadow in the south.
Sullea, Sulleah, Sullee, Sulleigh,
Sulley, Sulli, Sullie

Sulprice (French) one with the red
spotted face.
Sulpryce

Sultan (Swahili) ruler.
Sulten, Sultin, Sulton, Sultyn, Sum
(Thai)

Sulwyn (Welsh) fair-haired; sunny.
Sulwin, Sulwynn, Sulwynne

Summit (English) peak of a
mountain.
Sumet, Sumit, Summet, Summit,
Summyt, Sumyt

Sumner (English) summoner.
Summner

Sun (Chinese) bend. (Eng) sun.

Sundeep (Punjabi) enlightened.

S

Sunreep (Hindi) purity.
Sunrip

Surya (Sanskrit) sun.
Suria, Suriah, Suryah

Susi (Greek) one who works with horses.
Susee, Susie, Susy

Sutcliff (Old English) from the cliff in the south.
Suttclif, Suttcliff, Sutclif, Sutclyf, Sutclyff

Sutherland (Old Norse) from the southern land.
Southerland

Sutton (English) from the south town.
Suton

Svara (Sanskrit) mystical sound.
Svarah

Sven (Norse) youthful.
Svend, Swen, Swend

Svenbjorn (Norse) young bear.
Sveniborn

Swaggart (English) one who staggers.
Swaggert

Swain (English) attendant of the knight.
Swaine, Swayn, Swayne

Swaley (English) from the winding stream meadow.
Swalea, Swaleah, Swalee, Swaleigh, Swali, Swalie, Swaly

Swannee (Old English/Australian) swan.
Swanee, Swaney, Swani, Swanie, Swanney, Swanni, Swannie, Swanny, Swany

Sweeney (Irish/Gaelic) little hero. (O/Eng) strength.
Sweanee, Sweaney, Sweani, Sweanie, Sweany, Sweenee, Sweeni, Sweenie, Sweeny

Swindel (English) from the valley of the pigs.
Swindell, Swyndel, Swyndell

Swinfen (English) muddy pig.
Swynfen

Swinford (English) from the pig ford.
Swynford

Swinton (Old English) dweller at the farm of the pigs.
Swynton

Swithbert (Old English) strong; bright.
Swithbirt, Swithburt, Swithbyrt, Swythbert, Swythbirt, Swythburt, Swythbyrt

Swithin (Teutonic) strength.
Swithan, Swithen, Swithon, Swithun, Swithyn, Swythan, swythen, Swythin, Swython, Swythyn

Syed (Arabic) happy.
Sied

Sying (Chinese) star.

Symington (Old English) from Simon's town; from the listening town.
Simingtons

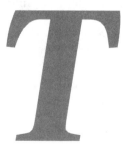

Ta (Chinese) great.
Tah

Taamiti (Lunyole) brave.
Taamit

Taaveti (Finnish) beloved.
Taavetie, Taavety, Taveti, Tavertie,
Tavery

Tab/Tabbener (Middle English/Old
French) drummer. (Ger) shining;
brilliant. (Gae) spring.
Tabar, Tabbner, Tabener, Taber,
Tabi, Tabie, Tabir, Tabner, Tabor
(Per), Taby, Tabyr

Tabari (Arabic) remember.
Tabaris, Tabarus, Tabary

Tabbai (Aramaic) good.
Tabbay

Tabib (Turkish) doctor.
Tabeeb, Tabyb

Tabulum (Australian Aboriginal) my
home.

Tadan (Native American) plentiful.
Taden, Tadin, Tadon, Tadyn

Tadao (Japanese) self-satisfying.

Tadashi (Japanese) serves faithfully.
Tadashee, Tadashie, Tadashy

Tadd (Old Welsh) father.
Tad

Taddia (Illyrian) praising God. A
form of Thaddeus.
Tadia, Tadiah, Taddiah, Tadias
(Lith), Taddya, Tadya, Tadyas

Tadeo (Spanish/Latin) praised.
Tadeas, Tades

Tadhg (Irish) poet.
Tadlee, Tadleigh, Teague, Teige,
Teyge, Tyegue

Tadi (Omaha) wind.
Tadee, Tadey, Tadie, Tady

Tadleigh (Irish/English) poet from
the meadow.
Tadlea, Tadleah, Tadlee, Tadley,
Tadli, Tadlie, Tadly

Tadzi (Carrier) moon.
Tadzie, Tadzy

Taffy (Welsh) beloved. The Welsh
form of David.
Taffee, Taffey, Taffi, Taffie, Taffy,
Tafy

Tafy (Old English) river.
Tafte

Tage (Danish) day.
Tag, Taig, Taige, Tayg, Tayge

Taggart (Gaelic) son of the priest.
Tagart, Tagert, Taggert, Taggirt,
Taggirt, Taggurt, Taggyrt, Tagirt,
Tagurt, Tagyrt

Taghee (Native American) chief.
Taghe

Tago (Spanish) day.
Tagot, Taio, Tajo (Span)

Taha (Polynesian) first born; one.
Tahah

Tahatan (Sioux) hawk.

Taheton (Sioux) crow.

T

Tahi (Tongan) sea.

Tahir (Arabic) purity.
Taher, Tahyr

Tai (Chinese) tribe; kin; weather; talented.

Taika (Tongan) tiger.
Tayka

Taima (Native American) born during a thunder storm.
Taimah, Tayma, Taymah

Tain (Gaelic) stream.
Taine, Tayn, Tayne

Tait (Old Norse) happy.
Taite, Taitt, Tate, Tayt, Tayte

Taiwan (Chinese) island dweller.
Taywan

Taiwo (Yoruba) first born of twins.
Taywo

Taj (Hindi) crown.
Taja, Taji

Tajuan (Hebrew/Spanish) God is gracious. A form of Juan.
Taijuan, Tayjuan

Takeishi (Japanese) bamboo.

Takeo (Japanese) strength.
Takeyo

Takoda (Lakota/Sioux) friend to everyone.
Takodah, Takota, Takotah

Tal (English) tall; fierce. (Heb) rain; dew.
Talbert, Talbot, Talford, Talmadge, Tall, Tallon

Tala (Tongan) seagull.
Talah

Talanoa (Tongan) story teller.
Talanoah

Talbert (German) from the bright valley.
Talberte, Talbirt, Talburt, Talburt, Talbyrt

Talbot (Teuntonic) commander; from the valley. (Fren) boot maker.
Talbert, Talbott, Talibot, Talibott, Talybot, Talybott

Talcott (Old English) from the tall cottage.
Talcolt, Talcot, Taldon, Talmadge

Taldra (Australian Aboriginal) kangaroo.
Taldrah

Tale (Tswana) green.
Tael, Tail, Tal, Tayl

Talfryn (Welsh) top of a hill.
Talfrin

Talib (Arabic) seeker.
Taleb, Talyb

Taliesin (Welsh) radiant top of the hill.
Talisan, Taliesen, Talieson, Taliesyn, Talyesin, Talyesyn, Tayliesin, Tayliesyn, Tallas, Tallis, Tallys

Talli (Native American) leader.
Talee, Taley, Tali, Tallee, Talley, Tallie, Tally, Taly

Tallis (Persian) wisdom.
Talis, Tallys, Talys

Talmai (Hebrew) small hills.
Talmay, Talmie, Telem

Talman (Aramaic) harsh.
Talmen, Talmin, Talmon, Talmyn

Talor (Hebrew) dew.
Talar, Taler, Tallar, Taller, Tallor

Talut (Arabic) borrowed; soul. A form of Saul.
Talu

Tam (Hebrew) twin. (Viet) heart.
Tamm

Tama (Maori) son.
Tamah, Tamma, Tammah

Taman (Slavic) dark; black-haired.
Tama, Tamann, Tamen, Tamin,
Tamon, Tamyn

Tamar (Hebrew) palm tree; date fruit.
The masculine form of Tamara.
Tamarr, Tamer, Tamir, Tamor,
Tamyr, Timar, Timarr, Timer, Timir,
Timor, Timur, Tymar, Tymarr,
Tymer, Tymir, Tymyr

Tamas (Hungarian) twin. A form of
Thomas.
Tamasa, Tamasah, Tamati (Maori)

Tambo (Swahili) vigorous.
Tambow

Tamir (Arabic) tall as a palm tree.
Tamirr, Tamyr, Tamyrr

Tammany (Delaware) friendly.
Tamany

Tamson (Scandinavian) son of
Thomas; son of the twin.
Tamsan, Tamsen, Tamsin, Tamsun,
Tamsyn

Tan (Burmese) million. (Viet) new.
Than

Tanaki (Polynesian) beat of a drum.
Tanakie, Tanaky

Tanay (Hindi) son.
Tanae, Tanai

Tancred (Teuntonic) giver of
thoughtful advice; counsellor.
Tancreda, Tancredi, Tancredie,
Tancredy, Tancrid, Tancryd

Tandie (African American) beloved;
masculine.
Tandee, Tandey, Tandi, Tandy,
Thandee, Thandey, Thandi, Thandie

Tane (Maori) husband.
Tain, Taine, Tayn, Tayne

Tanek (Greek) immortal.
Atek

Taneli (Finnish) God is my judge.
Tanel, Tanelie, Tanell, Tanella,
Tanelle, Tanely

Tanguy (French) warrior.
Tangui

Tangwyn (Welsh) peace that is
blessed.
Tangwin

Tani (Japanese) valley.
Tanee, Taney, Tanie, Tany

Taniel (Estonian/Hebrew) God is
my judge. A form of Daniel.
Daniel, Taniell, Tanyel, Tanyell

Tanjiro (Japanese) second-born son
who is highly valued.
Tanjyro

Tanne (Lettish) priceless. A form of
Anthony.
Tain, Taine, Tainn, Tainne, Tane,
Tayn, Tayne, Taynn, Taynne

Tanno (Spanish) camp of glory.
Tano

Tanner/Tanny (Old English) leather
worker; tanner of hides.
Tanar, Tani, Tanie, Tanna, Tanna,
Tannah, Tannar, Tannery, Tanni,
Tannie, Tannor, Tanny, Tany

Tano (Ghanian) river.
Tanno

Tanton (Old English) from the
quiet, still river near the town.
Tantan, Tantin, Tanton, Tantun,
Tantyn

Tanundra (Australian Aboriginal)
place of plentiful wild fowl.
Tanundrah

T

Tapani (Finnish) crowned.
Tapamn, Tapanee, Tapaney,
Tapanie, Tapany

Tapko (Kiowa) antelope.

Tarcoola (Australian Aboriginal)
river bend.
Tarcoolah

Taree (Australian Aboriginal) wild
fig tree.
Tarey, Tari, Tarie, Tary

Tareton (Old English) from the
town of the thunder ruler.
Taretan, Tareten, Taretin, Taretyn,
Tartan, Tarten, Tartin, Tarton,
Tartyn

Tarhe (Native American) tree.
Tarhee

Tarif (Arabic) uncommon.
Tareef, Taryf

Tarik (Arabic) one who comes by
night; conqueror.
Tareck, Tareek, Tarek, Tarick, Tariq,
Taryc, Taryck, Taryk, Tarreq, Tereik,
Teryc, Teryck, Teryk

Tarleton (Old English) from the
thunder ruler's town; from Thor's
town.
Tarletan, Tarleten, Tarletin, Tarletor,
Tarletyn

Tarn (Old Norse) from the
mountain pool.
Tarne

Taro (Japanese) first-born male; big
boy.
Tarot

Taron (English/Greek) the king's
courageous advisor.
Taeron, Tahron, Tarone, Tarran,
Tarren, Tarrin, Tarron, Tarrun,
Tarryn, Tarun, Taryn

Tarrance/Torrance (English/Latin)
smooth; good; gracious. (Ir) from
the place with the small rocky
hills. A form of Terence.
Tarance, Tarence, Tarince, Tarrence,
Tarrince, Tarrynce, Tarynce, Terance,
Terince, Terrance, Terrince,
Terrynce, Terynce, Torance, Torence,
Torrance, Torrant, Torrence, Torrent

Tarrant/Torrant (Welsh) thunder.
Tarant, Tarent, Tarrent, Terrant,
Torant, Torent, Torrant, Torrent

Tarril (Teutonic) belonging to Thor;
belonging to the thunder ruler.
Tarell, Terrail, Terral, Terrale,
Terrall, Terreal, Terrel, Terrell,
Terrelle, Terril, Terrill, Terryal,
Terryel, Terryl, Terryll, Tirel, Tirrel,
Tirrell, Turrell, Tyrel, Tyrell

Tarro (Australian Aboriginal) stone.
Taro

Tarver (Old English) softener of
whitened hide; from the tower
over the hills.
Terver

Tas (Gypsy) bird's nest. (Austra)
from Tasmania.
Tass, Taz, Tazz

Tashunka (Sioux) horse.
Tashunkah, Tasunke

Tatanka (Sioux) bull; buffalo.
Tatankah

Tate (Native American) long-winded
talker. (O/Eng) spirited; cheerful.
Tait, Taite, Tayt, Tayte

Tatius (Latin) ruler.
Tatianis, Tatianus, Tazio, Titis,
Titus, Tytius, Tytyus

Tatonga (Sioux) buck; male deer.

Tatum (Old English) from Tate's
homestead.
Taitam, Taitem, Taitim, Taitom,
Taitum, Taitym, Tatam, Tatem,
Tatim, Tatom, Taytam, Taytem,
Taytim, Taytom, Taytum, Taytym

Tau (Tswana) lion.

Taufa (Tongan) storm.
(Indo) hurricane.
Taufan

Taula (Tongan) priest.
Taulah

Tauno (Finnish) world leader.
Taunot

Taurean (Latin) like a bull;
stubborn strength; born under
the sign of Taurus.
Taurino, Taurion, Tauris, Taurus,
Tauryan, Tauryen, Tauryon, Toro

Tava (Polynesian) fruit tree.
Tavah

Tavares (Spanish) the hermit's son.
Tavar

Tavaris (Aramaic) misfortune.
Tavaris, Tarvarres, Tavar, Tavaras,
Tavares, Tavari, Tavarian, Tavarius,
Tavarres, Tavarri, Tavarris, Tavars,
Tavarse, Tavarus, Yavarys, Taveress,
Tevaris, Tevarus, Tevarys, Teverus,
Teverys

Tavas (Hebrew) peacock.

Taved (Estonian) beloved. A form of
David.
Tavad, Tavid, Tavod, Tavyd

Tavey (Latin) eighth-born child. The
short form of Octavio.
Tavee, Tavi, Tavie, Tavy

Tavi/Tavis (Scottish/Hebrew)
David's son; son of the beloved.
(Ara) good.
Tavee, Taveon, Tavey, Tavid, Tavie,
Tavin, Tavio, Tavion, Taviss, Tavon,
Tavy, Tavys, Tavyss, Tevin, Tevis,
Teviss, Tevys, Tevyss, Tuvia

Tavish (Gaelic) twin. A form of
Thomas.
McTavish, McTavysh, Tavis, Taviss,
Tavys, Tavysh, Tavyss

Tavor (Aramaic) misfortune.
Tarvoris, Tavaris, Tavores,
Tavorious, Tavoris, Tavorris,
Tavorrys, Tavorys, Tavuris, Tavurys

Tawa (Hopi) sun.
Tawah

Tawno (Gypsy) tiny.

Tayib (Sanskrit) delicate; good.

Taylor (Old English) tailor; repairer
of garments.
Taelor, Tailah, Tailar, Tailer, Talor,
Taylah, Taylar, Tayler, Taylon,
Taylour, Tayson, Teyler

Taz (Persian) goblet.
Tas, Tass, Tasswell, Taswell, Tazwell,
Tazz, Tazzwell

Teague (Native American) low rider.
(Eng) handsome. (Ir) poet.
Tadgh (Ir), Taggart, Teagan,
Teagun, Teak, Teeg, Teegue, Tegan,
Teig, Teigan, Teige, Teigen, Teigue,
Tighe, Tyg, Tygue

Teale (Middle English) water fowl.
Tadgh, Tadhgh, Taig, Teagan, Teak,
Teal, Teel, Teele, Teige, Teil, Teile,
Teyl, Teyle

Teangi (Australian Aboriginal)
earthy.
Teangie, Teangy

Tearlach (Gaelic) strong;
courageous. A form of Charles.
Tearlache, Tearloc, Tearloch,
Tearloche, Tearlock, Tearlock,
Tearlok

T

Tearle (English) stern.
Earl, Earle, Tearl

Teasdale (English) dweller at the river valley.
Tedail, Tedale

Tebes (Swiss) God is good.
Tobias, Tobyas

Tecwyn (Welsh) fair. (O/Eng) white-haired friend.
Tecwin

Ted/Teddy (Old English) wealthy ruling guardian; gift of God; bear. The short form of Edward/Theodore.
Tedd, Teddee, Teddey, Teddi, Teddie, Tedee, Tedey, Tedi, Tedie, Tedy

Tedmund (English) the land protector.
Tedman, Tedmand, Tedmon, Tedmond, Tedmondo, Tedmun

Tedorik (Polish) gift of God. A form of Theodore.
Tedoric, Tedorick, Tedoryc, Tedoryck, Tedoryk

Tedrick (English) gift of God; powerful ruler.
Tedric, Tedrik, Tedryc, Tedryck, Tedryk

Teeuw (Dutch/Hebrew) gift of God. A form of Matthew.

Tefere (Ethiopian) seed.
Tefer

Teiji (Japanese) second son who is righteous.

Tekea (Polynesian) king of the sharks.

Tekle (Ethiopian) plant.

Telek (Polish) one who works with iron.

Telem (Hebrew) mound.
Tellem

Telford (French) iron cutter. (O/Eng) from the iron ford.
Telforde, Tellford, Tellforde

Teller (English) story teller.
Tella, Tellah, Telli, Tellie, Telly, Tely

Tem (Gypsy) country.

Teman (Hebrew) to the right side; south.
Temani, Temanie, Temany, Temen, Temin, Temon, Temyn

Tembo (Swahili) elephant.
Tembeau

Tempest (French) storm.
Tempes, Tempess

Templar (Old French) knight who protected the Holy Land. (O/Eng) from the temple.
Tempal, Temple (Eng), Templer

Templeton (Old English) from the temple town.
Temple, Templetown

Tennant (English) renter of houses.
Tenant

Tennessee (Cherokee) mighty warrior; river.
Tennessee, Tennesy, Tennysee

Tennyson (Old French) tennant's son; son of the renter of houses; inhabitant.
Tenney, Tenneyson, Tennison, Tenyson

Tenoa (Tongan) tenor.
Tenoah

Teo (Spanish) God.
Tio, Tyo

Tepene (Maori) crowned. A form of Stephen.
Tepen

Terach (Hebrew) goat.
Tera, Terac, Terach

Teremun (Tiv) has his father's acceptance.

Terence (Latin) smooth; tender; gracious.
Tarrance, Temcio, Terencio (Span), Terrel, Terrance, Terrence, Terenz, Terril, Terrill, Terrince, Terrynce, Thierry, Torrance, Torrence, Torrince, Torrynce

Terran (English) of the earth.
Teran, Teren, Terin, Teron, Terone, Terrone, Terryon, Teryn, Terran, Terren, Terrin, Terron, Terryn

Terrel (English/German) strength.
Terral, Terrell, Terrelle, Terril, Terrill, Terryl, Terryll, Teryl

Terris (Latin) Terry's son; son of the smooth, tender, gracious one.
Teris, Terrys, Terys

Terry (Latin) smooth; tender; gracious. The short form of Terrence.
Teree, Terey, Teri, Terie, Terree, Terrey, Terri, Terrie, Terry, Tery

Tertius (Latin) third-born child; three.
Tertios, Tertyus

Teryl (African American) beloved who is smooth, tender and gracious. The combination of Daryl/Terry.

Tesher (Hebrew) one who donates.

Tete (Australian Aboriginal) kingfisher (bird).
Tet

Tetley (Old English) from Tate's meadow; from the long-winded talker's meadow; from the spirited, cheerful one's meadow.
Tatlea, Tatleah, Tatlee, Tatleigh, Tetli, Tetlie, Tetly

Teva (Hebrew) nature.
Tevah

Tevel (Yiddish) beloved.
Tevell, Tevil, Tevill, Tevyl, Tevyll

Tevis (Scottish) twin. A form of Thomas.
Tevish, Teviss, Tevys, Tevyss

Tevita (Polynesian) treasured.
Tevitah, Tevyta, Tevytah

Tex (American) from Texas.
Tejas, Texas, Texx, Texxas

Thabit (Arabic) firm.
Thabyt

Thabiti (Kenyan) man.

Thad (Greek) little courageous one.
Thadd

Thaddeus (Hebrew) praising God. (Grk) courageous.
Taddeo, Taddi, Taddia (Illy), Taddie, Taddy, Tadeo, Tadeusz (Pol), Tadi, Tadia, Tadias (Lith), Tadie, Tady, Thaddaus, Thaddaus, Thaddej (Russ), Thaddeo, Thaddeos, Thaddeys, Thadeas, Thadeis, Thadeos, Thadeus, Thadeys, Thadias, Thadios, Thadius, Thadiys, Thady (Ir), Thadyas, Thadyos, Thadyus

Thadford (Old English) from Thad's ford; from the little courageous one's ford.
Thadforde

T

Thai (Vietnamese) many. The short form of the country Thailand.
Thailan, Thailand

Thaiter (Irish/German) powerful warrior. A form of Walter.
Thai

Thalmus (Greek) flowering.
Thalmas, Thalmis, Thalmos, Thalmous, Thalmys

Thaman (Hindi) God-like.
Thamane, Thamen

Than (Burmese) million.
Tan

Thandiwe (Zulu) beloved.
Tandee, Tandey, Tandi, Tandie, Tandy, Thandee, Thandey, Thandi, Thandie, Thandy

Thane (English) attending warrior.
Thain, Thaine, Thayn, Thayne

Thang (Vietnamese) victorious.

Thanh (Vietnamese) tranquil; finished.
Than

Thaniel (Hebrew) gift of God.
Nathaniel, Thaneal, Thaneel, Thaneil, Thaneyl, Thaniell, Thanielle, Thanyel, Thanyell, Thanyelle

Thankful (Puritan) to give thanks.
Thank

Thanos (Greek) noble.
Athanasios, Thanasis, Thanus

Thatcher (Old English) roof mender.
Thacher, Thatch, Thaxter

Thaw (Old English) melting.
Thor

Thayer (Old French) belonging to the nation's army.

Thel (English) story above.

Thenga (Yao) to bring him.
Thengah

Theo/Theobald (German/Teutonic) the people's prince. The short form of Theobald/Theodore.
Dietbold (Ger), Fio, Tebaldo, Teo, Teobald, Teobalt, Teobaud, Thean (Fren), Theballd, Thebault (Fren), Theo, Theobaldo (Ital/Span/Port), Theobalt, Thibaud (Fren), Thibaut (Fren), Thio, Thyo, Thyobald, Thyobaldo, Thyobalt, Tibald, Tibalt, Tibold (Ger), Tiebout (Dut), Tioboid (Ir), Tybalt

Theodore (Greek) gift of God.
Fedor, Feodor (Slav), Feodore, Kwedders, Pheodor, Teodor, Teodorico, Teodoro (Span/Ital), Teudwer, Theodor (Ger/Dan/Swed), Theodric, Theorodus (Dut)

Theodoric (Teutonic) powerful ruler of the people.
Derek, Dieter, Dietrich, Tedric, Thedrick, Thedrik, Theodorick, Theodorik, Theodorio, Theodrick, Theodik, Theodryc, Theodryck, Theodryk, Thierry

Theon (Greek) Godly.
Feon

Theophilus/Thilo (Greek) dearest to God.
Fillo, Filo, Fiophilus (Ger), Filow, Thilow

Theron (Greek) one who hunts.

Theros (Greek) summer.
Theross

Thian (Vietnamese) smooth.
Thien

Thies (Swiss) gift of God.

Tho (Vietnamese) longevity.

Thoar (Australian Aboriginal) sunrise.
Thor

Thomar (Australian Aboriginal) small river.
Thom

Thomas (Aramaic/Hebrew) twin.
Didymus, Dummas, Foma, Tamas, Tamaso (Ital), Tamasz, Tamassa, Tamati, Tammeas, Tammen, Tavis, Tavish, Thoma, Thomasin, Thomaz, Thumas, Toma (Illy), Tomas (Span), Tomaso (Ital), Tomasino, Tomasz (Pol), Tomaz, Tomhas (Ir), Tuomas (Finn)

Thompson (English) Thomas' son; son of the twin.
Tompson

Thong (Vietnamese) clever.

Thor (Scandinavian/Old Norse) thunder.
Thorald, Thordis, Thore, Thorin, Thorkell, Thorley, Thorr, Thorsson, Thorvald, Thorwald, Thurman, Tor, Torald, Tore, Torre, Torrin, Torvald, Tyrus

Thorald (Old Norse) Thor ruler; thunder ruler.
Terrell, Thorold, Torald, Tyrell

Thorbert (Old Norse) brilliance of Thor; brilliant thunder.
Thorbirt, Thorburt, Thorbyrt, Torbert, Torbirt, Torburt, Tobyrt

Thorbjorn (Scandinavian) Thor's bear.
Thorborn, Thorborne, Thorburn, Thorburne, Thurborn, Thurborne, Thurburn, Thurburne

Thorburn (Old Norse) Thor's bear or thunder bear.
Thorborn, Thorborne, Thorburne, Thorbyrn, Thorbyrne

Thorgood (English/Scandinavian) Thor is good.

Thorleif (Scandinavian) Thor's beloved.
Thorlief, Thorleyf

Thorley (Old English) from the thorny meadow. (O/Eng) from Thor's meadow or thunder meadow.
Thor, Thorlea, Thorleah, Thorlee, Thorleigh, Thorli, Thorlie, Thorly, Tor, Torlea, Torleah, Torlee, Torleigh, Torley, Torli, Torlie, Torly

Thormond (Old English) under Thorn's protection.
Thormon, Thormondo, Thormun, Thormund, Thurmondo

Thorndike (Old English) from the place with the thorny embankment.
Thordike, Thordyke, Thorn, Thorndyck, Thorndyke, Thornedike, Thornedyke

Thorne (Old English) thorns.
Thorn, Thorni, Thornie, Thorny

Thornley (Old English) from the thorny meadow.
Thorn, Thorne, Thornlea, Thorleah, Thornlee, Thornleigh, Thornli, Thornlie, Thornly

Thornton (Old English) from the town near the thorny bushes.
Thornetan, Thorneten, Thornetin, Thorneton, Thornetyn, Thorntown, Thortan, Thorten, Thortin, Thorton, Thortyn

T

Thorpe (English) from the village farmstead.
Thorp

Thorvald (Old Norse) with the strength of Thor.
Thorvaldo

Thorwald (Scandinavian) from Thor's forest.
Thorvald, Thorvaldo, Thorwaldo

Thoth (Egyptian) mythological God of the moon; wisdom.

Thron (Greek) raised seat; important.
Throne

Thu (Vietnamese) born in autumn/ fall.

Thuc (Vietnamese) aware.

Thurlow (Old English) from the gapped hill; from Thor's hill.
Thurlo

Thurman (Old English) servant of Thor; servant of thunder.
Thirman, Thirmen, Thorman, Thornman, Thorold, Thorolo, Thorwald, Thunderbird, Thurgood, Thurlow, Thurmen, Thurnman, Thurnmen

Thurmond (English/Scandinavian) defended by Thor.
Thurmon, Thurmondo, Thurmun, Thurmund, Thurmundo

Thursday (Scandinavian/English) Thor's day.
Thordae, Thorsdai, Thorsday, Thurdae, Thurdsai

Thurstan (Scandinavian/Dutch) Thor's stone.
Thirstan, Thirsteen, Thurstein, Thirsten, Thirstin, Thirston, Thirstyn, Thorsteen, Thorstein, Thorsten, Thorstin, Thorstine,

Thorston, Thorstyn, Thursteen, Thurstein, Thursten, Thurstin, Thurstine, Thurston, Thurstyn

Thynne (Old English) slender.
Thinne

Tiarnach (Irish) devout.
Tiarnac, Tyarnach, Tyarnac

Tiba (Navajo) the colour grey.
Tibah, Tyba, Tybah

Tibb (Greek) God's gift.
Tibah, Tibba, Tibbah, Tyba, Tybah, Tybb, Tybba, Tybbah

Tibbot (Irish) bold person.
Tibbott, Tibot, Tibott, Tibout (Dut), Tybbot, Tybot

Tibor (Hungarian) holy place.
Tybor

Ticho/Tico (Latin/Spanish) noble.
Ticcho, Ticco, Tycco, Tyco

Tien (Chinese) heaven.
Tyen

Tiennan (French) crowned. A form of Stephen. (Ir) master.
Tyennan

Tierney (Irish) of royal decent; lordly.
Tiarnach, Tiernan, Tyrney

Tiger (Greek) tiger.
Tiga, Tigga, Tige, Tigger, Tyga, Tyger, Tygga, Tygger

Tiimu (Moquelumnan) caterpillar coming out of the ground.
Timu, Tymu

Tiki (Maori) greenstone ornament; carving. (Poly) a dead person's soul is taken by the Gods.

Tiktu (Moquelumnan) bird digging up potatoes.

T

Tilden (Old English) to cultivate a fertile valley.
Tildan, Tildin, Tildon, Tildyn

Till (German) the people's leader.
Til, Tyl, Tyll

Tillford (Old English) from the prosperous ford.
Tilford, Tilforde, Tillforde

Tilo (German) dear to God.
Tillo, Tylo

Tilon (Hebrew) from the hill.
Tylon

Tilton (Old English) from the hill town.
Tiltown, Tylton, Tyltown

Tim/Timmy/Timo (Greek) honouring God. The short form of Timothy.
Tim, Timee, Timey, Timi, Timie, Timm, Timmee, Timmey, Timmi, Timmie, Timmo, Timo (Finn), Tym, Tymee, Tymey, Tymi, Tymie, Tymm, Tymmee, Tymmey, Tymmi, Tymmie, Tymmo, Tymmy, Tymo, Tymy

Timin (Arabic) born near the sea.
Timyn, Tymin, Tymyn

Timon (Greek) honourable listener.
Timan, Timen, Timin, Timyn, Tyman, Tymen, Tymin, Tymon, Tymyn

Timothy (Greek) one who honours God.
Timathee, Timathey, Timathy, Timmothee, Timmothey, Timmothy, Timofee (Russ), Timofei, Timofey (Russ), Timon, Timotao (Span/Ital), Timotei (Ital), Timotejs, Timoteo (Ital/Span/Port), Timothee (Fren), Timotheus (Ger), Tiomoid (Ir), Tisha (Russ),

Tymmothee, Tymmothey, Tymothi, Tymothie, Tymothy

Timur (Hebrew) stately. (Russ) conqueror.
Tymur

Tin (Vietnamese) thinker.
Tyn

Tino (Spanish) majestic.
Tyno

Tinsley (Old English) defender of the meadow.
Tinslea, Tinsleah, Tinslee, Tinsleigh, Tinsli, Tinslie, Tinsly, Tynslea, Tynsleah, Tynslee, Tynsleigh, Tynsley, Tynsli, Tynslie, Tynsly

Tipu (Hindi) tiger.

Tiru (Hindi) devoted.
Tyru

Titan/Tite/Tito/Titus (French) great.
Titan, Tite (Fren), Tito (Ital/Span), Titus (Grk), Tiziano (Ital), Tyte, Tytan, Tyto, Tytus

Tivon (Hebrew) lover of nature.
Tyvon

Toa (Tongan) the casuarina tree.
Toah

Toafo (Polynesian) woods.

Toal (Irish) people of strength.

Tobar (Gaelic) fountain. (Eng) to tow. (Gyp) road.
Tobbar

Tobi (Yoruba) great.
Tobbee, Tobbey, Tobbi, Tobbie, Tobby, Tobee, Tobey, Tobie, Toby

Tobias (Hebrew) God is good.
Tebes, Tiveon, Tobej (Russ), Tobia (Ital), Tobiah, Tobiasz (Pol), Tobies (Swiss), Tobija (Russ),

T

Tobin, Tobit, Tobye, Tobyn, Tobyas, Tobysas (Lett)

Tobit (Hebrew) Tobias' son; son of the one whose God is good.
Tobin, Tobyn, Tobyt

Toby (Hebrew) God is good. The short form of Tobias.
Tobbee, Tobbey, Tobbi, Tobbie, Tobby, Tobee, Tobey, Tobie, Toby

Todd (Middle English/Norse/Latin) fox.
Tod, Todde

Toddhunter (Middle English) fox hunter.
Toddhunter

Tofe (Tongan) oyster.

Tofu (Tongan) calm.
Tofoo

Togar (Australian Aboriginal) smoke.
Tager, Togir, Togor, Togyr

Tohon (Native American) cougar.

Tohunga (Maori) priest.
Tohungah

Tohyah (Native American) walking past a river.
Tohya

Toivo (Finnish) hope.
Toyvo

Toka (Tongan) jellyfish.
Tokah

Tokala (Dakota) fox.
Tokalah

Tokoni (Tongan) helper.
Tokonee, Tokonie, Tokony

Tolan/Tolland (Old English) owner of land which is subject to a tax or a toll.
Tolen, Tolin, Tolon, Tolun, Tolyn

Tolbert (English) bright tax collector.
Talbert, Talberte, Talbirt, Talburt, Talburte, Talbyrt, Tolberte, Tolbirt, Tolburt, Tolburte, Tolbyrt

Toler (English) tax collector.
Toller

Tolman (Old English) tax man.
Tollman, Tollmen, Tolmen

Tom (Aramaic) twin. The short form of Thomas.
Teo, Teom, Thom, Thomee, Thomey, Thomi, Thomie, Thommee, Thommey, Thommi, Thommie, Thommy, Thomy, Tomee, Tomey, Tomi, Tomie, Tomm, Tommee, Tommey, Tommi, Tommie, Tommy, Tomy

Toma (Tongan) show off.
Tomah

Tomago (Australian Aboriginal) sweet water.
Toma

Tombe (Kakwa) from the north.
Tomba, Tombah

Tomer (Hebrew) tall.
Tomar, Tomir, Tomyr

Tomi (Japanese) wealthy.
Tomie, Tomy

Tomkin (Old English) little Tom; little twin.
Thomkin, Thomkyn, Tomkyn

Tomlin (English) little Tom; little twin from the pool.
Thomlin, Thomlyn, Tomlyn

Tommy (Hebrew) twin. The short form of Thomas.
Thomee, Thomey, Thomi, Thomie, Thommee, Thommey, Thommi, Thommie, Thommy, Thomy, Tom, Tomee, Tomey, Tomi, Tomie,

Tommy cont.
Tomm, Tommee, Tommey, Tommi,
Tommie, Tommy, Tomy

Tonda (Czech) priceless.
Tondah (Czech), Tone (Slav),
Toneek, Tonneli (Swiss)

Tong (Vietnamese) fragrance.

Tony (Latin/Italian) priceless. The
short form of Anthony.
Tonee, Toney, Toni, Tonie, Tonio
(Port/Ital), Tonye

Toolan (Australian Aboriginal)
wattle (small yellow flower balls
with a sweet scent).

Topper (English) top of the hill.
Toper

Tor (Celtic) rock. (Nor) thunder.
(Tiv) king.
Thor, Thorr, Torr

Torao (Japanese) tiger.

Torbert (Old English) rocky hilltop
with a sunny peak.
Thorbert, Thorbirt, Thorburt,
Thorbyrt, Torbirt, Torburt, Torbyrt

Torger (Scandinavian) Thor's spear;
thunder spear.
Tord

Torin (Irish/Gaelic) chief.
Thorfin, Thorin, Thorstein, Thoryn,
Torine, Torrin, Torrine, Torryn,
Torryne, Toryn

Torio (Japanese) bird's tail.
Torrio, Torryo, Toryo

Tormey (Irish/Gaelic) thunder
spirit; Thor's spirit.
Tormee, Tormi, Tormie, Tormy

Tormod (Scottish) from the north.
Tormed

Tormond (Scottish) north.
Thormon, Thormond, Thormondo,
Thormun, Thormund, Thormundo,
Tormon, Tormondo, Tormun,
Tormund, Tormundo

Torn (Irish) from the small round
hills. (Eng) to rip.
Torne

Torna (Irish) prince.
Tornah

Torr (Old English) tower on the
rocky peak.
Tor

Torrance (Irish/Gaelic) from the
place with the small, rocky hills.

Torsten (Old Norse) Thor's stone;
thunder stone.
Tawrence, Torance, Toreence,
Toren, Torin, Torn, Torr, Torren,
Torreon, Torrin, Torry, Torstan,
Torstin, Torston, Tory, Tuarence,
Turance

Toru (Japanese) sea.

Tory (Old Norse) Thor; thunder.
Toree, Torey, Tori, Torie, Torri,
Torrie, Torry, Tory

Toshiro (Japanese) intelligent;
talented; sincerity.

Tostig (Old Norse) harsh, severe
day.
Tostyg

Tove (Scandinavian) Thor's rules;
thunder rules.
Tov

Tovi (Hebrew) good.
Tovee, Tovey, Tovie, Tovy

Townley (Old English) from the
meadow town.
Tonlea, Tonleah, Tonlee, Tonleigh,
Tonley, Tonli, Tonlie, Tonly,
Townlea, Townleah, Townlee,
Townleigh, Townli, Townlie,
Townly

T

Townsend (Old English) from the edge; from the end of town.
Town, Towne, Towney, Townie, Townshend

Towrang (Australian Aboriginal) shield.
Towran

Tracy (Irish/Gaelic) warrior. (Lat) courageous.
Trace, Tracee, Tracey, Traci, Tracie, Treacey, Treaci, Treacie, Treacy

Trader (English) skilled worker.
Trade

Trahern (Welsh) possesses great strength; as strong as iron.
Ahern, Aherne, Traherne, Tray, Trayhern, Trayherne

Trai (Vietnamese) pearl.
Trae, Tray

Trant (Middle English/German) cunning.
Trent

Traugott (German) trust in God.
Traugot

Travell (English) traveller.
Traveler, Travelis, Travell, Travelle, Travil, Travill, Traville, Travyl, Travyll, Travylle, Trevel, Trevell, Trevelle, Trevil, Trevill, Treville, Trevyl, Trevyll, Trevylle

Travers (French) crossroads.
Travaress, Travaris, Travarius, Travarus, Traver, Traverez, Travis, Traviss, Travoris, Travorus

Travis (Old French) keeper at the crossroads; tax collector.
Travais, Traver, Travers, Traves, Traveus, Travious, Traviss, Travor, Travus, Travys, Travyss,Trevor, Trevus, Trevys, Trevyss

Traylor (English/Latin) crowned with trees; towed vehicle.
Trailor, Treilor, Treylor

Trayton (English) from the town with lots of trees.
Traiton, Treiton, Treyton

Treat (Latin) pleasure; swiftly moving stream.
Treet, Treit, Trentan, Trenten, Trentin, Trenton, TreytTre, Trea

Tredway (Old English) mighty warrior.
Treadway

Tremain (Scottish) from the big farm with the trees.
Tramain, Tramaine (Eng/Wel), Tramayn, Tramayne, Tremaine, Tremayn, Tremayne, Treymain, Treymaine, Treymayn, Treymayne

Trent/Trentan (English) cunning. (Lat) torrent, rapid stream. (Fren) thirty.
Trant, Trante, Trente, Trentine, Trentino, Trento, Trentonio

Trevelyan (Gaelic) from Elian's homestead; from the uplifting one's homestead.
Trevelian

Trevin (English/Welsh) from the uplifting one's village.
Travan, Traven, Traveon, Travin, Travien, Travion, Trevan, Treven, Trevian, Trevion, Trevyn

Trevor (Celtic) cautious. (Wel) large village home.
Travar, Traver, Travir, Trefor, Trevar, Trevares, Trevaris, Trevarus, Trever, Trevoris, Trevorus, Treyvor

Trey (Middle English) third-born child; three.
Trae, Traey, Trai, Traie, Tray, Traye, Trei, Treye

Trigg (Old Norse) trustworthy.
Trig

Trini (Latin) three.
Trinity, Triny, Tryny

Trinity (Latin/Hebrew) three; the
Father, the Son and the Holy
Spirit.
Trinitee, Trinitey, Triniti, Trinitie,
Trynity, Trynyty

Trip (Old English) traveller.
Tripp, Tryp, Trypp

Tristan (Old Welsh) loud. (Fren)
sorrowful. (Wel) bold knight.
Tristann, Tristen, Tristian, Triston,
Tristram, Trystan, Trystann,
Trystian, Trystion, Tryston, Trystyn

Tristram (Latin/Welsh) sorrowful
labour; mournful (given to a
child who's mother has died
during child birth).
Tristam, Tristan, Trystram, Trystran

Trot (English) from the trickling
stream.

Trowbridge (Old English) dweller
at the row of trees at the bridge.
Throwbridge

Troy (Irish/Gaelic) son of the warrior.
(Fren) curly-haired. (Eng) water.
Troi, Troye

True (Old English) faithful; loyal.
Tru

Truesdale (Old English) from the
beloved one's homestead in the
valley.
Trudail, Trudale, Trudayl, Trudayle

Truitt (English) little; honest.
Truet, Truett, Truit, Truyt, Truytt

Truman (Old English) faithful; true
man.
Trueman, Trumain, Trumann

Trumble (Old English) bold
strength.
Trumbal, Trumball, Trumbel,
Trumbell, Trumbul, Trumbull

Trung (Vietnamese) faithful.

Trustin (English) trustworthy.
Trusting

Tryg (Scandinavian) truth.
Trig, Trygve

Tryphon (Greek) dainty; elegant.
Triphon

Tse (Ewe) younger of twins.

Tsoai (Kiowa) rock tree.

Tu (Polynesian) man of war.
(Viet) tree.

Tuaco (Ghanian) eleventh-born
child.

Tuan (Australian Aboriginal) spear.
(Viet) unimportant.
Tuana, Tuane

Tuari (Laguna) young eagle.
Tuarie, Tuary

Tucker (English) tucker of cloth.
Tucka, Tuckar

Tudor (Welsh) God's gift. A form
of Theodore.
Tudore

Tui (Maori) handsome songbird.
(Tong) faith.

Tuketu (Moquelumnan) bear
running in the dust.

Tuki (Australian Aboriginal)
bullfrog.
Tukie, Tuky

Tukuli (Moquelumnan) caterpillar
crawling down a tree.

Tukupa (Tongan) promise.
Tukupah

Tullis (Latin) title.
Tullius, Tullos, Tulli, Tullie, Tully, Tullys

Tully (Irish/Gaelic) lives with the peace of God; mighty people.
Tulea, Tuleah, Tulee, Tuley, Tuli, Tulie, Tullea, Tulleah, Tullee, Tulley, Tulli, Tullie, Tuly

Tumaini (Mwera) hope.
Main, Maini, Mainie, Mainy, Tum, Tuma

Tumu (Moquelumnan) deer; buck thinking about eating some wild onions.

Tung (Vietnamese) dignified.
(Chin) everyone.

Tunu (Miwok) deer eating onions that are growing wild.
(Finnish) twin. A form of Thomas.

Tupi (Moquelumnan) to pull up.
Tupe, Tupee, Tupie, Tupy

Tupper (Old English) one who raises rams.

Turaku (Australian Aboriginal) comet.

Turlough (Irish/Norse) shaped like Thor; shaped like thunder.
Thorlough, Torlough

Turner (English) one who works with wood.
Terner

Turpin (Old Norse) Thor; thunder.
Thor, Thorpin, Torpin

Tut (Arabic) strong; courageous.
Tutt

Tutu (Spanish) just one.

Tuwile (Mwera) death is inevitable.

Tuxford (Old Norse) from the spear ford (shallow river crossing).
Tuxforde

Tuyen (Vietnamese) angel.
Tuien

Twain (English) separated into two parts; rope.
Tawaine, Twaine, Tway, Twayn, Twayne

Twia (Fanti) child born after twins.
Twiah

Twitchell (Old English) dweller at the narrow passage.
Twitchel, Twytchel, Twytchell

Twyford (Old English) from the double river crossing.
Twiford, Twiforde, Twyforde

Ty (English/American) from the enclosure. The short form of names beginning with 'Ti' or 'Ty' e.g. Tyler.
Ti, Tie, Tye

Tybalt (English) bold.
Tibalt, Tiboly, Tybolt

Tycho (German/Latin) furious.
Ticho

Tye (Old English) from the enclosure. The short form of names beginning with 'Ti' or 'Ty' e.g. Tyler.
Ti, Tie, Ty

Tyee (Native American) chief.

Tygrve (Norwegian) brave victory.
Tigrve

Tyke (Native American) chief.

Tyler (Old English) tile layer.
Tila, Tilar, Tiler, Tilor, Tyla, Tylar, Tyler, Tylor

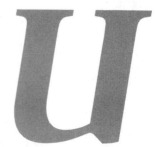

Tymon (Polish) sound.
Timon

Tynan (Irish/Gaelic) dark-haired.
Tinan, Tinane, Tynane

Tyr (Norse) born of war.
Tyre

Tyree (Scottish) island dweller.
Tyrey, Tyri, Tyrie, Tyry

Tyrone/Tyrus (Greek) monarch; royalty. (Ir/Gae) from Owen's land; from the well born one's land. (O/Per) sun; throne.
Teiron, Teirone, Terron, Tiron, Tirone, Tirown, Tirowne, Tirus, Tiruss, Tyron, Tyroney, Tyronn, Tyroun, Tyrown, Tyrowne, Tyrus, Tyruss

Tyshawn (Hebrew) God is gracious.
Tisean, Tishaun, Tishawn, Tysean, Tyshaun

Tyson (Old French) fire stick; firebird; son of Ty; son of the one from the enclosure.
Tison

Tzadok (Hebrew) righteous.
Tzadik, Zadok

Ualtar (Irish) army ruler.
Uailtar, Ualteir, Ualter

Ualusi (Tongan) walrus.
Ualusee, Ualusey, Ualusie, Ualusy

Uang (Chinese) great.

Uata (Polynesian) army leader.
Uatah

Ubadah (Arabic) server of God.
Ubada

Ubald/Ubaldus (Teutonic) peace of mind.
Ubaldas, Ubalde (Fren), Ublado (Ital), Ubaldus, Ubold, Uboldas, Uboldo, Uboldus

Ucal (Hebrew) powerful.

Ucello (Italian) bird.
Uccelo, Ucello, Ucelo

Uday (Hindi) showing up.
Udae, Udai

Udell (Old English) from the valley of the yew trees.
Udale, Udall, Udalle, Udel, Udele, Udelle

Udolf (Old English) courageous wolf.
Udolfe, Udolff, Udolph, Udolphe

Ueli (Swiss) noble ruler.
Uelie, Uely

Uffo (German) wild bear.
Ufo

U

Uggieri (Italian) holy.
Ugieri

Ugo (Teutonic) intelligent.
(O/Germ) heart; mind. A form of Hugo.
Hugo, Ugon (Illy), Ugues (Fren)

Uha (Tongan) rain.
Uhah

Uhila (Tongan) lightning.
Uhilah, Uhyla, Uhylah

Uniseann (Irish) conqueror.
Uinsean

Ujala (Hindi) shine.
Ujalah

Ulan (African) first born of twins.
Ulen, Ulin, Ulon, Ulyn

Uland (German) from the noble country.
Ulan

Ulbrecht (German) noble; bright.
Ulbright, Ulbryght

Uldericks (Lettish) noble ruler.
Uldric, Uldrics, Uldrik, Uldryc, Uldryck, Uldryk

Uleki (Hawaiian) wrathful.
Ulekee, Ulekie, Uleky

Ulf (Norse) wolf.
Ulfer, Ulph

Ulfer/Ulfred (Norse) warrior wolf; fierce warrior.
Ulf, Ulfer, Ulfrid, Ulfryd, Ulph, Ulpher, Ulphrid, Ulphryd

Ulger (Old English) wolf spearer.
Ulga, Ulgah, Ulgar

Ulick (Old Norse) rewarding mind.
Ulic, Ulik, Ulyc, Ulyck, Ulcyk

Ull (Norse) magnificent will.
Ul

Ullivieri (Italian) olive tree.
Oliver, Ulivieri

Ullock (Old English) wolf sport.
Uloc, Ulock, Uloch, Uloche, Ulok, Uloke, Ulloc, Ulloch, Ulloche, Ullok, Ulloke

Ulmer (Old Norse) famous wolf.
Ulmar, Ulmor, Ulmore

Ulric/Ulrich (Teutonic) ruling wolf.
(O/Nrs) wolf.
Oldrech, Oldrich, Olery, Olric, Olrick, Olrik, Olryc, Olryck, Olryk, Ulfa, Ulfah, Ullric, Ullrich, Ullrick, Ullrik, Ullric, Ullrich, Ullrick, Ullrik, Ullryc, Ullrych, Ullryck, Ullryk, Ulrech, Ulrich (Swiss), Ulrick (Nrs), Ulrico (Ital), Ulrik (Scand/Ger/Slav), Ulryc, Ulrych, Ulryck, Ulryk (Pol), Ulu

Ultan (Teutonic) noble stone.
(Ir) trouble stone.
Ulten, Ultin, Ulton, Ultyn

Ultra (Latin/English) extreme.
Ultrah

Uluka (Sanskrit) owl.
Ulukah

Ulysses (Latin/Greek) wrathful one who dislikes injustice.
Ulick, Ulises (Span), Ullioc (Ir), Uileos, Uluxe, Ulyses

Umar (Arabic) blooming.
Umer

Umberto (Spanish/Italian) bright of heart or mind.
Hughberto, Umberto, Umirto, Umburto, Umbirto

Umbra (Latin) shadow cast during an eclipse.
Umbrah

Umed (Hindi) desire.

Umi (Malawian) life.
Umee, Umie, Umy

Undolfo (Italian) noble wolf.
Adolffo, Adolfo, Adolpho,
Andolffo, Andolfo, Andolpho,
Undolfo

Uner (Turkish) famous.

Unger (German) from Hungary.
Unger

Unika (Malawian) shining.
Unikah

Unity (Latin/English) oneness.
Unitee, Unitey, Uniti, Unitie

Unkas (Native American) fox.

Uno (Latin) first-born child;
number one.
Unno

Unwin (Old English) not friendly.
Unwyn

Upravda (Slavic) upright.
Upravdah

Upton (Old English) from the estate
in the upper town.
Uptown

Upwood (Old English) from the
upper woods.

Urban (Latin) citizen of the town.
Urvan (Russ)

Urchin (Latin) mischievous child.

Ure/Uri (Hebrew) the light of God.

Uriah (Hebrew) God is my light.
Uriel, Yuri (Russ), Yuria, Yuriah,
Yurya, Yuryah

Urian (Welsh) born in the town.
Urien, Uryan, Uryen

Uriel (Hebrew) God is my flame,
my light.
Uri, Yuri (Russ), Yuriel, Yuryel

Ursan/Ursine/Ursus (Latin) bear.
Ursa, Ursah, Ursel, Urshell, Ursen,
Ursin, Ursyl, Ursyn, Urshyll, Ursus

Urvil (Hindi) sea.
Ervil, Ervyl, Urvyl

Usama (Arabic) lion.
Usamah

Useni (Malawian) telling.
Usenie, Useny

Usenko (Russian) son of the man
with the moustache.

Usher (English) people keeper.
Usha, Ushah

Usi (Malawian) smoke.

Usman (Arabic) owner of two
lights.

Ustin (Russian) righteous; just. A
form of Justin.
Usan, Usen, Uson, Usyn

Utatch (Native American) scratching
bear.
Utatci

Uthman (Arabic) best.
Uthmen, Uttam (Hin)

Utu (Polynesian) returning.

Uwe (German) inherited from birth.

Uyeda (Japanese) field of rice.
Uyedah

Uzair (Arabic) helper.
Uzaire, Uzayr, Uzayre

Uzi (Hebrew) strength.
Uzee, Uzey, Uzie, Uzy

Uziah (Hebrew) God is my strength.
Uzia

Uziel (Hebrew) strength.
Uzyel, Uzziah, Uzzyel

V

Uzoma (Nigerian) born while travelling.
Uzomah

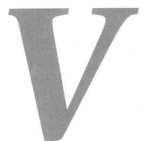

Vaal (Dutch) valley.
Val

Vachel (Old French) one who raises small cows.
Vachell, Vachelle

Vada (Latin) shallow area where water lies.
Vadah

Vaha (Tongan) open sea.
Vahaha

Vail (Old English) dweller in the valley.
Bail, Bale, Balle, Bayl, Bayle, Vale, Valle, Vayl, Vayle

Vaina (Finnish) from the mouth of the river.
Vain, Vainah, Vaino, Vayna, Vaynah, Vayno

Vaino (Finnish) builder of wagons.
Vayno

Vaitafe (Tongan) stream.
Vaytafe

Val (Latin) strength. The short masculine form of Valerie, strong; brave; healthy. The short form of Valentine.
Vala

Vala (Polynesian) loin cloth.
Valah

Valborg (Swedish) protection from the slaughter.
Valbor

Valdemar (German) famous, powerful ruler.
Vlademar, Vladimar, Vladymar

Valdus (Old German) possessor of power.
Valdis, Valdys

Vale (Old French) dweller in the valley.
Vael, Vail, Vaiel, Vayel, Vayl, Vayle

Valentine (Latin) powerful; strong; brave; healthy.
Bailintin (Irish), Balawyn, Valek, Valentijn (Dut), Valentin (Fren/Ger/Span/Swed), Valerius (Fren), Valentino (Ital), Valenty (Pol),Valentyn, Valentyne, Valentyno, Valerian, Valerij (Russ), Valerio (Ital), Valerius (Fren), Valery, Valerya, Valeryan, Walenty, Wallinsch, Waltinsch

Valgard (Norse) foreign spear.
Valgarde, Valguard

Vali (Tongan) paint.
Valea, Valeah, Valee, Valeigh, Valey, Valie, Valy

Valin (Hindi) mighty warrior.
Valan, Valen, Valon, Valyn

Vallis (Old French) Welsh one.
Valis, Vallys, Valys

Valmiki (Hindi) ant hill.

V

Valu (Polynesian) eighth-born child.

Vamana (Sanskrit) one who deserves praise.
Vamanah

Van (Dutch) of nobility; belonging to or from.
Vann

Vance (Middle English) from the very high place; from the swamp.
Vane, Vanne, Vanse, Von

Vanda (Lithuanian) the people rule.
Vandah

Vandan (Hindi) saved.
Vanden, Vandin, Vandon, Vandyn

Vander (Dutch) belonging to or of.
Vanda, Vandar, Vandir, Vandor, Vandyr, Venda, Vendar, Vender, Vendir, Vendor, Vendyr

Vandyke (Dutch) from the flood embankment.
Vandike

Vane (Dutch/German) belonging to.
Vain, Vaine, Van, Vayn, Vayne

Vanya (Russian) God is gracious.
Vanek, Vania, Vaniah, Vanja, Vanka, Vanyah

Vara (Illyrian) stranger; unknown.
Varah, Varra, Varrah

Varad (Hungarian) belonging to the fortress.
Vared, Varid, Varod, Varyd

Varde (Old French) dweller from the green hills.
Ardan, Ardant, Arden, Ardin, Ardon, Ardun, Ardyn, Vardan, Vardin, Vardon, Vardyn, Verdan, Verden, Verdin, Verdon, Verdyn

Varen (Hindi) better.
Varan, Varin, Varon, Varyn

Varesh (Hindi) God is better.
Vares

Varian (Latin) clever; intelligent.
Arian, Varien, Varion, Varyan

Varick (Icelandic) sea drifter.
Varic, Varik, Varyc, Varyck, Varyk

Varil (Hindi) water.
Varal, Varel, Varol, Varyl

Varnava (Russian) comfort in a time of grief.
Varnavah

Vartan (Armenian) rose.
Varten, Vartin, Varton, Vartyn

Varun (Hindi) water god.
Varan, Varen, Varin, Varon, Varyn

Varuna (Russian) one who sees all.
Varunah

Vasant (Hindi) born in the spring time.
Vasan

Vasil (Czech) royal; majestic; basil herb. A form of Basil.
Vasal, Vasel, Vasile, Vasilek, Vasili, Vasilios, Vasilis, Vasilos, Vasily, Vasol, Vassily, Vasyl

Vasilis (Greek) magnificent knight; warrior.
Vasileior, Vasos, Vasilys, Vasylis, Vasylys

Vasin (Hindi) leadership.
Vasan, Vasen, Vason, Vasun, Vasyn

Vassily (German/Russian/Slavic) protector; guardian.
Vasilea, Vasileah, Vasilee, Vasileigh, Vasilek, Vasiley, Vasili, Vasilie, Vasily, Vassilea, Vassileah, Vassilee, Vassileigh, Vassiley, Vassili, Vassilie, Vasya, Vasyuta

Vasu (Hindi) prosperous.

Vaughan (Celtic) small.
Vaughn, Vaughen, Vaun, Vaune,
Vauney, Vawn, Vawne, Vawney

Vaux (Old French) belonging to the
valley.

Vea (Polynesian) chief.

Veasna (Cambodian) lucky.
Veasnah

Vedie (Latin) I saw.
Vedi, Vedy

Veetini (Polynesian) all spearing.
Veetinie, Veetiny

Veiko (Finnish) brother.
Veyko

Veit (German/Swedish) wide.
Veyt

Vekoslav (Slavic) eternal glory.
Vekoslava

Vencel (Hungarian) wreath.
Vencal, Vencil, Vencyl

Venedict (Russian) blessed. A form
of Benedict.
Venedic, Venedick, Venedyc,
Venedyck, Venedyct

Venn (Irish/Gaelic) fair-haired.
(Eng) dweller at the marsh.
Ven

Verdun (Old French) from the hill
fort.
Virdun, Vyrdun

Vere (Latin) possessor of sacred
wisdom. (Lat) true. (O/Ger)
defender. The masculine form of
Verena.
Vear, Veer, Veere, Veir, Ver, Vir, Vyr

Vered (Hebrew) rose.
Verad, Verid, Verod, Veryd

Verge (Latin) twig; stick.
(Eng) edge.
Virge, Vyrge

Verill (Old French) truthful.
Veral, Verall, Veril, Verrall, Verrell,
Verroll, Veryl, Veryll

Verlie (French) (Geographical) from
Verlie in France.
Verlea, Verleah, Verlee, Verlei,
Verleigh, Verley, Verli, Verly

Verlin (Latin) flourishing; blooming
like a flower.
Verlan, Verlain, Verle, Verlinn,
Verlion, Verlon, Verlyn, Verlynn

Vermudo (Spanish) bear protection.
Ermond, Ermondo, Ermund,
Vermond, Vermondo, Vermund,
Vermundo

Verney (Old French) belonging to
the alder-tree grove.
Lavern, Laverne, Vernee, Verni,
Vernie, Verny, Virnee, Virney, Virni,
Virnie, Virny, Vurnee, Vurney,
Vurni, Vurnie, Vurny, Vyrnee,
Vyrney, Vyrni, Vyrnie, Vyrny

Vern/Vernon (Latin) like
springtime. (Fren) belonging to
the little alder grove.
Laverna, Laverne, Varney, Vern,
Vernan, Verne, Vernen, Vernice,
Vernin, Verrier, Vernun, Vernyn,
Virn, Virne, Vyrn, Vyrne

Verrill (French) loyal.
Veril, Verill, Veryl, Veryll

Veston (Latin) clothing. (O/Eng)
from the town of churches.
Vestan, Vesten, Vestin, Vestun,
Vestyn

Vibert (French) life. (Eng) one who
is shining brightly.
Viberte, Vybert, Vyberte

V

Vic/Victor (Latin) victory.
Buadhach (Irish), Vick, Vik,
Vikenty, Viktor (Ger/Slav), Vittorio
(Span), Vyc, Vyck, Vyctor, Vyk,
Vykk, Vyktor, Wiktor

Vicar (Old French/Old English)
clergy member.
Vica, Vicka, Vickar, Vicker, Vickor,
Vyca, Vicka, Vickar, Vika, Vikar,
Vyca, Vycar, Vycka, Vyckar, Vyka,
Vykar

Vida (English) loved.
Vidah, Vyda, Vydah

Vidal (Latin) life.
Vidale, Vidall, Vydal, Vydall

Vidkun (Scandinavian) experienced.
Vydkun

Vidor (Hungarian) happy.
Vidore, Vidoor, Vydoe

Vidya (Sanskrit) wisdom.
Vidyah, Vydya, Vydyah

Vijaya (Sanskrit) strength.
Vijayah, Vyjaya, Vyjayah

Vijnana (Sanskrit) intelligent
wisdom.
Vijnan, Vijnanah

Viking (Norse) viking.
Vikin, Vykin, Vyking, Vykyn,
Vykyng

Vila (Czech) wilful. A form of
William.
Vilah, Vyla, Vylah

Viliami (Polynesian) protector.

Vimal (Hebrew) purity.
Vylmal

Vinay (Hindi) polite.
Vynay

Vince/Vinnie (Latin/Australian)
victory. The short form of
Vincent.
Vinni, Vinnie, Vinny, Vinse, Vynce,
Vynse, Vynni, Vynnie, Vynny, Vyny

Vincent (Latin) victory.
Vicen, Vikenty (Russ), Vincante,
Vincence, Vincencio (Ital), Vincens
(Ger), Vincente (Span/Ital),
Vincentij (Slav), Vincentius (Dut),
Vincently, Vincents (Dan),
Vincenty (Pol), Vincentz (Ger),
Vincezio, Vincenz (Ger), Vineze,
Vinezio, Vinicent, Vinsin, Vinsint,
Vinson, Vinsyn, Vinsynt, Vinsynte,
Vyncen, Vyncent, Vyncente, Vyncin,
Vyncint, Vyncinte, Vyncyn,
Vyncynt, Vyncynte, Vynsynt

Vindo (Hindi) fun.
Vyndo

Vine (Old French) vineyard worker.
Vin, Viner, Vyn, Vyne, Vyner

Vinsun (Old English) Vincent's son;
son of the victorious one.
Vinsan, Vinsen, Vinsin, Vinson,
Vinsyn, Vynsan, Vynsen, Vynsin,
Vynson, Vynsyn

Viper (Latin) snake.
Vyper

Virgil (Latin) flourishing;
blooming; staff (stick) bearer.
Vergel, Vergill, Virgille (Fren),
Virgillion, Virgilo (Ital), Virgo,
Vurgil, Vurgyl, Vyrgil, Vyrgyl

Vishva (Sanskrit) one who has
everything.
Vishvah

Visvaldis (Latvian) ruler of all.
Visvaldya, Vysvaldis, Vysvaldys

Vitalis (Latin) alive; alert; life.
Vital, Vitale (Fren/Ger/Ital), Vitalij
(Russ), Vitaliss, Vitalys, Vitalyss,
Vjita (Boh), Vitus, Vyta, Vytal,
Vytalis, Vytalys

Vitas (Latin) full of life. The short
form of Davita, beloved. The
masculine form of Vita.
Vida, Vidal, Vidale, Viel, Vitalis,
Vyta, Vytas

Vito (Latin) alive.
Vitto, Vyto, Vytto, Witold (Pol)

Vitus (French) from the forest.
Vytus

Vivek (Hindi) wisdom.

Vivian (Latin) full of life. The
masculine form of Vivien.
Fithian, Fivian, Phythian, Vivien,
Vyvian, Vyvien, Vyvyan, Zivian,
Zyvian

Vlad/Vladimir/Vladislav (Slavic)
powerful prince.
Ladimir, Ladislas, Ladislaw,
Laidislaw, Valdemar (Fren/Ger/
Dan), Vladamar, Vladd, Vladimer,
Vladislau (Pol), Vladmir,
Vladymar, Vladymer, Vladymir,
Vladymyr, Vladyslau, Vladyslav,
Waldemar

Vladivoj (Russian) ruling army.
Vladivo, Vladyvoj

Vladlen (Russian/German) powerful
lion prince. A combination of
Lennard/Vladimir.
Vladan, Vladin, Vladon, Vladyn

Vlado (Slavic) to rule.

Vlas (Russian) one who stammers.

Vogel (German) bird.
Vogal, Vogil, Vogol, Vogyl

Voitto (Finnish) winner.
Voytto

Vojciech (Polish/Bohemian)
warrior.
Vojlech, Vojtech

Volker (German) folk person.

Volley (Latin) flying; soaring.
Volea, Voleah, Volee, Voleigh,
Voley, Voli, Volie, Vollea, Volleah,
Vollee, Volleigh, Voooli, Vollie,
Vollon, Volney, Voly

Volney (Old German) the people's
spirit.
Volnee, Volni, Volnie, Volny

Volo (Esperanto) will.

Volya (Russian) the people's ruler.

Von (German) of or from.
Vonn

Vortigern (Celtic) the great king.
Vortigerne, Vortygern, Vortygerne

Voshon (African American) the
grace of God.

Vova (Russian) ruler of the people.
Vovah

Vratislav (Slavic) brilliant; famous.
Vratislava

Vuc (Slavic) wolf.
Vuk

Vukmil (Slavic) wolf of love.
Vucmil, Vukmil, Vukmyl

Vyasa (Sanskrit) order.
Viasa, Vyasah

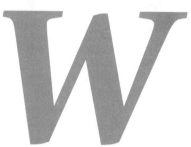

Waarrar (Australian Aboriginal) river.
Warrar

Waban (Native American) east wind.
Waben, Wabin, Wabon, Wabyn

Wachiru (Kenyan) law maker's son.

Waclaw (Polish) crowning glory.
Wencelas

Wade (English) dweller in the water; one who advances.
Waed, Waede, Waid, Waide, Wayd, Wayde

Wadley (English) from the meadow river crossing.
Wadlea, Wadleah, Wadlee, Wadlei, Wadleigh, Wadley, Wadli, Wadlie, Wadly

Wadsworth (English) from the estate with the wading pool.
Wadesworth

Wadud (Arabic) loving.
Wad

Wagner (Dutch) maker of wagons.
Waggoner, Wagnar, Wagnor, Wagoner

Wahhab (Arabic) presenter; one who gives.
Wahad, Wahib

Wahid (Arabic) unique.
Wahyd

Wahkan (Lakota) sacred.

Wahshee (Sioux) chubby boy.

Wahtsake (Osage) eagle.

Wai (Maori) water.
Wae, Way

Waine (English) wagon driver.
Wain, Wane, Wayn, Wayne

Wainwright (English) maker of wagons.
Wain, Waine, Wainright, Wainryght, Wayn, Wayne, Waynright, Waynryght

Waitangi (Maori) (Geographical) a place in New Zealand.

Waite (Middle English) guardian.
Wait, Wayt, Wayte

Wajid (Arabic) finder.
Wajyd

Wajih (Arabic) extraordinary.

Wake (English) alert.
Waik, Waike, Wayk, Wayke

Wakefield (Old English) dweller at the white field.
Waikfield, Waykfield

Wakeley (English) from the damp meadow.
Waklea, Wakleah, Waklee, Waklei, Wakleigh, Wakli, Waklie, Wakly

Wakeman (Old English) watcher; guardian.

Wakil (Arabic) advocate; supporter.
Wakyl

Wakiza (Native American) determined warrior.
Wakyza

Walaka (Hawaiian) the people's ruler.
Walakah

W

Walby (Old English) from the home near the wall.
Walbee, Walbey, Walbi, Walbie

Walcha (Australian Aboriginal) sun.
Walchah

Walcott (Old English) from the cottage with the walls.
Walcot

Waldemar (Teutonic) powerful. (O/Eng) famous ruler who is glorious.
Valdemar, Waldermar, Waldo

Walden (English) from the valley in the forest.
Waldan, Waldin, Waldon, Wadyn

Waldo (English) ruler.
Waldron, Waldryn

Waldron (Teutonic) ruling raven.
Waldran, Waldren, Waldrin, Waldryn

Waleed (Arabic) newborn child.
Walead, Waleyd

Waleliano (Hawaiian) strength.

Walena (Hawaiian) defending. A form of Warren, rabbit burrow.
Walenah

Walenty (Polish/Latin) strong, healthy. A form of Valentine.

Walerian (Polish) strong; brave.
Waleryan

Wales (English) (Geographical) from Wales in England.
Whales

Walfred (Teutonic) peaceful ruler.
Walfredd, Walfrid, Walfridd, Walfryd, Walfrydd

Wali (Arabic) servant of Allah.
Walea, Waleah, Walee, Waleigh, Waley, Walie, Waly

Walid (Arabic) newborn child.
Walyd

Walkara (Ute) yellow.
Walkarah

Walker (English) thickener of cloth.
Walka, Walkah

Wallace (English) Welsh; stranger.
Walach, Walice, Walise, Wallach, Wallache (Ger), Wallice, Wallis (Eng), Wallise, Walloch, Wallyce, Wallyse, Waloch, Walyce, Walyse, Walman, Walmen, Walsh, Welch, Welsh

Wallah (Australian Aboriginal) rain.
Walla

Waller (Old English) builder of walls. (O/Ger) army ruler.
Waler

Wallingford (Welsh) from the wall near the ford.
Walingford

Wallis (English) Welsh; stranger. A form of Wallace.
Walach, Walice, Walise, Wallach, Wallache (Ger), Wallice, Wallise, Walloch, Wallyce, Wallyse, Waloch, Walyce, Walyse, Walman, Walmen, Walsh, Welch, Welsh

Wally (English) Welsh. The short form of names starting with 'Wal' e.g. Wallace.
Walea, Waleah, Walee, Waleigh, Waley, Wali, Walie, Wallea, Walleah, Wallee, Walleigh, Walley, Walli, Wallie, Wally, Waly

Walsh (English) Welsh one; stranger. A form of Wallace.
Walshe, Walshi, Walshie, Walshy, Welsh

Walt/Walter (German) powerful warrior.
Bhaltair (Scott), Gaulter (Port), Gauthier, Gualter, Gualterio (Span), Gualtier (Fren), Gualtiero, Gaulterius (Lat/Dut), Ualtar (Ir), Walt, Walta, Waltah, Waltier, Waltir, Walther (Ger), Waltier (Fren), Waltor, Waltyr

Walther (German) ruling.
Walter, Waltier (Fren), Waltyer

Walton (English) from the town surrounded by walls.
Waltan, Walten, Waltin, Waltyn

Walwin (Welsh) hawk friend.
Alwin, Alwyn, Walwyn

Walworth (Old English) from the Welsh one's farm.
Wallworth, Wallsworth, Walsworth

Walwyn (Old English) Welsh friend.
Walwin

Wamba (Spanish) stomach.
Wambah

Wamblee (Lakota) eagle.
Wamblea, Wambleah, Wambleigh, Wambley, Wambli, Wamblie, Wambly

Wanbi (Australian Aboriginal) dingo (wild Australian golden/red-coloured dog).
Wanbee, Wanbey, Wanbie, Wanby

Waneta (Sioux) charger.
Wantetah

Wang (Chinese) king.
Wan

Wanikiya (Lakota) saviour.
Wanikiyah

Wapi (Native American) lucky.
Wapie, Wapy

Warburton (Old English) from the enduring town of the castle.

Ward (English) guardian.
Warde, Warden, Wardin, Wardon, Wardun, Wardyn

Wardell (Old English) from the hill of the guardian.
Wardel

Warden (Old English) guardian of valley.
Wardan, Wardin, Wardon, Wardun, Wardyn

Wardley (Old English) from the guardian meadow.
Wardlea, Wardleah, Wardlee, Wardleigh, Wardli, Wardlie, Wardly

Ware (Old English) wary. (O/Ger) defending.
Warey

Warfield (Middle English) from the war field. (O/Eng) from the field near the weir.
Warfyeld

Warford (Middle English) from the weir ford.

Warick (English) hero of the village.
Waric, Warick, Warik, Warric, Warrick, Warrik, Warryc, Warryck, Warryk, Waryc, Waryck, Waryk

Waring (German) shelter of protection.
Warin, Waryn, Waryng

Warley (English) from the meadow with the weir; from the war meadow.
Warlea, Warleah, Warlee, Warlei, Warleigh, Warli, Warlie, Warly

Warmond (Old English) true protector.
Warmon, Warmondo, Warmun, Warmund, Warmundo

Warner (German) warrior who protects.
Warnor, Wernar, Werner, Wernher

Warra (Australian Aboriginal) water.
Wara, Warah, Warrah

Warrack (Australian Aboriginal) the banksia tree.
Warrac, Warrak

Warren (German) defending; rabbit burrow.
Waran, Waren, Waring, Waringer, Warran, Warrin, Warron, Warrun, Warryn

Warrie (Australian Aboriginal) wind.
Wari, Warie, Warri, Warry, Wary

Warringa (Australian Aboriginal) sea.
Waringa, Waringah, Warringah

Warrun (Australian Aboriginal) sky.
Warun

Warton (Old English) from the weir town. (Eng) from the war town.
Wartan, Warten, Wartin, Wartyn

Warwick (English) from the house near the dam.
Warwic, Warwik, Warwyc, Warwyck, Warwyk

Washburn (Old English) from the burning stream.
Washbern, Washberne, Washbirn, Washbirne, Washborn, Washborne, Washbourn, Washbourne, Washburne, Washbyrn, Washbyrne

Washington (English) from the washing town; from the burning town.
Washintan, Washinten, Washingtin, Washingtyn

Wasi (Arabic) understanding.
Wasie, Wasy

Wasil (Arabic) divine.
Wasyl

Wasim (Arabic) graceful; handsome.
Wasym

Wassily (Russian/Greek) royal; majestic; basil herb. A form of Basil.
Wasily, Wassyly, Wasyly

Wata (Maori) powerful warrior. A form of Walter.
Watah, Watli (Swiss)

Watende (Nyakusa) revengeful.
Watend

Waterman (Old English) works on the water.
Watermen

Watford (Old English) from the white river crossing.
Wattford

Watkins (Old English) Walter's son; son of the powerful warrior.
Watkin, Watkyn, Watkyns, Wattkin, Wattkins, Wattkyn, Wattkyns

Watson (English) Walter's son; son of the powerful warrior.
Wattson

Wattan (Arapaho) black.
Watan

Waunakee (Algonquin) peace.

Waverley (Old English) from the meadow near the wavy sea; from the windy aspen meadow.
Waverlea, Waverleah, Waverlee, Waverleigh, Waverli, Waverlie, Waverly

Waya (Cherokee) wolf.
Waia, Waiah, Wayah

Wayamba (Australian Aboriginal) turtle.
Wayambah

W

Wayland (German) from the highway land.
Walan, Waland, Wailan, Wailand, Walylan, Waylan, Whalan, Whalen, Whalin, Whalon, Whalyn

Waylon (English) from the land by the highway.
Wailon, Wallen, Walon, Waylan, Wayland, Waylen, Waylin, Waylyn, Weylen, Weylin, Weylon, Weylyn

Wayne (English) maker of wagons.
Wain, Waine, Wayn

Wazire (Arabic) minister.
Wazyr

Webb (English) weaver.
Web, Webber, Weber

Webley (English) from the weaver's meadow.
Webblea, Webbleah, Webblee, Webbleigh, Webbley, Webbli, Webblie, Webbly, Weblea, Webleah, Weblee, Webleigh, Webli, Weblie, Webly

Webster (English) weaver.
Webstar

Weddell (Old English) from the advancer's hill.
Weddel, Wedel, Wedell

Weelya (Australian Aboriginal) parakeet (bird).
Weelyah

Weeronga (Australian Aboriginal) quiet.
Weerongah

Weiss (German) white.
Weis, Weise, Weisse, Weys, Weyse, Weyss, Weysse

Wekesa (Kenyan) born during harvest time.
Wekeasah

Welborne (Old English) born at the spring stream.
Welbern, Welberne, Welbirn, Welbirne, Welborn, Welburn, Welburne, Welbyrn, Welbyrne, Wellbern, Wellberne, Wellbirn, Wellbirne, Wellborn, Wellborne, Wellbourn, Wellbourne, Wellbyrn, Wellbyrne

Welby (Scandinavian) from the stream farm.
Welbee, Welbey, Welbi, Welbie

Weldon (English) from the willow trees on the hill near the stream.
Weldan, Welden, Weldin, Weldyn

Welford (English) from the ford by the well.
Wellford

Wellington (Old English) from the wealthy one's town.
Wellinton

Wells (English) from the stream.
Wels

Welton (Old English) from the town near the stream.
Welltan, Wellten, Welltin, Wellton, Welltyn, Weltan, Welten, Weltin, Weltyn

Wemilat (Native American) one who has everything.

Wemilo (Native American) everyone talks to him.

Wen (Chinese) cultured.

Wen Hu (Chinese) educated.

Wenceslaus (Slavic) crowning glory.
Vaacslav, Vaclav, Veleslav, Venceslav, Waclaw, Wenceslas, Wenzel

Wendel (German) wanderer.
Wenda, Wendah, Wendelin, Wendell, Wendil, Wendill, Wendyl, Wendyll

W

Wenlock (Old Welsh) from the lake at the holy monastery.
Wenloc, Wenloch, Wenlok

Wensley (Old English) from the meadow with the wood clearing.
Wenslea, Wensleah, Wenslee, Wensleigh, Wensli, Wenslie, Wensly

Wentworth (Old English) from the white one's estate.

Wenutu (Native American) clear sky.

Wenzel (Slavic) knowing.
Wensel, Wenzil, Wenzyl

Werner (Teutonic) warrior who defends.
Warner, Wernher

Wes (English) from the west.
West, Wess

Wescott (Old English) from the west cottage.
Wescot, Westcot, Westcott

Wesh (Gypsy) woods.

Wesley (Old English) from the westerly meadow.
Weslea, Wesleah, Weslee, Wesleigh, Wesli, Weslie, Wesly

Westbrook (English) from the westerly stream.
Wesbrook, Wesbrooke, Westbrook

Westby (Old English) from the westerly farmstead.
Wesbee, Wesbey, Wesbi, Wesbie, Wesby, Westbee, Westbey, Westbi, Westbie

Weston (Old English) from the westerly town.
Westan, Westen, Westin, Westyn

Wetherby (Old English) from the wether-sheep (male castrated sheep) farm.
Wetherbi, Wetherbie

Wetherell (Old English) from the wether-sheep (male castrated sheep) corner.
Wetheral, Wetherall, Wetherel, Wetheril, Wetherill, Wetheryl, Wetheryll

Wetherley (Old English) from the wether-sheep (male castrated sheep) meadow.
Wetherlea, Wetherleah, Wetherlee, Wetherleigh, Wetherli, Wetherlie, Wetherly

Wettriki (Finnish) king of peace. A form of Frederick.
Wetu (Finn)

Weylin (Celtic) the wolf's son lives near the pool.
Weilin, Weilyn, Weylyn

Weymouth (Celtic) mouth of the river.
Weimoth, Weimouth, Weymoth, Weymouth

Whalley (English) from the meadow near the hill.
Whalea, Whaleah, Whalee, Whaleigh, Whaley, Whali, Whalie, Whallea, Whalleah, Whallee, Whalli, Whallie, Whallie, Wahlly, Whaly

Wharton (English) from the town on the lake bank.
Warton

Wheatley (English) from the wheat meadow.
Whatlea, Whatleah, Whatlee, Whatleigh, Whatley, Whatli, Whatlie, Whatly, Wheatlea, Wheatleah, Wheatlee, Wheatli, Wheatlie, Wheatly

Wheaton (English) from the wheat town.
Wheatan, Wheaten, Wheatin, Wheatyn

Wheeler (English) maker of wheels.
Wheel, Wheela, Wheelah, Wheelar

Wherahiko (Maori) freedom.

Whetu (Polynesian) star.

Whistler (Old English) piper.
Whistla

Whitaker (Old English) from the white field.
Whitacker, Whitmaker, Whittaker, Whytaker, Whyttaker

Whitby (English) by the white house.
Whitbea, Whitbee, Whitbey, Whitbi, Whitbie

Whitcomb (English) from the white house.
Whitcombe, Whytcomb, Whytcombe

White (Old English) white-haired.
Whyte

Whitelaw (English) from the white, small hill.
Whitlaw, Whytlaw

Whitey (English) white-haired; white-skinned.
Whitee, Whiti, Whitie, Whity

Whitfield (English) from the white field.
Whytfield

Whitford (English) from the white ford.
Whytford

Whitley (English) from the white meadow.
Whitlea, Whitleah, Whitlee, Whitleigh, Whitli, Whitlie, Whitly

Whitlock (Old English) white lock of hair.
Whitloc, Whitloch, Whitlok, Whytloc, Whytloch, Whytlock, Whytlok

Whitman (English) white-haired man.
Whitmen, Whytman, Whytmen

Whitmore (English) from the white marsh land.
Whitmoor, Whitmoore, Whittemoor, Whittemoore, Whittemore, Whytmoor, Whitmoore, Whytmore, Whyttmoor, Whyttmoore, Witmore, Witmoor, Witmoore, Wittemoor, Wittemoore, Wittmore, Wytmoor, Wytmoore, Wytmore, Wyttmoor, Wyttmoore, Wyttmore

Whitney (Old English) from the white island.
Whittney, Whytney, Whyttney

Whittaker (English) from the white field.

Wicasa (Dakota) man.
Wicasah

Wichado (Native American) willing.

Wickham (Old English) from the enclosure in the village.
Wikham, Wyckham, Wykham

Wickley (English) from the willow meadow in the village.
Wicklea, Wickleah, Wicklee, Wickleigh, Wickli, Wicklie, Wickly, Wycklea, Wyckleah, Wycklee, Wyckleigh, Wyckley, Wyckli, Wycklie, Wyckly, Wyklea, Wykleah, Wyklee, Wykleigh, Wyklwy, Wykli, Wyklie, Wykly

Wid/Wido (English) wide.
Wid, Wyd, Wydo

W

Wies (German) warrior who is famous.
Wiess, Wyes, Wyess

Wikoli (Hawaiian) victory. A form of Victor.

Wiktor (Polish) victory.
Victor, Wyctor

Wilanu (Moquelumnan) to pour water onto flour.
Wylanu

Wilbert (German) brilliant.
Wilbirt, Wilburt, Wilbyrt, Wylbery, Wylbirt, Wylburt, Wylbyrt

Wilbraham (English) wilful father of the multitude. A combination of William/Abraham.
Abraham, Wylbraham

Wilbur (Teutonic) bright.
Wilber, Wilburn, Wilburne, Wilburt, Willber, Willbur, Wilver, Wylber, Wylbur, Wylbyr, Wyllber, Wyllbir, Wyllbyr

Wilder (English) from the wilderness.
Wild, Wilde, Wyld, Wylde

Wildon (English) from the hill in the woods.
Wildan, Wilden, Wildin, Wildyn, Willdan, Willden, Willdin, Willdon, Willdyn, Wyldan, Wylden, Wyldin, Wyldon, Wyldyn, Wylldan, Wyllden, Wylldin, Wylldon, Wylldyn

Wile (Hawaiian) wilful. A form of Willy.
Wilea, Wileah, Wilee, Wileigh, Wiley, Wili, Wilie, Wily, Wylea, Wyleah, Wylee, Wyleigh, Wyley, Wyli, Wylie, Wyly

Wiley (English) from the willows in the meadow.
Wile (Haw), Wilea, Wileah, Wilee,
Wileigh, Wili, Wilie, Wily, Wylea, Wyleah, Wylee, Wyleigh, Wyley, Wyli, Wylie, Wyly

Wilford (Old English) from the willow-tree river crossing.
Willford, Wylford, Wyllford

Wilfred (Old English) desired place.
Wilfredo (Span), Willfredo, Wilfried, Wilfrid, Wilfryd, Willfred, Willfrid, Willfryd

Wilhelm (German) determined, wilful guardian.
Wilhelmus, Willem, Wylhelm, Wyllhelm

Wilkins (English) William's son; son of the wilful one.
Wilken, Wilkens, Wilkes, Wilkie, Wilkin, Wilikes, Wilikins, Wylkin, Wylkins, Wylkyn, Wylkyns

Wilkinson (English) little William's son; son of the wilful one.
Wilkenson, Wylkenson, Wylkinson, Wylkynson

Will (English) wilful. A short form of names starting with 'Wil' e.g. William.
Wil, Wyl, Wyll

Willard (Teutonic) resolute; brave.
Wilard, Wylard, Wyllard

Willard (Old English) resolute; brave.
Wilard, Willard, Wylard, Wyllard

William (Old English) wilful.
Guillaume (Fren), Guglielmo (Ital), Guillermo (Span), Vasyl, Vilhelm (Ger), Viliam (Czech), Viljo (Finn), Ville (Swed), Welfel, Wilek, Willem, Wiliama (Haw), Wliame, Willaim, Willam, Willeam, Willem (Ger), Williams, Wim (Dut), Wyliam, Wyliams,

William cont.
Wylliam, Wylliams, Wyllyam,
Wyllyams, Wylyam, Wylyams,
Uilleam (Scott), Uilliam (Ir)

Williams (English) William's son;
son of the wilful one.
Wiliamson, Williamson,
Wyliamson, Wylliamson

Williamson (English) William's son;
son of the wilful one.

Willis (English) William's son; son
of the wilful one.
Wilis, Williss, Wylis, Wyliss, Wylys,
Wylyss

Willoughby (Old English) from the
willows by the farm.
Willobee, Willobey, Willowbee,
Willowbey, Willowbie, Willowby,
Wyllowbee, Wyllobey, Wyllobi,
Wyllobie, Wylloby, Wylobee,
Wylobey, Wylobi, Wylobie, Wyloby

Willy (English) wilful. A short form
of names starting with 'Wil' e.g.
William.
Wilea, Wileah, Wilee, Wileigh,
Wiley, Wili, Wilie, Willea, Willeah,
Willee, Willeigh, Willey, Willi,
Willie, Wily, Wylea, Wyleah, Wylee,
Wyleigh, Wyley, Wyli, Wylie, Wyll,
Wyllea, Wylleah, Wyllee, Wylley,
Wylleigh, Wylli, Wyllie, Wylly,
Wyly

Wilmer (Teutonic) famous.
Wylmer

Wilmot (English) from William's
moat. (O/Ger) resolute.
Wilmott, Wylmot, Wylmott

Wilny (Native American) flying,
singing eagle.
Wilni, Wilnie, Wylni, Wylnie,
Wylny

Wilson (English) William's son; son
of the wilful one.
Willsan, Willsen, Willsin, Willson,
Willsyn, Wilsan, Wilsen, Wilsin,
Wilsyn, Wyllsan, Wyllsen, Wyllsin,
Wyllson, Wyllsyn, Wylsan, Wylsen,
Wylsin, Wylson, Wylsyn

Wilstan (Teutonic) from the wolf
stone.
Wilsten, Wilstin, Wilstyn, Wylstan,
Wylsten, Wylstin, Wylstyn

Wilton (Old English) from Will's
town; from the wilful one's town.
Willtan, Willten, Willtin, Willton,
Willtown, Willtyn, Wiltan, Wilten,
Wiltin, Wiltown, Wiltyn, Wylltan,
Wyllten, Wylltin, Wyllton, Wylltyn,
Wyltan, Wylten, Wyltin, Wylton,
Wytyn

Wilu (Moquelumnan) squawking
chicken hawk.

Win (Cambodian) bright.
Winn, Wyn, Wynn, Wynne

Winchell (Old English) from the
corner.
Winchel, Wynchel, Wynchell

Windell (English) from the windy
valley.
Windel, Windlan, Wyndel,
Wyndell

Windham (English) from the
friendly town.
Winham, Wyndham

Windsor (German) from the river
bend.
Windsar, Windser, Wyndsar,
Wyndser, Wyndsor

Winfield (Old English) from the
friend's field.
Wynfield

Winfrid (English) friend of peace.
Winfred, Winfredd, Winfrid,
Winfryd, Wynfred, Wynfredd,
Wynfrid, Wynfryd

Wing (Chinese) glorious.

Wingate (English) divine protector.
Wyngate

Wingi (Native American) willing.
Wing, Wingie, Wingy, Wyng,
Wyngi, Wyngie, Wyngy

Winslow (Old English) from the hill of the friend.
Winslowe, Wynslow, Wynslowe

Winston (Old English) from the friendly town.
Winstan, Winsten, Winstin,
Winstyn, Wynstan, Wynsten,
Wynstin, Wynston, Wynstyn

Winter (Old English) born at winter time.
Winterford, Winters, Wynter,
Wynters

Winthrop (English) victory at the crossroads.
Wynthrop

Winward (Old English) from the friend and guardian's forest.
Wynward

Wirake (Australian Aboriginal) friend.
Wirak

Wiremu (Polynesian) wilful. A form of William.
Wir, Wire, Mu

Wirrin (Australian Aboriginal) tea tree.
Wirin, Wiryn

Wish (English) wished-for child.
Wishe, Wysh

Wistan (Teutonic) wise stone.
Wystan

Wit (Polish) life.
Witt, Wyt, Wytt

Witek (Polish) victory. A form of Victor.
Wytek

Witha (Arabic) handsome.
Wytha

Witt (Old English) wise; funny.
Wit, Wyt, Wytt

Witter (Old English) wise warrior.
Whiter, Whitter, Whyter, Whytter,
Wytter

Witton (Old English) from the wise one's town.
Whiton, Whyton, Whyton,
Whytton

Wladislav (Slavic) powerful glory.
Wladyslaw (Pol)

Wolcott (English) from the cottage in the woods.

Wolder (Dutch) ruler.

Wolf (German/English) wolf.
Wolff, Woolf

Wolfgang (German) leader of the wolf pack.
Wolfgans

Wolfram (German) wolf raven.
Wolfrem

Wollowra (Australian Aboriginal) eagle.
Wolloarah

Woodfield (English) from the field in the forest.
Woodfyeld

Woodford (English) from the ford in the forest.
Woodforde

Woodley (English) from the forest meadow.
Woodlea, Woodleah, Woodlee, Woodleigh, Woodli, Woodlie, Woodly

Woodrow (English) from the forest passage.
Woodroe

Woodruff (English) ranger from the forest.
Woodruf

Woodson (English) Woody's son; son of the one from the forest.
Woodsan, Woodsen, Woodsin, Woodsyn

Woodville (English) from the town on the edge of the forest.
Woodvil, Woodvill, Woodvyl, Woodvyll, Woodvylle

Woodward (English) guardian of the forest.
Woodard

Woody (English) from the forest.
Woodi, Woodie

Woolsey (English) victorious wolf; wool.
Woolsee, Woolsi, Woolsie, Woolsy

Worchester (English) from the army camp in the forest.
Worchester

Wordsworth (English) from the wolf guardian's farm.
Wordworth

Worippa (Australian Aboriginal) storm bird.
Woripa, Worypa, Woryppa

Worle (Ibo) born on market day.
Worl

Worrell (Old English) dweller at the true one's manor.
Worel, Worell, Woril, Worill, Worrel, Worril, Worryl

Worth (Old English) from the farmstead.

Worthy (English) from the enclosure.
Worthi, Worthie

Worton (English) from the farm town.
Wortan, Worten, Wortin, Wortyn

Wouter (German) powerful warrior.

Wray (English) accuser; crooked. (Scand) property on a corner.
Wrae, Wrai

Wren (Welsh) ruler. (O/Eng) the wren bird.
Ren

Wright (English) worker.
Right, Ryght, Wryght

Wriston (English) from the town near the shrubs.
Riston, Ryston, Wryston

Writer (Old English) writer.
Writer, Wryte, Wryter

Wulfram (Teutonic) wolf raven.
Wolfram, Wolfran, Wulfran

Wuliton (Native American) doing well.
Wulitan, Wuliten, Wulitin, Wulityn

Wullun (Australian Aboriginal) sky blue.
Wulun

Wunand (Native American) God is good.
Wunan

X

Wundurra (Australian Aboriginal) warrior.
Wundura

Wyatt (Middle English) Guy's son; son of the forest guide. (Fren) little warrior. (Amer) wide.
Whiat, Whyatt, Wiat, Wiatt, Wyat, Wyatte, Wye, Wyeth

Wybert (English) bright one in battle.
Wibert, Wibirt, Wiburt, Wibyrt, Wybirt, Wyburt, Wybyrt

Wyborn (Old Norse) war bear.
Wibjorn, Wiborn, Wybjorn

Wyck (Scandinavian) from the village.
Wic, Wick, Wik, Wyc, Wyk

Wycliff (German) from the village near the cliff.
Wiclif, Wicliff, Wicliffe, Wyche, Wycliffe, Wyck

Wyman (English) warrior.
Wiman, Wimen, Waiman, Waimen, Wayman, Waymen

Wymer (English) famous in battle.
Wimer

Wyn (Native American) first-born son. (Eng) friend. The masculine form of Wynonna.
Winono

Wyndham (Old English) from the winding path enclosure.
Winham

Wynn (English) white; fair-haired.
Win, Winn, Wyn, Wyne, Wynne (Wel)

Wystan (Teutonic) wisdom; stone.
Wistan

Wythe (Middle English) willow-tree dweller.
With, Withe, Wyth

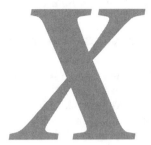

Xanthippus (Greek) light-coloured horse.
Xanthyppus, Zanthippus, Zanthyppus

Xanthus (Latin) golden-haired; blond.
Xanthius, Xanthyus, Zanthius, Zanthus, Zanthyus

Xaver/Xavier (Arabic) bright; brilliant.
Saveri, Savero, Xaver (Span), Xavery (Pol), Xaviero (Ital), Xavyer, Xever (Span), Zavier, Zavyer, Zever

Xayvion (African American) new home.
Xaivion, Xaivyon, Xayvyon

Xenophon (Greek) stranger's voice.
Xeno, Zeno, Zenophon

Xenos (Greek) stranger.
Xeno, Zeno, Zenos

Xerxes (Persian) royal ruler; king; prince.
Jerez, Xeres, Xerus, Xrus, Zerk, Zerzes

Xevach (Hebrew) sacrifice.
Zevach

Xevadiah (Hebrew) God will give.
Xevadia, Zevadia, Zevaddiah

Xeven (Slavic) lively.
Xyven, Ziven, Zyven, Zyvyn

Xevulun (Hebrew) home.
Zevulun

Xiaoping (Chinese) small bottle.
Xiaopin

Ximen/Ximenes (Spanish) listening.
A form of Simon.
Ximen, Ximene, Ximenes, Xymen,
Xymenes, Xymon, Zimen, Zimene,
Zimenes, Zymen, Zymene,
Zymenes, Xymon

Ximraan (Arabic) celebration.
Zimraan, Zymraan

Ximran (Hebrew) sacred.
Xymran, Zimran, Zymran

Xindel (Hebrew) protector of
humankind.
Xyndel, Zindel, Zyndel

Xing-Fu (Chinese) happy.

Xion (Hebrew) from the guarded
land.
Xyon, Zion, Zyon

Xitomer (Czech) living fame.
Xytomer, Zitomer, Zytomer

Xi-Wang (Chinese) desire.
Xi-Wpang

Xowie (Greek) life.
Xoe, Xoee, Xowee, Xowi, Xowy,
Zoe, Zoee, Zoey, Zoi, Zoie, Zoy

Xylon (Greek) from the forest.
Xilon, Zilon, Zylon

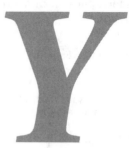

Yaar (Hebrew) forest.

Yabarak (Australian Aboriginal) sea.
Yabarac, Yabarack

Yadava (Sanskrit) descended.
Yadav

Yadid (Hebrew) God will judge.
Yadyd

Yael (Hebrew) mountain goat.
Yaell

Yafeu (Ghanian) bold.

Yagel (Hebrew) happiness.
Yagil, Yagyl, Yogil, Yogyl

Yahbini (Australian Aboriginal) star.
Yahbinie, Yahbiny

Yaholo (Creek) one who yells.

Yahya (Hebrew) God is good.

Yair (Hebrew) God will teach.
Jair, Jayr, Yayr

Yajna (Sanskrit) sacrifice.
Yajnah

Yakar (Hebrew) dear.

Yakecen (Native American) song
from the sky.

Yakez (Native American) heaven.

Yakim (Hebrew) God develops.
Jakim, Jakym, Yakym

Yakir (Hebrew) honoured; beloved.
Yakire, Yakyr, Yakyre

Yale (Welsh/Old English) elder.
Yael, Yaell, Yail, Yaill, Yayl, Yayll

Yama (Sanskrit) God of the setting sun.
Yamah

Yamal (Hindi) twin.

Yamin (Hebrew) right hand; helpful.

Yana (Hebrew) answer.

Yancy (Native American) English man.
Yance, Yancey, Yankee, Yantsey

Yandach (Hebrew) restful.

Yaphet (Hebrew) attractive.

Yaqub (Arabic) to grab at one's heel.

Yarb (Gypsy) herb.

Yardan (Arabic) king.

Yardley (Old English) from the enclosed meadow.
Yardlea, Yardleah, Yardlee, Yardleigh, Yardli, Yardlie, Yardly

Yarin (Hebrew) understanding.

Yarran (Australian Aboriginal) acacia tree.
Yaran

Yasar (Arabic) wealthy.

Yash (Hindi) famous.

Yashar (Hebrew) honourable; with high morals.
Yesher, Yeshurun

Yasuo (Japanese) calm.

Yates (English) gate keeper.
Yaits, Yayts

Yavin (Hebrew) God is understanding.
Jabin, Jehoram, Joram, Juti, Yadon, Yavnie, Yediel, Yehoram, Yehoshafat, Yekutiel, Yodin, Yoram

Yazid (Arabic) increasing; to grow.
Yazyd

Ye (Chinese) universe.

Yehoram (Hebrew) God will praise.

Yehoshua (Hebrew) God is my salvation.

Yehudi (Hebrew) teacher; praise to the Lord.
Jora, Jorah, Yehudit, Yehudie, Yehudy

Yelutci (Native American) quiet bear.

Yemon (Japanese) guardian.

Yen (Vietnamese) calm.
(Eng) wanted.
Yenn

Yeoman (Middle English) servant who has been in the family for a long period of time.
Yeomen, Yoman

Yered (Hebrew) Coming down.

Yeriel (Hebrew) found by God.

Yerik (Russian) God has praised.
Yeryk

Yestin (Old French/Welsh) righteous; just. A form of Justin.
Yestan, Yesten, Yeston, Yestyn

Yevgeny (Russian/Greek) noble; well born. A form of Eugene.
Yevgenyi

Yigael (Hebrew) God will redeem.
Yagel, Yigal

Yileen (Australian Aboriginal) dream.

Yitro (Hebrew) plentiful.

Yitzhak (Hebrew) laughter; happiness.
Itzaak, Itzaac, Itzaack, Itzaak, Itzac, Itzack, Itzak, Yitzaac, Yitzaack, Yitzaak, Yitzac, Yitzack, Yitzak, Yitzak

Yo (Chinese) bright.

Yogi (Sanskrit) one who practices yoga.
Yogee, Yogey, Yogie, Yogy

Yona (Native American) bear.
Yonah

Yonah (Hebrew) dove.
Yona, Yonas

Yonatan (Hebrew) gift of God.

Yong (Chinese) brave.

Yonus (Arabic/Hebrew) dove.
Yona, Yonah, Yonas, Yonos, Yonys

Yora (Hebrew) teacher.
Yorah

Yorath (English) worthy of God.

Yorick (English) farmer.
Yoric, Yorik, Yoryc, Yoryck, Yoryk

York (Celtic) from the farm with the yew trees.
Yorke, Yorick, Yorker

Yosef (Hebrew) God will increase; God has added a child. A form of Joseph.

Yosha (Hebrew) wisdom.
Yoshah

Yoshi (Japanese) quiet; respected.
Yoshee, Yoshie

Yotimo (Native American) bee flying into its hive.

Yottoko (Native American) mud.

Young (English) youthful.
Yung, Yunge

Yrjo (Finnish/Greek) farmer.

Yuan (Chinese) original; one of a kind.

Yucel (Turkish) noble; with high morals.
Yusel

Yudan (Hebrew) judgment.
Yuden, Yudin, Yudon, Yudyn

Yukiko (Japanese) snow.

Yukio (Japanese) snow boy.
Yukyo

Yul (Chinese) over the horizon.

Yule (Old English) born at Christmas time.
Eurl, Euell, Ewell, Yul, Yull

Yuma (Native American) son of the chief.
Yumah

Yunis (Arabic) dove.
Younis, Younys, Yunys

Yurchik (Russian) farmer.

Yuri (Russian/Greek) farmer.
Yuris (Latvi)

Yusha (Arabic) God is my help.
Yushua, Yushuah, Yasser

Yusuf (Arabic) God will increase; God has added a child. A form of Joseph.
Yussef

Yutu (Native American) coyote hunting.

Yvan (Russian) God is gracious. A form of Ivan.
Yven, Yvin, Yvyn

Yves (French) knight of the lion. The masculine form of Yvette/Yvonne, archer.
Eouan (Bret), Euzen

Ywain (Welsh/Greek) well born.
Ywyn

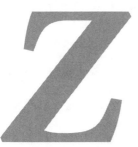

Zabad/Zabdi (Hebrew) gift.
Zabad, Zabdy, Zabi, Zavdi, Zavdiel. Zebdiel, Zebdy

Zabdiel (Hebrew) gift.
Zebdiel, Zabdi, Zabdil, Zabdyl, Zavdi, Zavdiel.

Zaccheus (Hebrew) purity.
Zacheus

Zachariah (Hebrew) God remembers.
Acarius, Benzecry, Chasija, Sachar, Zacaria, Zacarius (Span), Zaccaria (Ital), Zacchaeus, Zacharie (Fren), Zacharia (Fren), Zachariah, Zacharias (Heb), Zachary, Zacharyasz (Pol), Zacker (Bav), Zacko, Zaka, Zakah, Zakaria, Zakariah, Zakarias (Swed), Zakarius, Zakarya, Zakaryah, Zakaryas, Zakarys, Zakaryus

Zachary (English) God remembers.
Zacharee, Zacharey, Zachari, Zacharie, Zachery, Zacheri,
Zacherie, Zackaree, Zackarey, Zackari, Zackarie, Zackary, Zackery, Zackeri, Zackerie, Zakaree, Zakarey, Zakari, Zakarie, Zakary, Zakery, Zakiri, Zakirie, Zakery

Zac/Zack/Zak (Hebrew) God remembers.
Zacker (Bav), Zaker

Zadock (Hebrew) righteous; just.
Zadak, Zadoc (Fren)

Zafar (Arabic) winner.

Zahavi (Hebrew) gold.

Zahid (Arabic) self-denying; abstinent.
Zahyd

Zahir (Arabic) understanding.
Zahyr

Zahur (Swahili) flower.
Zaher, Zahir, Zahyr

Zaid (Arabic) growing; increasing.
Zaide, Zayd, Zayde

Zaim (Arabic) general.
Zaym

Zaki (Arabic) smart.
Zakie, Zaky

Zakiyya (Hindi) purity.
Zakiyyah

Zakkai (Hebrew) innocent; pure.
Zakai

Zako (Illyrian) God remembers.
Zacko, Zaco, Zak

Zakur (Hebrew) masculine.

Zale (Greek) power of the sea.
Zale, Zail, Zaile, Zayl, Zayle

Zales (English) salt.
Zail, Zails, Zale, Zayl, Zatle, Zayls

Z

Zalman (Hebrew) peace. A form of Solomon.
Salman, Salmen, Salmin, Salmon, Salmyn, Zalmen, Zalmin, Zalmon, Zalmyn

Zalmir (Hebrew) songbird.
Zalman, Zalmire, Zalmyr, Zelmir, Zelmire, Zelmyr, Zelmyre

Zamiel (German) God has heard.

Zamir (Hebrew) song.
Zamar, Zamer, Zamyr

Zan (Hebrew) well fed.
Zann

Zander (Greek) defender of humankind. A form of Alexander.
Alexander, Sander, Sanders, Xander, Zanda, Zandah, Zandar, Zanders, Zandor, Zandyr

Zane (English) God is gracious. A form of Shane/John.
Zandar, Zander, Zandor, Zain, Zaine, Zayn, Zayne

Zanthus (Greek) blond.
Zareb
African
Guardian.

Zared (Hebrew) ambush.
Zarad, Zarid, Zarod, Zaryd

Zarek (Slavic) God will protect.
Zarec, Zareck, Zaric, Zarick, Zaryc, Zaryck, Zaryk

Zavad/Zavao (Hebrew) present time.

Zavdiel (Hebrew) gift from God.

Zavier (Bohemian) bright; brilliant.
Xavier, Xavyer, Zavyer

Zayd/Zayn (Arabic) beautiful.
Zaid, Zain

Zayvion (African American) new home.

Zdzich (Polish) glorious.
Zdzis

Zeal (Latin) energy.
Zeel

Zebadiah (Hebrew) God's gift.
Zebadia, Zebadiah, Zebadya, Zebadyah, Zebedee, Zebedia, Zebediah, Zebedya, Zebedyah, Zubin

Zebedee (Greek) my gift.
Zebede

Zebulon (Hebrew) dwelling place; honourable.
Zebulen, Zebulun, Zevulum, Zubin, Zubyn

Zedekiah (Hebrew) God is mighty; God is right.
Zedekia, Zedekya, Zedekyah

Zeeman (Dutch) of the sea.
Zeaman, Zeman, Zemen, Ziman, Zimen, Zymen, Zymin, Zymyn

Zeev (Hebrew) wolf.

Zehariah (Hebrew) God's light.

Zeheb (Turkish) gold.

Zeira (Aramaic) small.
Zeirah, Zeyra, Zeyrah

Zeke (Arabic) intelligent.
Zeak, Zeake, Zek

Zeki (Turkish) clever.
Zekee, Zkey, Zekie, Zeky

Zelig (Yiddish) holy; blessed.
Zelyg

Zelimir (Slavic) peace is desired.
Zelimyr, Zelymir, Zelymyr

Zemariah (Hebrew) song.
Zemaria, Zemarya, Zemaryah

Zenas (Greek) living. A from Zeno.
Zena, Zeno, Zenos

Zenda (Czech) well born.
Zendah

Zenith (Latin) highest point.

Zeno/Zenobias (Greek) living; given life by Zeus.
Zenas, Zenobia, Zenobiah, Zenobya, Zenobyah, Zenon, Zenos, Zenus, Zenys

Zenphan/Zenphaniah (Hebrew) look out, guardian; protected treasure of God.
Zenphen, Zenphene, Zenphon, Zenphyn, Zevadia, Zevadiah

Zephyrus (Hebrew) wind from the west.

Zerach (Hebrew) light.
Zerac, Zerack, Zerak

Zerah (Hebrew) brightness of the morning.
Zera, Zira, Zirah, Zyra, Zyrah

Zerem (Hebrew) stream.

Zerika (Hebrew) rain storm.
Zerikah, Zeryka, Zerykah

Zero (Greek) empty.
Zerot

Zerxes (Persian) ruler.

Zesiro (Nigerian) first born of twins.
Zesyro

Zethan (Hebrew) shining.
Zethen, Zethin, Zethon, Zethyn

Zethus (Greek) son of Zeus, king of the gods.

Zeus (Greek) living; bright sky.
Zeon, Zous, Zus

Zev (Hebrew) living wolf.
Seef, Seff, Sif, Zeeb, Zeev

Zevach (Hebrew) sacrifice.
Zevac, Zevack, Zevak

Zevariah (Hebrew) God has given.
Zevaria, Zevarya, Zevaryah

Zevid (Hebrew) present.
Zevyd

Zeviel (Hebrew) gazelle of God.
Zevial, Zevyel

Zevulun (Hebrew) house.

Zhong (Chinese) second brother.

Zhu (Chinese) wish.

Zhuang (Chinese) strength.

Zia (Hebrew) light.
Ziah, Zya, Zyah

Ziggy (Teutonic) victorious protector. The short form of Sigmund.
Zigee, Zigey, Zigi, Zigie, Ziggee, Ziggey, Ziggi, Zigy

Zikomo (Malawian) thanks.
Zykomo

Zilpah (Hebrew) trickling water.
Zilpa, Zylpa, Zylpah

Zimen (Spanish) obedient.
Ziman, Zimin, Zimon, Zimyn, Zyman, Zymen, Zymin, Zymyn

Zimon (Hebrew) listening. A form of Simon.
Ziman, Zimen, Zimin, Zimyn, Zyman, Zymen, Zymin, Zymon, Zymyn

Zimraan (Arabic) celebration.
Zymraan

Zimri (Hebrew) valuable.
Zimry, Zymri, Zymry

Zinan (Japanese) second son.
Zynan

Zindel (Hebrew) protector of humankind.
Zyndel

Zinon (Greek) living.

Zion (Hebrew) the sign.
Zeeon, Zeon, Zione, Zyon

Zitomer (Czech) living fame.

Ziv (Hebrew) shining; bright with life.
Ziven, Zivon, Zivu, Zyv

Zivan (Hebrew) shining. (Slavic) lively.
Ziven, Zivin, Zivon, Zivyn, Zyvan (Slav), Zyven, Zyvin, Zyvon, Zyvyn

Ziya (Arabic) light.
Ziyah, Zyam Zyahm, Zyya, Zyyah

Ziyad (Arabic) increasing.

Zlatan (Czech) gold.

Zlatka (Slavic) gold.
Zlatkah

Zohar (Hebrew) radiant light.
Zohare

Zola (German) prince.
Zoilo, Zolah, Zollie

Zoltan (Arabic) sultan; great ruler.
Soltan, Zsolt, Zsoltan, Zolten, Zoltin, Zoltun, Zoltyn

Zoltin (Hungarian) life.
Zoltan, Zolten, Zolton, Zoltyn

Zomeir (Hebrew) tree pruner.
Zomer, Zomir, Zomyr

Zomelis (Lithuanian) asked of God.
Zomelys

Zonar (Latin) a sound.
Zonair, Zonayr, Zoner

Zooman (English) animal caretaker.
Zoomen

Zoomer (English) fast.
Zoomar, Zoomir, Zoomyr

Zoro (Persian) star.
Zorro

Zorya (Slavic) star.
Zoria, Zoriah, Zoryah

Zosime (French) lively.
Zosimus, Zosyme

Zosimus (Greek) full of life; lively.
Zosimos, Zosymos, Zosymus

Zotom (Kiowa) bitter.

Zowie (Greek) life.
Zoe, Zoee, Zoi

Zsiga (Hungarian) victorious, conquering protector. A form of Sigmund.
Zsigah, Zsyga, Zsygah, Zyga, Zygah

Zsolt (Polish) ruler.
Zoltan

Zuberi (Swahili) strength.
Zuber

Zubin (Hebrew) praised highly.
Zuban, Zuben, Zubon, Zubyn

Zuhayr (Arabic) young flower; bud.
Zuhair

Zuriel (Hebrew) God is my stone foundation.
Zurial, Zuryal, Zuryel

Zwi (Scandinavian) gazelle.
Zwie, Zwy

Zygfryd (Polish/Teutonic) victorious peace.
Sigfrid, Sigfryd, Sigismund, Sigmund, Sygfrid, Sygfryd, Zigamunt (Pol), Zigfrid, Zigfryd

Zygmunt (Polish) victorious protection.

Zylon (Greek) forest dweller.
Xylon, Zilon

Zymon (Hebrew) listening. A form of Simon.
Ziman, Zimen, Zimin, Zimon, Zimyn, Zyman, Zymen, Zymin, Zymyns